CURRENT PRACTICE UPDATES IN EMERGENCY MEDICINE

DR. NIDHI KAELEY
DR. ASHIMA SHARMA

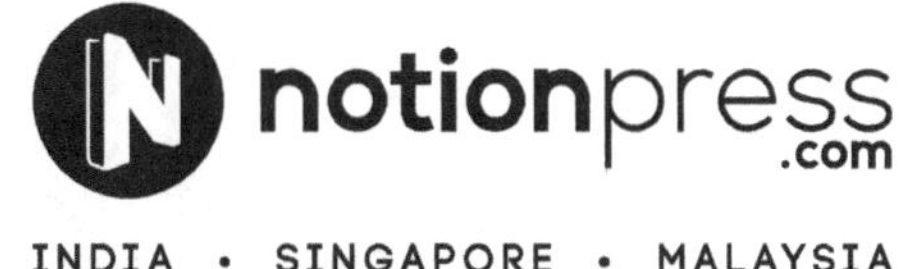

INDIA · SINGAPORE · MALAYSIA

ISBN 979-8-88704-380-7

Foreword

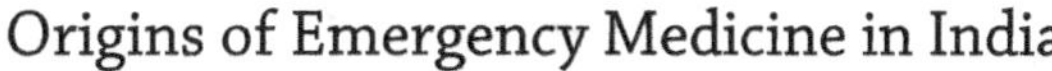

Origins of Emergency Medicine in India

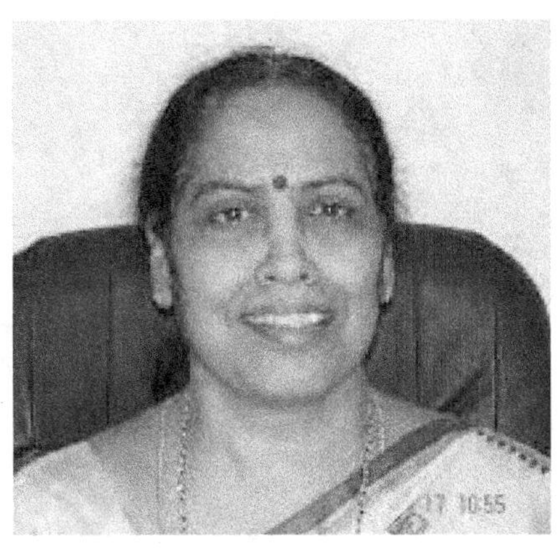

Emergency Medicine now is a full-fledged broad speciality in our Country. To get trained one has to undergo rigorous training for three years after completing basic MBBS. To get to where we are today the seeds were sown, in various institutions in the late eighties. Even in developed Countries, this speciality was referred to as casualty and later as Accident and Emergency department. There are different branches in the purview of Medicine aligned to acute care. Anaesthesiology was the primary medical branch which paved the way to both Emergency Medicine and Critical Care. The specialties must have the thinking that the hat of a Physician and the dextrous hands of a Surgeon as a lion's heart to manage acute and formidable cases taking split second decisions and have a very systematic approach.

Anaesthesiologists were called to resuscitate airway, breathing and circulation in the very beginning in all the countries but slowly it has given way to special training in both Critical Care and Emergency Medicine.

Looking at the need of the hour, the National Conference on Emergency Medicine was conducted in the year 2000 and an Emergency Medicine society was formed at the same time with many to follow. I remember the proceedings of the society as I was the Founder President .The commitment of members and young , dedicated minds to improve the care and training in Emergency Medicine with the starting of MD and DNB in the speciality.

The formation of the department is mandatory for every medical college by 2022 with well-trained Medical & Paramedical Personnel. The Emergency Department forms the face of the hospital and takes care of all people who come with acute problems be it minor, major or mass casualty 24/7.

It gives me a great pleasure to see the seeds which were sown 20 years back have made a great impact in this speciality to attend Critical Patients and give them a second chance to live.

Any book written for Emergency Medicine is welcome. In this book many aspects have been comprehensively reviewed. All the trials which made an impact for a day to day practice and particularly airway management both adult as well as Paediatric needs special mention written in a simple way. It would be an excellent book for anyone in Medicine, Anaesthesiology, Critical Care and Emergency Medicine in particular.

I congratulate the authors for their effort.

Dr. Manimala Rao

Prof. M. Bajpai
MS, MCh, PhD, FRCS, FACS, FAMS, National Board
Vice President & Hony. Executive Director
Fulbright Scholar (USA), Commonwealth Fellow (UK)
& Raja Ramanna Fellow (Science & Technology)

आयुर्विज्ञान में
राष्ट्रीय परीक्षा बोर्ड
स्वास्थ्य एवं परिवार कल्याण मंत्रालय, भारत सरकार
**National Board of Examinations
in Medical Sciences**
Ministry of Health & Family Welfare, Government of India

Ref. No: NBEMS/EDO/2022/ *2930*

Dated: 07.07.2022

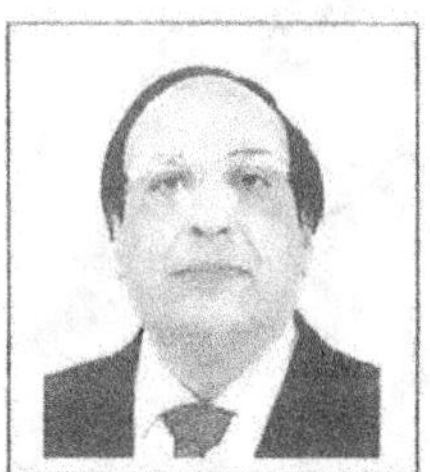

TESTIMONIAL

The practice of emergency medicine has the primary mission of evaluating, managing and providing treatment to these patients with unexpected injury or illness.

Doctors in emergency medicine carry out the immediate assessment and treatment of patients with serious and life-threatening illnesses and injuries.

This book "**Current Practice Updates in Emergency Medicine**" written by Dr. Nidhi Kaley & Dr. Ashima Sharma should prove to be of practical value to the practitioners.

My best wishes are with the authors.

(Prof. Minu Bajpai)
Honorary Executive Director

मेडिकल एनकलेव, अंसारी नगर, महात्मा गांधी मार्ग, नई दिल्ली-110029, दूरभाष: 91-11-45493091, ईमेल: edoffice@natboard.edu.in, वेबसाईट: www.natboard.edu.in
Medical Enclave, Ansari Nagar, Mahatma Gandhi Marg, New Delhi-110029, Tel.: 91-11-45493091, E-mail: edoffice@natboard.edu.in, website: www.natboard.edu.in

Testimonials

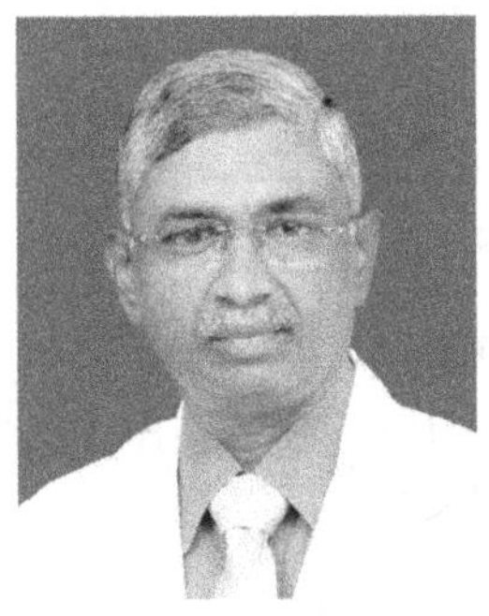

In the field of Medicine. Almost daily new trails and evidences get added for treating our patients. It is sometimes difficult to keep oneself updated with recent information. This book containing the Current Practice Updated will be a resource book for the newer guidelines and the algorithms of managing patients in Emergency Department. I extend my blessings and good wishes to Dr. Ashima Sharma and Dr. Nidhi Kaeley for their book. The book will be very helpful for the post graduate students for exam preparations also.

– Dr. K. Manohar
Director, NIMS

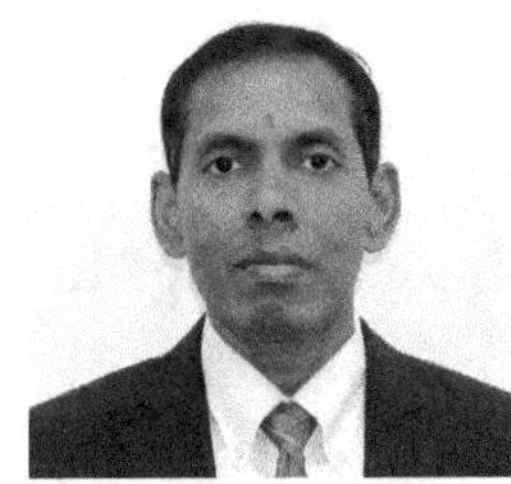

As a practicing emergency physician for the past 25 years in the USA, I Understand the importance of practice updates in emergency medicine. The field of emergency medicine is constantly changing and evolving with new technologies, practices, and innovations. Staying current with the latest developments in emergency medicine will enable physicians to provide the best possible care to their patients. Dr. Nidhi Kaeley and Dr. Ashima Sharma have been teaching emergency medicine and have many scientific publications and are ideal candidates to write this book. This book would benefit emergency physicians, postgraduate students, and all physicians and surgeons involved in emergency care. I express my deep appreciation to Dr. Nidhi Kaeley and Dr. Ashima Sharma for their commitment and hard work in helping to produce this book.

– Arunachalam Einstein
MD, FACEP, FAAEM

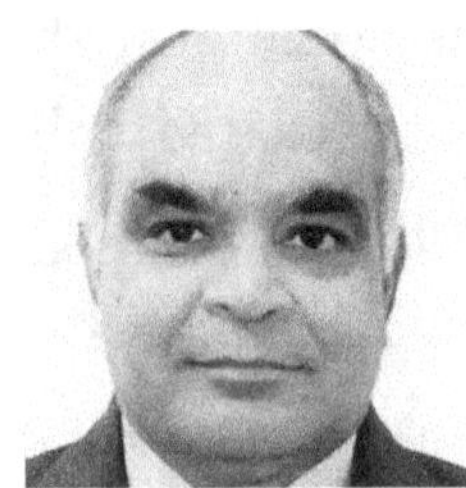

Emergency Medicine is a growing speciality across the word. The book titled **"Current Practice Updates in Emergency Medicine"** by Dr. Nidhi Kaeley and Dr. Ashima Sharma will be very useful for the doctors working in the filed of Emergency Medicine. I wish the authors best of luck and extend my blessing for the same.

– Dr. Arvind Rajvanshi
Director, AIIMS Rishikesh

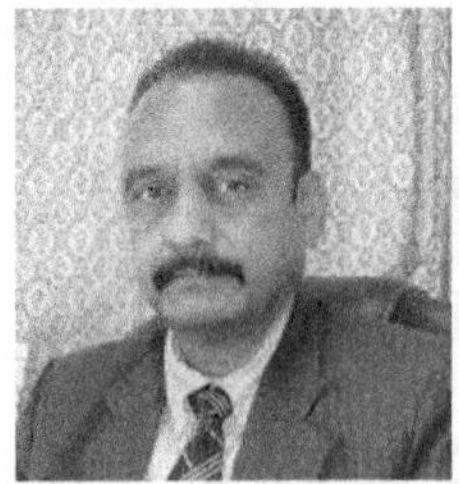

Emergency Medicine is a growing speciality across the world. This book titled "Current Practice updates in Emergency Medicine" by Dr. Nidhi Kaeley, and Dr. Ashima Sharma will be very useful for the doctors working in the field of Emergency Medicine. I wish the authors best of luck and extend my blessings for the same.

– Prof Manoj
Dean Academics, AIIMS Rishikesh

List of Authors

Dr. Ajay Kumar
MS Surgery
Associate Professor, Trauma Surgery
AIIMS Rishikesh

Dr. Akhil SL
MD Emergency Medicine
Resident, Emergency Medicine
Government Medical College, Kozhikode

Dr. Akshay Chipare
MD Medicine
Senior Resident, Emergency Medicine
B.J.G.M.C. & Sassoon General Hospital, Pune

Dr. Akula Hymavathi
MD Emergency Medicine
Senior Resident, Emergency Medicine
Nizam's Institute Of Medical Sciences, Hyderabad

Dr. Aman Verma
MS Orthopaedics,
Senior Resident, Orthopaedics
AIIMS Rishikesh

Dr. Anirban Ghosh Hazra
Junior Resident, Emergency Medicine
AIIMS, Rishikesh

Dr. Ankita Kabi
MD Anesthesiology, DNB
Associate Professor, Anesthesiology,
AIIMS, Gorakhpur

Dr. Aravind Ranjan CA
MD Emergency Medicine
Senior Resident, Emergency Medicine
Nizam's Institute Of Medical Sciences, Hyderabad

Dr. Archana Bairwa
Junior Resident, Emergency Medicine
AIIMS, Rishikesh

Dr. Aroop Mohanty
MD Microbiology
Assistant Professor, Microbiology
AIIMS, Gorakhpur

Dr. Arva Koushik
MD Emergency Medicine
Junior Resident, Emergency Medicine
Nizam's Institute Of Medical Sciences, Hyderabad

Dr. Ashima Sharma
MD Anesthesiology, MRCEM
Professor, Emergency Medicine,
Nizam's Institute Of Medical Sciences, Hyderabad

Dr. Austin Joju Mangaly
MD Emergency Medicine
Junior Resident, Emergency Medicine
Government Medical College, Kozhikode

Dr. Bhaskar Sarkar
MS Orthopaedics,
Associate Professor
AIIMS Rishikesh

Dr. Chandni R
MD Medicine, PhD, FICP, FRCP(Edin)
Professor and HOD, Emergency Medicine
Government Medical College, Kozhikode

Dr. Chidrupi Sharma
MBBS, DEM
Emergency Physician
Hyderabad

Dr. Deepali Rajpal
MD
Professor and HOD, Emergency Medicine
D.Y.Patil medical college, Navi Mumbai

Dr. Dharani G Reddy
MD Emergency Medicine
Senior Resident, Emergency Medicine
Nizam's Institute Of Medical Sciences, Hyderabad

Dr. Hannah Chawang
MD Emergency Medicine
Senior Resident, Emergency Medicine
AIIMS, Rishikesh

Dr. Hari Prasad
Junior Resident, Emergency Medicine
AIIMS, Rishikesh

Dr. Harsha Makwana
MD Anesthesia
Professor and Head of the Department
LG Hospital, Ahmedabad

Dr. Harshad Dongre
M.D. Anesthesia, FACEE
Associate Professor, Emergency Medicine
B.J.G.M.C. & Sassoon General Hospital, Pune

Dr. K. Sailaja
DA, DNB Anesthesia, FCCM
Consultant Anesthesiologist and HOD
Rainbow Hospital, Kondapur, Hyderabad.

Dr. Kavitha K P
MD Emergency Medicine
Senior resident, Emergency Medicine
Government Medical College, Kozhikode

Dr. Konda Sireesha
MS, McH Plastic surgery
Consultant, Rishikesh

Dr. Lubna Tarannum
MD Emergency Medicine
Senior Resident, Emergency Medicine
AIIMS, New Delhi

Dr. Mabel Vasnaik
MD Anaesthesiology
Senior Consultant and HOD Emergency Medicine
Manipal hospital, Bangalore

Dr. Madhur Uniyal
MS Surgery, MCh Trauma Surgery
Associate Professor, Trauma Surgery
AIIMS Rishikesh

Dr. Manisha Bisht
MD Pharmacology
Additional professor
AIIMS, Rishikesh

Dr. Monika Pathania
MD, Medicine
Associate Professor, General Medicine
AIIMS, Rishikesh

Dr. Mubashir Sohail
MD Emergency Medicine
Junior Resident, Emergency Medicine
Nizam's Institute Of Medical Sciences, Hyderabad

Dr. Nidhi Kaeley
MD Internal medicine
Associate Prof. and Head, Emergency Medicine
AIIMS Rishikesh

Dr. Nilesh Jagne
Senior Resident, Trauma Surgery
AIIMS Rishikesh

Dr. Nithya Shreya Meghana
DNB, Emergency Medicine
Emergency Medicine
AIG Hospitals, Gachibowli, Hyderabad

Dr. Priyanka Dwiwedi
MD, Anesthesiology
Assistant Professor, Anesthesiology
AIIMS, Gorakhpur

Dr. Rahul Rohan M
MD Emergency Medicine
Senior Resident, Emergency Medicine
AIIMS, New Delhi

Dr. Raj Binda Mishra
D.N.B. Emergency Medicine, FACEE
Senior Resident, Emergency Medicine
B.J.G.M.C. & Sassoon General Hospital, Pune

Dr. Rajeshwari Sanjay Vhora
M.D. Medicine/FACEE,
HOD Emergency Medicine
B.J.G.M.C. & Sassoon General Hospital, Pune

Dr. Rohan Bhatia
MD Anaesthesia
Associate Professor, Anaesthesia and Pain Medicine
Himalayan Institute Of Medical Sciences, Jolly Grant, Dehradun, Uttrakhand

Dr. Ruby Bhatia
M.D FICOG
Professor & HOD, Dept of Obst & Gynaecology
MMIMSR dmmu Mullana, Haryana

Dr. Ruhi
Junior Resident, Anaesthesia and Pain management
Himalayan Institute Of Medical Sciences, Jolly Grant, Dehradun, Uttrakhand

Dr. Sarat Chandra Uppaluri
MD Emergency Medicine
Senior Resident, Emergency Medicine
Nizam's Institute Of Medical Sciences, Hyderabad

Dr. Salva Ameena M S
Junior Resident, Emergency Medicine
AIIMS, Rishikesh

Dr. Shrirang Joshi
Resident Emergency Medicine
AIIMS, Rishikesh

Dr. Silpa. S
Junior Resident, Emergency Medicine
AIIMS, Rishikesh

Dr. Sree Sowjanya Patibandla
DNB, Emergency Medicine
Consultant, Emergency Medicine
Continental Hospitals, Hyderabad

Dr. Sukhdeep Somal
Junior Resident, Emergency Medicine,
AIIMS, Rishikesh

Dr. Tanve
Junior Resident, Psychiatry
AIIMS Rishikesh

Dr. Varsha Shinde
MD Anesthesiology
Professor And Head, Emergency Medicine
DY Patil, Pune

Dr. Vempalli Nagasubramanyam
MS General Surgery
Assistant Professor, Emergency Medicine
AIIMS Rishikesh

Dr. Vijeta Bajpai
MD, Anesthesia
Assistant Professor, Anesthesiology
AIIMS, Gorakhpur

Dr. Vikram Jain
Junior Resident, General Medicine
AIIMS, Rishikesh

Dr. Vikram Rawat
MD Psychiatry
Associate Professor, Psychiatry
AIIMS Rishikesh

Contents

Neurological Emergencies

Contributors

1. Dr. Nidhi Kaeley
2. Dr. Anirban Ghosh Hazra
3. Dr. Hannah Chawang

Chapters

1. Stroke
2. TIA
3. Subarachnoid Hemorrhage
4. Epilepsy
5. Coma
6. Dizziness

Stroke

Epidemiology

Stroke is the second cause of death worldwide as per the Global Burden of Diseases (GBD), with an estimated 6.5 million deaths and 113 million DALYs in 2013. India has witnessed a rise in stroke cases. It has become a major non-communicable disease (NCD) and is responsible for 3.5% of disability-adjusted life years (DALY). Recently, ICMR has come out with a report entitled "India: Health of the Nation's States," according to which stroke was the 4th leading cause of death and 5th Leading cause of Disability Adjusted Life Years (DALY) in 2016.

Definition

Stroke is defined as an abrupt onset of a neurological defect that is attributable to a focal vascular cause. The definition includes both clinical presentation and laboratory studies such as brain imaging to support the diagnosis.

Stroke is of two major types: ischemic (87%) and hemorrhagic (13%).

Ischemic stroke is further classified as thrombotic, embolic, and hypoperfusion related.

Vascular neuroanatomy

Stroke syndrome is classified as anterior and posterior circulation strokes.

Anterior circulation

Anterior circulation of the brain is contributed by the bilateral Internal carotid arteries (ICA). The ICA divides into the Anterior cerebral artery (ACA) and the Middle cerebral artery (MCA).

The cortical branches of MCA supply the lateral hemisphere, except for a strip along the superomedial border of the frontoparietal pole, which is supplied by ACA, and the lower temporal and occipital lobe are supplied by the Posterior circulation artery (PCA). *The proximal MCA* supplies the putamen, globus pallidus, posterior limb of the internal capsule, caudate nucleus, and corona radiata.

In the Sylvian fissure, MCA divides into *superior and inferior branches. The* superior branch supplies frontal and superior parietal lobes, and the inferior branch supplies inferior parietal and temporal lobes. Occlusion of the superior branch will result in *Broca's aphasia,* whereas occlusion of the inferior branch will cause *Wernicke's aphasia.* However, if both the cortical and proximal branches of MCA are occluded, the patient will develop contralateral hemiplegia, hemianesthesia, homonymous hemianopia, and aphasia (if the dominant lobe is involved). If the non-dominant lobe is involved, constructional apraxia, anosognosia, and hemineglect will be observed.

ACA is divided into *pre communal (A1) and post communal (A2) segments*. The A1 segment joins the anterior communicating artery with ICA. The A2 segment is distal to the origin of anterior communicating artery. The A1 segment supplies the anterior perforator substance, amygdala, anterior hypothalamus, and inferior part of the head of caudate nucleus. Occlusion of A1 segment is usually well tolerated as a result of collateral circulation. If both the A1 segments arise from single stem, it causes profound abulia, bilateral pyramidal signs with paraparesis and urinary incontinence.

<u>Posterior circulation</u>

Arterial branches of the vertebral arteries form Basilar arteries, which later divides to form the right and left Posterior cerebral arteries (PCA), all of which supply the posterior circulation of the brain.

Posterior circulation strokes are divided into P1 and P2 syndromes. Patients with *P1 syndrome* will have midbrain, subthalamic and thalamic signs, whereas those with *P2 syndrome* will have cortical temporal and occipital lobe signs. P1 syndrome includes Weber's syndrome, Claude's syndrome, and thalamic Dejerine-Roussy syndrome. Patients with P2 syndrome will present with contralateral hemianopia without macular sparing.

The right Vertebral artery arises from the innominate artery, whereas the left arises from the left subclavian artery. The vertebral artery is divided into four segments. The first segment (V1) arises from its origin till the 5th – 6th transverse foramina. The second segment (V2) traverses from C6 to C2. The third segment (V3) arches around the C1 vertebra and pierces the dura of the foramen magnum. The fourth segment (V4) joins the vertebral artery of the opposite side to form basilar artery.

The posterior inferior cerebellar artery (PICA) supplies the lateral medulla and the inferior surface of cerebellum. PICA syndrome results in ipsilateral facial palsy, ipsilateral face (trigeminal nerve) and contralateral trunk and limbs (lateral spinothalamic tract) impairment of pain and tempaerature, ipsilateral Horner's syndrome (descending sympathetic), nystagmus, dysphonia, dysarthria, and dysphagia (nucleus ambiguous), ipsilateral nystagmus, nausea, vomiting, vertigo (vestibular nucleus), ipsilateral ataxia (cerebellar involvement), ipsilateral absent gag reflex and hoarseness (glossopharyngeal reflex), deficit of reflex cough test (vagus nerve) and trismus due to masseter and temporals hyper connection (trigeminal nerve).

Management

Initial assessment

- Secure airway when threatened, maintaining saturation of more than 94% and correct dehydration with proper IV crystalloid fluids.

- Proper history and physical examination to rule out stroke mimics like hypoglycemia, hyponatremia, seizure, syncope, complicated migraine, and central nervous system (CNS) infections. Initial evaluation by the primary physician should not take more than 10 mins of arrival of patient.

- One stroke is suspected, the stroke team or the neurologic expertise contacted should be contacted within 15 mins of arrival of patient
- Brain imaging (CT scan or MRI brain) should be done ≤20 mins
- Interpretation of neuroimaging scan to be completed within 45 minutes from the time of arrival
- Determine if the patient is a candidate for intravenous thrombolytic therapy or endovascular therapy. Thrombolysis should be done ≤60 mins.

1. Blood pressure control in acute stroke

High blood pressure is common in acute stroke and is a predictor of poor outcome. Although lowering blood pressure in intracerebral hemorrhage is recommended, there is uncertainty over the optimal level of systolic blood pressure (SBP) in the setting of acute ischemic stroke (AIS).

Rapid Intervention with Glyceryl trinitrate in Hypertensive stroke Trial (RIGHT 2) was a study done to assess the safety and efficacy of transdermal Glyceryl trinitrate (GTN)when given very early after presumed stroke onset by paramedics before participants were admitted to the hospital. This was a multicentre, paramedic-delivered, ambulance-based, prospective, randomized, sham-controlled, blinded-endpoint, phase 3 trial in the UK done on adult patients with presumed stroke within 4 h of onset, face-arm-speech-time of 2 or 3, and systolic blood pressure of 120mmhg or higher. The result, however, showed that transdermal GTN did not improve the functional outcomes of the patients with presumed stroke within four hours of onset, the results however, are confounded by inclusion of patients with transient ischemic attack (TIA), intracerebral hemorrhage, and stroke mimics (1)

Early Manipulation of Arterial Blood Pressure in Acute Ischemic Stroke (MAPAS) aimed to study the efficacy of early manipulation of systolic blood pressure. This was a randomized control trial, where 218 patients were randomized within 12 h of AIS to maintain the SBP during 24 h within three ranges: 140-160 mmHg (Group 1), 161-180 mmHg (Group 2), or 181-200 mmHg (Group 3). Vasoactive drugs and fluids were used to achieve these targets. They observed that there were no clear benefit for blood pressure lowering within 12 hours of acute ischemic stroke onset, but an adjusted analysis suggested that a goal systolic blood pressure of 161 to 180 mmHg (group 2) increased the odds of a good outcome compared with higher or lower goal blood pressures. (2)

Blood pressure targets

- Acute ischaemic stroke
  - If the patient is a candidate for rtPA (recombinant tissue plasminogen activator) therapy, the target arterial blood pressures are systolic blood pressure ≤185 mm Hg and diastolic blood pressure ≤110 mm Hg.

- ○ If the patient is not a candidate for rtPA, rapid lowering of blood pressure is not indicated unless SBP and DBP are >220 mhg and >120 mmhg, respectively. This is to ensure protection of the penumbra. BP should be lowered slowly, by approximately 15% over 24 hours.

- Acute hemorrhagic stroke

  - ○ The optimum SBP target should be between 140-160 mmHg.

Table 1. Management of Hypertension Before Administration of Recombinant Tissue Plasminogen Activator (rtPA) or in Patients Awaiting Thrombectomy

Drug	Comments
Labetalol, 10–20 milligrams IV over 1–2 min, may repeat × 1	Use with caution in patients with severe asthma, severe chronic obstructive pulmonary disease, congestive heart failure, diabetes mellitus, myasthenia gravis
OR	
Nicardipine infusion, 5milligrams/h, titrate up by 2.5 milligrams/h at 5- to 15-min intervals; maximum dose: 15 milligrams/h; when desired blood pressure attained, reduce to 3 milligrams/h	Use with caution in patients with myocardial ischemia, concurrent use of fentanyl (hypotension), congestive heart failure, hypertrophic cardiomyopathy, portal hypertension, renal insufficiency, hepatic insufficiency (may need to adjust starting dose). Contraindicated in patients with severe aortic stenosis.

Table 2. Drug Treatment Of Hypertension During And After Administration Of Thrombolytics Or Other Acute Reperfusion Therapy

Drug	Comments
If systolic blood pressure is >180–230 mm Hg or diastolic blood pressure is >105–120 mm Hg	**Labetalol,** 10 milligrams IV followed by infusion at 2–8 milligrams/min. OR, **Nicardipine infusion,** 5 milligrams/h, titrate up by 2.5 milligrams/h at 5- to 15-min intervals; maximum dose 15 milligrams/h.
If blood pressure is not controlled by above measures, Consider **sodium nitroprusside infusion** (0.5–10 micrograms/kg/min). Continuous arterial monitoring; caution in patients with hepatic or renal insufficiency	

Table 3. Blood pressure monitoring

Time After Start of rtPA Infusion	Frequency of Blood Pressure Monitoring
0-2 h	Every 15 min
3-8 h Every 30 min	
9-24 h	Every 60 min

2. <u>Glycaemic control in acute stroke</u>

The current AHA/ASA guidelines recommend the maintenance of blood glucose between 140 milligrams/dL (7.77 mmol/L) and 180 milligrams/dL (9.99 mmol/L).

3. <u>Antiplatelet therapies in acute stroke</u>

Antiplatelet therapies reduce the relative risk of stroke by approximately 25 percent, or the absolute risk by 3.6 percentage over a period of 2 years, according to a meta-analysis from the Antithrombotic Trialists Collaboration. The only medical cost of this benefit is a slightly increased risk of major hemorrhage.

The current AHA/ASA guidelines recommend the administration of one antiplatelet agent to be started after 24 hours of receiving intravenous alteplase to minimize the risk of major intracranial bleeding in patients. Aspirin (at a dose of 160-300 mg), when administered within 48 hours of acute ischemic stroke, reduces the risk of recurrent stroke. Acute hemorrhagic stroke is a lifetime absolute contraindication to antiplatelet therapy.

There are no benefits from dual antiplatelet therapy (DAPT), as observed in the *MATCH trial (aspirin and clopidogrel compared with clopidogrel alone after recent ischaemic stroke or transient ischaemic attack in high-risk patients)*. It further increased the risk of intracerebral hemorrhage. (3)

However, the role of dual antiplatelet in high-risk Transient ischemic attacks (ABCD^2 >4) and small strokes (NIHSS ≤ 3) for short term use in the prevention of recurrent stroke has been studied. Two trials compared clopidogrel plus aspirin with aspirin alone in the early post ischaemic event period. The *CHANCE (Clopidogrel in High-Risk patients with Acute Non-disabling Cerebrovascular Events) and the POINT (Platelet Oriented Inhibition in New TIA and minor ischemic stroke) trial* showed a benefit of early DAPT after a high-risk TIA or small stroke, with longer duration of treatment in the POINT Trial resulting in a higher rate of hemorrhage. On the basis of these trials, short-term use of DAPT after a TIA or small stroke has been endorsed by recent guidelines. (4,5)

Genetic variation in clopidogrel metabolism due to loss-of-function *CYP2C19* variants may affect the efficacy of clopidogrel. The *CHANCE-2 Trial* took into account resistance to clopidogrel therapy based on genetic variation in the metabolism of drug. Clopidogrel being a prodrug, must be metabolized to an active drug by the hepatic CYP2C19 enzyme. Ticagrelor, like clopidogrel, works through the platelet P2Y12-ADP receptors, but does not require metabolic modification. Patients who carry one or both of the known loss of function of alleles of CYP2C19, can be expected to have a diminished response to clopidogrel. Such carriers make up an estimated 60 percent of the Asian population and 25 percent of the white population. In support of this hypothesis, there would be a decreased effect of clopidogrel in carriers of at least one CYP2C19 loss of function allele. Therefore, in patients with CYP2C19 loss of function alleles- single or both the copies, ticagrelor plus aspirin has superior benefits as compared to clopidogrel plus aspirin combination. (6)

The THALES trial found that the combination of ticagrelor and aspirin in patients with NIHSS score ≤5 and ABCD^2 score of 6-7 had a lower outcome of stroke or death within 30 days when compared to placebo(7). In conclusion from these three trials, DAPT with aspirin and clopidogrel or DAPT with aspirin and ticagrelor are both reasonable options for patients with high-risk TIA and minor stroke with an NIHSS score ≤5 for 21 days.

3. Role of anticoagulants in acute stroke

There is a limited role in early anticoagulant therapy in acute ischaemic stroke as compared to antiplatelet therapy due to the risk of bleeding complications and minimal efficacy. However, experts do use early anticoagulation therapy for acute cardioembolic ischemic stroke or TIA due to atrial fibrillation, large artery stenosis, intracardiac thrombus in the left ventricle or thrombus associated with mechanical or native heart valves who are at high short-term risk for recurrent stroke. Use of non-vitamin K Oral Anticoagulants (NOAC) like dabigatran, rivaroxaban, apixaban, and edoxaban provide more predictable anticoagulant activity than that of warfarin for prevention of stroke with a much lower risk of major bleeding.

4. Thrombolysis in acute stroke

The *NINDS (The National Institute of Neurological Disorders and Stroke rt-PA Study protocol)* trial in 1995 recommended that despite an increased incidence of symptomatic intracerebral hemorrhage, treatment with intravenous t-PA within three hours of the onset of acute ischemic stroke event improved clinical outcome at three months. (8)

The only FDA approved drug for thrombolysis to this day is *alteplase*; given intravenously at a dose of 0.9 mg/kg body weight (weight based), maximum dose of 90 mg; 10% of the total dose given as a bolus dose over 1 minute, and the remaining 90% given as a slow intravenous infusion over 1 hour. The door to needle time in case of acute ischemic stroke is 60 minutes.

Table 4. American Heart Association (AHA)/American Stroke Association (ASA) 2018 Inclusion/Exclusion Criteria for IV Alteplase in Acute Ischemic Stroke are as follows:

Inclusion criteria	
Onset of symptoms < 3h prior to thrombolytic administration	Defined as the time the patient was last known well or last known to be at their neurologic baseline
Measurable diagnosis of acute ischemic stroke	Use of NIHSS score recommended. There is no upper or lower limit of NIHSS score for thrombolytics, as the benefit may be seen with both mild but disabling stroke symptoms as well as in very severe strokes.
Age ≥18 y	No upper age limit for < 3h last well known time administration
Onset of symptoms from 3 to 4.5 h prior to rtPA administration	Must meet the above inclusion criteria, plus these additional inclusion criteria: Age ≤80 y; No history of diabetes mellitus and prior stroke; NIHSS score ≤25; Not taking oral anticoagulants; No brain imaging evidence of ischemic injury involving greater than one-third of the middle cerebral artery territory
Exclusion criteria	
1. Last known well time >3 or 4.5 hours	
2. Acute intracranial hemorrhage or history of intracranial hemorrhage	
3. Symptoms and signs suggestive of subarachnoid hemorrhage	
4. CT brain imaging that exhibits extensive regions of clear hypoattenuation	
5. Prior ischemic stroke or severe head trauma within 3 months	
6. Intracranial/intraspinal surgery within 3 months	
7. GI malignancy or GI bleeding within 21 days	
8. Pre-treatment systolic blood pressure >185 mm Hg or diastolic blood pressure >110 mm Hg despite therapy	

Two European trials, the *European Cooperative Acute Stroke Study (ECASS) and ECASS 2*, investigated a time window of up to 6 hours but failed to show the efficacy of thrombolytic therapy. Subsequently, the *ECASS 3 trial* showed that as compared to placebo, intravenous alteplase administered between 3 and 4.5 hours after onset of symptoms significantly improved clinical outcomes in patients with acute ischemic stroke. Alteplase was more frequently associated with symptomatic intracranial hemorrhage. *ECASS 4 trial* studied whether acute ischemic stroke patients with penumbral tissue identified in magnetic resonance imaging (MRI) 4.5-9 hours after symptom onset benefitted from intravenous thrombolysis compared to placebo. The study concluded that intravenous alteplase administered between 4.5 and 9 hours after onset of symptoms in patients with salvageable tissue did not result in a significant benefit over placebo.

Hence to this date, thrombolysis with intravenous alteplase is recommended only upto 4.5 hours from the onset of acute disabling ischemic stroke, if not otherwise contraindicated. (9–12)

About 25 percent of all strokes occur during sleep, i.e., without knowledge of the exact time of symptom onset. From clinical and imaging studies, there is evidence suggesting that many wake-up strokes occur close to awakening, and thus, patients might be within the approved time window of thrombolysis when presenting to the emergency department. Several imaging approaches are suggested to identify wake-up stroke patients likely to benefit from thrombolysis, including non-contrast CT, CT perfusion, penumbral MRI, and the recent concept of diffusion weighted imaging-fluid attenuated inversion recovery (DWI-FLAIR).

WAKE-UP trial sought to determine whether patients with stroke with an unknown time of onset and features suggesting recent cerebral infarction on MRI would benefit from IV thrombolysis. It was a multicenter, randomized, double-blind, placebo-controlled clinical trial involving patients with unknown time of stroke onset. All the patients otherwise met the clinical criteria of IV thrombolysis. Patients underwent randomization to receive either intravenous alteplase or a placebo. The study included all patients with an unclear time of onset of disabling acute ischemic stroke (>4.5 h from the time last known to be well), a diffusion restriction demonstrated in DW-MRI, but no abnormal parenchymal hyperintensities on FLAIR sequencing (i.e., mismatch), lesion not larger than one-third of the MCA territory, NIHSS score of 25 or less. All patients in whom thrombolysis was contraindicated, in whom thrombectomy was already planned, and NIHSS score >25 (severe stroke) were excluded from the study. The study inferred that there is a significantly better functional outcome and numerically more symptomatic intracranial hemorrhages amongst those who received IV thrombolysis than placebo at 90 days. (13)

For most patients with acute ischemic stroke, the odds of benefit from intravenous alteplase decline steeply over the first 4.5 hours. This decay curve is derived from trials in which all participants were selected on the basis of non-contrast computed tomography (CT), which is widely available and valuable to exclude hemorrhage or other structural contraindications to treatment. However, non-contrast CT has inherently low sensitivity to early ischemic changes and does not discriminate irreversibly damaged tissue from viable tissue.

Arrival at the hospital outside the 4.5-hour time window with uncertainty about the time of onset of symptoms, most commonly due to waking with stroke, has restricted a patients eligibility for intravenous thrombolysis. More advanced physiological imaging has suggested that this short time window may be too conservative for some, including those termed "slow progressors" with a favorable leptomeningeal collateral circulation who are able to sustain a small core/large penumbra perfusion pattern over longer periods of time. This has led to many studies studying the role of IV thrombolysis after 4.5 hours of symptom onset

Table 5. The table summarizes previous Randomized Clinical Trials of Intravenous Thrombolysis and Thrombectomy based on Imaging Biomarkers in Extended Time Windows (>4.5 hours since onset).

Trial	Year	Time window	Imaging method
Thrombolysis			
DIAS	2005	3-6h	MRI-diffusion perfusion mismatch
DEDAS	2006	3-9 h	MRI-diffusion perfusion mismatch
EPITHET	2008	3-9 h	MRI-diffusion perfusion mismatch
DIAS 2	2009	3-9 h	MRI-diffusion perfusion mismatch or CTP
DIAS 3	2015	3-9 h	Intracranial large vessel occlusion
DIAS 4	2016	3-9 h	Intracranial large vessel occlusion
EXTEND	2018	4.5-9 h	CTP
WAKE UP	2018	4.5 h after waking	MRI diffusion-FLAIR mismatch
ECASS 4	2019	4.5-9 h	MRI-diffusion perfusion mismatch
Mechanical thrombectomy			
MR RESCUE	2013	8 h	MRI-diffusion perfusion mismatch
DAWN	2018	6-24 h	CTP defined core or MRI DWI core
DEFFUSE 3	2018	6-16 h	Defined core and mismatch ratio on either CTP or MRI

5. <u>Mechanical thrombectomy in acute ischemic stroke</u>

Indications

- Neuroimaging (e.g., CT without contrast or diffusion-weighted MRI) is consistent with a small infarct core (ie, limited signs of early ischemic change) and excludes hemorrhage
- Angiography (e.g., CT angiography or magnetic resonance [MR] angiography) demonstrates a proximal large artery occlusion in the anterior circulation
- Thrombectomy is performed at a stroke center with appropriate expertise in the use of stent retrievers
- The patient has a persistent, potentially disabling neurologic deficit
- Thrombectomy can be started within 24 hours of the time last known to be well

Two randomized controlled trials have shown the benefit of mechanical thrombectomy performed ≥ 6 hours after onset of stroke in patients with an occlusion of the intracranial part of internal carotid artery, or the first segment of the middle cerebral artery.

The DAWN trial used the combination of patients in whom NIHSS score of 10 or higher and baseline infarct involving less than one-third of the territory of the MCA on CT or MRIselect patients who had an onset of stroke 6-24 hours earlier. (14)

The DEFUSE 3 trial included patients who had an onset of stroke 6-16 hours earlier and had a large mismatch profile on CT perfusion or MRI defined as an ischemic core volume <70 ml, a mismatch ratio (the volume of the perfusion lesion divided by the volume of the ischemic core) >1.8, and a mismatch volume (volume of perfusion lesion minus the volume of the ischemic core) >15 and NIHSS score of 6 or higher. (15)

Both the studies showed that patients with a score of 0-2 on the modified Rankin scale at 90 days were significantly higher among patients who underwent mechanical thrombectomy than amongst those who did not. Therefore, the studies concluded that mechanical thrombectomy that is done >6 hours of the onset of acute ischemic stroke proved to be beneficial in disability limitation and stroke outcome.

STICH II TRIAL

A randomized trial to identify the balance of risk and benefit from early neurosurgical intervention for conscious patients with superficial **supratentorial intracerebral hemorrhage** of 10–100 mL and no intraventricular hemorrhage admitted within 48 hrs.The trial was undertaken in 78 centers in 27 countries, compared early surgical haematoma evacuation within 12 h of randomisation plus medical treatment with initial medical treatment alone.The primary outcome was a prognosis-based dichotomised (favorable or unfavorable) outcome of the 8 point Extended Glasgow Outcome Scale (GOSE) obtained by questionnaires posted to patients at 6 months.

307 of 601 patients were randomly assigned to early surgery and 294 to initial conservative treatment, 298 and 291 were followed up at 6 months, respectively.174 (59%) of 297 patients in the early surgery group had an unfavorable outcome versus 178 (62%) of 286 patients in the initial conservative treatment group (absolute difference 3·7% [95% CI −4·3 to 11·6], odds ratio 0·86 [0·62 to 1·20]; p=0·367).

The **STICH II** results confirm that early surgery **does not increase the rate of death or disability** at 6 months and might have a small but clinically relevant survival advantage for patients with spontaneous superficial intracerebral hemorrhage without intraventricular hemorrhage.

Transient Ischemic Attack (TIA)

Definition

A transient ischemic attack (TIA) is a medical emergency. It is defined as a transient episode of neurologic dysfunction due to the focal brain, spinal cord, or retinal ischemia, without acute infarct or tissue injury. The definition of TIA has moved from time-based to tissue-based. The historical time-based definition of TIA was based on full resolution of all symptoms within 24 hours of onset. This time-based definition has been debated in light of diffusion-weighted MRI demonstrating relevant ischemic lesions in 30% to 50% of patients fulfilling the time-based definition of TIA.

TIA offers the greatest opportunity to prevent stroke that physicians encounter. A TIA should be treated as a medical emergency, as up to 80% of strokes after TIA are preventable.

Risk stratification score

1. *ABCD2 score-* is very important for predicting subsequent risks of TIA or stroke. It comprises factors including age, blood pressure, clinical symptoms, duration and diabetes.

A= Age more than 60 years/ score 1

B= SBP> 140 OR DBP> 90/ score 1

C= clinical features: Speech impairment without weakness/ score 1

Weakness with/without speech impairment/ score 2

D= Duration: More than 60 mins/ score 2

Between 10-59 mins/ score 1

D= Diabetes/ score 1

Low-risk (0-3), Medium risk (4-5), High-risk (6-7)

Patients with ABCD2 score of 6-7 have an 8% risk of stroke within 48 hours and those with a score of less than 5 have a 1% risk of stroke within 48 hours.

2. *ABCD3 score-* The $ABCD^3$-I score is derived by assigning 2 points for dual TIA (an earlier TIA within 7 days of the index event), 2 points for ipsilateral ≥50% stenosis of the internal carotid artery, and 2 points for acute DWI hyperintensity to the $ABCD^2$ score.

Low-risk (0–3), Medium-risk (4–7), and High-risk (8–13)

Table 6. Table summarizing risk stratification scores in TIA.

	ABCD2	ABCD3
Age ≥60 years	1	1
Blood pressure ≥140/90 mmhg	1	1
Clinical features		
Unilateral weakness	2	2
Speech impairment without weakness	1	1
Duration		
≥60 mins	2	2
10-59 mins	1	1
Diabetes mellitus present	1	1
Dual TIA (TIA prompting medical attention plus atleast another TIA in the preceding 7 days	NA	2
Imaging – Ipsilateral ≥50% stenosis of internal carotid artery	NA	2
Imaging – acute diffusion-weighted imaging hyperintensities	NA	2

Subarachnoid Hemorrhage

Introduction

Nontraumatic headache is one of the common complaints among patients presenting to the emergency department. Although many causes of headache are benign, subarachnoid hemorrhage (SAH) is one of the serious etiology and is a true medical emergency.

Common clinical presentation includes sudden severe headache (commonly referred to as thunderclap headache), neck stiffness, and altered mental status. Misdiagnosis occurs in 12% to 50% of patients and is more common in patients with atypical presentation.

Although trauma is the leading cause of SAH, the most common cause of atraumatic SAH is a ruptured cerebral aneurysm, accounting for 85% of cases, followed by non-aneurysmal venous "peri-mesencephalic" hemorrhages and arteriovenous malformations. Other less common causes of atraumatic SAH are amyloid angiopathy, hypertension, and reversible cerebral vasoconstriction syndrome. Risk factors for SAH owing to aneurysm rupture include smoking, hypertension, alcohol abuse, sympathomimetic drug use, having a first degree relative with a cerebral aneurysm, female sex, and polycystic kidney disease.

Patterns of hemorrhage

The location of the hemorrhage and pattern on a CT scan of the brain can be useful in predicting the presence of an aneurysm, location of the aneurysm, and whether or not it is traumatic. 70% of aneurysms occur in the anterior communicating artery, posterior communicating artery, and middle cerebral artery. Blood from a ruptured aneurysm typically surrounds the basal cisterns. In traumatic SAH, the blood is typically located in areas of coup or contrecoup force or higher up in the cerebral convexities. The difference in location may be particularly helpful in patients with SAH who may have fallen from syncope and present with a headache. Finally, convexal SAH has been described in various case series, and the etiologies are believed to be related to reversible cerebral vasoconstriction syndrome in younger patients or cerebral amyloid angiopathy as opposed to aneurysmal in origin.

Ottawa Subarachnoid rules

The rule can be applied to alert patients who are ≥15 years of age, have no recent head trauma, lack of new neurologic deficits, with no history of a prior aneurysm, brain tumor, or SAH.

If one or more criteria are present, SAH cannot be ruled out, and the patient requires a workup:

- Age greater than 40 years
- Complaint of neck pain or stiffness

- Witnessed loss of consciousness
- Onset with exertion
- Thunderclap headache
- Limited neck flexion on examination

Ottawa Subarachnoid rules have been internally and externally validated and are highly sensitive for ruling out SAH.

Emerald subarachnoid hemorrhage rule

If any one of the four criteria is present, patient needs further workup for SAH -

- Serum potassium< 3.9 mEq/L
- SBP> 150 mmHg
- DBP> 90 mmHg
- Blood glucose> 115 mg/dL

Diagnostic approach

In patients for whom SAH is suspected, the initial testing modality is brain imaging. This modality is most commonly a non-contrast CT scan because it is most readily available in most emergency departments. When performed in the first 24 hours of headache onset, the sensitivity of a CT scan for detecting subarachnoid blood ranges from 90% to 100% and approaches 100% when performed within the first 6 hours. The sensitivity decreases as time from onset to CT scan elapses owing to the dilution of blood by the normal flow of cerebrospinal fluid. Other factors that decrease the sensitivity include technical issues (i.e., older CT scanners with <32 slices or patient movements), interpretation error, small-volume bleeds, and anemia.

A negative head CT scan of more than 6 hours after the onset of headache can undergo a lumbar puncture to assess for the presence of red blood cells, or xanthochromia which will definitely rule out SAH. Both the number of RBCs and the presence of xanthochromia are a function of time from the bleed. Xanthochromia or the yellowish hue resulting from the breakdown of hemoglobin, is detected by visual inspection (in most North American laboratories) or spectrophotometry and is highly sensitive for SAH. RBCs appear very early in the course after the hemorrhage occurs, within the first few hours. Xanthochromia may take up to 12 hours to develop but is present by 6 hours. Thus, assessing CSF for both RBCs and the presence of xanthochromia is recommended. Emergency physicians must be aware of the possibility of a traumatic lumbar puncture when interpreting CSF results which can occur when blood from local trauma or a venous plexus contaminates the fluid. These are estimated to happen in 16% to 31% of lumbar punctures. There is no universally accepted method of evaluating RBC clearance to establish the likelihood of traumatic lumbar puncture versus

SAH. On the surface, a commonly held belief has held if there are fewer RBCs in the 4th tube than the first, the likelihood of a traumatic lumbar puncture is high, and the probability of SAH is lower.

For patients in whom the CSF analysis is suggestive of SAH, the next steps in the workup and management include vascular imaging and neurosurgical consultation. In the past several decades, CT angiography has become the imaging modality of choice because it is non-invasive and highly sensitive for cerebral aneurysms. If no source is visible on the CTA, then digital subtraction angiography should be considered.

Grading severity

Table 7. The grading system proposed by Hunt and Hess and that of the World Federation of Neurological Surgeons (WFNS) are among the most widely used.

Hunt and Hess scale	
Grade 1	GCS score 15, no motor deficit
Grade 2	GCS score 13 to 14, no motor deficit
Grade 3	GCS score 13 to 14, with motor deficit
Grade 4	GCS score 7 to 12, with or without motor deficit
Grade 5	GCS score 3 to 6, with or without motor deficit
World Federation of Neurological Surgeons (WFNS)	
Grade 1	Asymptomatic or mild headache and slight nuchal rigidity
Grade 2	Moderate to severe headache, stiff neck, no neurologic deficit except cranial nerve palsy
Grade 3	Drowsy or confused, mild focal neurologic deficit
Grade 4	Stupor, moderate or severe hemiparesis
Grade 5	Deep coma, decerebrate posturing

Table 8. Modified fisher score and VASOGRADE predicted the risk of delayed cerebral ischemia due to vasospasm after SAH.

Modified fisher score (Classen grading system)	
Grade 0	No SAH or IVH
Grade 1	Minimal SAH and no IVH
Grade 2	Minimal SAH with bilateral IVH
Grade 3	Thick SAH (completely filling one or more cistern or fissure) without bilateral IVH
Grade 4	Thick SAH (completely filling one or more cistern or fissure) with bilateral IVH
VASOGRADE	
Green	WFNS 1 or 2 and mFS 1 or 2
Yellow	WFNS 1 to 3 and mFS 3 or 4
Red	WFNS 4 or 5 and any mFS

Initial ED treatment

- Airway protection if this is compromised or for expected worsening clinical course
- Blood pressure control with a goal SBP of less than 160 mmHg or a mean arterial pressure (MAP) of less than 140 mmhg. Maintain euvolemic status
- Head end elevation to 30 degree and neutral head position
- Analgesia and sedation administration as needed
- Cardiac monitoring
- Nimodipine to prevent vasospasm (60 mg every 4 hours)
- Consideration of seizure prophylaxis and treatment
- Anticoagulant reversal if indicated.
- Neurosurgical opinion to be taken immediately

Epilepsy

Recent updates in epilepsy and its management

Definitions as per International League Against Epilepsy (ILAE)

Status epilepticus

A seizure that lasts longer than 5 minutes, or having more than one seizure within a 5 minutes period, without returning to a normal level of consciousness between episodes.

This is a medical emergency that may lead to permanent brain damage or death.

Established Status epilepticus

Status epilepticus that persists after treatment with a benzodiazepine (BZD, considered as the first line therapy).

Refractory Status epilepticus

Status epilepticus that persists or fails to terminate even after treatment with both first line agent (BDZ) and second line agents (phenytoin/levetiracetam/valproate).

Super refractory SE

Status epilepticus that persists or fails to terminate after treatment with first line, second line and third line agents (anaesthetic agents like midazolam or propofol infusion).

New-onset refractory SE (NORSE)

Defined as a condition and not a specific diagnosis where there isn't a clear or active structural, toxic or metabolic cause for the seizure in a patient without active epilepsy.

In up to half of the cases of NORSE, a possible or probable cause is ultimately found, most often autoimmune or paraneoplastic encephalitis. In remaining half of the cases of NORSE, no cause, whatsoever is identified, despite an extensive workup. These cases are referred to as *cryptogenic NORSE or NORSE of unknown etiology.*

Febrile Infection Related Epilepsy Syndrome (FIRES)

sub-category of NORSE, that requires a prior febrile infection starting between 2 weeks and 24 hours prior to onset of refractory SE, with or without fever at the onset of SE.

Recently ILAE has brought in two operational dimensions

Time point 1 (T1)

Actual length of the seizure and beyond which the seizure should be regarded as a continuous seizure activity.

Time point 2 (T2)

Time of ongoing seizure activity after which there is risk of long-term consequences.

Table 9. Time point 1 and 2 status epilepticus

Type of SE	Time point 1 (t1)	Time point 2 (t2)
Tonic clonic	5 minutes	30 minutes
Focal with impaired consciousness	10 minutes	>60 minutes
Absence	10-15 minutes	Inadequate data

Recent updates on the choice of antiepileptics

Established SE treatment trial (ESETT) in 2018 was a randomized trial that compared the efficacy and safety of levetiracetam, fosphenytoin, and sodium valproate.

The study concluded that in the context of benzodiazepine refractory SE, these three IV anticonvulsant drugs each led to the cessation of seizures, improved alertness at 60 minutes, and these drugs were associated with a similar incidence of adverse effects. No individual drug was found to be superior to another. (16)

Sanad II study (2021), an open-label, randomized controlled trial to compare levetiracetam with valproate as first-line treatment for patients with newly diagnosed generalized epilepsy and in epilepsy that is difficult to classify. Compared with valproate, levetiracetam was found to be neither clinically effective nor cost-effective. For girls and women of child-bearing potential, the results informed the risk-benefit assessment of sodium valproate with regard to teratogenic potentials. (17)

Newer drugs in the treatment of epilepsy

<u>Ketamine</u>

It is a non-competitive N-methyl D-aspartate (NMDA) receptor antagonist. In recent studies, it has been reported that the number and activity of glutamate-sensitive NMDA receptors significantly increased in refractory and super-refractory SE. Since ketamine acts by inhibiting NMDA, ketamine helps in abating seizure activity in refractory and super-refractory cases. It exerts neuroprotective action and is also not associated with significant cardiorespiratory depression.

<u>Brivaracetam (BRV)</u>

It is the N-propyl analogue of levetiracetam which is the latest antiepileptic drug to be licensed in Europe and the USA for adjunctive treatment of focal onset seizures with or without secondary generalization in patients aged 16 years and above. BRV is a highly selective and reversible SV2A ligand with a 15-30 fold higher affinity than levetiracetam.

Immunomodulators

The role of immunity and inflammation appears to be an integral part of the pathogenic process associated with some seizures, particularly refractory seizures. Prompt treatment with immunotherapy (such as corticosteroids, immunoglobulins, plasmapheresis, or steroid-sparing drugs like azathioprine) has been found to have a role in refractory and super-refractory SE.

Inhalational anesthetic agents

Isoflurane and, less commonly, desflurane has been found to be effective in refractory SE by obtaining burst suppression. The only documented side effect is significant hypotension.

Coma

Approach to coma in emergency medicine department

Introduction

Coma is defined as a state of prolonged unresponsive unconsciousness. The common pathway resulting in coma is thought to include the disruption of neuronal function or pathways from the ascending reticular activating system through the thalami to the cortex. Lesions only affecting the ascending reticular activating system or bilateral hemispheres result in coma. It should never be attributed to unilateral cortical lesions.

Treatment of coma is targeted toward immediate stabilization, identification of reversible underlying etiologies, and correcting alterations in normal physiological processes.

History

Relevant questions one must enquire are:

- Acuity and onset
- Was the patient showing earlier signs such as excessive sleepiness, confusion, or memory problems before coma onset?
- Was the patient experiencing other symptoms such as fevers, unusual movements, weakness, numbness or tingling, headaches, light sensitivity, or neck or back pain?
- What was the patient doing when this occurred?
- When was the last time they were seen in their usual state of health?
- History of brain surgery?

<u>Vascular risk factors</u>

Hypertension, hyperlipidemia, diabetes mellitus, coronary artery disease, smoking history, obstructive sleep apnea, atrial fibrillation, previous history of stroke or intracerebral hemorrhage, family history of aneurysms, or history of thrombosis or thromboembolism

<u>Seizure risk factors</u>

- Personal or family history of seizures or status epilepticus
- Febrile seizures as a child
- History of head trauma with loss of consciousness

- History of central nervous system infection
- History of psychiatric disease
- History of depression or suicidal ideations
- Prescribed psychiatric medications
- Compliant with medications
- the last refill of antiepileptics
- History of substance abuse
- Which substances
- How much
- Any use of injectable drugs

Physical examination

- Tachycardia
- Bradycardia
- Hypertension
- Hypotension may result in cerebral hypoperfusion and coma. It is nonspecific with a broad differential diagnosis that includes shock, End-stage renal disease, end-stage liver disease, an overdose of antihypertensive medication, spinal cord injury, and intoxication with opiates, barbiturates or benzodiazepine.
- Tachypnea may occur in response to a lesion in the midbrain, but more commonly as a result of a primary pulmonic process, a pain response, or as compensation for metabolic acidosis, in settings of sepsis and drug intoxication (Kussmaul's breathing).
- Apnea
- irregular breathing patterns like Cheyne-Stokes breathing because of metabolic encephalopathy, supratentorial lesions, and lesions of midbrain
- Apneustic breathing from pontine lesions
- Ataxic/biot's breathing from lesions in the medulla.
- Hiccups may be seen in medullary lesions.
- Important eye findings like papilledema, retinal hemorrhage and detachment suggestive of head trauma, and periorbital ecchymosis.

Neurologic examination

Table 10. Pupils and associated cranial nerve signs

Bilateral miosis "pinpoint pupils"	Opiates Benzodiazepines Barbiturates Cholinomimetic substances (pilocarpine, carbachol, etc.) Cholinesterase inhibiters (neostigmine, organophosphates, etc) Clonidine Phenothiazine Ergot derivatives Pontine lesion
Bilateral mydriasis	Anticholinergics (atropine, diphenhydramine, scopolamine) Sympathomimetics (cocaine, methamphetamines, MDMA, dopamine, phenylephrine, norepinephrine) Serotonergics (selective serotonin reuptake inhibitors, psilocybin, d-lysergic acid diethylamide, dextromethorphan) Opioid or benzodiazepine withdrawal Oxytocin Increased intracranial pressure with bilateral cranial nerve III compression (nonreactive) Botulinum toxin Post-traumatic iridoplegia Diabetic neuropathy
Anisocoria	May be a normal finding, especially if minimal difference in size and both reactive Unilateral cranial nerve III compression (herniation) Midbrain lesion affecting the cranial nerve III nucleus Posterior communicating artery aneurysm Horner's syndrome Adie's tonic pupil Post-traumatic irido plegia Diabetic neuropathy
Conjugate gaze deviation	Structural lesion involving the frontal lobe ipsilateral to direction of gaze Rarely, can be caused by pontine lesion Seizure involving the frontal lobe contralateral to direction of gaze
Skew	Brain stem or cerebellar lesion
Nystagmus	Bidirectional and sustained, vertical or rotatory - brain stem or cerebellar lesion
Sunset Sign	Loss of vertical gaze - dorsal midbrain lesion or hydrocephalus
Ocular bobbing	Extensive pontine lesion, associated with poor prognosis

<u>Other cranial nerve finidngs</u>

The absence of the corneal, cough or gag reflexes is another sign of severe diffuse cerebral dysfunction, but the etiology is nonspecific. Central facial asymmetry seen with cortical or subcortical injury. The Head version may be indicative of a focal seizure originating from the contralateral hemisphere.

<u>Motor and sensory findings</u>

Increased tone because of serotonin syndrome, malignant hyperthermia, neuroleptic malignant syndrome, subacute or chronic brain injury, and seizure. Response to noxious stimulation in the upper extremities can be categorized as localization, withdrawal, decorticate, or decerebrate posturing. Triple flexion is a non-sustained, stereotyped flexion at the hip, knee, and ankle and is a brain stem mediated response reflecting a loss of cortical involvement.

<u>Reflex testing</u>

Hyperreflexia or clonus are seen in serotonin syndrome, neuroleptic malignant syndrome, malignant hyperthermia, or tetanus. Hyporeflexia is seen in the acute brain or spinal cord injury.

Differential diagnosis of coma and discussion

Structural causes of coma

- <u>Ischemic causes</u>

  Bilateral anterior cerebral artery strokes
  Basilar occlusion
  Vasculitis

- <u>Hemorrhagic causes</u>

  SAH
  Thalamic hemorrhage
  Pontine hemorrhage

- <u>Others</u>

  Traumatic brain injury
  Hydrocephalus
  Midbrain tumour
  Central pontine myelinolysis
  Supratentorial mass causing herniation
  Multiple sclerosis

Initial management

Comatose patients will have a compromised airway and therefore need endotracheal intubation to ensure safety for neuroimaging. Since neuroimaging requires prolonged supine positioning, any patient with over evidence of elevated intracranial pressure must be treated with empiric osmotic therapy before neuroimaging.

Any lesion causing substantial mass effect, herniation, or suspicion for globally elevated intracranial pressure to be treated with osmotic therapy such as mannitol or hypertonic saline while awaiting neurosurgical consultation.

Steroid administration should be confined to vasogenic cerebral edema due to an underlying tumor and is not recommended for edema surrounding hemorrhages. In cases of intracranial hemorrhages, targeting systolic blood pressure to less than 160 mmHg has been shown to limit hematoma expansion. There is no evidence for the use of prophylactic antiepileptic drugs.

Some conditions are discussed below

1. **Non-convulsive status epilepticus versus postictal state**

   Status epilepticus is further divided into convulsive or nonconvulsive. Generalized convulsive status epilepticus is characterized by tonic or tonic–clonic movements accompanied by an altered mental status. In contrast, non-convulsive status epilepticus does not have any obvious signs suggesting prolonged seizures but rather is defined electrographically. Patients who present with non-convulsive status epilepticus have underlying comorbidities and are acutely ill. The differentials are broad and include toxic or metabolic derangements, infection, or structural brain lesions. Non-convulsive status epilepticus is generally more refractory to treatment.

   <u>Diagnosis</u>

   A non-contrast CT of the head is the initial imaging to rule out acute structural etiologies. MRI brain can be considered once the patient is stabilized.

   An electroencephalogram (EEG) is the only definitive method of making the diagnosis of non-convulsive SE and helps in differentiating non-convulsive SE from postictal state.

   Serum prolactin levels is a non-specific test for the diagnosis of SE which helps to differentiate patients with epileptic seizures from psychogenic nonepileptic seizures. Blood sample must be drawn within 20 minutes from the time of the seizure.

   A lumbar puncture is of value to exclude central nervous system infections.

   <u>Treatment</u>

   • Primary survey and initial securing of airway.

Benzodiazepines are the first line treatment – lorazepam IV 0.1mg/kg, or midazolam 0.2mg/kg

- Second line treatment – levetiracetam 20-60mg/kg; lacosamide 200-400 mg; phenytoin 20mg/kg loading dose may be repeated by 5-10mg/kg after 5-10 mins; valproate 20-40mg/kg,

- Anaesthetic agents – third line treatment (refractory SE)- propofol 1-2mg/kg loading dose followed by infusion 20 mcg/kg/min; midazolam 0.2mg/kg loading followed by infusion starting 0.05-2mg/kg/h.

- Super-refractory SE induced barbiturate coma with phenobarbital 5-15mg/kg loading dose followed by continuous infusion at 0.5-5mg/kg/h, at a maximum rate of 50mg/h.

2. **Encephalitis**

Meningoencephalitis is one important differential among patients in a comatose state. Both infectious and non-infectious causes are to be considered.

Meningitis does not present with altered mental status and instead presents with meningismus: headache, neck stiffness, and photosensitivity.

Encephalitis, in contrast, affects the brain focally or diffusely and may present with a myriad of signs, including confusion, lethargy, personality changes, motor or sensory deficits, or seizures.

Diagnosis

A CT scan of the head may not be abnormal in meningitis or encephalitis, but may have a localized area of hypodensity reflecting vasogenic edema surrounding an abscess. It is also necessary to exclude a mass lesion to ensure a safe lumbar puncture. An MRI of the brain with and without contrast may be considered once the patient has been treated empirically for potentially reversible causes.

Treatment

If an infectious cause is of high suspicion, steroids and empiric antimicrobial therapy should be started without delay. Recommended empiric regimen:

- Dexamethasone 0.15mg/kg every 6 hours for 2-4 days

- Vancomycin 15-20 mg/kg every 8-12 hours

- Third-generation cephalosporin- ceftriaxone 2g every 12 hourly

- Acyclovir 10mg/kg every 8 hours

- Consider ampicillin to cover atypical organisms in elderly patients >50 years and immunocompromised patients.

- Use fourth-generation cephalosporin- cefepime instead of third-generation in case of recent neurosurgical procedures.

3. Metabolic causes

Hypoglycemia is one of the most common and immediately reversible causes of coma. All comatose patients with initial finger prick suggestive of hypoglycemia with history of alcohol abuse should be treated with immediate IV dextrose preceded by IV thiamine.

Among diabetic patients on treatment, an underlying explanation for hypoglycemia such as insulin overdose should always be sought; in the case of accidental overdose of short-acting insulin. Emergency department observation and discharge may be all that is indicated, whereas patients with intentional overdoses, overdoses of long-acting insulin, and unexplained hypoglycemia should be admitted for more prolonged monitoring and further workup.

Other important causes include hypercarbic respiratory insufficiency (COPD, neuromuscular disorders, opiate intoxication causing central hypoventilation), electrolyte abnormalities, including calcium, magnesium, and sodium. Consider written documentation of core body temperature of all comatose patients as hypothermia is an important environmental cause of coma.

4. Thyroid dysfunction

Thyroid dysfunction in the form of severe decompensated hypothyroidism can result in an entity termed "myxedema coma." This syndrome includes hypoactive delirium or coma, hypoventilation, bradycardia, hypotension, hypothermia, thick coarse skin, and thinning hair. Seizures may occur as well, especially in the setting of severe metabolic derangements. It is important to also investigate precipitating factors such as infection, cold exposure, and recent trauma. An association exists between decompensated hypothyroidism and intoxication with opioids or other classes of sedating medications, as well as with amiodarone use.

<u>Diagnosis</u>

The mainstay of diagnosis is laboratory confirmed thyroid function test; raised TSH levels suggestive of primary hypothyroidism, whereas a normal or low TSH level points toward secondary hypothyroidism. Decreased cortisol levels occur secondary to adrenal insufficiency. Euvolemic hyponatremia can cause AMS. ABG reveals hypoxia and hypercapnia. ECG may show sinus arrhythmia and QT prolongation. EEG monitoring will help excluding nonconvulsive status epilepticus.

<u>Treatment</u>

- IV hydrocortisone 100 mg 8 hourly till exclusion of adrenal insufficiency
- Levothyroxine 200-300mcg IV, followed by daily doses of 1.6mcg/kg

- Tri-iodothyronine 10-25mcg IV followed by 2.5-10mcg every 8 hours
- Supportive care- ventilatory and circulatory support
- Treatment of underlying infections
- Treatment of arrhythmias

5. Toxicologic causes

<u>Opiate toxicity</u> is associated with miosis and bradypnea. IV naloxone, a competitive opiate antagonist, helps in the reversal of opiate toxicity besides having a benign side-effect profile and may help avoid intubation. Naloxone has a short half-life, often shorter than opiate; therefore, continuous infusion is started after initial reversal of symptoms.

<u>Benzodiazepine,</u> another class of drug have the potential to cause coma, particularly in intentional or suicidal ingestions. Physical findings include severe depressed mental status with silent EEG. Flumazenil, competitive antagonist, can be used to reverse the effects of a known benzodiazepine. However, it should be best avoided in unknown or chronic benzodiazepine administration to avoid withdrawal and intractable seizures.

<u>Barbiturate</u> ingestion causes a similar presentation as benzodiazepine, but it does not have a specific reversal agent, and therefore supportive treatment is the primary treatment modality available to this day.

<u>Acute alcohol intoxication</u> mandates management of hypotension and bradycardia. Elevated levels of osmolar gap and anion gap metabolic acidosis should raise suspicion of methanol and ethylene glycol toxicity. When clinical suspicion exists, fomepizole- an alcohol dehydrogenase inhibitor is administered so as to prevent breakdown into toxic metabolites. Wernicke's encephalopathy causes reversible global confusion and coma. Thiamine should be administered empirically to comatose patients with suspicion of alcohol use disorders.

<u>Severe carbon monoxide poisoning</u> may result in coma. MRI brain showing restricted diffusion, particularly in the globus pallidus is strongly suggestive of CO poisoning. Besides supportive care, specific treatment includes oxygen supplementation and consideration of hyperbaric oxygen therapy.

6. Psychogenic causes

Catatonia, psychogenic nonepileptic seizures, conversion disorders, factitious disorders, or malingering should be considered as a possible underlying cause of coma once other medical conditions are considered and ruled out. The patient's physical examination is the most telling diagnostic test for these entities and consultation with an experienced neurologist may be helpful.

Dizziness

Diagnostic approach in patients with acute dizziness

In an analysis of 9472 patients from a large National Hospital Ambulatory Medical Care Survey database of ED patients, the causes of dizziness listed by the attending emergency physicians were as follows:

- General medical- toxic, metabolic, and infectious conditions
- Otologic or vestibular conditions
- Cardiovascular causes
- Respiratory conditions
- Neurologic diseases
- Cerebrovascular causes.

ATTEST diagnostic approach

A= associated symptoms

TT= timing and triggers

ES= examination signs

T= (confirmatory) testing

The ATTEST algorithm uses an evidence-based systemic approach to diagnose patients with acute dizziness. Associated symptoms, timing, and triggers refer to historical information. (For example, what happened? When? Is the dizziness continuous or intermittent? Are there associated symptoms?)

Patients without an obvious general medicine cause usually fall into one of any three categories:

- acute vestibular syndrome (AVS),
- the triggered episodic vestibular syndrome (t-EVS) and
- the spontaneous episodic vestibular syndrome (s-EVS).

History and vital signs help in identifying patients in whom dizziness is caused by general medical causes. Special consideration has to be taken for those who present with dizziness along with any of the following:

- Heavy ibuprofen uses and black stools
- New antihypertensive or anticonvulsant medication use
- Moderate mechanism motor vehicle crash

- Abdominal pain, vaginal bleeding, and positive pregnancy test
- Chest pain and dyspnea in a patient with factor V Leiden.

If a general medical cause is likely, a brief diagnostic **"STOP"** is recommended that takes less than one minute to perform. The three components of "STOP" are:

- testing for worrisome nystagmus,
- arm dysmetria
- truncal ataxia.

To test for truncal ataxia, have the patient sit up in the stretcher without holding onto the side rails.

If the "STOP" is reassuring, proceed with management of the presumed condition. If it is worrisome, consider various vestibular or central conditions. The next question that should be asked: is the dizziness persistently present and still present at the time of ED evaluation? A "yes" identifies all patients with AVS, who have an abrupt or rapid onset of dizziness that has lasted hours to days, and is still present at the time of examination even when the patient is in a supine position. The dizziness may decrease when lying still and worsen with head movement, a common occurrence that does not mean that the dizziness has a peripheral cause.

5 questions should be asked in the following sequence for the diagnosis of patients with acute-onset persistent dizziness while performing physical examination:

- Is there a central pattern of nystagmus?
- Is skew deviation present?
- Is the head impulse test (HIT)worrisome for a central process?
- Are there central nervous system findings on the targeted posterior circulation examination?
- Can the patient sit up or walk without assistance?

Since none of these tests is 100% sensitive, patients with a YES answer to any one of the questions mean the cause is central (likely stroke) and should be admitted to the hospital for further management. However, if the answer to all of the five questions is no, then the patient likely has neuritis and can be safely discharged on oral prednisolone with the advice of outpatient follow-up.

To test for nystagmus, ask the patient to open their eyes and look forward. Then observe for any jerk nystagmus with eyes drifting in one direction. Next, ask the patient to follow the examiner's finger, going 30 degrees to the right, then the left. This known as gaze-evoked nystagmus. At the same time, observe for vertical nystagmus. In patients with AVS, nystagmus, which is vertical, torsional, or that changes direction with the direction of gaze, is central.

Check for skew deviation using the alternate cover test where you stand in front of the patient, instructing them to focus on the tip of your nose, and then alternately cover one eye then the other multiple times. A small vertical correction in the eye when it is uncovered indicates a brainstem localised lesion.

The third component of the examination is the HIT (head impulse test). The patient is asked to relax their head and neck; and focus on the examiner's nose. The examiner holds the patient's head on both sides and very rapidly snaps it in one direction or the other over a small arc of 15 degrees. The normal or negative HIT is worrisome for stroke, whereas an abnormal or positive HIT is reassuring for neuritis.

The fourth component of AVS evaluation is to look for any CNS finding due to posterior circulation ischemia where in addition to the motor and sensory examination, cranial nerve, cerebellar function, and visual field examination are also taken into consideration. Any abnormality indicates a central finding and, therefore would be inconsistent with neuritis. Anisocoria and ptosis suggest a lateral medullary infarct. The unilateral facial sensory loss in lateral medullary stroke involves pain and temperature, not light touch. Although associated with a peripheral process, acute hearing loss can also occur with an acute cerebrovascular event involving AICA or the labyrinthine artery.

Gait should always be tested in patients with dizziness. Patients who are unsteady cannot be discharged from ED. Greater degrees of gait abnormalities are seen in stroke as compared to patients with neuritis.

Patients with an s-EVS endorse one or more episodes of dizziness of variable duration not triggered by head or body position changes. Since, by definition, these patients are no longer symptomatic and are not triggerable, physical examination are not useful to distinguish the 2 most common diagnoses (vestibular migraine and posterior circulation TIA). If a patient with vestibular migraine or TIA were still symptomatic at the time of evaluation, one would proceed as if they had an AVS just as if a patient with an anterior circulation TIA still had symptoms at the time of presentation, they would be assumed to be having a stroke. For vestibular migraine, there is a strong female preponderance. Patients having multiple episodes of dizziness with or without headaches that may not occur with the dizziness. When headache occurs, they are usually similar to migraine that occurs without dizziness. Dizziness may last from minutes to days. Associated nystagmus will be of central type as migraine is a central phenomenon. Patients with Meniere disease also present with an s-EVS and will usually have buzzing in the ear and over time progress to hearing loss.

The physical examination is very helpful in patients with a t-EVS and will usually establish a specific diagnosis. Patients with dizziness on standing up with orthostatic vital signs likely have orthostatic hypotension as a cause of the dizziness, and the evaluation should be directed at finding its underlying cause. Benign paroxysmal positional vertigo (BPPV) should be suspected in patients with a very brief episode of dizziness, generally lasting less than a minute. Episodes of dizziness that wake a patient from sleep are nearly always due to BPPV. In patients with suspected BPPV, bedside testing can confidently establish the diagnosis. The most commonly affected canal is the posterior (pc-BPPV), which is tested by the Dix-Hallpike maneuver. If this test is negative on both sides, then the horizontal canal (hc-BPPV) should be tested by the supine head roll test. Patients with occasional BPPV have no nystagmus. Possible causes are a small number of otoliths in the canal, use of vestibular suppressants at the time of diagnosis, or small amplitude nystagmus that the examiner does not perceive due to visual fixation by the patient. In addition, some patients with hc-BPPV will have spontaneous (or more persistent) nystagmus, normally not seen with BPPV. This occurs because, depending on the orientation of the patient's head, otoliths in the horizontal canal may be moving in a patient sitting up and looking forward. Finally, very rarely, patients with CPPV, caused by structural lesions (usually a tumour, multiple sclerosis plaques, or small brainstem stroke) adjacent to the fourth ventricle, will exhibit nystagmus or other features that are atypical for BPPV, such as headache or diplopia, atypical nystagmus or poor response to therapeutic maneuvers.

Diagnostic testing

Diagnostic tests among patients who are suspected of having some general medical condition causing their dizziness will depend on suspected diagnosis, for example, blood glucose for hypoglycemia, stool guaiac, and hematocrit for gastrointestinal bleeding.

In cases of AVS, physical examination helps in distinguishing between stroke and vestibular neuritis or labyrinthitis. CT is unreliable in diagnosing acute ischemic stroke and even worse in diagnosing posterior circulation stroke. Approximately 10% to 20% of patients with the AVS who present within 48 hours of onset will have a false negative MRI, even with DWI. Delayed MRI with DWI-MRI after 72 hours should reliably diagnose stroke and is considered the gold standard.

In patients with the s-EVS, there is no specific test that distinguishes vestibular migraine from posterior circulation TIA, and thus, the decision-making must be individualized based on history, epidemiology, and context. In patients with t-EVS who likely have BPPV, no diagnostic testing beyond physical examination is needed. A therapeutic repositioning maneuver (Epley) might be considered a diagnostic test.

References

1. Bath PM, Woodhouse LJ, Krishnan K, Appleton JP, Anderson CS, Berge E, et al. Prehospital Transdermal Glyceryl Trinitrate for Ultra-Acute Intracerebral Hemorrhage: Data From the RIGHT-2 Trial. Stroke. 2019 Nov;50(11):3064–71.

2. Nasi LA, Martins SCO, Gus M, Weiss G, de Almeida AG, Brondani R, et al. Early Manipulation of Arterial Blood Pressure in Acute Ischemic Stroke (MAPAS): Results of a Randomized Controlled Trial. Neurocrit Care. 2019 Apr;30(2):372–9.

3. Diener H-C, Bogousslavsky J, Brass LM, Cimminiello C, Csiba L, Kaste M, et al. Aspirin and clopidogrel compared with clopidogrel alone after recent ischaemic stroke or transient ischaemic attack in high-risk patients (MATCH): randomised, double-blind, placebo-controlled trial. Lancet (London, England). 2004 Jul;364(9431):331–7.

4. Wang Y, Wang Y, Zhao X, Liu L, Wang D, Wang C, et al. Clopidogrel with Aspirin in Acute Minor Stroke or Transient Ischemic Attack. N Engl J Med [Internet]. 2013 Jun 26;369(1):11–9. Available from: https://doi.org/10.1056/NEJMoa1215340

5. Johnston SC, Easton JD, Farrant M, Barsan W, Conwit RA, Elm JJ, et al. Clopidogrel and Aspirin in Acute Ischemic Stroke and High-Risk TIA. N Engl J Med [Internet]. 2018 May 16;379(3):215–25. Available from: https://doi.org/10.1056/NEJMoa1800410

6. Wang Y, Meng X, Wang A, Xie X, Pan Y, Johnston SC, et al. Ticagrelor versus Clopidogrel in CYP2C19 Loss-of-Function Carriers with Stroke or TIA. N Engl J Med [Internet]. 2021 Oct 28;385(27):2520–30. Available from: https://doi.org/10.1056/NEJMoa2111749

7. Johnston SC, Amarenco P, Denison H, Evans SR, Himmelmann A, James S, et al. Ticagrelor and Aspirin or Aspirin Alone in Acute Ischemic Stroke or TIA. N Engl J Med [Internet]. 2020 Jul 15;383(3):207–17. Available from: https://doi.org/10.1056/NEJMoa1916870

8. Tissue Plasminogen Activator for Acute Ischemic Stroke. N Engl J Med [Internet]. 1995 Dec 14;333(24):1581–8. Available from: https://doi.org/10.1056/NEJM199512143332401

9. Amiri H, Bluhmki E, Bendszus M, Eschenfelder CC, Donnan GA, Leys D, et al. European Cooperative Acute Stroke Study-4: Extending the time for thrombolysis in emergency neurological deficits ECASS-4: ExTEND. Int J stroke Off J Int Stroke Soc. 2016 Feb;11(2):260–7.

10. Hacke W, Kaste M, Bluhmki E, Brozman M, Dávalos A, Guidetti D, et al. Thrombolysis with Alteplase 3 to 4.5 Hours after Acute Ischemic Stroke. N Engl J Med [Internet]. 2008 Sep 25;359(13):1317–29. Available from: https://doi.org/10.1056/NEJMoa0804656

11. Hacke W, Kaste M, Fieschi C, von Kummer R, Davalos A, Meier D, et al. Randomised double-blind placebo-controlled trial of thrombolytic therapy with intravenous alteplase in acute ischaemic stroke (ECASS II). Second European-Australasian Acute Stroke Study Investigators. Lancet (London, England). 1998 Oct;352(9136):1245–51.

12. Boysen G. European Cooperative Acute Stroke Study (ECASS): (rt-PA-Thrombolysis in acute stroke) study design and progress report. Eur J Neurol. 1995 Jan;1(3):213–9.

13. Thomalla G, Simonsen CZ, Boutitie F, Andersen G, Berthezene Y, Cheng B, et al. MRI-Guided Thrombolysis for Stroke with Unknown Time of Onset. N Engl J Med [Internet]. 2018 May 16;379(7):611–22. Available from: https://doi.org/10.1056/NEJMoa1804355

14. Nogueira RG, Jadhav AP, Haussen DC, Bonafe A, Budzik RF, Bhuva P, et al. Thrombectomy 6 to 24 Hours after Stroke with a Mismatch between Deficit and Infarct. N Engl J Med [Internet]. 2017 Nov 11;378(1):11–21. Available from: https://doi.org/10.1056/NEJMoa1706442

15. Albers GW, Lansberg MG, Kemp S, Tsai JP, Lavori P, Christensen S, et al. A multicenter randomized controlled trial of endovascular therapy following imaging evaluation for ischemic stroke (DEFUSE 3). Int J stroke Off J Int Stroke Soc. 2017 Oct;12(8):896–905.

16. Kapur J, Elm J, Chamberlain JM, Barsan W, Cloyd J, Lowenstein D, et al. Randomized Trial of Three Anticonvulsant Medications for Status Epilepticus. N Engl J Med. 2019 Nov;381(22):2103–13.

17. Marson A, Burnside G, Appleton R, Smith D, Leach JP, Sills G, et al. The SANAD II study of the effectiveness and cost-effectiveness of valproate versus levetiracetam for newly diagnosed generalised and unclassifiable epilepsy: an open-label, non-inferiority, multicentre, phase 4, randomised controlled trial. Lancet (London, England). 2021 Apr;397(10282):1375–86.

Airway Updates

Contributors

1. Dr. Ashima Sharma
2. Dr. Harsha Makwana
3. Dr. Akula Hymavathi
4. Dr. Arva Kousik
5. Dr. Mubashir Ahmed Sohail

Chapters

1. Assessment of Airway
2. Drugs and Equipments
3. Pediatric airway
4. Techniques to conquer a difficult airway

Assessment of Airway in Emergency Departments

Introduction- Airway control is an important skill to be learnt and practiced by emergency physicians. It is expected that emergency medicine trained doctors should be able to effectively assess, oxygenate, ventilate and stabilize the airway of the patient. There is no room for laxity in this area of specialization because a poorly managed airway has led to disastrous complications like hypoxic brain insults and cardiorespiratory arrests in the past.

The term patent or non threatened airway refers to a conscious patient who is able to talk clearly and has no upper airway anatomical reasons (due to trauma or anaphylaxis) for a breach in the safety of the airway. Sometimes, this definition can also be extended to a drowsy patient who is arousable to verbal command and has not lost his ability to swallow his secretions. A threatened airway on the other hand needs to be early protected with a definitive airway device. It is a crucial step in patient management where a step by step algorithm can prove to be the best help to secure the airway. These steps are majorly divided into assessment, preparation, procedure and post event stabilization. An airway is classified as difficult based on the level at which difficulty arises which means it can be difficult to ventilate with a Bag mask, difficult to insert LMA and keep it in the correct position, difficult to perform laryngoscopy and ultimately difficult to intubate. Traditionally, if an experienced airway provider cannot intubate in three attempts, it is labeled as a difficult airway.

Epidemiologically, it is noted that the incidence of failed intubation is highest in emergency situations i.e., 1 in 100 in comparison to obstetric 1in 250 and other elective cases 1 in 1000 to 2000.

The recent updates over the last 2 to 3 years on this topic has focussed on newer techniques of assessment of difficult airway, newer indications for intubation drugs, redefining the technique of Rapid sequence intubation and algorithms of managing airway.

Neither all anticipated difficult airways prove to be difficult intubations nor can all difficult intubations be accurately predicted.

Studies -

1. Kuzmack E et al. A Novel Difficult-Airway Prediction Tool for Emergency Airway Management: Validation of the **HEAVEN Criteria** in a Large Air Medical Cohort. JEM 2018. PMID: 29331494

   - Predicting a difficult airway is quite challenging as there are not merely one parameter to predict it. Historically, difficult airway prediction tools (ie;LEMON criteria, MOANS, RODS, and SHORT criteria) have just focused on anatomical threats and ignored physiological threats as they are derived in the elective surgical patient population (Table 1).

<table>
<tr><td>

Difficult intubation = LEMON
Look externally
Evaluate 3-3-2 rule
Mallampati score
Obstruction
Neck Mobility

</td><td>

Difficult LMA = RODS
Restricted mouth opening
Obstruction
Distorted airway
Stiff lungs or c-spine

</td></tr>
<tr><td>

Difficult BMV = BONES
Beard
Obese
No teeth
Elderly
Sleep Apnea / Snoring

</td><td>

Difficult surgical airway = SHORT
Surgery
Hematoma
Obesity
Radiation distortion or other deformity
Tumour

</td></tr>
</table>

Figure 1- The 3-3-2 rule requires head extension which is not possible in patients with traumatic injuries until cervical spine injury is ruled out.

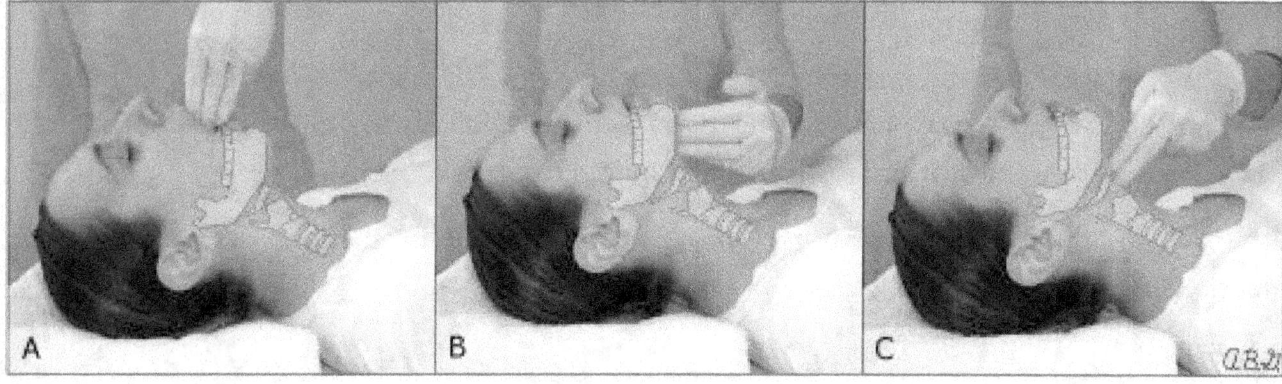

Figure 2- depicts the traditional Mallampati grading which can be remembered by a mnemonic PUFA that implies structures seen from Class IV to I airway. P is for palate, U for uvula base, F for fauces and A for all.

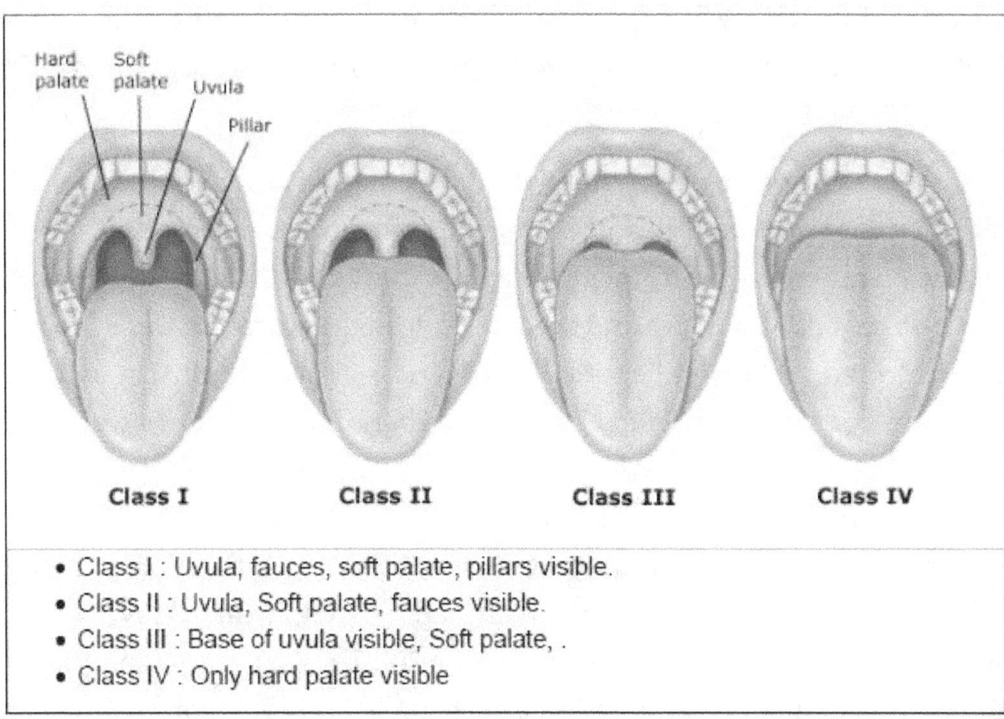

- Class I : Uvula, fauces, soft palate, pillars visible.
- Class II : Uvula, Soft palate, fauces visible.
- Class III : Base of uvula visible, Soft palate, .
- Class IV : Only hard palate visible

As the Emergency physicians receive patients in critically ill states, there has to be a criteria which should predict difficult airways having both anatomical and physiological challenges.

A new criteria called HEAVEN criteria was developed to predict difficult airways in emergency settings. The parameters of the criteria are outlined in Table 2.

The authors did an internal validation of the criteria in 2419 patients undergoing RSI and they have reported a 92% success rate in first attempt intubation and 97% success in overall intubation success rate.1363 (56.3%) of patients had at least one HEAVEN criteria identified. There was an inverse relationship observed between HEAVEN criteria and intubation success with each additional HEAVEN criteria.

H- *Hypoxemia (Spo2 ≤ 93% At The Time Of First Laryngoscopy)*
E- *Extremes Of Size (Pediatric Patient < 8 Years Of Age And Clinical Obesity)*
A- *Anatomic Challenge Including Trauma, Mass,Swelling, Foreign Body Or Any Other Structural Abnormality Limiting Laryngoscopic View*
V- *Vomit / Blood / Fluid - Clinically Significant Amount Present In Pharynx, Hypopharynx At Time Of Laryngoscopy*
E- *Exsanguination- Suspected Anemia That Can Accelerate Desaturation During Rsi Associated Apnea*
N- *Neck Mobility Is Limited Due To Cervical Spine Trauma Or Arthritis*

2. Nausheen F et al. **The HEAVEN Criteria Predict Laryngoscopic View and Intubation Success for Both Direct and Video Laryngoscopy**: A Cohort Analysis. Scand J Trauma Resusc Emerg Med 2019. PMID: 31018857

The investigators did a retrospective analysis including air medical RSI patients. A checklist was used to assess HEAVEN criteria prior to RSI, and Cormack-Lehane (CL) laryngoscopic view was recorded for the first intubation attempt. The incidence of a difficult (CL III/IV) laryngoscopic view as well as failure to intubate on first attempt with and without oxygen desaturation were determined for each of the HEAVEN criteria and total number of HEAVEN criteria. In addition, the association between HEAVEN criteria and both laryngoscopic view and intubation performance were quantified using multivariate logistic regression for direct laryngoscopy (DL) and video laryngoscopy (VL) configured with a Macintosh #4 non-hyperangulated blades. Results from a total of 5137 RSI patients over 24 months were included. Overall intubation success was 97%. A CL III/IV laryngoscopic view was reported in 25% of DL attempts and 15% of VL attempts. Each of the HEAVEN criteria and total number of HEAVEN criteria were associated with both CL III/IV laryngoscopic view and failure to intubate on the first attempt with and without oxygen desaturation for both DL and VL. These associations persisted after adjustment for multiple co-variables including the other HEAVEN criteria.

3. Rachel Munn, Jarrod Mosier, Darren Braude, Calvin A. Brown III, and Fred Ellinger, Jr.,. **CRASH, a Mnemonic for the Physiological Difficult Airway** | ACEP on July 21, 2020.

CRASH CRITERIA

It is similar to the HEAVEN mnemonic which adds consideration of hypoxemia and blood loss to traditional anatomical markers. Other major physiological variables to be considered include increased oxygen consumption, right heart dysfunction, severe metabolic acidosis, and hypotension. We believe that the physiologically difficult airway deserves its own mnemonic, CRASH, to help recognize and modify the critical physiological variables in advance of intubation. CRASH can be memorized as in Table 3 below.

	Physiological abnormality	Response
C	Consumption increase	Preoxygenation, apneic oxygenation, anticipate short apnea times
R	Right ventricular failure	Preoxygenation, inhaled pulmonary vasodilators, choice of induction agents, early use of vasopressors
A	Acidosis- Metabolic	Correct underlying issues, avoid mechanical ventilation, if possible, minimize apnea time, consider awake intubation, maintain increased minute ventilation
S	Saturation	Preoxygenation, consider NIV / HFNO
H	Hypotension, Volume	Volume resuscitation, vasopressors

4. Barret Zimmerman, Hannah Chason, Alexandra Schick, Nicholas Asselin, David Lindquist, Nicholas Musisca. Assessment of the **Thyromental Height Test as an Effective Airway Evaluation Tool.** Annals of Emergency Medicine. 2021; 77(3): 305-314.

In 2013, the thyromental height test was first described by Etezadi et al in 314 patients aged 16 years or older and undergoing planned elective direct laryngoscopy in an operative setting. Thyromental height (TMH)describes the distance from anterior borders of the chin to thyroid cartilage while the patient is supine with mouth closed. Therefore, it measures purely in the anterior-posterior plane, unlike thyromental distance, sternomental distance, mouth opening, etc, which have significant superior-inferior contributions. The authors hypothesized that thyromental height measures the anterior positioning of the larynx and degree of mandibular protrusion/retrognathia. Shorter measurements, commonly defined as less than or equal to 50 mm, predict difficult laryngoscopy. They found that 7.3% of the patients had Cormack-Lehane grade III to IV, with no failed intubations with short TMH. They also compared the thyromental height test with 3 of the most common examinations: the modified Mallampati test, thyromental distance, and sternomental distance. The thyromental height test correctly predicted 19 of 23 difficult views (sensitivity 83%), generated only 2 false-positive results (specificity 99%), had strong interrater reliability, and vastly outperformed all other examinations. The second best examination, the modified Mallampati test, predicted only 4 of 23 difficult views (sensitivity 26%) and generated 40 false-positive results (specificity 86%).

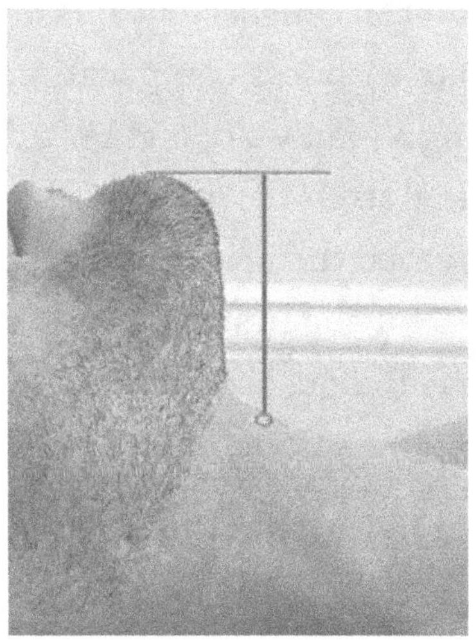

With the background of Mallampati grading requiring a conscious and cooperative patient who can sit up and open his mouth wide for assessment, it is a wise change to use HEAVEN criteria instead. This criteria also emphasizes the need to improve oxyg\enation and blood pressures before proceeding for intubation. It is important for preoxygenation and fluid infusion to be started before or simultaneously with the intubation for avoiding cardiorespiratory mishaps during the procedure. One should understand that poor vitals or crashing patients can make a seemingly easy intubation also very difficult.

Equipments and Drugs for Airway Control

<u>Introduction</u>- Uneventful airway control requires proper drugs and equipment. An emergency physician is required to learn a set of skills aka anesthesiologist in intubation of a difficult airway with help of basic and advanced equipment and newer and safer drugs. This chapter discusses the new equipment and drugs available as well as their remodeled indications and techniques. The rule should be to use what one is more comfortable to use especially in difficult scenarios. Trying out newer gadgets in an emergency difficult airway scenario can be disastrous.

Studies and Trials

1. Arulkumaran N, Lowe J, Ions R, Mendoza M, Bennett V, Dunser MW. **Videolaryngoscopy versus direct laryngoscopy for emergency orotracheal intubation outside the operating room**: a systematic review and meta-analysis. Br J Anaesth 2018; 120: 712-24.

Traditionally, Macintosh laryngoscope has been used during intubation with few centers using MCCoy for anteriorly placed larynx. Miller blade is a straight blade used in infants to lift up epiglottis which hinders the view of glottis. Fiberoptic bronchoscopy is a special skill which is more suitable to be used in elective scenarios with attending anesthesiologist. Video laryngoscopes (VL) have gained major advantage in recent times for direct laryngoscopy. It is reported to have a higher first pass oral intubation rate and overall success rate with less complications. The emphasis on appropriate size and type of blade for example choosing a Mac-VL or a HA-VL (Highly angulated VL) is emphasized. Few authors have also pointed out a final attempt with HA-VL before deciding to proceed for surgical airway access. Use of VL has also decreased the incidence of esophageal intubations. For the ease of remembering, consider using a HA-VL for the first attempt if the airway is predicted to be difficult whereas for patients with soiled airway (blood, secretions) a Mac-VL is better.

2. Driver BE et al. Effect of Use of a Bougie vs Endotracheal Tube with Stylet on Successful Intubation on the First Attempt Among Critically Ill Patients Undergoing Tracheal Intubation: A Randomized Clinical Trial **(BOUGIE Trial)**. JAMA 2021. PMID: 34879143

Apart from recommending VL, a lot of recent attention has been focussed on the use of bougie or stylet during the first attempt at laryngoscopy itself. This is in stark contrast to using these gadgets after the first or second attempt has failed. The bougie is an inexpensive device that has gained considerable attention in the last ten years. Prior to this trial, a single center study demonstrated that use of the bougie resulted in a massive benefit in terms of first attempt success. These remarkable results convinced many to adopt the bougie as standard operating procedure (SOP) for all intubations. Bougie trial authors enrolled 1102 patients with a median age of 58 years to compare the first pass intubation success with use of the gum-elastic bougie versus endotracheal tube with stylet in critically ill patients. These results were shocking as it did not support the use of bougie routinely for all intubations. Stylet loaded ETT performed marginally better than bougie and also had an equivalent number of critical hypoxemia events.

The authors concluded that the operator skill is most important in intubation and a trained personnel can make difference in airway control.

3. Driver BE et al. Effect of Use of a **Bougie vs Endotracheal Tube and Stylet** on First-Attempt Intubation Success Among Patients With Difficult Airways Undergoing Emergency Intubation: A Randomized Clinical Trial. JAMA 2018.

BEAM Trial- This was a single center, randomized clinical trial of consecutive patients, requiring orotracheal intubation with a Macintosh laryngoscope blade, comparing bougie first intubation vs ETT + stylet first intubation among patients with difficult airways undergoing emergency intubation performed by ED physicians.757 patients randomized to Macintosh laryngoscope blade intubation for respiratory arrest, difficulty breathing, or airway protection were enrolled with 380 of the patients randomized having at least one difficult airway characteristic. In their exploratory analysis, the bougie appeared to be superior compared to ETT + stylet for first pass success (FPS) in patients with cervical in-line immobilization (100% vs 78%), obese patients (96% vs 75%), and patients with incomplete glottic views on laryngoscopy (97% vs 60%).31 patients or 7% of the intubations with bougie met resistance from the arytenoid cartilages, but a simple maneuver with the ETT overcame this.

4. Jaber S, Rollé A, Godet T, Terzi N, Riu B, Asfar P, Bourenne J, Ramin S, Lemiale V, Quenot JP, Guitton C, Prudhomme E, Quemeneur C, Blondonnet R, Biais M, Muller L, Ouattara A, Ferrandiere M, Saint-Léger P, Rimmelé T, Pottecher J, Chanques G, Belafia F, Chauveton C, Huguet H, Asehnoune K, Futier E, Azoulay E, Molinari N, De Jong A; STYLETO trial group. Effect of the use of an **endotracheal tube and stylet versus an endotracheal tube alone** on first-attempt intubation success: a multicentre, randomized clinical trial in 999 patients. Intensive Care Med. 2021 Jun;47(6):653-664. doi: 10.1007/s00134-021-06417-y. Epub 2021 May 25. PMID: 34032882.

A multicentre randomized controlled trial was conducted in 32 intensive care units (999 patients) in which the authors had randomly assigned patients to tracheal tube + stylet or tracheal tube alone (i.e. without stylet). The primary outcome was the proportion of patients with first-attempt intubation success. The secondary outcome was the proportion of patients with complications related to tracheal intubation. Serious adverse events, i.e., traumatic injuries related to tracheal intubation were evaluated. First-attempt intubation success occurred in 392 patients (78.2%) in the tracheal tube + stylet group and in 356 (71.5%) in the tracheal tube alone group. A total of 194 patients (38.7%) in the tracheal tube + stylet group had complications related to tracheal intubation, as compared with 200 patients (40.2%) in the tracheal tube alone group. The incidence of serious adverse events was 4.0% and 3.6%, respectively. The conclusion was that among critically ill adults undergoing tracheal intubation, using a stylet improves first-attempt intubation success.

5. Sonia Vaida. Airway Management of the **Obstetric Patient**: What's New? Anesthesiology news. com. August 29,2018

The airway in pregnant females is difficult anatomically and physiologically. Upper airway edema is more pronounced in pre eclampsia. There is a major danger of hypoxia and its adverse consequences in emergency obstetric airway control. A recent study has supported the use of video laryngoscopes during intubation. The benefits of VL are less lifting force is needed and there is less cervical spine movement, a lower incidence of sore throat, and a faster learning curve. In addition, it reduces the risk of intubation failure and makes intubation easier in patients with an anticipated difficult airway. It is also suggested that an airway doctor should learn the skill of insertion of at least two supraglottic devices particularly one being LMA and other from second generation SADs like LMA supreme etc. Effective use of LMA in difficult situations is very rewarding. Ultrasound evaluation of airway in obstetrics is also recommended especially for the CTM depth for front of neck access.

Drugs- Studies and Trials

Intubation of trachea requires supplementation of sedative and paralyzing agents in predetermined doses especially in RSI. A critically ill patient in the emergency room may be hemodynamically unstable and it maynot be possible to give them a full dose of induction agent. Traditionally, the dose of an induction agent is titrated to loss of eyelash reflex, which is not practiced in RSI. Therefore, the emergency physician takes a decision on the choice and dose of drug based on the physiological response of the patient. In other words, it can be said that the RSI is tailor made to the patient. Drugs like thiopentone which cause major cardiovascular adverse effects were never popular in ED. Propofol in a dose of 1.5-2 mg/kg with a supporting fluid bolus has been extensively used during RSI. Etomidate, due to its inherent property to cause adrenal suppression, was debated for many years. The present status of the drug is that due to its stable hemodynamic profile it can be used in patients with low BP. Ketamine is another drug which was controversial to be used in neurosurgical emergencies especially traumatic brain injuries, however there has been a recent resurgence in its use in ED. Propofol, ketamine, and etomidate can all induce hypotension. With propofol, hypotension is predictable and usually short-lived and depends on the dosage of the drug, the degree of hypovolemia, and underlying heart failure. It is possible that clinicians are familiar with the hemodynamic effects of propofol and thus carefully plan their intubations and peri intubation interventions to prevent significant hypotension. It is also possible that dose adjustments may mitigate some of the hemodynamic effects of propofol. With etomidate, hypotension can be related to transient adrenal insufficiency which may have contributed to the higher risk of mortality and prolonged ICU length of stay, at times. In septic patients, the deleterious effect of etomidate remains unclear. A single dose of etomidate was not associated with increased mortality in ICU patients. The coadministration of hydrocortisone with etomidate was associated with decreased risk of mortality in septic shock. With ketamine, hypotension is less predictable; this is a rare and less well-recognized phenomenon. Ketamine is typically associated with a transient increase in blood pressure and heart rate. Clinicians accustomed to the positive hemodynamic effects of ketamine may not anticipate the risk of paradoxical hypotension in certain unstable patients.

1. Driver, BE. Prekker, ME. Reardon, RF. Sandefur, BJ. April MD. Walls RM, Brown CA. Success and Complications of the **Ketamine-Only Intubation** Method in the Emergency Department. *J Emerg Med.* 2021; 60(3): 265-272.

The authors compared first attempt intubation success and adverse events for patients who underwent intubation using ketamine-only or topical anesthesia vs traditional RSI, utilizing both a sedative agent and neuromuscular blocking agent. A subgroup analysis of successful intubation on the first attempt for patients with ≥ 1 difficult airway characteristics. A total of 12,511 eligible intubations were analyzed. The results of the study are tabulated below.

Parameter	Ketamine only	Topical anesthesia	Traditional RSI
% successful first time intubation	61	85	90
% of patients with ≥ 1 difficult airway characteristics	72	80	50
First attempt results for difficult airways	51	86	87
Successful intubation on the first attempt without any adverse events	55	78	83
≥ 1 adverse events	32	19	13
NMBA after first failed attempt	58	42	-
Hypoxemia	16	13	8
Median dose of ketamine, mg/kg	1.3(0.8-1.9)	0.6 (0.3-1.3) in 34/80 patients	

It was clear that ketamine-only intubations were found to have a lower first attempt success rate and more adverse events when compared with an approach facilitated by topical anesthesia or traditional RSI. However, the ideal patient population and procedural logistics for ketamine-only intubation have not yet been clearly accepted.

2. Breindahl et al. **Ketamine versus propofol for rapid sequence induction** in trauma patients: a retrospective study. Scand J Trauma Resusc Emerg Med (2021) 29:136.

Ketamine versus Propofol as induction agents in Trauma RSI have recently been compared once again for 30 day mortality after hospital admission. Historically, ketamine has been associated with increase in blood pressures and therefore was considered safer than Propofol which causes myocardial depression and peripheral vasodilatation in patients who are in hemorrhagic shock.

The authors found no difference between 30-day mortality for trauma patients intubated with RSI using ketamine compared to propofol. There were statistically significant differences between the ketamine and propofol group regarding systolic blood pressure and GCS score before intubation. However, we did not observe any significant haemodynamic difference between the two agents in terms of SBP after intubation or change in SBP after intubation. No significant difference regarding hospital and ICU length of stay or duration of mechanical ventilation was identified either. The 30-day mortality for patients intubated with ketamine (N=228) compared to patients intubated with propofol (N=320) was 20.2% and 22.8%, respectively. The study concludes ketamine is safe and effective in the emergency department. Concerns regarding increased myocardial ischemia or increased intracranial pressure from intubation with ketamine have been rejected and it may actually be considered neuroprotective.

3. Levin NM, Fix ML, April MD, Arana AA, Brown CA 3rd, NEAR Investigators. The association of **rocuronium dosing and first-attempt intubation success** in adult emergency department patients. CJEM. 2021;23(4):518. Epub 2021 Apr 10.

Traditional rocuronium dosing for emergency rapid sequence intubation (RSI) in adults has been 1 to 1.2 mg/kg intravenously (IV), but the optimal dose is unclear. An observational study of data from the multicenter National Emergency Airway Registry (NEAR) evaluated over 8000 emergency department intubations of patients >14 years to determine whether a higher dose of rocuronium (≥1.4 mg/kg IV) during RSI would improve first-pass success rate. Compared with three other dosing ranges (<1 mg/kg, 1 to 1.1 mg/kg, or 1.2 to 1.3 mg/kg), a dose of ≥1.4 mg/kg was associated with higher first-pass success rates when RSI was performed with direct laryngoscopy or in patients with pre-intubation hypotension. Across all doses, first-pass success was similar when video laryngoscopy was used. The frequency of peri-intubation adverse events did not significantly differ among the groups. These findings support our suggested rocuronium dose of 1.5 mg/kg IV when performing emergency RSI in adults.

It has always been the anesthesiologist which has been considered as the airway doctor but the real airway emergencies are faced by the ED doctor. Therefore, it is important to stay updated with the newer equipment and drugs. The first attempt is always considered as the best attempt and to ensure high FPS using a bougie and VL seems to be attractive options. Each instrument has a learning curve. A postgraduate student should practice macintosh laryngoscope and direct laryngoscopy for intubation during his initial 50 (atleast) intubations. The technique of inserting VL from the center of mouth and not from the corner is also different. It is always important to keep the suction ready in emergency airways during intubation. Drugs like Etomidate have a cardiovascular stable profile and should be frequently used in ED for intubations.

Pediatric Airway

<u>Introduction-</u> Pediatric airway management requires a high level of updated knowledge and key skill. As pediatric patients are not small adults, the smaller the child, higher the skill required for airway management. Pediatric airway has significant differences compared to the adult so it has unique challenges during management. Emergency physicians are required to be updated about anatomical and physiological differences, important pathological conditions affecting children, and a knowledge of the available airway techniques and tools. This helps in safe and effective management of the pediatric airway and also reduces morbidity and mortality.

The primary goal of pediatric airway management is to ensure oxygenation and ventilation, not intubation. Recently fiberoptic intubation in expert hands is considered as the gold standard of difficult pediatric airway management. Based on scientific literature over the past few years, changing practice in the pediatric airway is highlighted.

<u>Journey of pediatric airway from 2010 to 2020-</u>

1. Pediatric airway reconsidered
2. Neuromuscular relaxant added in difficult airway algorithm
3. ECMO introduced in resuscitation protocol
4. Vortex protocol
5. Airway ultrasound
6. Mass use of apneic oxygenation
7. Pediatric airway protocols
8. Covid-19 pandemics

<u>Whats new in Pediatric airway assessment:</u> Poor airway assessment leads to poor planning and poor outcome of a child but there is no universal single screening test or combination of tests that can be applied for airway assessment in pediatric patients and also, we do not have much time in emergency to do so.

<u>Pointers towards Difficulty-</u>

1. Absolute measurements are changing with child growth so predictors in adults (Mallampati, thyromental distance, mouth opening) are not implicated in pediatrics. Mallampati classification is valid above 5 years of age.
2. The information about a potentially difficult airway has to be seeked from past history of difficult management is highly sensitive and specific. Past history of tracheostomy, prolonged

intubation and post-extubation dysphonia are warning signs of potential difficulties during airway management.

3. Respiratory infections like active flu or flu episode within the past three weeks; a history of epiglottitis, bronchospasm, rhinitis, obstructive sleep apnea syndrome, adenoid or tonsillar hypertrophy are associated with DA. Even a child with an apparently normal airway may develop complications such as laryngospasm and bronchospasm resulting in rapid arterial desaturation that requires immediate diagnosis and management.

4. Abnormalities of the lower third of the face, low-set ears, limited neck mobility and inability to open the mouth at least 3 of the child's finger breadths are associated with DA. In a cooperative child, the inability to project the mandible farther than the maxilla (inability to bite the upper lip with the lower teeth) is a finding associated with DA. A higher body mass index (obesity) is associated with high incidence of airway complications

Classification of the pediatric airway:

a. Normal airway: Healthy airway without past history of physical and anatomical disorders and routine airway management is normally easy.

b. Altered airway: previously healthy and normal airway but due to the foreign body, trauma, burns, allergies, and inflammation (epiglottitis, croup, submandibular/perimandibular abscess) airway may be impaired and becomes difficult. They require complete management of difficult airway with trained personal and minimum standard equipment. Child has no apparent anatomical abnormalities but has physiological respiratory disorders or history of prolonged airway manipulation, e.g., intubation in ICU, history of tracheostomy or flu episode. These children can be managed in the emergency room but inform expert persons that their help may be required and be ready for it.

c. Anticipated difficult airway: Expected or apparently abnormal anatomy. In this, child has congenital abnormalities and syndromes. They should be handled and observed with experienced personnel and immediate availability of appropriate specific equipment required to handle the case

B. Pediatric airway anatomy-Previously, the shape of the pediatric larynx was described as tapered while the adult airway was described as cylindrical. This "dogma" in pediatric anesthesia emerged more than half a century ago from various studies with mummified pediatric anatomical models. Recent in vivo studies with CT, MRI and fiber-optic bronchoscopy with spontaneous breathing suggest that the pediatric larynx has the same cylindrical shape of the adult larynx, even somewhat elliptical and the anteroposterior diameter is longer than the lateral diameter. The controversy is still open as some experts challenging these findings by arguing that these measurements should be compared between cadaver models and live children and also between spontaneous and controlled breathing, or between inspiratory and expiratory phases, making consensus difficult

A useful recommendation is the use of tubes with pneumo plug, taking care not to exceed a balloon pressure of 20 mmHg, which has shown to be associated with a lower incidence of re intubations from tube exchanges.

POCUS in pediatric airway

Initially Ultrasound was used to assess the adult airway only, but over 5 years, many publications on the assessment of the pediatric airway have been done for amplitude of the retrolingual space and the ability to measure the distance between the arytenoid cartilages in order to select the right endotracheal tube diameter and predict a difficult approach to the airway. A superficial neck scan can identify the location of the cricothyroid membrane and tracheal rings for guidance should the need for emergency percutaneous access arise. Correct endotracheal intubation as well as selective ventilation due to endobronchial intubation can be detected by the US through comparison of bilateral "pleural movement".

What is new in Approaches of airway management and oxygenation:

Three techniques that have been reintroduced over the past decade are described.

1. Apneic oxygenation: An old technique consisting of the use of high flow nasal cannula (up to 15 litres per minute in adolescents) besides the conventional facial mask during oxygenation to achieve longer safe apnea time and reduce the possibility of arterial desaturation which is faster and more severe in pediatric patients because of their lower functional residual capacity (oxygen reserve) and higher tissue oxygen consumption. Isolated cases of pneumothorax have been described with the use of high flow devices in children

2. ECMO: It allows for longer periods of pulmonary and/or cardiac support, even over several days, without the acute problems associated with the extracorporeal circulation pump used in cardiovascular surgery. The use of ECMO in pediatrics has been described since the 1970s, has been expanded and has been incorporated in cardiopulmonary resuscitation algorithms, for example, it offers management option in child when pediatric airway is lost completely as injury to trachea or obstruction by foreign body. It provides adequate oxygenation of blood and removes CO_2. However, a specialized center with the necessary resources and staff training is required for its implementation.

3. Fetal EXIT (Ex Uteri intrapartum treatment): It is used mainly in cesarean section delivery in emergency operation theater and not much useful in emergency rooms. First described in 1997 where fetal abnormalities compromising the airway are identified on prenatal visits. This procedure consists of maintaining the fetus attached to the placenta during cesarean delivery while the fetal airway is approached with the most appropriate technique for each individual case, ranging from traditional laryngoscopy to flexible fiberoptic bronchoscopy assistance or tracheostomy. Once the airway is secured, the umbilical cord is ligated and delivery can proceed. There is always the possibility of placental detachment or interruption of blood flow to the umbilical cord, requiring either faster maneuvers on the fetal airway or delivery and traditional neonatal airway management in an adjacent room.

What's new in devices-Grouped under three categories.

- **Basic or first-line** (for ventilation)- For appropriate ventilation and oxygenation in the vast majority of children, the use of the face mask, with or without support of an oral or nasal cannula, is the cornerstone for management of pediatric airway. Endotracheal intubation is secondary, except in specific conditions such as risk of aspiration which requires securing the airway as soon as possible. There are no new considerations to discuss in this regard.

- **Intubation devices-**

Laryngoscopes. With technological advancement whatever available for adults is also available for children starting from traditional laryngoscopes (different blade sizes and styles) to modern video laryngoscopes.

Video Laryngoscopes: Video laryngoscopy uses the principles of indirect laryngoscopy. Unlike direct laryngoscopy, alignment of the oral, pharyngeal, and laryngeal axes is not required for successful visualization of the glottis (GlideScope and Storz C-MAC and Airtraq optical laryngoscope). Success rates of first attempts in pediatric difficult airway population is higher in video than in direct laryngoscopy.

Vendors offer blade sizes ranging from 00 to adult sizes and even devices that can be connected to smartphone screens. Some of the most common video laryngoscopes are the Storz®, GlideScope®, Truview®, Pentax AWS®, Airtraq®, McGrath®, and kingVission®, among others. The choice depends on the preference of each work team, budget availability and experience.

While selecting a blade one should choose one size smaller than weight base recommendation for a better view.

Supraglottic devices: There is a wide range of supraglottic devices available for pediatric use. They have certain advantages like easy placement, less dislodgement, ease of ventilation and oxygenation and they form a seal in the periglottic area. Few allow suction of gastric contents and few incorporate bite protectors. In all, they allow time to prepare other airway maneuvers, passage of traditional tubes for endotracheal intubation and helps in navigation and visualization of the glottis with a fiberoptic bronchoscope. When SGA is used for ETT insertion, microlaryngoscopy tubes, available in sizes 4.0, 5.0, and 6.0 mm are preferred as they are few centimeters longer than a standard ETT.

LMA is a useful and powerful supraglottic airway device for management of both routine and difficult pediatric airways. Over the years, various designs (1st, 2nd, and 3rd generation) and insertion techniques have been described, accepted widely, and incorporated into difficult pediatric airway algorithms.

Fiberoptic bronchoscope: It is considered a gold standard approach to anticipated or apparently difficult airway (limited mouth opening) where direct and indirect laryngoscopies are not feasible. It is also frequently preferred by experienced hands in elective airway management of pediatric patients with a known or suspected unstable cervical spine. Recently flexible fiberoptic bronchoscopes of different sizes, even in diameters as small as 1.8 mm are available which allow the passage of a 2.5 mm internal diameter endotracheal tube. The 2.8 mm fiberoptic bronchoscope is the most commonly used in pediatrics and passes through 3.5 mm internal diameter tubes and larger. In "cannot ventilate, cannot oxygenate" scenarios, it can be used before front-of-neck access (e-FONA). Rigid fiberoptic bronchoscopy is the choice for removal of foreign bodies lodged in the airway and obstructing it. Visualization is affected by secretions or blood in the airway. It's not routinely used in all pediatric patients so it is not handy in the emergency room and takes more time to arrange its set-up and perform the procedure compared to indirect video laryngoscopes. Experience and competence with fiberoptic bronchoscopy have diminished after introduction of indirect video laryngoscopes.

Role of the fiberoptic bronchoscopy is debatable in the management of the emergent and unanticipated difficult airway. However, it is still used frequently at tertiary care hospitals for indirect visualization and placement of an ETT through a SGA.

- **Front-of-neck surgical access (FONA)**

A debate is going on for its usefulness in very young children, because of its very high incidence of complications and failed procedures and in hospital mortality due to issues of location of cricothyroid membrane and incorrect approach. When there is a scenario of "cannot ventilate, cannot intubate" any other option is not working and child develops acute hypoxemia, bradycardia, cardiac arrest and impending death, then FONA is started.

In children under 8 years of age it is done through tracheal rings as identifying the cricothyroid membrane is very difficult. This procedure may be performed through puncture- percutaneous or open cricothyroidotomy (in older children) or through an incision - percutaneous or open tracheostomy.

- **Difficult Airway Cart**

A dedicated pediatric difficult airway cart can facilitate quick and organized equipment retrieval and is recommended for any institution caring for children. The difficult airway cart should be stored adjacent to locations of pediatric beds in the emergency room.

- **Vortex protocol**

Described by an emergency physician and anesthetist in Australia, consists of a funnel visual schematic that begins, at the top, with airway management using three of the four "life lines" - facial mask, endotracheal intubation and supraglottic devices. They are applied and altered depending on individual case to maintain the patient in a green safety zone, with adequate oxygenation and ventilation. The fourth "life line", i.e., neck access is activated when the other 3 have failed. The protocol highlights nontechnical skills and teamwork and includes other important considerations besides the mere implementation of a sequence of steps contained in the algorithms. It can be accessed for free at http://vortexapproach. org where a more thorough description of the components and uses is available.

What is new in algorithm-

1. Facial mask ventilation has given priority over endotracheal intubation by different algorithms because it is usually easier to ventilate children with the adequate facial seal technique which allows, with positive pressure, to create an air column that acts like a "splint" to maintain an open patent airway..

2. The basic algorithm of facial mask ventilation followed by attempted intubation and/or placement of a supraglottic device continues to prevail, and if a "cannot ventilate, cannot oxygenate" emergency occurs, access through the neck would be considered.

3. In pediatrics, strategies of combining fiberoptic bronchoscopy with supraglottic devices are valid.

4. The possibility of arousing the child to allow spontaneous breathing must be considered depending on each particular case.

5. In neonates, intubation without muscle relaxation using "gentle" ventilation (high frequency and low volume) should be done in anticipation of rapid desaturation.

Considerations during the COVID-19 pandemic: The incidence of asymptomatic carriers among children is high, requiring great care during their management. Crying should be avoided as far as possible in view of abundant droplet production and to avoid it excellent premedication and peaceful arousal are required. Positive pressure ventilation is allowed in neonates considering that low volumes result in minimal droplet scatter-less than 10 cm radius. Whenever possible, tubes with adequately inflated pneumoplugs should be used over supraglottic devices. The most important recommendations are summarized in Table 1, based on the recommendation of the Colombian Neonatology Association (ASCON) and the consensus guidelines of the Pediatric Difficult Intubation Collaborative and the Canadian Pediatric Anesthesia Society.

During preparing for airway management	Personal protection elements Prepare and implement check-lists Prepare and have all things ready before initiation of airway management Prepare closed suction system Provide sufficient premedication and control crying and coughing Avoid nasal premedication Do not allow family members in the covid area Use a negative pressure operating room
Intubation	Prefer intravenous rapid sequence induction Do not use rapid sequence induction in neonates Use muscle relaxant Use clear plastic to cover the airway during the procedure The airway must be approached by the person with most expertise Use the facial mask quickly (to limit droplets) Avoid high flow nasal cannula Prefer endotracheal tube with pneumoplug Avoid laryngeal masks, but if needed, use second generation masks (better seal) Avoid oral suction if possible and do only after giving sedation and muscle relaxant
Extubation and post extubation	Apply suction before extubation Place facial mask promptly after extubation (limits droplets) Maintain adequate distance between patients in the recovery room Avoid nebulization
Avoid unreliable, unfamiliar or repeated techniques during airway management	
Team persons and role Person 1- Doctor: Team leader Person 2- Nurse Person 3- Doctor/ Nurse	Manual ventilation and intubation, Oxygen and suction Ventilator and circuit - Cricoid pressure – Compressor Medication - Equipment - Defibrillation - Timer/Recorder
HEPA filters	Choice is limited, as most of are designed for adults (require a tidal volume of at least 200-300 ml)
Video laryngoscope	longer distance can be maintained between the intubation field and the operator, reducing the risk of transmission

Techniques to Control a Difficult Airway

<u>Introduction</u>- One failed airway is enough for the lifetime of a doctor. The consequence of failed intubation and inability to ventilate and oxygenate can cause hypoxic brain injury to the patient and early death. It is very important to practice airway algorithms in a simulated environment. There is a saying " the more one slogs in peace, the less he bleeds in war". This statement is very apt in CVCI scenarios where inability to perform a surgical airway or providing nonoptimal oxygenation and ventilation can be catastrophic to a patient's life. The airways are potentially more difficult in ED as there is less time to assess and even lesser means to intervene. All advanced equipment is under the armamentarium of the Anesthesiology department and it may take time to retrieve them in emergencies.

Studies:

1. Pascale Avery, Sarah Morton, James Raitt, Hans Morten Lossius and David Lockey. **Rapid sequence induction: where did the consensus go?** Scandinavian Journal of Trauma, Resuscitation and Emergency Medicine (2021) 29:64.

RSI was revisited in2021 in a review by P Avery et al. in which a *facelift* was given to the original technique of RSI. The traditional method describes: denitrogenation of the lungs with 100% oxygen for at least 2 min, induction with a pre-determined dose of thiopentone, application of cricoid pressure, administration of a predetermined dose of suxamethonium, a period of apnoea with no positive pressure ventilation, tracheal intubation with a cuffed tracheal tube, and the release of cricoid pressure when tube placement is successfully confirmed. The concept of 'critical care without walls' – where key critical care interventions are delivered wherever required – has resulted in RSI frequently being performed outside the operating theater in the emergency department (ED), intensive care unit (ICU) and in pre-hospital settings. The purpose of RSI is to achieve rapid intubation without aspiration of gastric contents. The indications have been refined in ABCDE format.

Airway – loss of airway patency

Breathing – inadequate ventilation, respiratory failure or hypoxia

Circulation – improve oxygen delivery in hypovolaemia or allow hemorrhage control procedures

Disability – neuroprotection particularly in traumatic brain injury, reduced Glasgow Coma Score, status epilepticus, post cardiac arrest protection

Everything else – e.g. emergency surgery, humanitarian indications, temperature control (e.g. serotonin syndrome), to facilitate safe transfer.

The other new changes are addition of opioid at induction and replacing the original thiopentone with propofol, ketamine and etomidate. The most common opioids are fentanyl and sufentanil. Suxamethonium is also getting replaced with rocuronium slowly, especially so with sugammadex available in the market. The early reversal of neuromuscular blockade is possible in times of failed intubation.

Application of cricoid pressure is clinically known to hamper the view of glottis and this has deterred many non anesthesiologists from practicing the traditional RSI. It is increasingly being realized that there are instances when aspiration has occurred even with application of cricoid pressure and therefore almost all new difficult airway guidelines except for UK guidelines have suggested for release of cricoid in patients with poor CL grades 3b and 4. The critical time for aspiration to occur during intubation is the time between administration of drugs to intubation. The following are the suggested methods of apneic oxygenation are - 1).Delivery of high flow oxygen (10-15 L/min) through nasal cannulae, 2) Transnasal humidified rapid insufflation ventilatory exchange (THRIVE) which is although more suitable in the operating theater environment, 3) gentle BMV during the time which does not practically increase risk of aspiration and, 4) a ramp up position of 25 degrees which can make intubation difficult.

The required monitoring for RSI has expanded to essentially cover capnography and also invasive BP monitoring to avoid hypo- or hypertension.Overall, it is important to be very safe in conduct of RSI in the chaotic ED environment.

2. Brewster DJ, Begley JL, Marshall SD. **Rise and fall of the aerosol box;** and what we must learn from the adoption of untested equipment*Emergency Medicine Journal* 2021;38:109-110.

The list of equipment for the airway were refined over the last few years and one of which is an intubation box. This is a transparent acrylic box which allows intubations for covid afflicted patients with negligible risk to the operator. The box was designed keeping its utility in mind but however, within a few months an intubation study under simulated environment on manikins could prove that there was an unwanted but significant increase in intubation time. Also, there was major contamination of PPE and risk to healthcare workers was not as less as it was thought. The author suggests *THE END* for the intubation box.

3. Takahashi J, Goto T, Funakoshi H on behalf of the Japanese Emergency Medicine Network Investigators, et al. Association of **advanced age with intubation-related adverse events** in the emergency department: a multicentre prospective observational study*Emergency Medicine Journal* 2021;38:874- 881.

It has been always believed that geriatric populations have a higher incidence of intubation related addverse effects and more so when the procedure is taking place in ED. JEAN 2 study from Japan has analyzed data in 9714 patients with primary exposure being age and primary outcome being overall intubation-related adverse events during or immediately after an intubation. Adverse events were further categorized into major (hypotension, hypoxaemia, oesophageal intubation, cardiac arrest, dysrhythmia and death) and minor (endobronchial intubation, oesophageal intubation with early recognition, dental/lip trauma, airway trauma and regurgitation) adverse events. 15% of patients were aged ≥85 years and 16% had adverse events. The most significant adverse effect seen was hypotension while advanced age was not associated with minor adverse events.

4. J. Adam Law et al. **Canadian Airway Focus Group updated consensus-based recommendations** for management of the difficult airway: part 1. Difficult airway management encountered in an unconscious patient.Can J Anesth.2021; 68:1373 –1404.

The <u>face mask ventilation</u> (FMV) has been revised by authors with proper clinical scenarios expected in these situations. Grade 0-2 of mask ventilation are those patients where it was easy to perform FM ventilation, without or with use of airway adjuncts like guedel oral airway. Each delivered breath will show a chest rise and a plateau phase of capnography on monitor. Grade 3 airways have difficult FM ventilation with inadequate ventilation despite trying optimizing maneuvers. Consequently, capnograph will not show a plateau phase and there will be poor chest rise. The grade 4 is a failed mask ventilation wherein no matter which technique is employed, it is impossible to ventilate the patient. A flat or majorly attenuated capnogram is seen and the patient shows low SPO_2 with minimal or no perceivable chest rise.

As for the difficult laryngoscopy grading, the original **Cormack lehane classification** is very important for grading the glottis look on direct laryngoscopy. Figure 3 shows the original version of cormack lehane's airway grading. This has been revised to subdivide grade 3 airway into 3a and 3b. 3a are described as moderately difficult intubations where though only epiglottis is visible but it can be lifted off from the posterior pharyngeal wall. This means that intubation is possible with use of bougies and stylets. Grade 3b are failed airways where lifting of epiglottis from posterior pharyngeal wall is not easy and therefore use of above mentioned adjuncts may not help in intubation and an alternative device or technique is required.

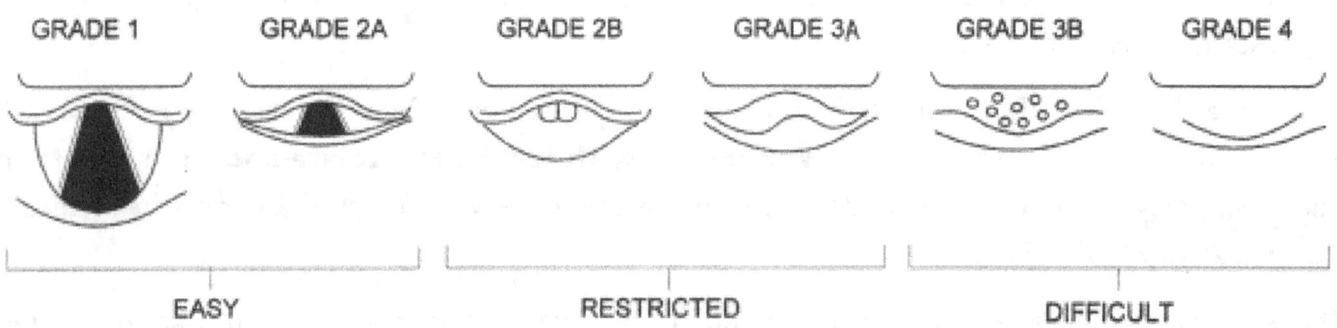

Strategies for appropriate airway control in real time difficult airways.

A. *Options for responding to difficult face-mask ventilation* - can be applied independently or as a bundle. It is clinically observed that an adequately sedated patient allows airway manipulations for proper mask seal..

1. Routine use of an oropharyngeal airway or a nasopharyngeal airway as an alternative if the mouth cannot be accessed but not if there is suspicion of base of skull fracture or nasal bone fractures.

2. A two-handed mask hold with exaggerated jaw lift will significantly improve mask seal; positive pressure ventilation can be performed by an assistant or a ventilator set to pressure control ventilation at ≥ 15-cm H2O.

3. Use a thenar eminence ("V-E") grip for two-handed mask seal/jaw lift. This is also known as C-E grip if one hand is used for mask holding.

4. Ensure neuromuscular blockade.for the final try on holding the mask.

5. Consider an alternate size or type of face mask to improve the airway seal.

6. Perform additional head extension or lateral head rotation (if not contraindicated)

7. Release any applied cricoid pressure or sellicks maneuver.

8. Consider head-up patient positioning in patients with stable hemodynamics.

9. Consider gastric decompression via an orogastric tube if significant gastric distention is suspected especially if both hands are used for AMBU Bag compression.. This generates pressures above 20 cm of H2O and opens the esophageal sphincter.

10. Exclude presence of a physical obstruction or compression (e.g., foreign body, tumor, or stenosis) in the upper airway or trachea.

11. Progress to an alternate mode of ventilation, e.g LMA or tracheal intubation.

B. *Options for responding to difficult supraglottic airway (SGA) insertion-* also have been collectively bundled.

1. It is essential to maintain an adequate depth of general anesthesia for SGA insertion. This may not be possible in an emergency room which requires the provider to titrate the drug doses to the vital signs of the patient.

2. Unless contraindicated as in suspected spinal injuries, use a "sniff" position for SGA insertion, with lower neck flexion and head extension.

3. Consider rotating the SGA 90 degrees during advancement around the tongue. This technique requires more practice skill

4. Use an alternate size or design of SGA, including one with a different cuff material. These refer to use of Igel, Air Q, Supreme LMA and Proseal LMA based on the availability.

5. In the context of failed tracheal intubation, release any applied cricoid pressure for SGA insertion.

6. Consider neuromuscular blockade - no benefit, no harm reported in clinical trials

7. Consider SGA insertion facilitated by direct or video laryngoscopy.

8. With a second-generation SGA, a tracheal tube introducer ("bougie") placed through the SGA's esophageal drainage port can first be advanced into the esophagus to subsequently help guide the SGA into position. These require higher practice skill as they have a potential for airway injury

9. Progress to an alternate mode of ventilation, e.g., tracheal intubation or FMV.

C. *Options for response to difficulty with glottic exposure* using direct laryngoscopy (DL) have been expanded to include Macintosh geometry blade video laryngoscopy (Mac-VL) or intermediate geometry blade video laryngoscopy. The previous conditions like ensuring adequate sedation and neuromuscular blockade is evidence proven.

1. Apply external laryngeal manipulation (not cricoid pressure).

2. Ensure the Macintosh blade is inserted sufficiently deep into the vallecula to engage the hyoepiglottic ligament.

3. Consider directly lifting the epiglottis (applies to both Macintosh and straight blades).

4. Exaggerate head lift and "sniff" positions, if not contraindicated.

5. If using Mac-VL, switch to indirect, videoscopic viewing if direct eye-to-glottis viewing is suboptimal.

6. For continued difficulty with glottic exposure, if the patient remains well-oxygenated, strongly consider progressing to HA-VL.

D. *Options for response to difficulty with tracheal tube passage* during DL or Mac-VL requires use of bougie. The bougie is an effective adjunct when Mac-VL or DL results in a limited (e.g Cormack–Lehane 2b or 3a) view. If not using a bougie, use a stylet to optimally shape the tracheal tube.

<u>Situation of failed intubation</u>

This happens when after three attempts, the patient is still not tracheally intubated, though oxygenation is maintained using FMV or SGA device. In emergency patients, it is not possible to awaken the patient and plan for intubation and general anesthesia another time. Here, we have a *"do or die" situation*. Therefore, sending a call to an experienced anesthesiologist and considering the use of fiberoptic bronchoscope guided intubation is important. Intubating oral airway, a SGA or VL blade can help fiberoptic guided intubation.

The CVCO- eFONA recommendation:

The main catastrophe occurs when there is Cannot ventilate, cannot oxygenate. Recent trials have shown a good success rate for Front of neck access surgical cricothyroidotomy or tracheotomy as life saving procedures. This technique is called eFONA which is a short form of emergency Front of neck access technique. Surgical cricothyroidotomy is preferred by emergency physicians and scalpel bougie-tube approach is preferred for cricothyrotomy. The procedure involves a liberal longitudinal skin incision, laryngeal handshake, transverse incision on cricothyroid membrane, holding the scalpel in cephalad caused orientation through the incision, passing bougie into trachea and railroading a 6.0-mm internal diameter cuffed tube (adult patient) over the bougie.

5. Ghaffar S, Blankenstein TN, Patel D, *et al*Quantification of the effect of **body mass index on cricothyroid membrane depth**: a cross-sectional analysis of clinical CT images*Emergency Medicine Journal* 2021;38:355-358

The recommended front of neck access procedure in can't intubate, can't oxygenate scenarios relies on palpation of the cricothyroid membrane (CTM), or dissection of the neck down to the larynx if CTM is impalpable. CTM palpation is particularly challenging in obese patients, most likely due to an increased distance between the skin and the CTM (CTM depth). Sadia Gaffar et al measured CTM depth in a representative clinical sample of 355 clinical CT scans, and to quantify the relationship between body mass index (BMI) and CTM depth. Median CTM depth was 8.12 mm. There was no association between CTM depth and sex, height or age. Increasing weight and BMI were strongly associated with CTM depth. Predicted CTM depth increased from 6.4 mm at a BMI of 20 kg/m2 to 16.8 at BMI 40 kg/m2. This is an important study to guide the emergency physicians to consider before proceeding to cricothyroidotomy in CVCO situations.

Preparedness to deal with an unanticipated difficult airway is an important skill in learning to be an emergency physician. The guidelines and algorithms support us to develop our plan for stabilizing the airway of the patient. It is important to formulate your own protocols based on the availability of resources and trained personnel.

Respiratory Emergencies

Contributors

1. Dr. Anita Kabi
2. Dr. Aroop Mohanty
3. Dr. Vijeta Bajpai
4. Dr. Priyanka Dwiwedi
5. Dr. Sree Sowjanya Patibandla
6. Dr. Ashima Sharma

Chapters

1. ARDS
2. Pneumonia
3. Acute Asthma
4. COPD
5. Pulmonary thromboembolism

Acute Respiratory Distress Syndrome

Introduction

Acute Respiratory Distress Syndrome (ARDS), a life-threatening inflammatory lung injury, was first described in 1967 by Ashbaugh.[1] It is characterized by bilateral pulmonary infiltrates and acuity of onset. ARDS is characterized by acute onset of hypoxaemia with bilateral chest radiographic opacities due to non cardiogenic pulmonary edema. The COVID-19 pandemic highlighted the challenges associated with this syndrome especially the high mortality rate and the lack of effective pharmacotherapy. The wide spectrum of causes, manifestations and the supportive management of this syndrome still continues to drive the clinicians and scientists for further research.

Definition

The definition of ARDS was updated in 2012 and is called the Berlin definition. It differs from the previous American European Consensus definition by excluding the term acute lung injury; it also removed the requirement for wedge pressure <18 and included the requirement of positive end-expiratory pressure (PEEP) or continuous positive airway pressure (CPAP) of greater than or equal to 5. The Berlin Definition of Acute Respiratory Distress Syndrome is illustrated in the table 1.[2]

Table 1: The Berlin definition of ARDS

Acute Respiratory Distress Syndrome	
Timing	Within 1 week of a known clinical insult or new or worsening respiratory symptoms
Chest Imaging[a]	Bilateral opacities—not fully explained by effusions, lobar/lung collapse, or nodules
Origin of edema	Respiratory failure not fully explained by cardiac failure or fluid overload Need objective assessment (eg, echocardiography) to exclude hydrostatic edema if no risk factor present
Oxygenation[b]	
Mild	200 mm Hg< $PaO_2/FIO_2 \leq$ 300 mm Hg with PEEP or CPAP $\geq$ 5 cm H_2O
Moderate	100 mm Hg < $PaO_2/FIO_2 \leq$ 200 mm Hg with PEEP $\geq$5 cm H_2O
Severe	$PaO_2/FIO_2 \leq$ 100 mm Hg with PEEP$\geq$ 5 cm H_2O

Abbreviations: CPAP, continuous positive airway pressure; FIO_2, fraction of inspired oxygen; PaO_2, partial pressure of arterial oxygen; PEEP, positive end-expiratory pressure.

[a]Chest radiograph or computed tomography scan.

[b]If altitude is higher than 1000 m, the correction factor should be calculated as follows: [PaO_2/FIO_2 X (barometric pressure/ 760)].

[c]This may be delivered noninvasively in the mild acute respiratory distress syndrome group.

The PaO_2/FIO_2 ratio is estimated after putting a patient on CPAP or PEEP ≥5 cm H_2O using a ventilator. However, the Berlin criterion is not suitable in the scarcity of resources where access to mechanical ventilation, chest radiography, and arterial blood gas data is difficult. The ARDS defined by Kigali keeps the same criteria of 1 week of insult and origin of edema as that of the Berlin definition. The minimum Positive End-Expiratory Pressure (PEEP) requirement is excluded, and hypoxemia, the ratio of arterial oxygen saturation (SpO_2)/inspiratory oxygen fraction (FiO_2), as measured by pulse oximetry is equal to or less than 315 with S_pO_2 ≤97%.[3]

An international panel of experts convened the Pediatric Acute Lung Injury Consensus Conference (PALICC) to establish new definitions and guidelines for pediatric acute respiratory distress syndrome (PARDS). The 2015 PALICC definition broadens the radiographic requirement to include any new parenchymal infiltrate(s). Additional key differences in the PARDS definition include allowing use of pulse oximetry to avoid underestimating ARDS prevalence in children if arterial blood oxygenation measurements are not available and SpO_2 ≤ 97%, and utilization of the oxygenation index (OI) [(FiO_2 × mean airway pressure × 100)/PaO_2] and oxygenation saturation index (OSI) [(FiO_2 × mean airway pressure × 100)/SpO_2] rather than the PaO_2/FiO_2 (P/F) ratio to assess hypoxemia.[4]

In the year end of 2019, a sudden outbreak of a new primarily pulmonary disease was first reported in Wuhan located in China. Researchers of the Chinese Center for Disease Control and Prevention evaluated the lower respiratory tract of infected patients and discovered a novel coronavirus named COVID-19.[5] A COVID-19 patient with ARDS (CARDS)[6] was described as patients who presented to hospital at any stage of their pulmonary illness and vary in responses to standard treatment. If they are inadequately managed, can lead to multiple organ failure, thromboembolism and eventually death. The criteria for the PaO_2/FIO_2 ratio were modified in COVID-19 ARDS to improve detection of mild-moderate disease between 150 mmHg and 200 mmHg, and moderate-severe disease <150 mmHg. The differences in the ARDS and CARDS is exemplified in the table 2.

Table 2: Differences between ARDS and CARDS

Features	ARDS	CARDS
Genes	More than 40 genes associated including VEGF, MIF, ACE etc.7	ACE gene 2 protein
Onset	Within 1 week	8-12 days

Lung compliance	Reduced	May be relatively normal
PaO_2/FIO_2 ratio with PEEP ≥5 cm H2O	As per Berlin criterion	mild-moderate - 150 mmHg and 200 mmHg, moderate-severe disease - <150 mmHg
Management	Mechanical ventilation (non invasive or invasive)	HFNO can be useful in some cases of moderate-severe disease Timing of invasive ventilation is crucial Due to normal compliance of lungs in many patients, recruitment manoeuvres are not used unless progressed to severe disease
Proning	Severe ARDS / refractory cases	Instituted early in the disease
Mortality	35.3 – 40 %	21- 65% even higher if the patient is put on invasive ventilation

Epidemiology

The incidence and mortality of ARDS in a large international cohort was undertaken as a part of the Large Observational Study to Understand the Global Impact of Severe Acute Respiratory Failure (LUNG SAFE).[8] It was done to address the large regional differences within the developed countries for example, the incidence of ARDS in Europe was reported to be 10-fold lower than in the United States.[9]

This investigation, which was an international, multicenter, prospective cohort study enrolling 459 ICUs in 50 countries was undertaken to assess the ICU epidemiology and outcomes from ARDS (as well as to evaluate clinical recognition of the disease and its management). One of the strengths of this study was that the patients were enrolled from all over the world, in the same period of 4 consecutive winter weeks (February–March 2014 in the Northern hemisphere and June–August 2014 in the Southern hemisphere). The overall incidence of ARDS was 10.4% of ICU admission and 23.4% of all patients requiring mechanical ventilation. Geographic variations were confirmed, with Europe having an incidence of 0.48 cases/ICU bed over 4 weeks; North America, 0.46; South America, 0.31; Asia, 0.27; Africa, 0.32; and Oceania, 0.57 cases/ICU bed per 4 weeks. Taking into account that the Berlin definition was adopted for all cases and the low availability of ICU beds in the developing world, it was conceivable to suppose that ARDS was underestimated in low-income countries. In other worlds, the results of the LUNG SAFE study strengthens the rationale for the Kigali modification of the Berlin definition.[8]

Mortality for ARDS remains sobering; observational studies consistently report greater than 30% hospital mortality.8 The proportion of ARDS mortality that is attributable to the syndrome itself (as opposed to risk factors and comorbidities) has been challenging to determine, but was estimated for sepsis-associated ARDS at 27–37%.[10]. As given in the Berlin definition report of 2012, the mortality of ARDS was commensurate to the severity of the disease; it was 27%, 32%, and 45% for mild, moderate, and severe disease, respectively.[2]

The cause of death is more commonly sepsis and multiple organ failure than respiratory failure. Although most ARDS survivors recover normal or near-normal pulmonary function, many remain burdened by functional limitations related to muscle weakness, deconditioning, or psychological sequelae of severe illness. Cognitive impairment is also distressingly common, affecting almost half of survivors at 2 years. [11]

Pathophysiology

ARDS is characterized by increased vascular permeability, protein-rich edema, diffuse alveolar infiltrate, and loss of aerated lung tissue, leading to decreased lung compliance, tachypnea, and severe hypoxemia. The pathophysiological mechanism can lead to three phases: a) exudative phase, b) proliferative phase, and c) fibrotic phase.[12]

The early phase that occurs within 72 hours is the exudative phase (0–7 days), characterized by an increase in the permeability of membranes, leakage of protein-rich fluid, inflammatory cellular infiltrates (predominantly neutrophils), and gradual refractory hypoxemia.[4]

Due to diffuse alveolar damage there is pooling of the inflammatory cells and fibroblasts. These in turn produce cytokines like TNF-α, IL-1β, IL-6, and chemokines such as IL-8. Cytokines increase the infiltration of neutrophils, which activates and releases toxic mediators such as reactive oxygen species and nitric oxide. These toxic mediators damage the epithelium of alveoli and capillary endothelium, resulting in increased permeability, allowing protein-rich fluid and blood cells to move into the interstitium and alveoli.[13]

The air spaces become filled with fluid and cellular debris. Eosinophilic depositions termed hyaline membrane is the histopathological hallmark of ARDS. Also, the coagulation pathway becomes disrupted, leading to micro thrombus formation. The impaired surfactant-producing cells, ie, alveolar type II cells, lead to alveolar atelectasis and lung stiffness. These changes and hyaline membrane deposition impair gas exchange.[14]

The fibro-proliferative/proliferative phase (7–21 days) is characterized by proliferation and architectural changes. The repair process is initiated during this phase, and surfactant production is restored because of type II alveolar cells' proliferation. Aside from that, the epithelium rejuvenates as a consequence of type I pneumocyte proliferation, culminating in the reabsorption of alveolar edema. The proliferative phase may progress to the fibrotic stage, marked by extensive diffuse fibrosis, obliteration of the typical lung architecture, and patchy emphysematous alterations.[15]

Causes and risk factors

The exact etiology of ARDS are indeed not ascertainable. It can develop in the presence of various causes and risk factors as shown in Table 3. Notably, severe bacterial infections, such as pneumonia, non pulmonary sepsis and aspiration of gastric contents are the most common cause of ARDS.[8] Factors such as age, gender, genetics, external factors (cigarette smoke), chronic pulmonary diseases, and concomitant diseases increase ARDS risk. ARDS affects individuals of all ages, although the incidence of ARDS increases with age because the elderly are more susceptible to the primary risk of sepsis. Also, apart from COVID-19 disease, there is emergence of new cause such as e-cigarette or vaping product use associated lung injury (EVALI).[16]

Table 3: Classic precipitants of ARDS

Common precipitants
Pneumonia (bacterial and viral are the most common, whereas fungal, mycobacterial, and parasitic pneumonia are less common
Non-pulmonary sepsis
Aspiration of gastric contents
Non-cardiogenic shock
Pancreatitis
Severe trauma or high-risk surgery (eg, esophagectomy)
Drug overdose
Ischaemia-reperfusion injury
Less common precipitants
Smoke inhalation
Drowning
Vape or e-cigarette use
Multiple transfusion of blood products
Diagnoses not typically classified as ARDS
Vasculitis
Diffuse alveolar haemorrhage
Drug-induced pneumonitis
Organising pneumonia
Hypersensitivity pneumonitis
Acute eosinophilic pneumonia
Acute exacerbation of interstitial lung disease
Acute chest syndrome (ie, sickle cell disease)
Alveolar proteinosis
Malignancy

Table taken from "Acute respiratory distress syndrome" published by Meyer N J et al in Lancet 2021.[11]

Management

There is no single test to identify or exclude the diagnosis. The heterogeneity of ARDS is evident in its causes, manifestations, and response to therapy.

Some biomarkers have been identified in plasma, bronchoalveolar lavage fluid (BALF), and exhaled gas of ARDS patients. The purpose is to diagnose development of ARDS in at risk individuals and monitor their response to therapeutic interventions.

Most of the biomarkers in the blood reflect inflammation. Biomarkers investigated in blood for the exudative phase include endothelial protein angiopoietin-1, thrombomodulin, von Willebrand factor (vWF), protein C, intercellular adhesion molecule-1 (ICAM-1), and plasminogen activator inhibitor-1.[17] Biomarkers, investigated both in blood and BALF, are receptor for advanced glycation endproducts (RAGE), Krebs von den Lungen-6 (KL-6), Clara cells (CC16), interleukins (IL-1β, IL-6, IL-8, IL-10), tumor necrosis factor-α (TNF-α), surfactant protein, matrix metalloproteinases (MMPs), vascular endothelial growth factor (VEGF).[17,18]

Biomarkers for the fibroproliferative phase include keratinocyte growth factor (KGF), hepatocyte growth factor (HGF), N-terminal procollagen peptide-III (N-PCP-III), and Fas/FasL.[18] The benefit of BALF is that it is the closest sample to the site of injury. In the exhaled breath, three volatile organic compounds (VOCs) such as octane, acetaldehyde, and 3-methylheptane are potential markers of ARDS.[19]

In order to hasten the development of effective therapy for ARDS, the National Heart, Lung, and Blood Institute (NHLBI), National Institutes of Health (NIH), initiated a clinical network to carry out multi-center clinical trials of ARDS treatments. The ARDS Network was established as a contract program in 1994 that ended in 2014. During its 20 years of service, 5,527 patients were enrolled in 10 randomized controlled trials and one observational study. These included the landmark trials like ARMA, FACTT, ALVEOLI, EDEN and more. 20 Mostly the management of ARDS is derived from the observations made from these studies.

The treatment of ARDS is mainly supportive (Figure 1). The search for the underlying cause and it's treatment should be aggressively done

A. General measures includes nutritional support, prevention of stress ulcers and venous thromboembolism

B. Ventilation: Low Tidal Volume Ventilation (LTVV) or lung protective ventilation is recommended. Any mode can be chosen like volume assist keeping Inspiratory: Expiratory ratio of 1:1 to 1:3; PEEP and FiO_2 to be set in accordance with ARDSNet protocol; Respiratory rate of <35 breaths per minute and initial tidal volume of 6 ml/kg. Prevent patient ventilator asynchrony and hence ventilator induced lung injury (VILI).

C. Monitoring:

    a. Arterial pH 7.30-7.45

    b. SpO_2 of 88-95%

    c. PaO_2 of 55-80 mmHg

    d. Plateau pressure <= 30 cm H_2O

D. Conservative fluid therapy: including diuresis if needed to reach net negative fluid status, once shock has resolved (off vasopressors)

E. Daily spontaneous breathing trials to assess for ventilator liberation beginning when the patient can tolerate FiO_2 ≤0·5 and PEEP ≤8 cm H_2O

F. For patients with moderate to severe ARDS (PaO_2/FiO_2 ratio <150 mm Hg), consider:

    – Neuromuscular blockade, with goal duration <48 h

    – Prone positioning for at least 12-18 hours per day

Clinical practice guidelines recommend maintaining an arterial pH of 7.30 to 7.45, although patients in some research trials have tolerated permissive hypercapnia and a pH as low as 7.15.[21]

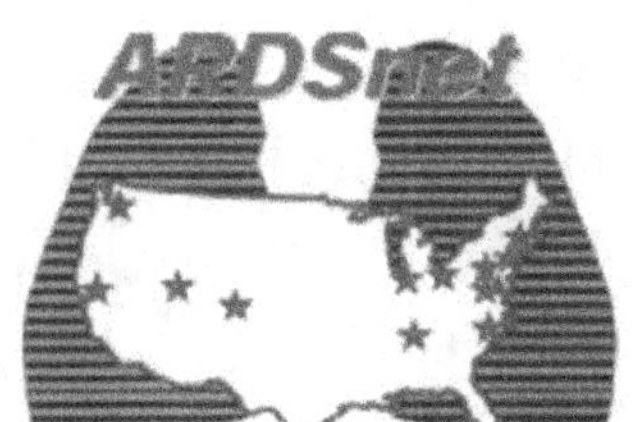

NIH NHLBI ARDS Clinical Network
Mechanical Ventilation Protocol Summary

INCLUSION CRITERIA: Acute onset of
1. PaO_2/FiO_2 ≤ 300 (corrected for altitude)
2. Bilateral (patchy, diffuse, or homogeneous) infiltrates consistent with pulmonary edema
3. No clinical evidence of left atrial hypertension

PART I: VENTILATOR SETUP AND ADJUSTMENT
1. Calculate predicted body weight (PBW)
   Males = 50 + 2.3 [height (inches) - 60]
   Females = 45.5 + 2.3 [height (inches) -60]
2. Select any ventilator mode
3. Set ventilator settings to achieve initial V_T = 8 ml/kg PBW
4. Reduce V_T by 1 ml/kg at intervals ≤ 2 hours until V_T = 6ml/kg PBW.
5. Set initial rate to approximate baseline minute ventilation (not > 35 bpm).
6. Adjust V_T and RR to achieve pH and plateau pressure goals below.

OXYGENATION GOAL: PaO_2 55-80 mmHg or SpO_2 88-95%
Use a minimum PEEP of 5 cm H_2O. Consider use of incremental FiO_2/PEEP combinations such as shown below (not required) to achieve goal.

Lower PEEP/higher FIO2

FiO_2	0.3	0.4	0.4	0.5	0.5	0.6	0.7	0.7
PEEP	5	5	8	8	10	10	10	12

FiO_2	0.7	0.8	0.9	0.9	0.9	1.0
PEEP	14	14	14	16	18	18-24

Higher PEEP/lower FIO2

FiO_2	0.3	0.3	0.3	0.3	0.3	0.4	0.4	0.5
PEEP	5	8	10	12	14	14	16	16

FiO_2	0.5	0.5-0.8	0.8	0.9	1.0	1.0
PEEP	18	20	22	22	22	24

PLATEAU PRESSURE GOAL: ≤ 30 cm H_2O
Check Pplat (0.5 second inspiratory pause), at least q 4h and after each change in PEEP or V_T.
If Pplat > 30 cm H_2O: decrease V_T by 1ml/kg steps (minimum = 4 ml/kg).
If Pplat < 25 cm H_2O and V_T< 6 ml/kg, increase V_T by 1 ml/kg until Pplat > 25 cm H_2O or V_T = 6 ml/kg.
If Pplat < 30 and breath stacking or dys-synchrony occurs: may increase V_T in 1ml/kg increments to 7 or 8 ml/kg if Pplat remains ≤ 30 cm H_2O.

Acidosis Management: (pH < 7.30)
If pH 7.15-7.30: Increase RR until pH > 7.30 or $PaCO_2$ < 25 (Maximum set RR = 35).

If pH < 7.15: Increase RR to 35.
If pH remains < 7.15, V_T may be increased in 1 ml/kg steps until pH > 7.15 (Pplat target of 30 may be exceeded).
May give $NaHCO_3$
Alkalosis Management: (pH > 7.45) Decrease vent rate if possible.

I: E RATIO GOAL: Recommend that duration of inspiration be ≤ duration of expiration.

PART II: WEANING
A. **Conduct a SPONTANEOUS BREATHING TRIAL daily when:**
   1. FiO_2 ≤ 0.40 and PEEP ≤ 8 OR FiO_2 ≤ 0.50 and PEEP ≤ 5.
   2. PEEP and FiO_2 ≤ values of previous day.
   3. Patient has acceptable spontaneous breathing efforts. (May decrease vent rate by 50% for 5 minutes to detect effort.)
   4. Systolic BP ≥ 90 mmHg without vasopressor support.
   5. No neuromuscular blocking agents or blockade.

spontaneous breathing with FIO2 ≤ 0.5 and PEEP ≤ 5:
   1. Place on T-piece, trach collar, or CPAP ≤ 5 cm H_2O with PS ≤ 5
   2. Assess for tolerance as below for up to two hours.
      a. SpO_2 ≥ 90: and/or PaO_2 ≥ 60 mmHg
      b.   Spontaneous V_T ≥ 4 ml/kg PBW
      c.   RR ≤ 35/min
      d.   pH ≥ 7.3
      e.   No respiratory distress (distress= 2 or more)
         ➢ HR > 120% of baseline
         ➢ Marked accessory muscle use
         ➢ Abdominal paradox
         ➢ Diaphoresis
         ➢ Marked dyspnea
   3. If tolerated for at least 30 minutes, consider extubation.
   4. If not tolerated resume pre-weaning settings.

> Definition of <u>UNASSISTED BREATHING</u>
> **(Different from the spontaneous breathing criteria as PS is not allowed)**
>
> 1. Extubated with face mask, nasal prong oxygen, or room air, OR
> 2. T-tube breathing, OR
> 3. Tracheostomy mask breathing, OR
> 4. CPAP less than or equal to 5 cm H_2O **without pressure support or IMV assistance.**

Figure 1: Ventilator protocol card[22] taken from: http://www.ardsnet.org/files/ventilator_protocol_2008-07.pdf

Patients who remain hypoxemic despite LTVV, supportive measures, and alternative ventilator settings/modes will continue to worsen, with development of severe and refractory hypoxaemia, hypercapnia or acidosis, elevated plateau pressures, or a combination. In these patients, rescue therapies whose benefits have not been conclusively shown for all patients but could show benefit in individualised circumstances

Options include the following:

a. Extracorporeal Membrane Oxygenation (ECMO)

b. Higher PEEP strategies

c. Recruitment manoeuvre

d. Inhaled pulmonary vasodilators

e. Corticosteroids

f. Continuous Renal Replacement Therapy

This disease continues to challenge clinicians and scientists to provide impeccable supportive care and discover new therapies

Recent updates

1. Results of the landmark ARMA study found the use of low (6 ml/kg predicted weight) rather than "standard" (12 ml/kg predicted weight) tidal volumes reduced mortality from 40 to 30%. These results provide much of the basis for use of low- stretch/low tidal volume ventilation strategy in acute lung injury.[23]

2. Report on symptoms, demographic data, and management of patients with EVALI[16] during 2019 outbreak - As of November 13, 2019, 49 states, the District of Columbia, and two U.S. territories (Puerto Rico and U.S. Virgin Islands) have reported 2,172 EVALI cases to CDC, including 42 (1.9%) EVALI-associated deaths. Among 2,016 EVALI patients with available data on hospitalization status, 1,906 (95%) were hospitalized, and 110 (5%) were not hospitalized.[24]

3. Writing Group for the Alveolar Recruitment for Acute Respiratory Distress Syndrome Trial (ART) Investigators - Multicenter trial of 1010 patients with moderate to severe ARDS randomized to low PEEP (control) or a lung recruitment maneuver and PEEP titration according to the best respiratory-system static compliance (intervention). The intervention group had increased mortality at 28 days (55% vs 49%; p=0.041), and increased risk of pneumothorax requiring draining (3.2% vs 1.2%; p=0.03). ART is noteworthy for being the first major study of the "open lung approach" to show harm. Concerns raised about the study include the relatively high mortality in both groups as well as the method of recruitment. On the whole, these studies pointed toward the greatest benefit of high PEEP among patients with severe ARDS.[25]

4. LUNG SAFE study[8] described the management of patients with ARDS. A substudy examined the current practice of NIV use in ARDS, the utility of the PaO_2/FiO_2 ratio in classifying patients receiving NIV, and the impact of NIV on outcome. Of 2,813 patients with ARDS, 436 (15.5%) were managed with NIV on Days 1 and 2 following fulfillment of diagnostic criteria. Classification of ARDS severity based on PaO_2/FiO_2 ratio was associated with an increase in intensity of ventilatory support, NIV failure, and intensive care unit (ICU) mortality. NIV failure occurred in 22.2% of mild, 42.3% of moderate, and 47.1% of patients with severe ARDS. Hospital mortality in patients with NIV success and failure was 16.1% and 45.4%, respectively. NIV use was independently associated with increased ICU (hazard ratio, 1.446 [95% confidence interval, 1.159-1.805]), but not hospital mortality. In a propensity matched analysis, ICU mortality was higher in NIV than invasively ventilated patients with a PaO_2/FiO_2 lower than 150 mm Hg. Hence they concluded that NIV seemed to be associated with higher ICU mortality in patients with a PaO_2/FiO_2 lower than 150 mm Hg.[26]

5. In a multicenter, randomized trial, patients with ARDS were assigned to receive either conservative oxygen therapy (target PaO_2, 55 to 70 mm Hg; oxygen saturation as measured by pulse oximetry [SpO_2], 88 to 92%) or liberal oxygen therapy (target PaO_2, 90 to 105 mm

Hg; SpO_2, ≥96%) for 7 days. The same mechanical-ventilation strategies were used in both groups. The primary outcome was death from any cause at 28 days. Enrollment was stopped for futility after 205 subjects. There was no difference in 28-day mortality (primary outcome) and 5 episodes of mesenteric ischemia occurred in the O_2 conservative group.[27]

6. PROSEVA trial - In contrast to previous studies of prone positioning, this group found significantly decreased (and strikingly low) mortality at 28 (32.8 vs.16%) and 90 (41% vs. 23.8%) days without an increase in adverse events among 466 patients with severe ARDS (PaO_2/FIO_2 < 150 mmHg). The treatment group was placed in the prone position sessions of at least 16 hours within the first 3-4 days. Normal ICU beds were used.[28]

7. The multicenter EOLIA randomized 249 patients with very severe ARDS to immediate veno-venous ECMO vs standard care. Although patients randomly assigned to ECMO had an 11% absolute risk reduction for 60-day mortality compared with the control group (35% *vs* 46%, p=0·09), this outcome did not meet the predetermined criteria for statistical significance. The study was stopped early for futility despite a trend toward benefit. Of note, 28% of control patients crossed over to ECMO due to refractory hypoxemia, with 43% of this group surviving. ECMO appeared to be safe by comparison with conventional treatment, although with higher incidences of thrombocytopenia and bleeding requiring transfusion. The benefit of ECMO could partly be attributed to the reduced plateau pressures required by the ECMO protocol, the resulting lower tidal volumes, or both. These data suggest that ECMO should be strongly considered in patients with very severe ARDS who are early in the course of disease (mechanical ventilation ≤7 days) and with potentially reversible respiratory failure.[29]

8. A RCT to evaluate NMB in 1006 patients with moderate to severe ARDS found no difference in 90 day mortality with early use of a 48 hour infusion of neuromuscular blockade compared to usual care. This trial was similar to the ACURASYS trial except for the use of lighter sedation targets in the usual care group. There was no difference in rates of ICU-acquired weakness or recall of paralysis. Trial was stopped early for futility.30

9. 91 Patients with severe early ARDS (< 72 hours) were randomized (2:1 fashion) to methylprednisolone infusion (1 mg/kg/d) vs placebo. The duration of treatment was up to 28 days. In intention-to-treat analysis, the response of the two groups (63 treated and 28 control) clearly diverged by day 7, with twice the proportion of treated patients achieving a 1-point reduction in LIS (69.8% vs 35.7%; p = 0.002) and breathing without assistance (53.9% vs 25.0%; p = 0.01). Treatment was associated with a reduction in the duration of mechanical ventilation (p = 0.002), ICU stay (p = 0.007), and ICU mortality (20.6% vs 42.9%; p = 0.03). 31

10. RECOVERY trial - a large pragmatic randomised open-label study in the UK, reported that dexamethasone 6 mg daily for 10 days was associated with a lower 28-day mortality for hospitalised patients with COVID-19, with the largest effect seen in patients receiving mechanical ventilation. A total of 2104 patients were assigned to receive dexamethasone and

4321 to receive usual care. Overall, 482 patients (22.9%) in the dexamethasone group and 1110 patients (25.7%) in the usual care group died within 28 days after randomization (age-adjusted rate ratio, 0.83; 95% confidence interval [CI], 0.75 to 0.93; P<0.001). The proportional and absolute between-group differences in mortality varied considerably according to the level of respiratory support that the patients were receiving at the time of randomization. In the dexamethasone group, the incidence of death was lower than that in the usual care group among patients receiving invasive mechanical ventilation (29.3% vs. 41.4%; rate ratio, 0.64; 95% CI, 0.51 to 0.81) and among those receiving oxygen without invasive mechanical ventilation (23.3% vs. 26.2%; rate ratio, 0.82; 95% CI, 0.72 to 0.94) but not among those who were receiving no respiratory support at randomization (17.8% vs. 14.0%; rate ratio, 1.19; 95% CI, 0.92 to 1.55).[32]

11. A trial randomized 277 ARDS patients with PaO_2/FIO_2 < 200 despite PEEP ≥ 10 and FIO_2 ≥ 0.5 to 10 days of dexamethasone or routine care. Mean ventilator-free days was 4.8 days higher (95% CI 2.57 to 7.03) in the dexamethasone group and 60 day mortality was lower in the dexamethasone group (21% vs 36% with 95% CI -25.9 to – 4.9). Slow rate of patient recruitment and lack of blinding were the limitations.33

12. Sivelestat is a neutrophil elastase inhibitor, which induces competitive inhibition of neutrophils, inhibition of neutrophil activation, and reduction of inflammation in the lungs. Currently, the use of sivelestat is already approved in Japan. Several RCTs have indicated that sivelestat therapy can improve ventilation days and PaO_2/FiO_2. Hence a metanalysis was conducted whereby 6 RCTs involving a total of 804 patients with ALI/ARDS were included. Moreover, five trials included patients who received 0.2 mg/kg/h sivelestat, and one trial included those who received 0.16 mg/kg/h sivelestat. The study quality was assessed using the Jadad score. The findings of this study suggested that sivelestat therapy might play an important role on the PaO_2/FiO_2 level, while it had no significant effect on 28–30 days mortality, ventilation days, and ICU stays.[34]

13. CITRIS-ALI trial - investigated high dose vitamin C versus placebo in 167 patients with early sepsis and ARDS; although no difference was observed in the primary outcome of modified sequential organ failure assessment score at 96 h, patients treated with vitamin C had a significant reduction in 28-day all-cause mortality, compared with placebo (30% *vs* 46%, p=0·03). Vitamin C was intravenously infused in the treatment group at 50 mg/kg actual body weight every 6 hours for 96 hours. Infusion bags (50 mL) containing the calculated vitamin C dosage in dextrose 5% in water or placebo (dextrose 5% in water alone). Vitamin C is also being studied in sepsis and might have beneficial effects on systemic inflammation, coagulopathy, alveolar fluid clearance, and formation of neutrophil extracellular traps.[35]

14. The H1N1 influenza A virus is known to be associated with high morbidity and mortality. The infection can cause a severe acute respiratory failure or ARDS with multiorgan failure.

The H1N1 pandemic of 2009 saw many cases of severe ARDS with refractory hypoxemia that needed the veno-venous extracorporeal membrane oxygenation as a rescue therapy. Recently, the interferon-inducible transmembrane (IFITM3) protein has shown in models to have a pivotal role in defending the host from pathological virus such as influenza A. In human individuals hospitalized for influenza H1N1/2009 virus it has been found elevated expression of a minor IFITM3 allele and in vitro minor CC genotype IFITM3 has reduced influenza virus restriction.[18,36]

15. Official American Thoracic Society/European Society of Intensive Care Medicine/Society of Critical Care Medicine Clinical Practice Guideline regarding High Frequency Oscilatory ventilation (HFOV)[37]– This type of ventilation uses novel mechanisms of alveolar ventilation, permitting the delivery of very small tidal volumes at higher mean airway pressures. By simultaneously recruiting collapsed lung units and minimizing tidal stress and strain, HFOV offers a theoretically attractive mode of lung protection. The panel of experts considered all six RCTs, whereby no significant difference in mortality between groups (six studies, 1,705 patients; RR, 0.94; 95% CI, 0.71–1.24; low confidence). However, their recommendation was strongly based on considered evidence from the RCT that used LTV with higher PEEP in the control group that reported significantly higher mortality with HFOV (RR, 1.41; 95% CI, 1.12–1.79)[38] as well as a large pragmatic RCT that showed no benefit with HFOV (adjusted odds ratio, 1.03; 95% CI, 00.75-1.40)[39]

16. In the Fluid and Catheter Treatment Trial (FACTT) of the National Institutes of Health Acute Respiratory Distress Syndrome Network, a conservative fluid protocol (FACTT Conservative) resulted in a lower cumulative fluid balance and better outcomes than a liberal fluid protocol (FACTT Liberal). Subsequent ARDSNet studies used a simplified conservative fluid protocol (FACTT Lite). FACTT Conservative targeted a central venous pressure (CVP) of less than 4 mm Hg or a pulmonary artery occlusion pressure (PAOP) of less than 8 mm Hg, whereas FACTT Liberal targeted a CVP of 10–14 mm Hg or PAOP of 14–18 mm Hg. Management with the FACTT Conservative protocol resulted in a significantly lower cumulative fluid balance over 7 days. While there was no difference in 60-day mortality, the FACTT Conservative group had more ventilator-free days and an improved oxygenation index and lung injury score. Wherein FACTT Lite excluded instructions for ineffective circulation because the clinical examination findings of ineffective circulation did not correlate with cardiac index FACTT Lite. It provides three possible instructions determined by the CVP and urine output: furosemide administration, fluid bolus, or no intervention.

In a retrospective comparative study analyzed 1,124 subjects from the ARDS Network studies managed with the FACTT Lite protocol excluded 40 subjects on chronic dialysis from ARDS Network studies using FACTT Lite. They analyzed a total of 497 subjects in the FACTT Liberal group and 503 subjects in the FACTT Conservative group. Both the FACTT Lite and FACTT Conservative groups had significantly lower daily fluid balance than FACTT Liberal ($p < 0.001$ on all days)

Fluid management with FACTT Lite resulted in a significantly greater cumulative fluid balance by 2,054 mL over 7 days than FACTT Conservative, but a significantly lower cumulative fluid balance by 5,074 mL over 7 days than FACTT Liberal

After adjustment for age and APACHE III score, 60-day mortality was similar between groups ($p = 0.84$). The FACTT Lite and FACTT Conservative groups had similar ventilator-free days ($p = 0.61$), and FACTT Lite had higher ventilator-free days than FACTT Liberal ($p < 0.001$). Similarly, FACTT Lite had the same ICU-free days as FACTT Conservative and more than FACTT Liberal ($p < 0.001$).

Although the FACTT Lite protocol had a greater cumulative fluid balance than FACTT Conservative, the results of this study indicate that the FACTT Lite protocol is safe and has equivalent ventilator-free days, ICU-free days, acute kidney injury, and adjusted 60-day mortality to FACTT Conservative.[40]

References

1. Hussain M, Khurram Syed S, Fatima M, Shaukat S, Saadullah M, Alqahtani AM, Alqahtani T, Bin Emran T, Alamri AH, Barkat MQ, Wu X. Acute Respiratory Distress Syndrome and COVID-19: A Literature Review. J Inflamm Res. 2021 Dec 21;14:7225-7242.

2. Ranieri VM, Rubenfeld GD, Thompson BT, et al. Acute respiratory distress syndrome: the Berlin definition. JAMA 2012; 307: 2526–33.

3. Riviello ED, Kiviri W, Twagirumugabe T, et al. Hospital incidence and outcomes of the acute respiratory distress syndrome using the Kigali modification of the Berlin definition. *Am J Respir Crit Care Med*. 2016;193(1):52–59

4. Matthay MA, Zemans RL. The acute respiratory distress syndrome: pathogenesis and treatment. Annu Rev Pathol 2011; 6:147–163

5. Tan W, Zhao X, Ma X, et al. A novel coronavirus genome identified in a cluster of pneumonia cases - Wuhan, China 2019–2020. *China CDC Weekly*. 2020;2(4):61–62

6. Marini JJ. Dealing With the CARDS of COVID-19. Crit Care Med. 2020 Aug;48(8):1239-1241.

7. Liu C, Li J. Role of genetic factors in the development of acute respiratory distress syndrome. *J Transl Int Med*. 2015;2(3):107–110.

8. Bellani G, Laffey JG, Pham T, et al. Epidemiology, Patterns of Care, and Mortality for Patients With Acute Respiratory Distress Syndrome in Intensive Care Units in 50 Countries. *JAMA*. 2016;315(8):788–800

9. Villar J, Blanco J, Añón JM, et al; ALIEN Network. The ALIEN study: incidence and outcome of acute respiratory distress syndrome in the era of lung protective ventilation. *Intensive Care Med.* 2011;37(12):1932-1941

10. Auriemma CL, Zhuo H, Delucchi K. Acute respiratory distress syndrome-attributable mortality in critically ill patients with sepsis. *Intensive Care Med.* 2020;46:1222–1231.

11. Meyer NJ, Gattinoni L, Calfee CS. Acute respiratory distress syndrome. Lancet. 2021 Aug 14;398(10300):622-637.

12. Thompson BT, Chambers RC, Liu KD. Acute Respiratory Distress Syndrome. *N Engl J Med.* 2017;377(6):562–572

13. Ware LB. Pathophysiology of acute lung injury and the acute respiratory distress syndrome. *Semin Respir Crit Care Med.* 2006;27(4):337–349.

14. Greene KE, Wright JR, Steinberg KP, et al. Serial changes in surfactant-associated proteins in lung and serum before and after onset of ARDS. *Am J Respir Crit Care Med.* 1999;160(6):1843–1850

15. Ware LB. Pathophysiology of acute lung injury and the acute respiratory distress syndrome. *Semin Respir Crit Care Med.* 2006;27(4):337–349.

16. Layden JE, Ghinai I, Pray I, et al. Pulmonary illness related to e-cigarette use in Illinois and Wisconsin—final report. N Engl J Med 2019; 382: 903–16

17. Calfee CS, Janz DR, Bernard GR, May AK, Kangelaris KN, Matthay MA et al. Distinct molecular phenotypes of direct versus indirect ARDS in single and multi-center studies. *Chest.* 2015;147:1539–1548

18. Spadaro S, Park M, Turrini C, Tunstall T, Thwaites R, Mauri T et al. Biomarkers for Acute Respiratory Distress syndrome and prospects for personalised medicine. J Inflamm (Lond). 2019 Jan 15;16:1. doi: 10.1186/s12950-018-0202-y. PMID: 30675131; PMCID: PMC6332898.

19. Cronin WA, Forbes AS, Wagner KL, Kaplan P, Cataneo R, Phillips M et al. Exhaled Volatile Organic Compounds Precedes Pulmonary Injury in a Swine Pulmonary Oxygen Toxicity Model. Front Physiol. 2019 Dec 3;10:1297. doi: 10.3389/fphys.2019.01297. PMID: 31849689; PMCID: PMC6901787.

20. ARDSNet[Internet]. Massachusetts General Hospital Biostatistics Center: NHLBI ARDSNet. [reviewed 2022 Apr15; cited 2022 Apr 17]: Available from: http://www.ardsnet.org/index.shtml

21. Dellinger RP, Levy MM, Carlet JM, et al.; International Surviving Sepsis Campaign Guidelines Committee. Surviving Sepsis Campaign: international guidelines for management of severe sepsis and septic shock: 2008. *Crit Care Med.* 2008;36(1):296–327

22. ARDSNet Ventilator protocol Tool[Internet]. Massachusetts General Hospital Biostatistics Center: NHLBI ARDSNet. [reviewed 2022 Apr15; cited 2022 Apr 17]: Available from: http://www.ardsnet.org/files/ventilator_protocol_2008-07.pdf

23. ARDS Network. Ventilation with lower tidal volumes as compared with traditional tidal volumes for ALI and ARDS. N Engl J Med. 2000;342:1301-8

24. Chatham-Stephens K, Roguski K, Jang Y, et al. Characteristics of hospitalized and nonhospitalized patients in a nationwide outbreak of e-cigarette, or vaping, product use-associated lung injury - United States, November 2019. MMWR Morb Mortal Wkly Rep. 2019; 68:1076-1080

25. Cavalcanti AB, Suzumura EA, Laranjeira LN, et al. Effect of lung recruitment and titrated positive end-expiratory pressure (PEEP) vs low PEEP on mortality in patients with acute respiratory distress syndrome: a randomized clinical trial. JAMA. 2017; 318:1335-1345.

26. Bellani G, Laffey JG, Pham T, Madotto F, Fan E, Brochard L et al; LUNG SAFE Investigators; ESICM Trials Group. Noninvasive Ventilation of Patients with Acute Respiratory Distress Syndrome. Insights from the LUNG SAFE Study. Am J Respir Crit Care Med. 2017 Jan 1;195(1):67-77. doi: 10.1164/rccm.201606-1306OC. PMID: 27753501.

27. Barrot L, Asfar P, Mauny F, et al. LOCO$_2$ Investigators and REVA Research Network. Liberal or Conservative Oxygen Therapy for Acute Respiratory Distress Syndrome. N Engl J Med. 2020;382(11):999-1008.

28. Guerin C, Reignier J, Richard JC, et al. Prone positioning in severe acute respiratory distress syndrome. N Engl J Med. 2013; 368:2159-2168.

29. Combes A, Hajage D, Capellier G et al. Extracorporeal membrane oxygenation for severe acute respiratory distress syndrome. N Engl J Med. 2018; 378:1965-1975.

30. Moss M, Huang DT, Brower RG, et al. Early neuromuscular blockade in acute respiratory distress syndrome (ROSE). N Engl J Med. 2019;380:1997-2008.

31. Meduri GU, Golden E, Freire AX, et al. Methylprednisolone infusion in early severe ARDS: results of a randomized controlled trial. *Chest*. 2007;131(4):954–963.

32. RECOVERY Collaborative Group, Horby P, Lim WS, Emberson JR, Mafham M, Bell JL, Linsell L et al. Dexamethasone in Hospitalized Patients with Covid-19. N Engl J Med. 2021 Feb 25;384(8):693-704.

33. Villar J, Ferrando C, Martínez D, et al. Dexamethasone treatment for the acute respiratory distress syndrome: a multicentre, randomised controlled trial. Lancet Respir Med. 2020; 8:267-276.

34. Pu S, Wang D, Liu D, Zhao Y, Qi D, He J et al. Effect of sivelestat sodium in patients with acute lung injury or acute respiratory distress syndrome: a meta-analysis of randomized controlled trials. BMC Pulm Med. 2017 Nov 21;17(1):148..

35. Fowler AA, Truwit JD, Hite RD, et al. Effect of Vitamin C Infusion on Organ Failure and Biomarkers of Inflammation and Vascular Injury in Patients With Sepsis and Severe Acute Respiratory Failure: The CITRIS-ALI Randomized Clinical Trial. *JAMA*. 2019;322(13):1261–1270.

36. Everitt AR, Clare S, Pertel T, John SP, Wash RS, Smith SE et al. IFITM3 restricts the morbidity and mortality associated with influenza. *Nature*. 2012;484:519–523.

37. Fan E, Del Sorbo L, Goligher EC, Hodgson CL, Munshi L, Walkey AJ et al; American Thoracic Society, European Society of Intensive Care Medicine, and Society of Critical Care Medicine. An Official American Thoracic Society/European Society of Intensive Care Medicine/Society of Critical Care Medicine Clinical Practice Guideline: Mechanical Ventilation in Adult Patients with Acute Respiratory Distress Syndrome. Am J Respir Crit Care Med. 2017 May 1;195(9):1253-1263.

38. Ferguson ND, Cook DJ, Guyatt GH, Mehta S, Hand L, Austin P *et al.*; OSCILLATE Trial Investigators; Canadian Critical Care Trials Group. High-frequency oscillation in early acute respiratory distress syndrome. *N Engl J Med* 2013;368:795–805.

39. Young D, Lamb SE, Shah S, MacKenzie I, Tunnicliffe W, Lall R et al OSCAR Study Group. High-frequency oscillation for acute respiratory distress syndrome. *N Engl J Med* 2013;368:806–813

40. Grissom CK, Hirshberg EL, Dickerson JB, Brown SM, Lanspa MJ, Liu KD et al; National Heart Lung and Blood Institute Acute Respiratory Distress Syndrome Clinical Trials Network. Fluid management with a simplified conservative protocol for the acute respiratory distress syndrome*. Crit Care Med. 2015 Feb;43(2):288-95.

Pneumonia

Table 1. Definitions

Community acquired pneumonia
Infection of the lung parenchyma acquired outside the hospital setting
Nosocomial pneumonia
Acute infection of the lung parenchyma acquired during hospital stay it can be of two types – Hospital acquired pneumonia (hcp) - acquired more than or equal to 48 hours after hospital admission Ventilator acquired pneumonia - occurs after more than or equal to 48 hours after endotracheal intubation
Health care associated pnuemonia
It is acquired in health care facilities such as nursing homes and haemodialysis centres.

Classification of pneumonia by aetiology

- Atypical Pneumonia

It is caused by typical organisms such as legionella pneumonia, mycoplasma pneumonia, chlamydia pneumoniae, chlamydia psittaci and Coxiella burnetti.

- Aspiration Pneumonia

It is caused by aspiration of gastric or esophageal contents, which may contain bacteria and /or be of low pH or exogenous substances such as ingested food particles, mineral oil or fresh water.

- Chemical Pneumonitis
- Bacterial Aspiration Pneumonia

Community Acquired Pneumonia (CAP)

It is one of the common presentations in ED. These patients usually present with acute onset fever, shortness breath, cough with and without expectoration.

Radiologically, it appears as lobar consolidations, interstitial infiltrates and or cavitations.

<u>Following parameters indicate the need for inpatient treatment:</u>

1. Septic shock with need for vasopressor support
2. Respiratory failure requiring mechanical ventilation.
3. History of substance abuse, mental illness, concerns regarding adherence to treatment, cognitive impairment.

4. Pneumonia severity index – it was validated by pneumonia patient outcomes research team (PDRT) prospective cohort study.

<u>2 score that are widely used</u>

<u>Pneumonia severity score</u>

sub-classified all patients of pneumonia with radiological evidence into five classes for risk of death assessment at 30 days of presentation.

Risk Class 1

- Age < 50years
- Absence of other co-existing conditions such as neoplastic diseases, heart failure, cerebrovascular diseases, renal and hepatic diseases.
- Absence of other physical findings such as altered mental status, pulse ≥ 125/minute, respiratory rate ≥30/minute. Systolic blood pressure <90mmhg. Temperature < 35c or ≥40 c.

The risk classes II, III, IV or V, include laboratory and radiographic parameters.

The recommendation is to treat patients as inpatient for class IV and V.

<u>CURB-65 scores</u>

- Confusion
- Urea (BUN >20mg/dl)
- Respiratory rate ≥30 breaths /min
- Blood pressure (SBP <90mmhg, DBP≤60mmhg)
- Age ≥65 years

A score of 0 can be managed as outpatient, A score of 1 or 2 can be admitted in general medical ward and score of 3 to 5 with clinical criteria requiring ICU level of care should be admitted to ICU (intensive care unit)

<u>SMART -COP criteria</u> – Risk stratify patients who will require intensive respiratory or vasopressor support (IRVS)

- Systolic blood pressure < 90mmhg
- Multilobar pneumonia
- Hypoalbuminemia (<3.5 g/dL)
- respiratory rate

  o ≤50 years ≥25 breaths/minute
  o ≥50 years ≥30 breaths/min

- Tachycardia ($\geq$125/min)
- Confusion (new onset)
- poor oxygenation
    - $\leq$50 years PaO_2 <70 mmhg and O_2 saturation $\leq$ 93%
    - >50 years PaO_2 <60 mmhg and O_2 saturation $\leq$90%
- low arterial pH (<7.35)

<u>IDSA/ATS severity criteria</u> –

- Altered mental status
- Hypotension requiring fluid support
- Temperature <36°C (96.8F)
- Respiratory rate $\geq$30 breaths/min
- PaO_2/fiO_2 ratio $\leq$250
- BUN $\geq$20mg/dl
- Leucocyte count <4000 cells /microL
- Platelet count <100000/ml
- Multilobar infiltrate

The presence of three of these criteria warrants ICU admission

Differential Diagnosis

- Acute bronchitis
- Influenza
- Interstitial lung disease
- Upper respiratory tract infection
- Corona virus disease
- Acute exacerbation of COPD
- Acute exacerbation of asthma
- Acute exacerbation of bronchiectasis
- Heart failure with pulmonary edema
- Pulmonary embolism
- Atelectasis
- Lung cancer

Diagnostic Tests

- Chest x-ray
- CT chest
- Blood cultures – to enhance the diagnostic yield, blood culture to be sent prior to antibiotic administration.
- Sputum gram stain and culture
- Urinary pneumococcal antigen testing for Strep Pneumonia.
- Diagnostic tests for legionella include urinary antigen test, culture and PCR.
- PCR for COVID-19

Empiric Antibiotic Treatment – For Community Acquired Pneumonia

- For healthy patients aged <65 years with no recent antibiotic use – high dose Amoxicillin (1gm orally three times a day) plus either a macrolide or doxycycline.
- For patients with comorbidities, aged 65years or older or with history of recent antibiotic use –
  - Extended-release Amoxicillin–clavulanate plus a macrolide or doxycycline, or
  - Third generation cephalosporins plus macrolides or doxycycline, or
  - Fluoroquinolones, or
  - Lefamulin monotherapy

Antimicrobial - resistant gram-negative bacilli are important causes of both VAP and HAP

Antimicrobial resistance-

- MDR means acquired non-susceptibility to atleast *one agent* in three different antimicrobial classes.
- Extensively drug resistant (XDR) means resistance to atleast *one agent but two antimicrobial classes.*
- Pan drug resistant means resistance to all the agents that can be utilized for treatment

Risk factors for MDR pathogens in a patient include –

- History of antibiotic used in last 90 days
- Septic shock in a patient with VAP
- ARDS
- History of previous hospitalization of more than 5 days
- History of renal replacement therapy prior to development of VAP

Risk factors of MDR pseudomonas along with other gram-negative bacilli –

- History of treatment in ICU with more than 10 percent isolates as gram-negative organisms being resistant to an antimicrobial agent considered for monotherapy.
- History of treatment in ICU with unknown susceptibility rates.
- Colonization with MDR pseudomonas or other gram negative bacilli

Risk factors for MRSA include –

- History of treatment in a unit with more than 10 to 20 % methicillin resistant staphylococcus aureus isolates.
- History of treatment in a unit with unknown prevalence of MRSA.
- History of prior colonization of MRSA

Patients without risk factors of MDR organisms should receive

- Piperacillin-tazobactam 4.5gm IV every 6th hourly.
- Cefepime 2gm IV 8th hourly
- Levofloxacin 750mg IV

The following patients with any of the following risk factors should receive two agents active against Pseudomonas aeruginosa

- IV antibiotic use within previous 90 days
- Septic shock
- ARDS
- ≥5 days of hospitalization
- Acute renal replacement therapy

Patients should receive following

- Piperacillin – Tazobactum, or
- Ceftazidime, or
- Imipenem, or
- Meropenem, or
- Aztreonam

Plus any one of the following -

- Amikacin (15-20 mg/kg IV daily)
- Gentamicin (5-7mg/kg IV daily)
- Tobramycin (5-7mg /kg IV daily)

In patients with highly resistant pseudomonas spp, Enterobacteriaceae, addition of an alternative agent such as polymyxin B or colistin is suggested

Inhaled colistin can be added in highly resistant cases

Injection ceftazidime avibactam, ceftolozane-tazobactum and imipenem -cilastin -relebactam provide alternative single agent options with potential against MDR gram-negative bacteria.

Plus

Linezolid, vancomycin, or Telavancin.

Recent advances

1. APEKS-NP trial (2021)

- Compared Cefiderocol versus high-dose, extended-infusion meropenem for the treatment of Gram-negative nosocomial pneumonia.
- They included adult patients who were older than 18 years with hospital-acquired pneumonia, ventilator-associated pneumonia, or health-care-associated Gram-negative pneumonia, and were assigned randomly (1:1 by interactive response technology) to 3-h iv infusions of either cefiderocol 2 g or meropenem 2 g every eight hourly for 7–14 days. All patients also received open-label iv linezolid (600 mg every 12 h) for at least five days.
- The study showed that Cefiderocol was non-inferior to high-dose, extended-infusion meropenem in all-cause mortality after 14 days in patients with Gram-negative nosocomial pneumonia, with similar tolerability.
- The results suggested that cefiderocol is a potential option for treating patients with nosocomial pneumonia, including those caused by multidrug-resistant Gram-negative bacteria. (1)

2. CREDIBLE-CR trial (2021)

Studied the efficacy and safety of cefiderocol versus best available therapy in adults with serious carbapenem-resistant Gram-negative infections.

It was a randomized, open-label, multicentre, pathogen-focused, descriptive, phase 3 study done in 95 hospitals in 16 countries. Adult patients were admitted to the hospital with nosocomial pneumonia, bloodstream infections or sepsis, complicated urinary tract infections (UTI), and evidence of a carbapenem-resistant gram-negative pathogen.

The patients were randomly assigned to receive either a 3-h iv infusion of cefiderocol 2 g every eight hour or best available therapy (pre-specified by the investigator before randomization) comprised of a maximum of three drugs) for 7–14 days.

The primary endpoint was clinical cure at the test of cure (7 days [plus or minus 2] after the end of treatment). Mortality was reported after the study visit (28 days [plus or minus 3] after treatment).

Cefiderocol had similar microbiological and clinical efficacy to best therapy available in the heterogeneous patient population with carbapenem-resistant Gram-negative bacterial infections. Overall, the findings from this study supported cefiderocol as an option for treating carbapenem-resistant infections in patients with limited treatment options. (2)

3. LEAP 2 trial (2019)

Evaluated the efficacy and adverse events of a 5-day oral lefamulin regimen in patients with community acquired pneumonia (bacterial).

Adult patients with PORT risk classes II, III, or IV radiographically documented pneumonia, acute illness (≤7 days), three or more CABP symptoms (dyspnea, new or increased cough, purulent sputum production, and chest pain) were included in the study. Patients were classified as responders, non-responders, or indeterminate.

Patients were randomized 1:1 to receive per oral tablets of either Lefamulin 600 mg q12 hours for five days or moxifloxacin 400 mg q24 hours for seven days.

The primary outcome was the early clinical response at 96 hours after receiving the first dose of either study drug which resulted to be the same in both groups. The overall incidence of adverse events was lefamulin (32.6%) and moxifloxacin (25.0%).

This study showed the noninferiority of oral lefamulin to oral moxifloxacin to treat community-acquired bacterial pneumonia. (3)

4. Novel Severity Scoring System for Pneumonia in Intensive Care Unit

- A prospective cohort study was done in general ICUs in Brazil. ICU severity scores like (Simplified Acute Physiology Score 3 [SAPS 3] and Sepsis-Related Organ Failure Assessment [qSOFA]), pneumonia prognostic scores (CURB-65 and CRB-65), and clinical and epidemiological variables in the first 6 hours of hospitalization were analyzed.

- 200 patients were included in the study who were admitted from the emergency department (65%) with community-acquired pneumonia (CAP, 80.5%). SAPS 3, CURB-65, CRB-65, and qSOFA showed poor performance in mortality prediction.

- Multivariate regression found few variables that independently were associated with mortality. A novel pneumonia-specific ICU severity score (Pneumonia Shock score) that outperformed SAPS 3, CURB-65, and CRB-65 was developed. The pneumonia shock scoring system was validated in an external multicenter cohort of critically ill patients admitted with CAP.

- Pneumonia SHOCK Score included the following parameters –

  - Age more than 75 years old

  - Heart rate≥ 110 beats per minute

  - Hematocrit ≤38%

  - WBC ≥15x103

  - Serum Na ≥145 mmol/L

  - FiO_2 ≥30%

  - Use of vasopressors, and

  - Presence of obtundation by GCS less than 15.

- This score outperformed prior scores analyzed in their cohort and demonstrated robust discriminate function in a distinct validation cohort.

5. ANTHARTIC trial

- studied the role of empirical antibiotics to prevent ventilator associated pneumonia in out of hospital cardiac arrest patients (due to a shockable rhythm) treated with targeted temperature management at 32 to 34°C.

- It was a multicenter, double-blind, randomized, placebo-controlled trial which involved adult patients in the intensive care units (ICUs)

- The patients were either given intravenous amoxicillin-clavulanate (1 g and 200 mg, respectively) or placebo, three times a day for 2 days which started less than 6 hours after the cardiac arrest.

- A lower incidence of early (within seven days) ventilator associated pneumonia was seen in the intervention group. However, there is no difference in the rate of late VAP, other nosocomial infections, 28-day mortality, and length of ICU stay.

- This trial showed that by using short-course antibiotics in OOHCA patients due to a shockable rhythm resulted in a decreased rate of VAP. (4)

6. Are macrolides as effective as fluoroquinolones in Legionella pneumonia?

- The current Infectious Diseases Society of America guidelines recommends either a fluoroquinolone or a macrolide as a first-line antibiotic treatment for Legionella pneumonia, but it is still unclear which antibiotic leads to optimal clinical outcomes.

- A systematic review and meta-analyisis was done which included 21 studies of randomised control studies and observational studies that compared the two drugs. The study showed that there was no differences in the effectiveness of either fluoroquinolones or macrolides in reducing mortality (the primary endpoint).

- In addition, post ad hoc analyses found no differences in the type of macrolide (clarithromycin vs. azithromycin) or quinolone used (levofloxacin vs. moxifloxacin). (5)

7. Ceftazidime-Avibactam for Carbapenemase–Producing *K. pneumoniae* Infections

- A retrospective observational study was done to investigate the use of Ceftazidime-avibactam (CAZ-AVI) in managing infections caused by Klebsiella pneumoniae carbapenemase-producing *K.pneumoniae* (KPC-Kp) strains. All received treatment with CAZ-AVI alone or with ≥1 other active antimicrobials.

- The all-cause mortality rate 30 days after infection onset was 25% (146/577). There was no significant difference in mortality between patients managed with CAZ-AVI alone and those treated with combination regimens.

- In multivariate analysis, mortality was positively associated with a presence at infection onset of septic shock (P =.002), neutropenia (P <.001), or an INCREMENT score ≥8 (P =.01); with lower respiratory tract infection (LRTI) (P =.04); and with CAZ-AVI dose adjustment for renal function (P =.01).

- Mortality was negatively associated with CAZ-AVI administration by prolonged infusion (P =.006).

- CAZ-AVI is an essential option for treating severe KPC-Kp infections, even when used alone. (6)

References

1. Wunderink RG, Matsunaga Y, Ariyasu M, Clevenbergh P, Echols R, Kaye KS, et al. Cefiderocol versus high-dose, extended-infusion meropenem for the treatment of Gram-negative nosocomial pneumonia (APEKS-NP): a randomised, double-blind, phase 3, non-inferiority trial. Lancet Infect Dis. 2021 Feb;21(2):213–25.

2. Bassetti M, Echols R, Matsunaga Y, Ariyasu M, Doi Y, Ferrer R, et al. Efficacy and safety of cefiderocol or best available therapy for the treatment of serious infections caused by carbapenem-resistant Gram-negative bacteria (CREDIBLE-CR): a randomised, open-label, multicentre, pathogen-focused, descriptive, phase 3 trial. Lancet Infect Dis. 2021 Feb;21(2):226–40.

3. Alexander E, Goldberg L, Das AF, Moran GJ, Sandrock C, Gasink LB, et al. Oral Lefamulin vs Moxifloxacin for Early Clinical Response Among Adults With Community-Acquired Bacterial Pneumonia: The LEAP 2 Randomized Clinical Trial. JAMA. 2019 Nov;322(17):1661–71.

4. François B, Cariou A, Clere-Jehl R, Dequin P-F, Renon-Carron F, Daix T, et al. Prevention of Early Ventilator-Associated Pneumonia after Cardiac Arrest. N Engl J Med [Internet]. 2019 Nov 6;381(19):1831–42. Available from: https://doi.org/10.1056/NEJMoa1812379

5. Jasper AS, Musuuza JS, Tischendorf JS, Stevens VW, Gamage SD, Osman F, et al. Are Fluoroquinolones or Macrolides Better for Treating Legionella Pneumonia? A Systematic Review and Meta-analysis. Clin Infect Dis an Off Publ Infect Dis Soc Am. 2021 Jun;72(11):1979–89.

6. Tumbarello M, Raffaelli F, Giannella M, Mantengoli E, Mularoni A, Venditti M, et al. Ceftazidime-Avibactam Use for Klebsiella pneumoniae Carbapenemase-Producing K. pneumoniae Infections: A Retrospective Observational Multicenter Study. Clin Infect Dis an Off Publ Infect Dis Soc Am. 2021 Nov;73(9):1664–76.

Acute Severe Asthma

Introduction

Asthma is a major non-communicable disease (NCD), affecting 1-18% of the children and adult population in different countries across the world.[1] It is characterized by narrowing and inflammation of the small airways in the lungs which leads to variable symptoms, which can be any combination of cough, wheeze, shortness of breath and chest tightness. It is a long-term condition which has a substantial impact on quality of life as it is often under-diagnosed and under-treated, particularly in low- and middle-income countries.

Exacerbation of asthma is an emergency condition which requires timely intervention and if untreated can lead to life threatening situations and death. It may exacerbate preexisting asthma or as a first presentation of asthma. It usually presents as a change in patient's symptoms and lung functions from the usual status.

Epidemiology

Globally, asthma is ranked as 16th leading cause of years lived with disability and 28th leading cause of burden of disease, as measured by disability-adjusted life years. Asthma affected an estimated 262 million people in 2019 and caused 461000 deaths.[2] Currently around 300 million people have asthma worldwide, and by 2025 a further 100 million people may be affected.[3] There is a large geographical variation in asthma prevalence, severity, and mortality. While prevalence of asthma is higher in high income countries, asthma-related mortality occurs mostly in low middle income countries.[4] In adults, it is more common in females (9.8%) than men (6.1%). However, in children, the occurrence is higher in boys (8.3%) than in girls (6.7%), with the highest incidence in teenagers.[5-7]

The current evidence suggests that asthma is a complex multifactorial disorder and its etiology is increasingly attributed to interactions between genetic susceptibility, host factors, and environmental exposures. These include environmental factors (air pollution, pollens, mold and other aeroallergens, and weather), host factors (obesity, nutritional factors, infections, allergic sensitization), and genetic factors (asthma susceptibility loci on genes). Although underlying mechanisms of asthma are not yet fully understood, they may include airway inflammation, control of airway tone and reactivity.[8] It is also now recognized that asthma may not be a single disease but a group of heterogeneous phenotypes with different etiologies demographic, clinical or pathological characteristics and prognoses.[8] Some of the common phenotypes are[9]:

Allergic asthma: mostly commence in childhood and is associated with past and /or family history of allergic disease such as eczema, allergic rhinitis, or food or drug allergy. Sputum examination usually reveals eosinophilic airway inflammation and usually respond well to inhaled corticosteroids.

Non allergic asthma: is not associated with allergy and usually less responsive to inhaled corticosteroids. Sputum examination of patients reveals paucigranulocytic picture (neutrophilic, eosinophilic or contain only a few inflammatory cells).

Adult-onset asthma: usually appears first time in adult life. These patients often require high doses of inhaled corticosteroids and are relatively refractory to steroid treatment.

Asthma with persistent airflow limitation: these long-standing asthma usually presents with airflow limitation due to airway remodeling that is persistent or incompletely reversible.

Asthma with obesity: some obese patients with asthma have prominent respiratory symptoms and little eosinophilic airway inflammation.

Def/about the disease

According to the GINA guidelines 2021, "Asthma is a heterogeneous disease, usually characterized by chronic airway inflammation. It is defined by the history of respiratory symptoms such as wheeze, shortness of breath, chest tightness and cough that vary over time and in intensity, together with variable expiratory airflow limitation".

Exacerbation of asthma are episodes characterized by a progressive increase in symptoms of shortness of breath, cough, wheezing or chest tightness and progressive decrease in lung function, i.e. they represent a change from the patient's usual status that is sufficient to require a change in treatment.[10]

Pathophysiology

The airway obstruction in asthma is widespread but uneven in its distribution. It is caused by a combination of thick tenacious mucous plugging of the smaller airways, bronchial mucosal inflammation, edema and smooth muscle spasm. The increase in lung volume raises the static trans pulmonary pressure and results in an increased outward radial traction on the airways that attempts to keep them open. The airway obstruction is reflected in falling peak expiratory flow (PEF) and forced expiratory volume in one second (FEV1), whilst the increasing lung volume is recognized clinically and radiologically by a hyper inflated chest and physiologically by a markedly increased residual volume (RV), functional residual capacity (FRC), total lung capacity (TLC), and RV/TLC. The combination of advanced airway obstruction and hyperinflation results in markedly increased work of breathing. The extreme dyspnea experienced by an asthmatic is a reflection of the difficulty experienced in breathing at a high lung volume for prolonged periods of time. The work of breathing during severe attack of asthma increases several times than that done by normal adults at rest.

During the initial phase of a severe exacerbation, the primary presentation is hypoxemia due to poor gas exchange accompanied by hypocapnia due to increased alveolar ventilation induced by hypoxia and anxiety. As the obstruction evolves and exacerbation worsens, the $PaCO_2$ starts to rise leading to hypercapnia. Whilst the incidence of hypercapnia is low, prompt identification is critical because of the frequent need for mechanical ventilation at this stage. Respiratory acidosis and lactic acidosis are also a grave prognosis.

Clinical features

Onset of acute exacerbation of asthma can be dramatic. Patients can present to the emergency department with extreme chest tightness and inability to breath. More often the exacerbation may have been building up over several hours, days or even weeks before the patient is hospitalized. A history of wheeze at night, bad enough to wake the patient up, must always be elicited. Worsening of exertional dyspnea and increasing requirement of inhaled beta-agonist with less relief after each puff, are also pointers to severe attacks.

On examination, the patients are distressed and able to speak in short sentences or words only. They gasp and struggle for breath and each breath being accompanied by loud wheezing and sometimes uncontrollable coughing. They may be unable to lie flat and usually sit upright or leans forward using accessory muscles. Tachypnea >30/mint is a bad prognostic sign. On auscultation of chest most patients have loud, widespread inspiratory and expiratory rhonchi, but the occasional patients with severe asthma has a silent chest with hardly any audible breath sound or rhonchi. A silent chest is another grave prognostic sign and denotes obstruction so severe that is hardly any air flow. Tachycardia is always present and may be worsened by the medication the patient has already taken or received to ward off the attack. The presence of a significant pulsus paradoxus due to lung hyperinflation combined with wide fluctuations in intrathoracic pressure, reflects a severe attack.

Table 1: symptoms and signs of acute exacerbation of asthma

Symptoms	
Wheezing	
Cough	
Chest tightness	
Shortness of Breath	Physical Exam
Tachypnea	
Tachycardia	
Retractions	
Use of accessory respiratory muscles	

Speaking in short sentences or unable to speak	
Sitting upright or leaning forward while sitting, or unable to lie flat	
Expiratory rhonchi	
Decreased breath sound or silent chest	

Investigations

Diagnosis of acute exacerbation of asthma requires objective assessment regarding lung function as the physical examination alone may not indicate the severity of the exacerbation.[11,12]

Measurement of lung function is strongly recommended and if possible, should be done prior to the initiation of treatment. Changes in lung functions (PEF and FEV1) are more reliable indicator of severity of exacerbation while symptoms are a sensitive indicator of onset of exacerbation. Measurement of PEF can establish peak flow variability and quantify asthma severity. A PEF <50% of the predicted or patients best is usually considered as severe exacerbation of asthma. Lung function should be monitored at one hour and until a clear response to treatment has occurred or a plateau is reached.

Oxygen saturation measurement can be conveniently assessed using pulse oximetry. It is especially useful in children as they are unable to perform PEF measurement. In children, oxygen saturation is normally >95%, and saturation <92% is a predictor of the need for hospitalization. Saturation levels <90% in children and adults signal the need for aggressive management. It should be assessed prior to the initiation of oxygen therapy.

Arterial blood gas (ABG) measurements are routinely required. They should be considered for patients with PEF or FEV1 < 50% predicted or for those who do not respond to the initial treatment and are deteriorating. Usual findings in exacerbation are increase in A-a gradient, decrease in PaO_2, increase in $PaCO_2$ and respiratory alkalosis due to tachypnea. Supplemental controlled O_2 should be continued while obtaining ABG sample. During an asthma exacerbation $PaCO_2$ is often below normal (<40 mmHg). Features of fatigue, dizziness and altered mental conditions suggest that $PaCO_2$ may be increasing and airway intervention may be needed. PaO_2 < 60mmHg and normal or increased $PaCO_2$ (especially >45mmHg,) indicate respiratory failure.

Chest x-ray is not routinely recommended and should be considered for patients who are not responding to treatment or are complicating due to suspected cardiopulmonary involvement or pneumothorax. similarly, in children, routine chest x-ray is not recommended unless there are physical signs suggestive of pneumothorax, parenchymal disease or an inhaled foreign body. The usual finding is hyper inflated lungs. A complicating consolidation or collapse secondary to mucous plugging or allergic pulmonary aspergillosis may also be detected.

Table 2: Diagnosis of asthma based on symptoms, signs and change in lung function

Mild to moderate asthma exacerbation
Severe exacerbation
Life threatening asthma exacerbation
Talks in phrases, not agitated, avoid lying flat and prefer sitting
Respiratory rate <30/min, no use of accessory muscle
Heart rate 100-120/min
O_2 saturation @ room air 90-95%
PEF >50% of predicted or personal best
Talks in words, agitated, leaning forward while sitting
Respiratory rate >30/min, active use of accessory muscle
Heart rate >120/min
O_2 saturation @ room air <90%
PEF <50% of predicted or personal best
Alert mental status (confusion, drowsiness)
silent chest (overall decreased breath sounds)
cyanosis may or may not present
pulsus paradoxus may or may not present

Differential diagnosis:

They can be due to upper or lower airway disorders, Acute left ventricular failure (cardiac asthma), pulmonary embolism, and psychiatric disorders. Foreign body obstruction should always be suspected in children presenting for the first episode of asthma in emergency department.

Table 3: Differential diagnosis:

Vocal cord paralysis or spasm
Vocal dysfunction syndrome
Foreign body aspiration
Laryngotracheal mass
angioedema
Airway edema (inhalational injury)
Tracheomalacia
COPD (chronic bronchitis/ bronchiectasis)
Allergic bronchopulmonary mycosis
Sarcoidosis
Cystic fibrosis
Carcinoid syndrome

Bronchiolitis obliterans
Eosinophilic pneumonia
Conversion disorders
Emotional laryngeal wheezing

Management-

Management of asthma should be initiated as soon as the patient arrives to the health care facility because the longer the delay in initiating effective therapy, and the more protracted the attack, the worse the prognosis in acute severe asthma.

Inhaled short acting beta2 agonist (SABA):

Inhaled short acting beta2 agonist (albuterol, levalbuterol) are the mainstay of treatment of acute exacerbation of asthma. It should be administered rapidly and frequently with a pressurized metered dose inhaler (pMDI) for effective and efficient delivery[13,14]. For mild to moderate exacerbation, repeated administration of inhaled SABA (up to 4-10 puffs every 20 min for first hour and then 4-10 puffs every 3-4 hours or more often) is recommended. Once there is improvement in the lung function i.e. PEF >68-80% of the predicted or personal best after inhaled SABA, no further additional doses of SABA are required. Use of (pMDI) is preferred over nebulized SABA as it can generate and disseminate aerosols and potentially contribute to viral infection.

Current evidence does not support use of intravenous beta2 agonist for management of asthma exacerbation.[15] (Evidence A)

Oxygen:

In majority of asthma exacerbations, hypoxemia of varying severity present at the time of visit to the hospital. Controlled low flow oxygen therapy should be started as early as possible either with nasal cannula or with mask. The oxygen should preferably be well humidified to minimize bronchial irritation and drying of secretion. The target for arterial oxygen saturation should be 93-95% in adults and 94-98% for children aged 6-11 years and can also be monitored with pulse oximetry to maintain a saturation of 93-95%. Oxygen therapy should not be withheld if pulse oximetry or ABG monitoring is not available.

Systemic steroids:

Since asthma is an inflammatory airway disease, early administration should be utilized in all but the mildest exacerbations in adults, adolescents and children 6-11 years. Whenever possible, it should be administered within 1 hour of onset of symptoms. Use of systematic corticosteroids is particularly important if

- inhales SABA fail to achieve improvement in symptoms

- patient already taking OCS developed exacerbation
- patients having history of previous exacerbation managed with OCS

Oral steroids are preferred over intravenous steroid although both routs are equally effective. If the patient does not have very severe exacerbation, is not vomiting and can swallow, preferably oral steroids should be given in following doses and to be continued for 5-7 days in adults and 3-5 days in children, however dexamethasone should not be continued beyond 2 days because of the concerns of metabolic effects.

Prednisolone: 40-50 mg in adult (max 60 mg) and 1-2 mg/kg, in children 6-11 years (max 40 mg) oral

Methylprednisolone: 1 to 2 mg/kg (maximum 125 mg/day) IV

Dexamethasone: 0.6 mg/kg (maximum 16 mg/day) by mouth, IM, or IV

Critically ill asthmatic patients, requiring mechanical ventilation should be given intravenous corticosteroids in dose of 200 mg of hydrocortisone every 6-8 hours.????

Inhaled steroids:

High dose inhaled corticosteroids given within the first hour after presentation reduces the need for hospitalization in patients not receiving systemic corticosteroid. In children, administration of ICS in addition to corticosteroids within the first hours of attendance to emergency department might reduce the risk of hospital admission. Even while discharging the patient from emergency department continuing ICS treatment along with other prescription should be done as it significantly reduces the risk of future asthma exacerbations and asthma related death.

Ipratropium bromide:

Ipratropium is a Short-Acting Muscarinic Antagonists (SAMA) which may have an additive effect when combined with SABA. For adults and children with moderate to severe exacerbations, addition of ipratropium bromide, a short acting anticholinergic to SABA is associated with greater improvement in lung function compared to SABA alone. An advantage of ipratropium bromide over beta 2 agonist is that it does not cause tachycardia.

Dose:

Ipratropium bromide nebulizer solution (250 micrograms/mL)

Ipratropium bromide MDI with spacer (18 micrograms/puff) 4 to 8 puffs every 20 minutes as needed for up to 3 hours.

Epinephrine: is not routinely recommended in asthma exacerbation and should be reserved for exacerbations associated with anaphylaxis and angioedema (1 mg/mL (1:1000) solution subcutaneously).

Magnesium Sulphate: is also not recommended for routine use and should be used in adults and children who fail to respond to initial treatment and have persistent hypoxemia or in children whose FEV1 could not improve (>60% of predicted or personal best) despite of treatment in one hour. Standard dose 50 mg/kg (0.2 mmol/kg) IV, with a range of 25 to 75 mg/kg IV (0.1 to 0.3 mmol/kg), given over 20 minutes (up to 2 grams approximately equal to 8 mmol)

Leukotriene receptor antagonists: Limited supportive evidence is available for use of Leukotriene receptor antagonists in acute exacerbation of asthma.

Inhaled corticosteroid and long acting beta2 agonist combination (ICS-LABA): role of this medication in management of acute exacerbation is yet unclear and needs to be studied further.

Antibiotics are not recommended for routine use in acute exacerbation unless there is strong evidence of lung infection.

Helium oxygen therapy: can be considered in patients who do not respond to standard therapy however its role is not proven in routine care.

Sedatives should be strictly avoided in acute exacerbation as they may cause respiratory depression and hypoxemia leading to death.

Table 3: Management of asthma based on severity

Mild to moderate asthma exacerbation
Severe exacerbation
Life threatening asthma exacerbation
Inhaled SABA 4-10 puffs by pMDI + spacer, repeat every 20 min for 1 hour
Controlled low flow O_2 to maintain saturation 93-95% (94-98% in children)
Systemic corticosteroids (oral or IV) Prednisolone 40-50 mag adult and 1-2 mg/kg, max 40 mg in children
Inhaled SABA 4-10 puffs by pMDI + spacer, repeat every 20 min for 1 hour
Ipratropium bromide
Controlled low flow O_2 to maintain saturation 93-95% (94-98% in children)
Systemic corticosteroids (oral or IV) Prednisolone 40-50 mag adult and 1-2 mg/kg, max 40 mg in children
Consider high dose inhaled corticosteroids
Consider IV magnesium
Start inhaled SABA
O_2 therapy via mask or nasal cannula
Prepare for intubation and transfer to ICU for further management

Assessment and hospitalization after initial management:

After initial management, patient should be assessed for improvement in symptoms and lung function one hour after initiation of treatment.

Factors associated with increased likelihood of hospital admission are female sex, older age, use of more than eight beta2 agonist puffs in the previous 24 hours, severity of the exacerbation (e.g. need for resuscitation or rapid medical intervention on arrival, respiratory >22 breaths/min, oxygen saturation <95%, final PEF < 50% predicted), past history of severe exacerbation.

Following lung function criteria can be considered for admission or discharge from emergency department.16,17

If pre-treatment FEV1 or PEF is <25% predicted or personal best, or post treatment FEV1 or PEF is <40% predicted or personal best, hospitalization is recommended.

If post treatment lung function is 40-60% predicted, discharge may be possible after considering the patients risk factors and availability of follow-up care.

If post treatment lung function is >60% predicted or personal best, discharge is recommended after considering risk factors and availability of follow-up care.

Recent advances

As per the current GINA 2021 guidelines1:

Intravenous beta2 agonist are not recommended

Aminophylline and theophylline are not recommended.

Antibiotics are not recommended for routine use unless any infective etiology suspected.

Magnesium Sulphate is also not recommended for routine use and should be reserved for refractory cases.

Only limited evidence supports Leukotriene receptor antagonists

Biologicals- Although, ICS have been the foundation for asthma treatment; inhaled or systemic corticosteroids can be ineffective in many patients with asthma. For patients with steroid-resistant asthma, recent development of a new class of biological agents that target airway type 2 inflammation has provided an opportunity for treatment in the past decade. These biologicals provide a targeted approach for difficult to treat asthma, including monoclonal antibodies against IgE, blockage of IL-4 and IL-13 signaling, and anti-IL-5 and anti-IL-5 receptor therapies.18-20 Currently, there are five biologicals approved for difficult-to-control asthma, targeting IgE (omalizumab), IL-5 (mepolizumab and reslizumab), IL-5Rα (benrali-zumab), and IL-4Rα (dupilumab). These drugs were shown to have steroid-sparing effects and reduce asthma exacerbations, as well as hospital admissions, in randomized control trials.[21] although higher cost of treatment is a major concern.

Arginase inhibitors- Another new approach is the use of arginase inhibitors which lead to an increase in nitric oxide levels, thereby promoting bronchodilation and inhibiting airway inflammation. Currently, these drugs are under development[22].

Allergen-specific immunotherapy (AIT). The role of Allergen-specific immunotherapy in allergic asthma has been largely explored in recent years in experimental research and they are under development.[23]

Role of epithelial cell–derived cytokines (eg, IL-33 or TSLP), kinases (eg, JAK and Pi3K), and the PGD2 (acts as a pro-inflammatory mediator) are also under trial for management of asthma and allergy.[18,24] A comprehensive review by an EAACI task force174 highlighted the complex roles of eicosanoids in asthma and allergy.[25]

Asthma and COVID 19

The currently available data suggest asthma is not a risk factor for the development of severe forms of COVID-19. Yet, COVID-19 can be a severe disease in chronic asthma and COPD patients. More data are required from controlled clinical trials to fully understand the impact of asthma and asthma therapies on the prevalence and the course of COVID-19. Meanwhile, considering the current emergency, asthmatic patients should take all necessary precaution against SARS-CoV-2 infection and should receive the SARS-CoV-2 vaccine. In the present situation, prevention and proper asthma control, including continuation of the background controller treatment, are the most efficacious way to assure the safety of asthma patients.

References

1. Global initiative for asthma. Global strategy for asthma management and prevention, 2021. Available from www.ginasthma.org

2. Global burden of 369 diseases and injuries in 204 countries and territories, 1990-2019: a systematic analysis for the Global Burden of Disease Study 2019. Lancet. 2020;396(10258):1204-22

3. Network GA. The Global Asthma Report, Auckland, New Zealand. (2018).

4. To T, Stanojevic S, Moores G, Gershon AS, Bateman ED, Cruz AA, et al. Global asthma prevalence in adults: findings from the cross-sectional world health survey. BMC Public Health. (2012) 12:5. doi: 10.1186/1471-2458-12-204

5. Centers for Disease Control and Prevention. COVID-NET preliminary data May 30, 2020. 2020. https://gis.cdc.gov/grasp/COVIDNet/COVID19_5.html.

6. Centers for Disease Control and Prevention. National health interview survey. 2018. www.cdc.gov/asthma/nhis/2018/table2-1.htm.

7. American Lung Association. Current asthma demographics. 2021. www.lung.org/research/trends-in-lung-disease/asthma-trends-brief/current-demographics.

8. Eder W, Ege MJ, von Mutius E. The asthma epidemic. N Engl J Med. (2006) 355:2226–35. doi: 10.1056/NEJMra054308

9. Wenzel SE. Asthma phenotypes: the evolution from clinical to molecular approaches. Nature Medicine2012;18:716-25.

10. Reddle HK, Taylor DR, Bateman ED, et al. An official American Thoracic Society/ European Respiratory Society Statement: asthma control and exacerbations: standardizing endpoints for clinical asthma trials and clinical practice. Am J Respir Crit Care Med 2009;180:59-99

11. Shim CS, Willium MH, Jr. Evaluation of severity of asthma: patients versus physicians. Am J Med 1980;68:11-3.

12. Atta JA, Nunes MP, Fonseca-Guedes CH, et al. Patient and physician evaluation of severity of acute asthma exacerbations. Braz J Med Biol Res 2004;37:1321-30

13. Cates CJ, Welsh EJ, Rowe BH. Holding chambers (spacers) versus nebulisers for beta-agonist treatment of acute asthma. Cochrane Database Syst Rev 2013.

14. Selroos O. Dry powder inhalers in acute asthma. Therapeutic Delivery 2014;5:69-81.

15. Trevers AH, Milan SJ, Jones AP, Camargo CA, Jr Rowe BH. Addition of intravenous beta(2)-agonist to inhaled beta(2)-agonists for acute asthma. Cochrane Databas Syst Rev 2012;12:CD010179.

16. Kelly A-M, Kerr D, Powell C. is severity assessment after one hour of treatment better for predicting the need for admission in acute asthma? Respir Med 2004;98:777-81.

17. Wilson MM, Irwin RS, Connolly AE, Linden c, Manno MM. A prospective evaluation of the 1-hour decision point for admission verse discharge in acute asthma. J Intensive Care Med 2003;18:275-85.

18. Seys SF, Quirce S, Agache I, et al. Severe asthma: entering an era of new concepts and emerging therapies: Highlights of the 4th international severe asthma forum, Madrid, 2018. Allergy 2019;74(11):2244–2248

19. Papadopoulos NG, Barnes P, Canonica GW, et al. The evolving algorithm of biological selection in severe asthma. Allergy 2020;75(7):1555–1563.

20. Israel E, Reddel HK. Severe and Difficult-to-Treat Asthma in Adults. N Engl J Med. 2017;377(10):965–976.

21. Fokkens WJ, Lund V, Bachert C, et al. EUFOREA consensus on biologics for CRSwNP with or without asthma. Allergy 2019;74(12):2312–2319

22. Meurs H, Zaagsma J, Maarsingh H, van Duin M. Recent patents in allergy/immunology: use of arginase inhibitors in the treatment of asthma and allergic rhinitis. Allergy 2019;74(6):1206–1208

23. Schmitt J, Wüstenberg E, Küster D, Mücke V, Serup-Hansen N, Tesch F. The moderating role of allergy immunotherapy in asthma progression: Results of a population-based cohort study. Allergy 2020;75(3):596–602

24. Eyerich S, Metz M, Bossios A, Eyerich K. New biological treatments for asthma and skin allergies. Allergy 2020;75(3):546–560

25. Maun HR, Jackman JK, Choy DF, et al. An allosteric anti-tryptase antibody for the treatment of mast cell-mediated severe asthma. Cell 2020;180(2):406

Chronic Obstructive Pulmonary Disease

Introduction:

Chronic obstructive pulmonary disease is one of the top three causes of death.More than 3 million people die of COPD accounting for 6% of all deaths globally.COPD represents an important public health challenge which is preventable and also treatable.

Definition:

COPD is a common preventable and treatable disease that is characterized by persistent respiratory symptoms and airflow limitation that is due to airway and alveolar abnormalities caused by significant exposure to noxious particles or gases and influenced by host factors including abnormal lung development.

Pathogenesis Or Etiology:

COPD is the result of complex interplay of long term cumulative exposure to noxious gases and particles combined with host factors like genetics, airway hyper responsiveness and poor lung growth during childhood.

The risk of developing COPD is due to following factors:

- Tobacco smoking: High prevalence of respiratory symptoms, lung function abnormalities, greater decline of FEV.
- Indoor air pollution: Resulting from burning wood and other biomass fuels used for cooking and heating in poorly vented dwellings.
- Occupational exposures: Organic and inorganic dusts, chemical agents and fumes under appreciated risk factors for COPD.
- Outdoor air pollution: Association between ambient levels of particulate matter and incidence of COPD.
- Genetic factors: severe hereditary deficiency of alpha 1 antitrypsin(AATD) the gene encoding matrix metalloproteinase 12(MMP-12) and Glutathione transferase related to a decline in lung function or risk of COPD.
- Age and sex: Aging and female sex increased risk of COPD.
- Lung growth and development: low birth weight, Respiratory infections in early childhood are potential risks of developing COPD.
- Socio economic status: poverty is consistently associated with airflow obstruction and low socioeconomic status is associated with increased risk of developing COPD.

- Asthma and airway hyperreactivity: Asthma may be a risk factor for development of airflow limitation and COPD..

- Chronic bronchitis: Increase the frequency of total and severe exacerbation.

- Infections: Severe childhood respiratory infections have been associated with reduced lung infection and increased respiratory symptoms in adulthood.

PATHOGENESIS:

Inhalation of cigarette smoke and other noxious particles such as smoke from biomass fuels causes lung inflammation. This chronic inflammatory response may induce parenchymal tissue destruction (resulting in emphysema) and disruption of normal repair and defense mechanisms resulting in small airway fibrosis. These Pathological changes lead to air trapping and progressive airflow limitation. The inflammation observed in the respiratory tract of COPD is a modification of the normal inflammatory response of the respiratory tract to chronic irritants such as cigarette smoke. The mechanisms responsible for inflammatory changes in COPD are Oxidative stress, protease-Antiprotease imbalance, Inflammatory mediators, Peribronchiolar and interstitial fibrosis and telomere shortening. These changes are responsible for pathological changes in COPD.

PATHOPHYSIOLOGY:

AIRWAY LIMITATION & GAS TRAPPING: The Extent of inflammation, fibrosis, and luminal exudates in small airway correlates with reduction in FEV1 and FEV1/FVC ratio. The peripheral airway progressively traps gas during expiration resulting in hyperinflation. Static hyperinflation reduces inspiratory capacity and dynamic hyperinflation during exercise leads to increased dyspnea and limitation of exercise capacity. Hyperinflation develops early in the disease and is the main mechanism for exertional dyspnea.

GAS EXCHANGE ABNORMALITIES: Gas exchange abnormalities leads to hypoxemia and hypercapnia. Gas transfer for O_2 and CO_2 worsens as the disease progresses. reduced ventilation may also be due to reduced ventilatory drive (or) increased dead space ventilation. This may lead to carbon dioxide retention. The abnormalities in alveolar ventilation and reduced pulmonary vascular bed further worsen VA/Q abnormalities.

MUCUS HYPERSECRETION: Mucus hypersecretion leads to productive cough, which is a feature of chronic bronchitis. mucus hypersecretion is due to an increased number of goblet cells and enlarged submucosal glands. It happens because of chronic airway irritation by cigarette smoke and other noxious agents.

PULMONARY HYPERTENSION: Pulmonary hypertension may develop late in the course of COPD and is mainly due to hypoxic vasoconstriction of the small pulmonary arteries leading to structural changes like intimal hyperplasia and smooth muscle hyperplasia/hypertrophy. The loss of pulmonary capillary bed in emphysema may further contribute to increased pressure in pulmonary circulation. Progressive pulmonary hypertension leads to Right ventricular hypertrophy and eventually right heart failure.

DIAGNOSIS:

A clinical diagnosis of COPD should be considered in any patient with dyspnea, chronic cough, sputum production and a history of recurrent lower respiratory tract infections and history of exposure to risk factors for the disease. COPD has a slow progressive course of the disease and may have absence of symptoms with gradual narrowing of airway indices. hence spirometry is required to make the diagnosis.

Key indicators for considering a diagnosis of COPD:

- Dyspnea - progressive overtime characteristically worsen with exercise persistent
- Chronic cough - May be intermittent, may be unproductive recurrent wheeze.
- chronic sputum production - Any pattern of chronic sputum production may indicate COPD or recurrent lower respiratory tract infections.
- history of risk factors - Host factors (genetic factors congenital development abnormalities)
  - Tobacco smoke
  - smoke from home cooking & heating fuels
  - occupational dusts, vapors fumes, gases and other chemicals.
- Family history of COPD (or) childhood factors - low birth weight, childhood respiratory infections.

Consider COPD and perform spirometry if any of these indicators are present in an individual over age 40. These indicators are not diagnostic but presence of multiple key indicators increase the probability of diagnosis of COPD. spirometry is required to establish the diagnosis of COPD.

Clinical Features:

Dyspnea - A cardinal symptom of COPD is a major cause of disability and anxiety Dyspnea is described as a sense of increased effort to breathe, chest heaviness, air hunger or gasping. COPD Patients frequently report dyspnea during exertion. This symptom is more prominent in women.

Cough - Chronic cough is often the first symptom of COPD. Initially cough may be intermittent but slowly progress to be present everyday often throughout the day. chronic cough may be productive (or) unproductive.

Sputum production - COPD patients commonly raise small quantities of tenacious sputum with coughing. Regular production of sputum for 3 to more months in 2 consecutive years is the classical definition of chronic bronchitis. Sputum production can be intermittent with periods of flare up interspersed with periods of remission. Patients producing large volumes of sputum may have underlying bronchiectasis. The presence of purulent sputum reflects an increase in inflammatory mediators and its development may identify onset of bacterial exacerbation.

Wheezing and chest tightness: Wheezing and chest tightness are symptoms that may vary between days and over the course of a single day. audible wheeze may arise at the laryngeal level and need not be associated with auscultation abnormalities in the chest. Wide spread inspiratory or expiratory wheeze can be heard on auscultation.Chest tightness occurs after exertion and it is muscular in nature. It occurs due to isometric contraction of the intercostal muscles. An absence of wheezing or chest tightness does not exclude diagnosis of COPD nor does the presence of these symptoms confirm diagnosis of asthma.

Fatigue: It is a subjective feeling of tiredness or exhaustion. It is one of the most common and distressing symptoms experienced by people with COPD. Fatigue is experienced as a feeling of generalized tiredness or a feeling drained of energy. Fatigue impacts patients ability to perform activities and their quality of life.

Additional features: Syncope during cough occurs due to rapid increase in intrathoracic pressure during prolonged attacks of coughing. Coughing spells may cause rib fractures and may be asymptomatic. Ankle swelling may be the sign of cor-pulmonale. Fatigue, weight loss, muscle loss, and anorexia are common problems seen with patients of severe and very severe COPD

Severity of airflow limitation: A forced expiratory volume in 1 second (FEV)/ Forced vital capacity (FVC) less than 0.70 measured by spirometry is required to make the diagnosis of COPD.

Classification of Airflow limitation severity in COPD (based on post bronchodilator FEV) in patients with FEV/FVC<0.70.

Gold 1	Mild	FEV> 80% PREDICTED
Gold 2	Moderate	50% <= FEV1 <80% PREDICTED
Gold 3	Severe	30% <=FEV1 <50% PREDICTED
Gold 4	Very severe	FEV1 < 30% PREDICTED

These grades can be predictive of an increased frequency of exacerbations as well as an increased risk of death.

Physical examination:

Physical examination is rarely diagnostic of COPD. physical signs of airflow limitation are usually not present until significant impairment of lung function has occurred. In patients with chronic bronchitis findings of chronic respiratory failure and cor pulmonale with air hunger, anxiety may be present and the combination of polycythemia and hypoxemia, Plethoric and cyanotic appearance may be seen.

If acute ventilatory failure is present, the patient's consciousness is clouded and leads to irritability, somnolence and asterixis may be present. chronic ventilatory failure and cor pulmonale leads to peripheral edema and jugular venous distension. The presence of severe bronchopulmonary secretions gives rise to scattered rhonchi and rales especially at lung bases. These patients may have chronic carbon dioxide retention requiring close monitoring of oxygen therapy because of relative dependency of hypoxic drive for ventilation.

In patients with emphysema they are often thin, anxious, alert and oriented dyspneic and tachypneic and use accessory muscles of breathing. They often self administer positive end expiratory pressure (PEEP) by using a pursed lip exhalation pattern to increase intra luminal bronchial pressure and provide internal support for collapsed bronchial walls. Patients usually assume sedentary existence and chronically hunched forward. Gross lung over inflation occurs with low immobile diaphragm and increased antero-posterior diameter of thorax. Percussion of the chest reveals hyper resonance and auscultation demonstrates diminished breath sounds with faint end expiratory rhonchi. Despite air hunger and extensive lung parenchyma destruction patients maintain adequate oxygen saturation and often have near normal ABG levels. Heart is small and hypodynamic and blood pressure is usually low.

Differential Diagnosis:

The differential diagnosis of actually dyspneic and hypoxic patients is broad. The differential diagnosis and the suggestive features are summarized below,

Diagnosis	Suggestive features
COPD	Onset in mid life symptoms slowly progressive History of tobacco smoking or exposure to other types of smoke.
Asthma	Onset early in life (often childhood) Symptoms vary widely from day to day Symptoms worse at night/early morning allergy, rhinitis and eczema also present Obesity co existence
Congestive heart failure	C X R shows dilated heart, pulmonary edema, pulmonary function tests indicate volume restriction and not airflow air limitation.
Bronchiectasis	Large volume of purulent sputum Commonly associated with bacterial infection, C X R/CT Shows bronchial dilation and bronchial wall thickening
Tuberculosis	Onset all ages C X R shows lung infiltrates, microbiological confirmation, high local prevalence of tuberculosis.

Obliterative bronchiolitis	Onset at younger age, non smokers May have h/o RA/Acute fume exposure, seen after lung or bone marrow transplantation CT on expiration- hypo dense areas.
Diffuse panbronchiolitis	Predominantly seen in patients of aside descent, most patients are male and non smokers almost all have chronic sinusitis CXR and HRCT chest show diffuse small centrilobular nodular opacities and hyperinflation.

These features tend to be characteristic of the respective disease but not mandatory.

Diagnostic Testing:

The diagnosis of COPD is clinical and based on increase in dyspnea, cough, sputum production that is beyond normal day to day variation. Pulse oximetry helps in identifying hypoxia and helps in monitoring the response to emergency therapy. Arterial blood gases reveal hypoxia, respiratory failure and hypercapnia based on the severity of the disease. Chest radiograph showed hyper inflated lungs decreased vascular markings and a small cardiac silhouette enlarged right ventricle can be seen on the lateral chest film. Spirometry plays a key role in making a diagnosis of COPD, its role is limited in ED as the air flow limitation during acute exacerbation is inaccurate. Sputum examination may not be of true value in the emergency setting. ECG and Cardiac Monitoring shows classic description of P pulmonale (peaked P wave in leads V2, V3 and aVF), low QRS voltage, clockwise rotation and poor R wave progression are interesting correlations of COPD but are insensitive and non-specific. Blood tests may reveal polycythemia and leukocytosis. The measurement of BNP may be useful as a diagnostic adjunct of patients with severe dyspnea. Troponin assay can guide the cause of disproportionate dyspnea in patient of COPD with concomitant cardiac disease

CAUSES OF ACUTE DECOMPENSATION IN PATIENTS WITH COPD

ACUTE EXACERBATIONS -

Infections -

Viral - Rhinovirus, Respiratory Syncytial Virus, CoronaVirus, Influenza virus

Bacterial - Haemophilus influenzae, Streptococcus pneumoniae, Moraxella Catarrhalis, Pseudomonas aeruginosa

Atypical - Chlamydia pneumonia, Legionella

Air pollution - Nitrogen dioxide, Ozone particulate, dust

Other critical events - Pneumothorax, Pulmonary Embolism, Lobar atelectasis, Congestive Heart Failure, Pneumonia, Pulmonary compression (due to Obesity, Ascites, Gastric distention, Pleural effusion)

Trauma - Rib fractures, Pulmonary contusion

Non compliance with prescribed treatment regime

MANAGEMENT -

The three classes of medication often used in Acute exacerbation of COPD are short acting bronchodilators, steroids and antibiotics, along with appropriate oxygenation and ventilation. Depending on the severity of the disease, the general therapeutic guidelines are summarized below.

General therapeutic guidelines for COPD exacerbation -

Life threatening	Moderate (or) Severe	Mild
Address ABC	Oxygen to maintain saturation near 90%	Oxygen to maintain saturation near 90%
Bag valve ventilation Pre oxygenation	Nebulized with Beta-agonist, Anticholinergic	Nebulized Beta agonist / Anticholinergic
Intubation with or without Rapid Sequence Intubation	Noninvasive ventilation if severe	Consider oral or IV corticosteroid
IV Beta agonist, Anticholinergic, IV Corticosteroid, IV Antibiotic	IV Corticosteroid, IV Antibiotics	Consider Oral Antibiotic on discharge

OXYGENATION AND VENTILATION -

All COPD patients win acute respiratory distress require continuous ECG and pulse oximetry monitoring. Patients who are hypoxemic should receive controlled oxygen therapy, with a goal of oxygen saturation of 88% - 92% RA or PaO_2 of above 60mmHg. It is recommended to avoid uncontrolled high flow oxygen in dyspneic COPD patients even in prehospital settings.

The patient in terminal ventilatory failure may be cyanotic, speechless, lethargic or confused and has gasping, ineffective respirations. These patients require immediate endotracheal intubation with mechanical ventilation. Rapid sequence intubation should be performed with a goal of rapid paralysis and unconsciousness. Using Etomidate or Ketamine and Succinylcholine (Rapid acting paralytic) are the appropriate regimen.

Initial ventilatory settings should include a fraction of inspired oxygen FiO_2 OF 100% tidal volume 6-8ml.kg and respiratory rate of 8-10 breaths/minute in an assist control mode with inspiratory flow rate of 80-100 L/min. Sedation and analgesia are indicated to facilitate ventilation. Permissive hypercapnia is essential to the ventilatory treatment of these patients.

Non-invasive ventilation is an effective and accepted alternative to invasive ventilation in many patients with ventilatory failure. BiPAP is highly beneficial in avoiding ventilation by decreasing respiratory rate, work of breathing, improving respiratory acidosis and reducing mortality rates. It also helps in preventing Ventilator Associated Pneumonia and length of stay in the hospital.

PROPOSED INDICATIONS FOR MECHANICAL VENTILATION -
Respiratory Arrest
Worsening level of consciousness despite maximal therapy
Cardiovascular Instability (Shock, Heart Failure)
NIV Fatigue
Severe dyspnea with use of accessory muscles and paradoxical abdominal motion
Severe Tachypnea
Life threatening hypoxia
Severe acidosis and Hypercapnea
Other complications - Metabolic abnormalities, Sepsis, Pneumonia, Pulmonary Embolism, Barotrauma, Massive Pleural Effusion

INDICATIONS AND CONTRAINDICATIONS FOR NIV IN COPD PATIENTS

INDICATIONS	CONTRAINDICATIONS
Moderate to Severe dyspnea, with use of accessory muscles and paradoxical abdominal motion	Respiratory Arrest
Respiratory Rate > 25/min	Cardiovascular instability
Moderate to Severe Acidosis (pH < 7.35)	Uncooperative patient (agitated or severly somnolent)
Hypercapnia - $PaCO_2$ > 45mmHg	Upper airway obstruction
	High aspiration risk
	Recent facial or gastro-esophageal surgery
	Craniofacial trauma
	Fixed nasopharyngeal abnormalities
	Non fitting mask

DRUG THERAPY -

BRONCHODILATORS Although bronchospasm is not the primary inciting events in Acute COPD exacerbation, both short acting Beta agonist and Anticholinergic agents are considered first line agents

Inhaled Albuterol (2.5mg - 5mg) is a short acting, selective Beta 2 receptor agonist of choice. Most of the patients tolerate it safely. Side effects associated with nebulized albuterol are tremors, tachycardia and ventricular ectopy

Anticholinergic block muscarinic receptors and prevent smooth muscle contraction while decreasing the release of secretions from submucosal glands. Ipratropium bromide - a quaternary ammonium compound has been used for nebulization in dose of 0.5mg, repeated up to 3 times successively and every 4th hourly. Caution to be exercised with pre existing arrhythmias and cardiac disease.

Magnesium sulphate causes bronchial smooth muscle relaxation and there by causes bronchodilation. It has synaptic effect when used along with Beta-agonist

Methylxanthines like Aminophylline has controversy for its use as bronchodilators due to the risk of their toxicity

CORTICOSTEROIDS -

The anti-inflammatory effects of steroids provide a strong rationale for their use in patients with COPD. They help in improving dyspnea and decrease the relapse rate of acute exacerbation. Prednisolone 40 mg PO or Methyl prednisolone 1-2mg/kg IV are acceptable initial steroid doses.

It is recommended to use the lowest effective dose and shortest effective duration of therapy to minimize the adverse effects like hyperglycemia, Myopathy and Immunosuppression

ANTIBIOTICS -

Antibiotics are recommended in patients with an increase in sputum purulence, increased dyspnea or increased sputum volume or patients requiring invasive or non invasive ventilation.

Broad spectrum antibiotics like Respiratory fluoroquinolones or Macrolides are preferred. Short course (3-5 days) of antibiotics is preferred over longer course of antibiotics (7-14 days)

OTHER THERAPEUTIC AGENTS -

Heliox - Helium-oxygen mixture decreases the work of breathing and improve airflow by virtue of their low density

Respiratory stimulants - Doxapram works by stimulating chemoreceptors in the carotid bodies, stimulating the brain stem respiratory center

PREVENTION OF COPD EXACERBATIONS -

Roflumilast, a selective phosphodiesterase-4-inhibitor may be of benefit in the outpatient setting to prevent exacerbations

Macrolide antibiotics - Erythromycin and Azithromycin exhibit immunomodulatory and anti inflammatory properties in addition to their antibiotic effect

FUTURE THERAPIES FOR COPD EXACERBATION -

Bedoradrine - is a highly selective Beta adrenergic agent for management of exacerbations. This is in phase II trial and not yet recommended for routine therapy till further studies are completed

Disposition:

Mild COPD and Moderate COPD patients after being stabilized in the Ed can be discharged home safely. Severe and Life threatening COPD patients and those requiring advanced airway or Non invasive ventilation are required to admit as in patients for further management.

GUIDELINES FOR ADMISSION OF PATIENT WITH COPD -

- Significant worsening of symptoms from baseline
- Inadequate response of symptoms to ED management
- Significant comorbid condition (Pneumonia, Heart Failure)
- Worsening hypoxia or hypercarbia
- Inability to cope at home or insufficient home resources

SUMMARY:

- Acute Exacerbation of COPD is defined as worsening of patient respiratory symptoms that is beyond normal day-to day variations requiring a change in medication.

- Consider other life-threatening diagnoses in the acute exacerbation of COPD such as acute heart failure, pulmonary thromboembolism, pneumothorax or lung malignancy

- The most common dysrhythmias associated with COPD are atrial fibrillation and multi focal atrial tachycardia.

- The most important factor in the decision to intubate is the patient's clinical status and not arterial blood gas measurement.

- The three classes of medication used in the treatment of acute COPD exacerbations are bronchodilators, steroids and antibiotics.

- Currently there is no role for methylxanthines, heliox, or respiratory stimulants in the management of COPD in the emergency department

Pulmonary Thromboembolism in Non Covid Patients

Pulmonary embolism (PE) refers to obstruction of the pulmonary artery or one of its branches by material (eg, thrombus, tumor, air, or fat) that originated elsewhere in the body. The diagnosis of PE is challenging as the clinical presentation is variable and nonspecific. The ED physicians should keep a high degree of suspicion and get the workup done for PE so that it gets diagnosed early and there is no delay in initiation of treatment.

The incidence of PE is dependent on -

Increased	Reduced
D dimers	Use of statins
CTPA	Regular exercise
Females above age of 75 years	Low BMI
Male sex	

The special population with higher incidence of VTE and PE are-

1	Patients with malignancy
2	pregnancy
3	stroke
4	Hospitalized critically ill patients
5	Nephrotic syndrome
6	Acute traumatic spinal cord injury
7	Total joint replacement
8	Inherited thrombotic disorders

Pathophysiology:

Virchow's triad- venous stasis, endothelial injury and hypercoagulable state.

Risk factors-

Genetic		Factor V leiden, prothrombin gene mutation
Acquired	provoking	Recent trauma or surgery, immobilization, initiation of hormonal therapy, active cancer
	non provoking	Obesity, heavy cigarette smoking

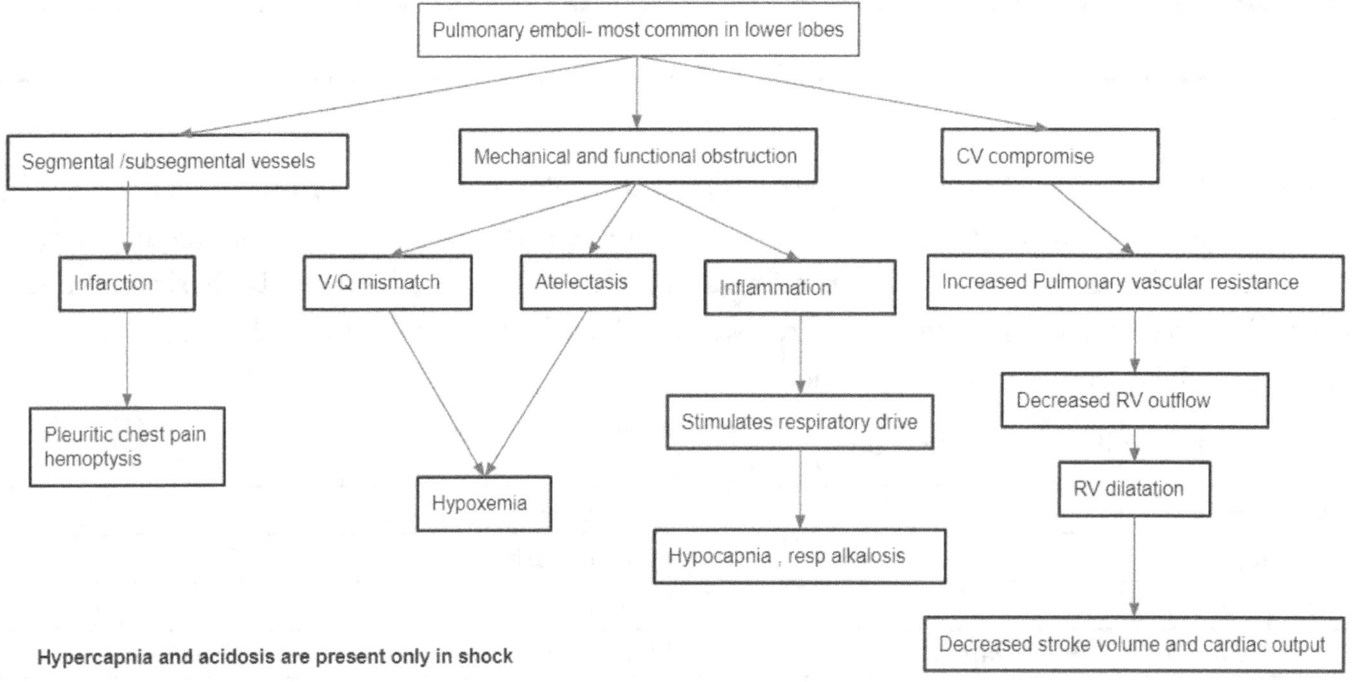

There are many ways of classifying PE.

1	Temporal pattern of presentation	Acute – when symptoms develop immediately after obstruction of pulmonary vessels.
		Subacute – Some patients also present subacutely within days or weeks following the initial event.
		Chronic – Patients slowly develop symptoms of pulmonary hypertension over many years
2	Hemodynamic stability	Hemodynamically unstable PE is that which results in hypotension (SBP <90 mmHg or a drop in SBP of ≥40 mmHg from baseline for a period >15 minutes or hypotension that requires vasopressors or inotropic support and is not explained by other causes such as sepsis, arrhythmia, left ventricular dysfunction from acute myocardial ischemia or infarction, or hypovolemia).
		Hemodynamically stable PE is called "submassive" or "intermediate-risk" PE if there is associated right ventricular strain, or "low-risk" PE if there is no evidence of right ventricular strain.
3	The anatomic location (saddle, lobar, segmental, subsegmental).	Saddle PE (3-6%) lodges at the bifurcation of the main pulmonary artery, often extending into the right and left main pulmonary arteries - mortality 5%
		Most PE move beyond the bifurcation of the main pulmonary artery to lodge distally in the main lobar, segmental, or subsegmental branches of a pulmonary artery
		Clot that is "in transit" through the heart is often classified as a form of PE, even though the thrombus has not yet lodged in a pulmonary artery - mortality 40%

4	The presence or absence of symptoms (symptomatic or asymptomatic)	Symptomatic PE refers to the presence of symptoms that usually leads to the radiologic confirmation of PE, whereas asymptomatic PE refers to the incidental finding of PE on imaging (eg, contrast-enhanced computed tomography performed for another reason) in a patient without symptoms.

Proximal veins Iliac, femoral and popliteal are the common sources for PE. Embolization is less common if DVT is seen in renal and upper extremity veins.

Clinical presentation: ranges from no symptoms to shock or sudden death. The most common symptoms are dyspnea, chest pain (mostly pleuritic but not always), cough and symptoms of DVT. The unusual symptoms are hemoptysis whereas shock, syncope and arrhythmias are indicators of severe PE.

Wells criteria for PE-

1	Clinical symptoms of DVT(leg swelling, pain with palpation)	3
2	Other diagnosis less likely than PE	3
3	HR >100	1.5
4	Immobilization ≥ 3 days or surgery in last one month	1.5
5	Previous DVT/PE	1.5
6	Hemoptysis	1
7	Malignancy	1

TOTAL SCORE-

TRADITIONAL WELLS		MODIFIED WELLS	
LOW PROBABILITY OF PE	<2	PE LIKELY	>4
MODERATE	2-6	PE UNLIKELY	≤ 4
HIGH	>6		

Initial resuscitation and stabilization-

1. Limited IV fluid therapy asit can further distend RV
2. As much as possible, try to avoid intubation and mechanical ventilation as it can decrease preload further.
3. For patients with Wells score more than 6, start anticoagulation before making a diagnosis.

Algorithms for further workup of patients -

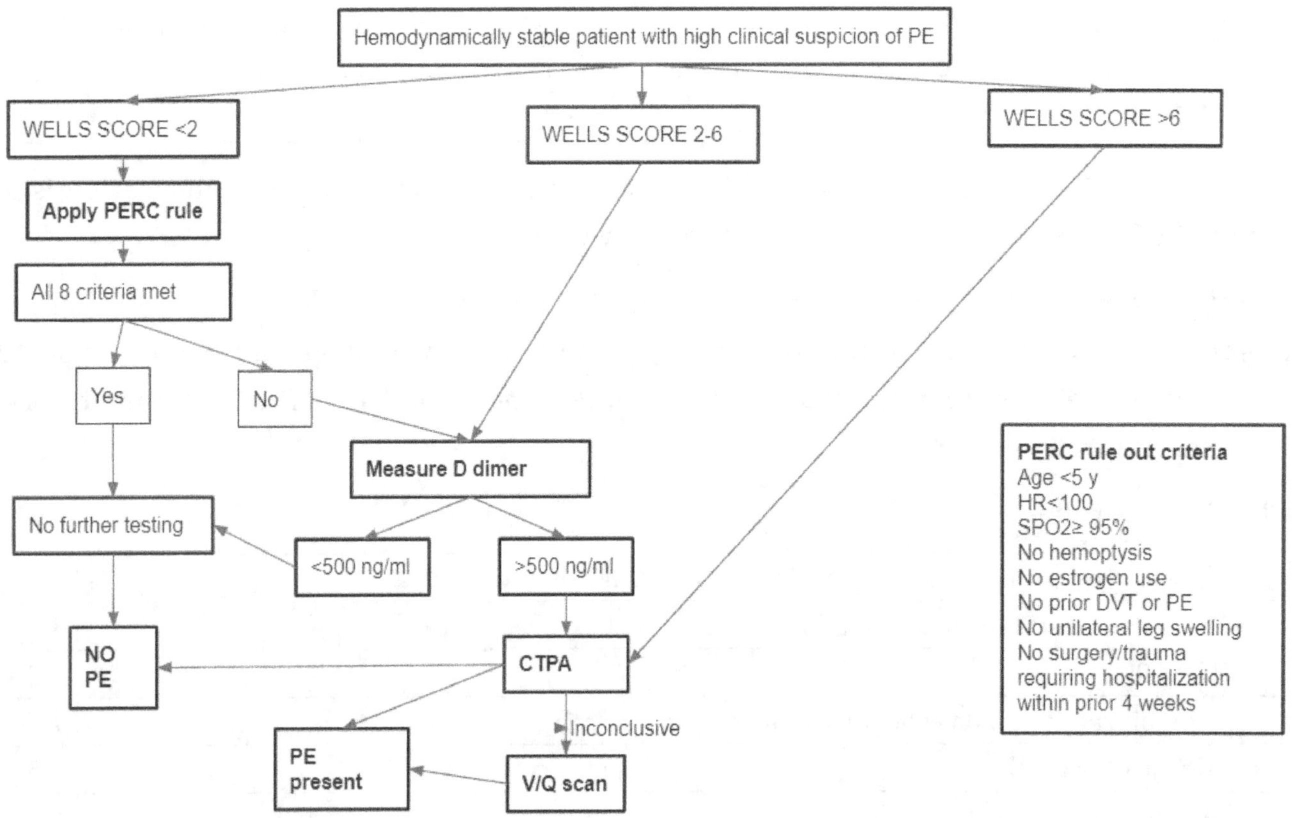

For patients who are hemodynamically unstable, bedside POCUS or venous compression ultrasonography are the modalities of further workup as shifting patients for CTPA can be unsafe.

YEARS algorithm-

1. Hemoptysis
2. PE is the most likely diagnosis
3. Clinical signs of DVT

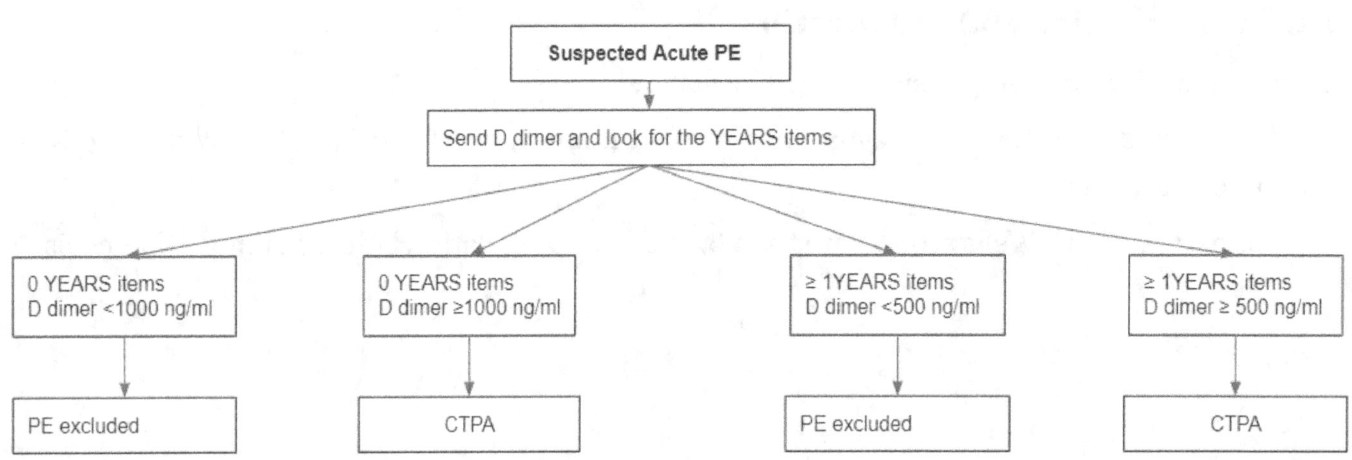

Investigations-

1. CBP- Raised TLC and ESR

2. Liver function tests- Raised lactate, LDH, AST

3. Kidney function tests- serum creatinine to determine safety of contrast studies

4. ABG- Hypoxemia with normal CXR findings. Approx. 18% of PE patients can have a normal ABG. Other abnormalities are widened alveolar-arterial gradients for oxygen, respiratory alkalosis and hypocapnia. Hypercapnia, respiratory, and/or lactic acidosis are uncommon but can be seen in patients with massive PE associated with obstructive shock and respiratory arrest.

5. BNP- limited diagnostic value in patients suspected of having PE. However, elevated BNP or its precursor, N-terminal (NT)-proBNP may be useful prognostically for risk stratification.

6. Troponin- Serum troponin I and T levels are useful prognostically but not diagnostically. As markers of right ventricular dysfunction, troponin levels are elevated in 30-50% of patients who have a moderate to large PE and are associated with clinical deterioration and death after PE. Troponin elevations usually resolve within 40 hours following PE, in contrast to the more prolonged elevation after acute myocardial injury.

7. D dimer- the role is discussed above in the algorithms.

8. ECG- common in patients with suspected PE but are nonspecific. The most common findings are tachycardia and nonspecific ST-segment and T-wave changes (70%). Abnormalities historically considered to be suggestive of PE (S1Q3T3 pattern, right ventricular strain, new incomplete right bundle branch block) are uncommon (less than 10%). Those who have a poor prognosis are atrial arrhythmias (eg, atrial fibrillation), bradycardia (<50 beats per minute) or tachycardia (>100 beats per minute), new right bundle branch block, inferior Q-waves (leads II, III, and aVF), anterior ST-segment changes and T-wave inversion and S1Q3T3 pattern.

9. CXR- Normal is upto 20%of patients. Atelectasis and effusion are non-specific findings. A Hampton's hump and Westermark's sign are rare but, when present, should raise suspicion for PE.

10. CTPA- CTPA is >90% sensitive and specific for the diagnosis of PE especially in the low and intermediate clinical risk groups. The highest sensitivities (≥96 percent) are reported when CTPA is combined with a moderate to high clinical probability assessment for PEA CTPA result may be indeterminate for a number of reasons. The most common include patient motion, large body habitus, beam hardening artefacts from metallic foreign bodies, and suboptimal enhancement of the pulmonary artery usually due to abnormal cardiac output. CTPA may be relatively contraindicated in patients with a history of moderate to severe iodinated contrast allergy or renal insufficiency (eGFR <30 mL/min per 1.73 m2). The approximate effective radiation dose from CTPA is 10 mSv. CT venogram (CTV) of the lower extremities and pelvis

with contrast to evaluate for DVT is not routinely performed concurrently with the CTPA. CTV, when added to CTPA, may marginally improve diagnostic yield. However, the added effective radiation dose from CTV is approximately 6 mSv, thereby significantly increasing the radiation dose over the entire patient population.

Studies-

1. 1. Stals MAM, Takada T, Kraaipoel N, van Es N, Büller HR, Courtney DM, Freund Y, Galipienzo J, Le Gal G, Ghanima W, Huisman MV, Kline JA, Moons KGM, Parpia S, Perrier A, Righini M, Robert-Ebadi H, Roy PM, van Smeden M, Wells PS, de Wit K, Geersing GJ, Klok FA. **Safety and Efficiency of Diagnostic Strategies for Ruling Out Pulmonary Embolism** in Clinically Relevant Patient Subgroups: A Systematic Review and Individual-Patient Data Meta-analysis. Ann Intern Med. 2022;175(2):244. Epub 2021 Dec 14.

   The authors evaluated the safety and efficiency of the Wells and revised Geneva scores combined with fixed and adapted D-dimer thresholds, as well as the YEARS algorithm, for ruling out acute PE in subgroups of age, sex, cancer and previous VTE.in 20 553 patients. Efficiency was defined as the proportion of individuals classified by the strategy as "PE considered excluded" without imaging tests. Across all strategies, efficiency was highest in patients younger than 40 years (47% to 68%) and lowest in patients aged 80 years or older (6.0% to 23%) or patients with cancer (9.6% to 26%). However, efficiency improved considerably in these subgroups when pretest probability-dependent D-dimer thresholds were applied. Predicted failure rates were highest for strategies with adapted D-dimer thresholds, with failure rates varying between 2% and 4% in the predefined patient subgroups. From an efficiency perspective, this individual-patient data meta-analysis supports application of adapted D-dimer thresholds.

2. Freund Y, Chauvin A, Jimenez S, Philippon AL, Curac S, Fémy F, Gorlicki J, Chouihed T, Goulet H, Montassier E, Dumont M, Lozano Polo L, Le Borgne P, Khellaf M, Bouzid D, Raynal PA, Abdessaied N, Laribi S, Guenezan J, Ganansia O, Bloom B, MiróO, Cachanado M, Simon T Effect of a Diagnostic Strategy Using an Elevated and **Age-Adjusted D-Dimer** Threshold on Thromboembolic Events in Emergency Department Patients With Suspected Pulmonary Embolism: A Randomized Clinical Trial.JAMA. 2021;326(21):2141.

   The investigators prospectively validated the safety of a strategy that combines the YEARS rule with the pulmonary embolism rule-out criteria (PERC) rule and an age-adjusted D-dimer threshold.. In the intervention period (726 patients), PE was excluded without chest imaging in patients with no YEARS criteria and a D-dimer level less than 1000 ng/mL and in patients with 1 or more YEARS criteria and a D-dimer level less than the age-adjusted threshold (500 ng/mL if age<50 years or age in years×10 in patients≥50 years). In the control period (688 patients), PE was excluded without chest imaging if the D-dimer level was less than the age-adjusted threshold. PE was diagnosed in the ED in 100 patients (7.1%). At 3 months, VTE was diagnosed in 1 patient in the intervention group vs 5 patients in the control group. Among ED patients with suspected PE, the use of the YEARS rule combined with the age-adjusted D-dimer threshold in PERC-positive patients, compared with a conventional diagnostic strategy, did not result in an inferior rate of thromboembolic events.

3. Prandoni P et al. Prevalence of **Pulmonary Embolism Among Patients Hospitalized for Syncope**. NEJM 20165(16): 1; 37524 – 31.

   It was a multicenter, cross-sectional study from 11 Hospitals in Italy including 560 patients. It was observed that Pulmonary embolism was identified in nearly one of every six patients hospitalized for a first episode of syncope.

4. Piazza G et al. A prospective, Single-Arm, Multicenter Trial of **Ultrasound-Facilitated, Catheter-Directed, Low-Dose Fibrinolysis** for acute Massive and Submassive Pulmonary Embolism: The SEATTLE II Study. JACC 2015; 8(10): 1382 – 92.

   This was a prospective multicenter trial from 22 sites across the United States to evaluate the safety and efficacy of ultrasound-facilitated, catheter-directed, low-dose Fibrinolysis. The patients with proximal PE and Right Ventricle to Left Ventricle Ratio (RV:LV) ≥9 on Chest CT were given initiation of anticoagulation + 24mg of tissue-plasminogen activator (t-PA) at 1mg/hr with single catheter for 24hrs or 1mg/hr/catheter for 12hrs with bilateral catheters. The Modified Miller Index Score was used to assess clot burden seen on CT. This score goes from 0 – 16, with 16 being the highest. The breakdown is that there are 9 segmental branches of the right lung and 7 segmental branches in the left lung totaling 16 segments. For each segment that has a filling defect, one point is assigned. If there is a more proximal filling defect then the number of segmental branches affected distally would be totaled up. For example a filling defect in the right main pulmonary artery would score 9 points. The results indicated decrease in mean RV/LV diameter ratio, mean pulmonary artery systolic pressure and Modified Miller Index Score. Also, compared to systemic thrombolytic reports minimized intracranial hemorrhage in patients with acute massive and submassive PE.

5. Sharifi M et al. Pulseless Electrical Activity in Pulmonary Embolism Treated with Thrombolysis (from the **"PEAPETT" study**. American Journal of Emergency Medicine 2016; 34: 1963 – 1967.

   This was a single center case series including 23 patients with PEA and cardiopulmonary arrest due to confirmed massive PE who received 50mg of tPA as intravenous push over 1 minute. Subsequently, patients were given between 2000 – 5000 Units of heparin as a bolus and then started on an initial maintenance drip of 10U/kg/hr.ROSC occurred in 2 – 15 minutes after tPA administration in all but 1 patient. there were no minor or major bleeding, 2/23 died in the hospital and 20/23 patients (87%) were alive at 22 +/- 3 months of follow-up. the RV/LV ratio and pulmonary artery systolic pressure dropped within the first 48 hours indicating that rapid administration of 50mg of tPA is safe and effective in restoration of spontaneous circulation in PEA due to massive PE leading to enhanced survival and significant reduction in pulmonary artery pressures.

6. Kearon C et al. Diagnosis of Pulmonary Embolism with **D-dimer Adjusted to Clinical Probability.** NEJM 2019; 381(22): 2125-34.

The authors included (Emergency Department patients or outpatient clinics) > 18 years of age with symptoms or signs suggestive of PE to study the role of probability based D-dimer threshold safely for excluding the diagnosis of PE without further imaging. They concluded that in a group of low pre-test probability patients for pulmonary embolism based on a Wells < 4, the D-dimer threshold can be safely set to 1000 ng/ml FEU (500 ng/ml DDU).

Summary- Always keep a high index of suspicion for the diagnosis of PE. Early and interim anticoagulation can save many lives.

Cardiac Emergencies

Contributors-

1. Dr. Rajeshwari Sanjay Vhora
2. Dr. Harshad Dongre
3. Dr. Raj Binda Mishra
4. Dr. Nidhi Kaeley
5. Dr. Shrirang Joshi
6. Dr. Akshay Chipare

Chapters-

1. ACS
2. Acute Heart failure
3. Atrial fibrillation
4. Emergency cardiac care
5. Hypertensive emergency/ urgency
6. Syncope

Acute Coronary Syndromes

Acute coronary syndrome is applied to patients with suspected and confirmed cases of myocardial ischemia or infarction.

It is further classified as

1. STEMI (ST-elevation myocardial infarction)
2. NSTEMI (Non-ST-elevation myocardial infarction)
3. Unstable angina

STEMI and NSTEMI are defined as clinical features characteristics of myocardial infarction along with elevated troponin levels. They present different electrocardiographic findings.

Traditionally, patients with unstable angina present with clinical and electrographic features of myocardial ischemia without raised cardiac biomarkers. However, with the advent of the high sensitivity troponin test, the diagnosis of unstable angina has changed to NSTEMI as the patients with unstable angina have abnormal troponin levels. Hence, the terms unstable angina and NSTEMI are often used indistinguishably.

The 3 clinical characteristics of the acute coronary syndrome are

1. Rest angina, usually more than 20 minutes in duration
2. New-onset angina that limits physical activity
3. Angina, more frequent, longer in duration and occurs with lesser exertion as compared to previous angina

Diagnosis- ECG and cardiac biomarkers have been a primary determinant factor in activation of cath-lab. Hence, causing delay in cath lab activation for NSTEMI patients, who had equally worse outcomes as STEMI patients is no longer accepted. So, Meyer, Weingart and Smith in 2018 suggested a new paradigm namely Occlusion MI (OMI) and Non-Occlusion MI (NOMI). It was defined as:

OMI - A branch of the ACS algorithm representing near or total occlusion with insufficient collateral circulation causing active infarction

NOMI - No occlusion, or sufficient collateral circulation to avoid active infarction (1)

In 2020, DIFFOCULT study had identified that 25-35% of NSTEMI patients had significant coronary occlusion on delayed cardiac catheterisation.(2) The ECGs initially classified as NSTEMI or not fitting the classical STEMI criteria were reviewed by expert cardiologists and were identified to have evidence of at least one major vessel occlusion in electrical distribution. The ECG criteria for OMI include:

1. <u>OMI and STEMI:</u>

Classic STEMI criteria:

- Leads V2 & V3 (age/sex specific)

  - Women: ≥ 1.5 mm
  - Men ≥ 40 years old: ≥ 2.0 mm
  - Men < 40 years old: ≥ 2.5 mm

- Right sided leads V3R & V4R (RV STEMI)

  - Women: ≥ 0.5 mm
  - Men ≥ 30 years old: ≥ 0.5 mm
  - Men < 30 years old: ≥ 1.0 mm

- Posterior leads V7-V9 (Posterior STEMI)

Women: ≥ 0.5 mm

  - Men ≥ 40 years old: ≥ 0.5 mm
  - Men < 40 years old: ≥ 1.0 mm

- ST segment depression ≥ 1.0 mm in six or more surface leads, which may be associated with ST-segment elevation in leads aVR or V1, and hemodynamic compromise, is suggestive of multivessel disease or left main disease
- Modified Sgarbossa criteria in patients with LBBBs or paced rhythms for acute MI(1)

  - Concordant ST segment elevation ≥ 1 mm in any lead
  - Concordant ST segment depression ≥ 1 mm in V1, V2, V3
  - Excessively discordant STE (STE/S wave ratio > 25%)

2. <u>OMI but not STEMI</u>

- ST depression of any amount that is maximal in anterior leads (V1-V4)
- Hyperacute T waves:

  - Straightening of the upslope (initial part) of the T-waves
  - Excessively large T waves relative to the size of the preceding QRS

- Abnormal Q waves

  - Any Q wave in leads V1-V3

- ○ Q waves > 40ms (1 small box) in leads I, II, aVL, aVF, V4-V6
- ○ Q wave MI - abnormal Q waves in at least 2 contiguous leads and > 1 mm in depth

- Reciprocal changes

  - ○ New STD or T-wave inversions in lead aVL can be the first sign of an inferior STEMI
  - ○ "Checkmark sign"- QRS complexes that lead straight into the T-wave with abnormal ST-segment morphology
  - ○ New upright T-wave in V_1 (loss of precordial T-wave balance)
  - ○ Inverted U waves- Usually occurs in lateral leads, associated with LAD or LMCA disease

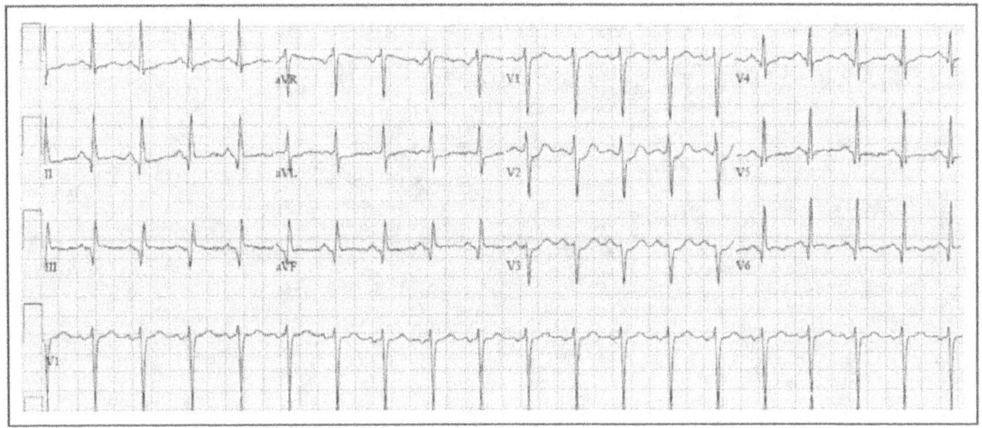

- The Aslanger pattern (3)

  - ○ ST segment elevation in V1 > V2
  - ○ Inferior ST elevation isolated to lead III
  - ○ Concomitant ST depression in any of V4-V6 with a positive/terminally positive T wave

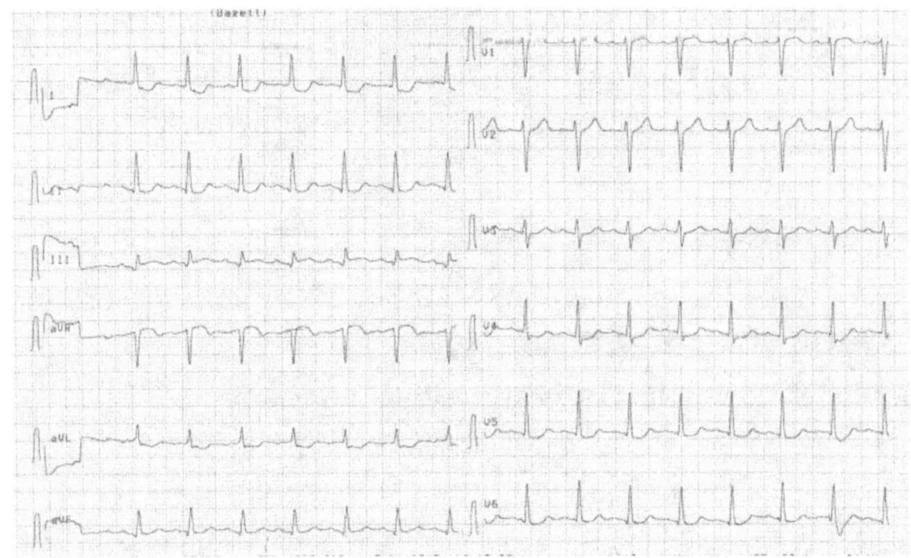

- Bilateral bifascicular bundle branch blocks

    ○ RBBB + LAFB (seen in large anteroseptal infarction)
    ○ RBBB + LPFB

- Subtle lengthening of the QT interval
- Terminal QRS distortion: Absence of S wave or J wave in V2 or V3

Such patients were further subjected to cardiac catheterization and classified into OMI defined as

1. acute TIMI 0–2 flow culprit or
2. TIMI 3 flow culprit with peak troponin T ≥1.0 ng/mL or I ≥10.0 ng/mL

On comparison of the STEMI/NSTEMI vs OMI/NOMI paradigm, OMI/NOMI paradigm was found to have more sensitivity and specificity in detecting acute MI. (4)

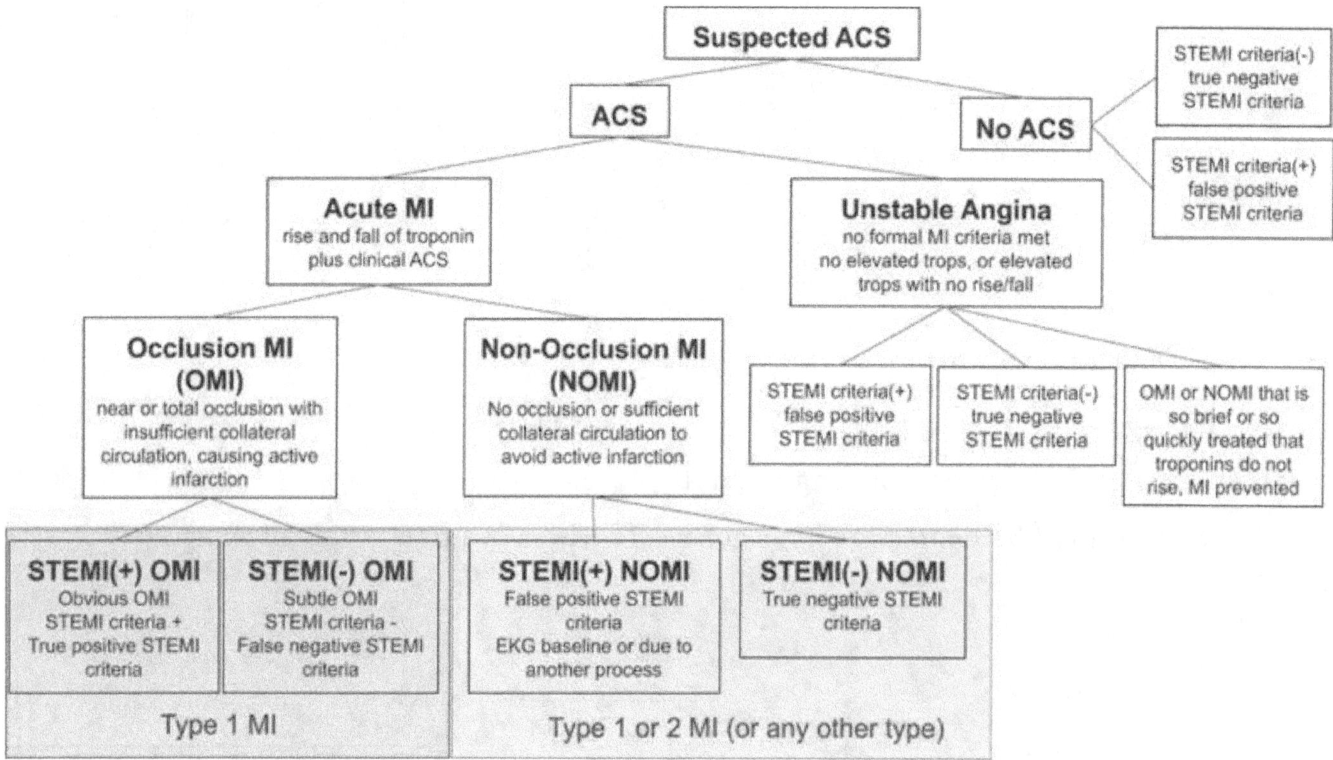

<u>Types of Myocardial infarction</u>

According to the Joint Task force of the European Society of Cardiology Foundation, the American Heart Association, and the World Heart Federation, the clinical classification of myocardial ischemia has been developed in relation to the proximate cause of myocardial ischemia.

	Type	Remark
Type 1	Spontaneous MI	Due to plaque rupture
Type 2	MI secondary to Ischemic imbalance	e.g. Anemia, Thyrotoxicosis , respiratory failure , LVH
Type 3	Sudden cardiac death	Cardiac death with ischemic symptoms (Biomarkers N/A)
Type 4a	PCI related MI $\leq$48hrs	Biomarkers > 5 x the 99th percentile or >20 % rise
Type 4b	Stent thrombosis	Thrombus detected by angio/autopsy with rise in Tn
Type 4c	In-stent restenosis	MI detected by CAG or autopsy
Type 5	CABG related MI	Cardiac biomarkers ↑ > 10x the 99th percentile

Treatment of ACS - updates

Definitive Treatment of acute coronary syndrome focuses on reperfusion of the ischemic area of the muscle along with prevention of further muscle damage. Reperfusion strategies include PCI, fibrinolysis and CABG which are selected on the basis of time since onset of pain and hospital capacity.

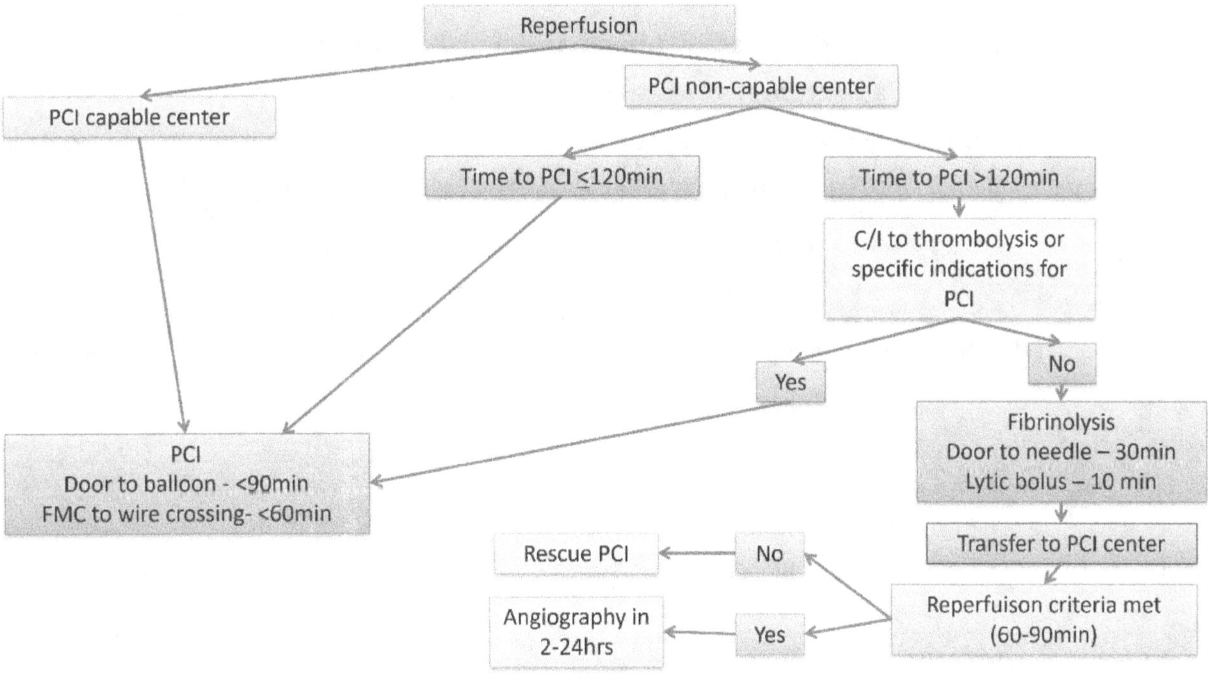

Primary percutaneous coronary intervention should be performed within 120 minutes of medical contact preferably within 90 minutes.

Multiple trials such as DANAMI-2, PRAGUE-2, AIRPAMI, STAT, ATOPAMI-1, STOPAMI-2 have documented evidence of better outcome with primary PCI over fibrinolysis in lowering risk of mortality as well as risk of recurrent myocardial infarction. Additionally, primary PCI is considered a choice over fibrinolysis in patients in whom initial diagnosis is in doubt, increased risk of bleeding exists and those with late presentation that is more than 12 hours in high-risk patients such as those in cardiogenic shock, severe heart failure or pulmonary edema.

<u>Fibrinolysis</u>

Fibrinolytic therapy should be initiated within 10 minutes of diagnosis; it is preferred over primary PCI when PCI is expected to be delayed more than 90 minutes. However, if fibrinolysis is preferred, subsequent angiography and PCI of infarct-related arteries is recommended. This is termed as a pharmaco-invasive strategy. Subsequent angiography and PCI is recommended within 2 -24 hours of fibrinolytic therapy.

In STREAM trial, patients who presented within 3 hrs of chest pain were randomly distributed to the 2 groups- bolus Tenecteplase and primary PCI group, although there was no difference in primary composite endpoints (death, shock, congestive heart failure, reinfarction) time to Reperfusion, was shortened.

<u>Types of PCI</u>

1. <u>Rescue PCI</u>: in patients who develop failed fibrinolysis or threatened re occlusions, rescue PCI is recommended

2. <u>Facilitated PCI</u>: It is defined as use of pharmacological treatment as soon as possible after the onset of STEMI in an attempt to establish only reperfusion followed by transport to an interventional laboratory for emergent mechanical reperfusion in an attempt to maximise the frequency of TIMI 3 flow in the infarct artery and to stabilize the ruptured plaque with PCI.

FIBRINOLYTIC AGENTS	DOSE	FIBRIN SPECIFICITY	RISK OF BLEEDING	PATENCY RATE
Tenecteplase	0.53mg/kg bolus (half dose in >75yr)	++++	++	85%
Reteplase	10U + 10U i.v bolus 30 minutes apart	++	++	84%
Alteplase (t-PA)	15mg i.v. bolus f.b. 50 mg i.v. over 30 min f.b. 35 mg i.v. over 60 min	++	++	73-84%
Streptokinase	1.5 million units i.v. over 30-60 minutes	No	++	60-68%

Routine medical therapy

1. Aspirin- Loading dose of 162- 325 milligram now enteric unquoted to be chewed for better absorption followed by 75 to 81 milligrams. In the case of aspirin, P2Y12 receptor blockers agents, prasugrel or ticagrelor are preferred over clopidogrel.

   Dual antiplatelet therapy has been a major part of emergency department therapy for ACS patients as it decreases the risk of reinfarction and stent thrombosis. Along with Aspirin the options include: Clopidogrel, Ticagrelor and Prasugrel.(5)

As per CLARITY-TIMI-28 trial it is recommended to give clopidogrel in patients younger than 75 years who are planned for Fibrinolytic therapy. TRITON-TIMI 38 trial considers Prasugrel to replace clopidogrel in patients undergoing PCI more than 24 hours after Fibrinolytic therapy. Another trial (TREAT Trial) had compared Ticagrelor and Clopidogrel After Fibrinolytic Therapy in Patients With ST-Elevation Myocardial Infarction where they found both to be equal in terms of major bleeding events. (7)

One recent trial (Intracoronary Stenting and Antithrombotic Regimen: Rapid Early Action for Coronary Treatment (ISAR-REACT) 5) had compared Ticagrelor and Prasugrel in ACS. Patients were given Ticagrelor: Loading dose 180 mg f/b 90 mg PO BID and Prasugrel: Loading dose of 60 mg f/b 10mg PO qD (5mg in patients > 75 years of age or body weight of <60kg). They found that in patients undergoing PCI Prasugrel was superior to Ticagrelor in terms of decreasing incidence of death, myocardial infarction or stroke, however, incidence of major bleeding was same.(6)

2. Nitrates target chest discomfort and hypertension

3. Beta-blockers

4. Anticoagulation in addition to antiplatelet agent: in patients undergoing PCI should receive anticoagulation heparin, bivalirudin) prior to PCI

5. Statins are recommended as early as possible along with a loading dose of aspirin.

6. Morphine use is only recommended in patients with chest discomfort, not relieved with nitrates.

7. Oxygen therapy is not recommended in patients with oxygen saturation more than or equal to 94% without signs of respiratory distress.

    DETO2X-AMI found no added benefit of giving 6 litre per minute supplemental oxygen in terms of primary endpoint such as mortality re-hospitalization and hospitalization for heart failure. Similarly, the 2015, AVOID trial concluded no added benefit of oxygen therapy.

8. Currently, attempts are being made to develop or discover agents that can decrease myocardial damage in patients with initial ischemic insult. One such agent in trials these days is colchicine. However, In COVERT MI trial patients with a first episode of STEMI and occluded culprit coronary artery, high dose colchicine given orally at the time of reperfusion for a short period did not reduce myocardial damage induced by ischaemia reperfusion injury compared with placebo.(8) However, in patients with a recent myocardial infarction, low dose colchicine significantly reduced ischaemic cardiovascular complications. (COLCOT trial)(9)

Acute MI and anemia

Anemia in Acute coronary syndromes have shown worse outcomes. It is not known if transfusing patients with anaemia and AMI ameliorates this risk and often patients with acute coronary syndromes are excluded from trials. REALITY trial comparing liberal(transfusion triggered by Hb≤10g/dL) and restrictive (Transfusion triggered by hemoglobin ≤8g/dL) transfusion strategies found that both had same degree of MACE at 30 days.(10) Myocardial Ischemia and transfusion (MINT) trial is underway with regards to this subject.(11)

<u>Complications of Myocardial infarction</u>

Myocardial infarction can lead to acute LV/RV dysfunction, ventricular free wall rupture, ventricular septal rupture, papillary muscle rupture and ischemic MR, ventricular pseudoaneurysm and arrhythmias all of which can lead to cardiogenic shock. Cardiogenic shock requires intensive cardiac care management and has poor outcomes. Treatment is supportive with inotropes or inodilators. Options include, noradrenaline, dopamine, adrenaline, amrinone, milrinone etc. One comparison study between Dopamine and milrinone (DOREMI trial) in cardiogenic shock has shown both to be equally efficacious. (12)

<u>Updates specific to NSTEMI/USA-</u>

1. Advice Fondaparinux to people with USA/NSTEMI who do not have a high bleeding risk unless they are undergoing immediate CAG.

2. Offer immediate CAG to people with USA/NSTEMI if their clinical condition is unstable.

3. Consider CAG with follow up PCI if indicated within 72 hours of first admission for people with USA/NSTEMI who have an intermediate or high risk of MACE and no contraindications to CAG (active bleeding or comorbidity)

4. Consider CAG with follow up PCI, if indicated for people with USA / NSTEMI who are initially assessed to be at low risk of MACE if ischaemia is subsequently experienced or is demonstrated on ischaemia testing.

5. Offer systematic UFH in cardiac cath lab to patients with USA / NSTEMI who are undergoing PCI whether or not they have received fondaparinux.

6. If stenting is indicated, offer a drug eluting stent to people with USA or NSTEMI undergoing revascularization.

Right heart failure - update

Heart failure is defined as inability of the heart to pump blood effectively. It can either be left heart failure or right heart failure. Acute Right heart failure is usually a feature of obstructive shock caused by either pericardial tamponade, pulmonary embolism or tension pneumothorax which warrant immediate diagnosis and urgent treatment. For a long time, differentiating between acute vs chronic right heart failure was a topic of debate. Point of care ultrasound is an excellent tool that has emerged in recent times. It can accurately diagnose pericardial tamponade and tension pneumothorax bedside. Diagnosis of acute pulmonary embolism requires determining the presence of acute heart strain. The features in echocardiography which favour presence of an acute right heart strain include:

1. <u>RV free wall thickness < 5mm</u>

In 2D Subcostal view, measure RV free wall thickness at Mid-point in End diastole

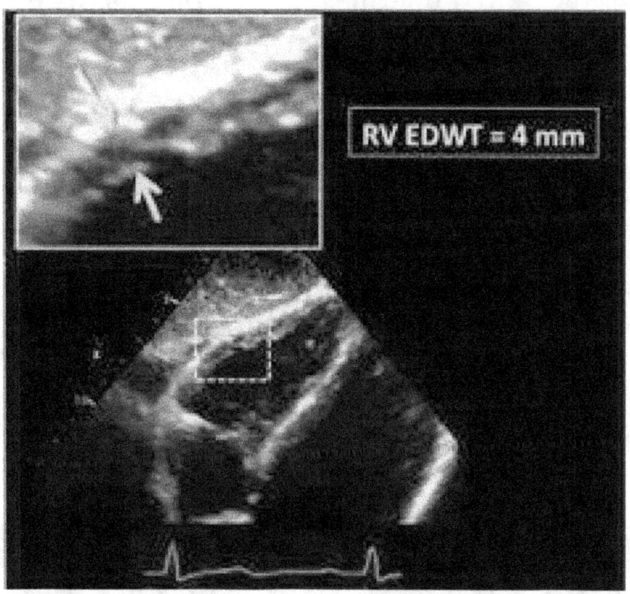

2. <u>Pulmonary artery systolic pressure (PASP) <60mm Hg</u>

In 2D A4C view, find the TR jet and measure the peak velocity (VTR Max) with CW doppler at TV. Estimate the pressure gradient (ΔP) between the right ventricle and the right atrium using the modified Bernoulli equation ($\Delta P = 4VTR\ Max2$). Add ΔP to the RAP to obtain the estimated PASP.

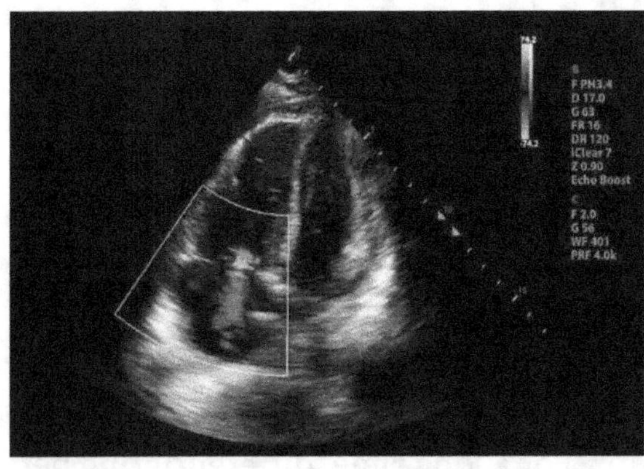 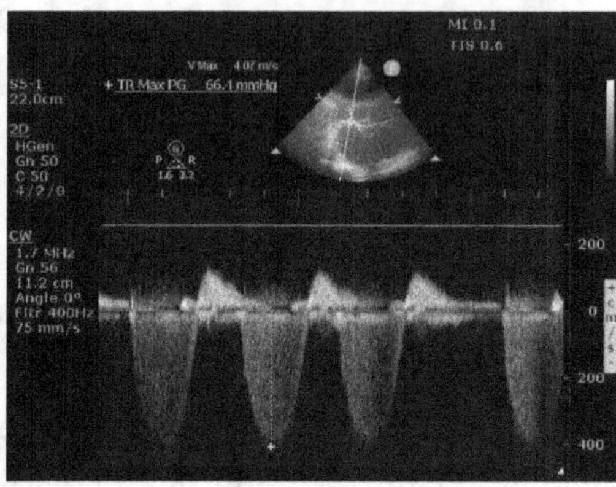

a. RVSP ≈ PASP (assuming no pulmonic stenosis)

b. PASP = ΔP + RAP

c. ΔP = 4V2 = Pressure gradient across tricuspid valve (Modified Bernoulli equation)

d. V = VTR Max = Peak Tricuspid Regurgitant Jet Velocity

e. RAP ≈ CVP

• CVP ≈ IVC diameter/variability

CVP	Normal 0-5(3)mmHg	Intermediate 5-10(8)mmHg	Intermediate 5-10(8)mmHg	High (≥15)mmHg
IVC diameter	≤ 2.1cm	≤ 2.1cm	≥ 2.1cm	≥ 2.1cm
Collapse with sniff	>50%	<50%	>50%	<50%

3. <u>Pulmonic valve Acceleration Time (PAT) <60msec</u>

Obtain PSAX view at MV, fan the probe towards base until RVOT is seen. (This view is characterized by visualization of the tricuspid valve, the pulmonic valve, and the "Mercedes Benz" shaped aortic valve). Place a PW gate centered over the pulmonic valve and toggle to spectral display. To obtain the PAT, measure the time interval from the start of blood flow to its peak velocity.

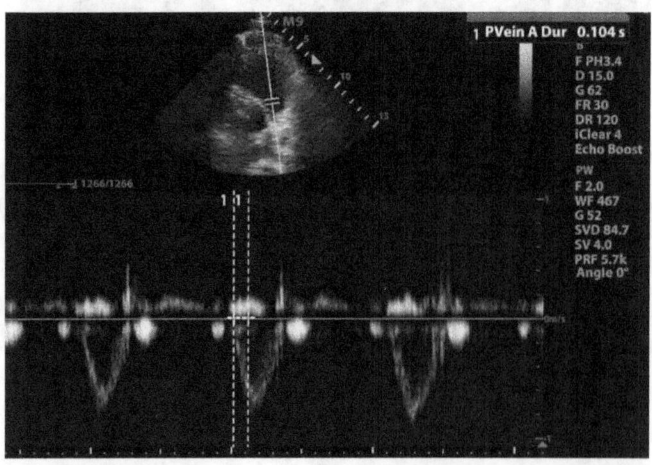

Right ventricular (RV) failure remains a major cause of global morbidity and mortality for patients with advanced heart failure, pulmonary hypertension, or acute myocardial infarction and after major cardiac surgery. Over the past 2 decades, percutaneously delivered acute mechanical circulatory support pumps specifically designed to support RV failure have been introduced into clinical practice. RV acute mechanical circulatory support now represents an important step in the management of RV failure and provides an opportunity to rapidly stabilize patients with cardiogenic shock involving the RV. As experience with RV devices grows, their role as mechanical therapies for RV failure will depend less on the technical ability to place the device and more on improved algorithms for identifying RV failure, patient monitoring, and weaning protocols for both isolated RV failure and biventricular failure.

Left heart failure- updates

Acute left heart failure is defined as an impaired ability of the heart to pump blood effectively either due to structural or due to a functional aetiology. Ischemic heart disease as an aetiology

<u>Terminology</u> – makes the major chunk of heart failure patients.

1. <u>Acute decompensated heart failure</u> - ADHF is a clinical syndrome characterised by new or worsening signs and symptoms of heart failure, which frequently necessitates hospitalisation or a visit to the emergency room.

2. <u>Advanced heart failure</u> - Advanced heart failure (HF) occurs when patients with HF have persistent severe symptoms that interfere with daily life despite receiving the most effective evidence-based medical treatment.

Left heart failure can be classified as –

- Heart failure with preserved ejection fraction (HFpEF) - EF>50%
- Heart failure with mildly reduced ejection fraction (HFmrEF) - EF 40-49%
- Heart failure with reduced ejection fraction HFrEF - EF <40%

Acute decompensated heart failure can present as one of the following clinical or hemodynamic syndrome –

- Mild to moderate ADHF (de novo or as decompensation of chronic HF) with no hypertensive crisis or cardiogenic shock and no or mild to moderate pulmonary edema

  ○ Manifest as progressive dyspnea, abdominal and peripheral congestion.

- Hypertensive ADHF

  ○ Rapid onset of HF with systolic blood pressure >140 mmHg;

- ADHF with severe pulmonary edema
- Cardiogenic shock
    - Acutely decompensated HF with at least one sign of cardiogenic shock (eg, blood pressure <90 mmHg, cutaneous pallor, mental confusion)
- High-output HF
    - Caused by anemia, thyrotoxicosis, advanced liver failure, and skeletal conditions such as Paget disease
- Right HF

Evaluation of acute decompensated heart failure in ED is based on determining the cardiopulmonary instability, presence of respiratory failure or shock, and presence of acute coronary syndrome. Point of care investigations include ECG, NT-proBNP, chest imaging and lung and cardiac ultrasound.

ECG can be diagnostic for acute coronary syndrome showing the ST-T changes. An NT-pro BNP level of more than 400pg/ml is highly suggestive of acute heart failure. Cardiomegaly on chest radiograph along with pleural effusion and pulmonary edema suggest the presence of heart failure. A recent study has shown that Addition of Lung ultrasound to look for B-Lines along with left ventricular function assessment can improve the diagnostic accuracy for ADHF.

Other investigations that can be done include the

- Renal function tests to determine the presence of acute kidney injury,
- Complete blood count,
- Lactic acid levels to look for shock and peripheral perfusion
- Troponin levels to look for an acute myocardial infarction

Treatment goals for patients with acute decompensated heart failure are:

- Improve congestion and low-output symptoms
- Restore normal oxygenation
- Optimize volume status
- Identify etiology
- Identify and address precipitating factors
- Optimize chronic oral therapy
- Minimize side effects
- Identify patients who might benefit from revascularization
- Identify patients who might benefit from device therapy

- Identify risk of thromboembolism and need for anticoagulant therapy
- Educate patients concerning medications and self-management of HF
- Consider and initiate a disease-management program

Primary treatment modality for acute heart failure includes use of diuretics, inotropes or vasodilators and mechanical circulatory support if required.

Supplemental oxygen therapy should be initiated for patients having saturation below 90%. A non-rebreather mask is an appropriate therapy for patients not in respiratory distress. However, those in respiratory distress with a good level of consciousness can be given non-invasive ventilation with BiPAP or CPAP. Those with altered level of consciousness or severe respiratory distress should be managed with invasive ventilation with lung protective strategy.

Loop diuretics (furosemide, torsemide, bumetanide) are most commonly used. Diuretics should be administered to patients with heart failure as they are in a fluid overload state. Diuretics should be administered with careful hemodynamic monitoring, intake output monitoring and electrolyte monitoring. A recent study (DRAIN trial) has found that furosemide infusion had a better outcome over intermittent dosing in patients with acute heart failure.

Vasodilators may be required to correct elevated filling pressures and/or LV afterload in patients with ADHF. The selection of vasodilators depends on the underlying hemodynamics. Nitrates are the most commonly used vasodilators.

Other therapies include

- Sodium restriction - The 2013 ACC/AHA guidelines suggest some degree (eg, <3 g/d) of sodium restriction in patients with symptomatic HF
- Water restriction - Fluid restriction (eg, 1.5 to 2 L/d) may be helpful in patients with refractory HF and hyponatremia, as suggested by the 2013 ACC/AHA guidelines
- In patients admitted with ADHF who are not already anticoagulated and have no contraindications to anticoagulation, prophylaxis against venous thromboembolism (deep vein thrombosis and pulmonary embolism) with low-dose unfractionated heparin or low molecular weight heparin, or fondaparinux, is indicated.
- Vasopressin receptor antagonists have been studied as an adjunct to diuretics and other standard therapies in patients with ADHF to counteract arterial vasoconstriction, hyponatremia, and water retention.

In hypotensive patients the approach to acute HF differs for HF with reduced ejection fraction (HFrEF) and HF with preserved ejection fraction (HFpEF). Inotropic agents like milrinone, dobutamine and dopamine are indicated in patients with reduced ejection fraction. Whereas, vasopressors are indicated in patients with preserved ejection fraction.

The treatment of HFpEF is based on the following general principles: control of systolic and diastolic hypertension, control of heart rate (particularly in patients with atrial fibrillation), control of pulmonary congestion and peripheral edema with diuresis (with caution to avoid hypotension and/ or LV outflow obstruction), and treatment of associated conditions. Evidence-based pharmacologic therapy to reduce morbidity and mortality for patients with chronic HFrEF includes a renin-angiotensin system antagonist, beta blocker, mineralocorticoid receptor antagonist (MRA), sodium-glucose co-transporter 2 (SGLT2) inhibitor, and maintenance diuretic therapy as needed.

<u>Treatment recommendations are:</u>

- For patients with HFrEF, an ACE inhibitor or ARNI or ARB is a mainstay of chronic therapy. Maintenance of oral therapy should be cautiously continued. However, the dose should be decreased, or the drug discontinued if hypotension, worsening renal function, or hyperkalemia is present. Do not initiate the therapy in acutely decompensated heart failure patients.

- Beta blockers reduce mortality when used in the long-term management of patients with HFrEF, but must be used cautiously in patients with decompensated HFrEF because of the potential to worsen acute HF.

- MRA therapy (spironolactone or eplerenone) reduces mortality when included in long-term management of selected patients with systolic HF. These include patients who have New York Heart Association (NYHA) functional class II HF and an LVEF ≤30 percent.

- ACE-I, Beta blockers, MRAs, sacubitril/valsartan have shown to reduce mortality and hospitalisation in HFmrEF patients.

- Ivabradine reduces the risk of hospitalization in patients with chronic HFrEF but has no proven role in acute HF.

- SGLT2 inhibitors are recommended for HFrEF patients, especially in diabetics. (Dapagliflozin, empagliflozin). In general, patients who are already on an SGLT2 inhibitor can continue on that therapy during an episode of acute decompensation. We prefer to initiate SGLT2 inhibitors prior to or shortly after discharge in patients who are not currently taking one.

- Long term anticoagulation to be started in patients having heart failure with atrial fibrillation and CHA2DS2VASc score of ≥1 in men and ≥2 in women.

- Iron deficiency anemia should be treated in symptomatic patients having EF<50% and features of iron deficiency (ferritin<100ng/ml or 100-200 with TSAT<20%) (14)

Atrial Fibrillation

It is characterised by an irregularly irregular ventricular rhythm and absence of distinct P waves. Ischemic heart disease and hypertensive heart disease are the most common causes of AF in developed countries. In developing countries RHD makes its mark.

<u>Hallmark ECG features of AF include:</u>

Atrial rate 300-600bpm

Irregularly irregular rhythm

No isoelectric baseline

No distinct P waves

Fibrillatory "f" waves present

Narrow QRS complex

Ventricular rate:

Slow ventricular response - <60 bpm

Controlled ventricular response – 70 to 110 bpm

Rapid ventricular response - >120 bpm

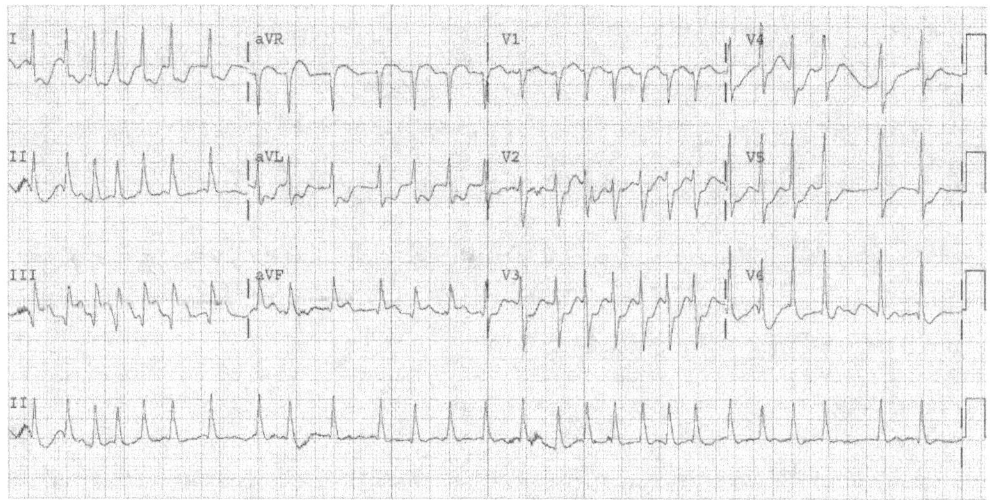

AF is classified as:

1. Paroxysmal AF – Spontaneously terminate within 7 days of onset
2. Persistent AF – Do not terminate spontaneously within 7 days
3. Long standing persistent AF – AF that has lasted for more than 12 months
4. Permanent AF – A persistent AF for which Rhythm control is no longer warranted (15)

Treatment strategies in AF include rate control and rhythm control. Both can be achieved pharmacologically as well as electrically. The decision for rate control vs rhythm control depends on patient characteristics. Although studies have shown that both strategies are equivalent to each other in terms of mortality and morbidity, but a rhythm control strategy is preferred over rate control in acute onset AF in a young patient where long standing AF can cause remodelling in the heart, conversely in a patient with long standing or persistent AF with symptoms, a rate control strategy is good enough to provide symptomatic relief.

Pharmacological strategies and drugs:

> Rate control: CCB(Verapamil, Diltiazem), Beta Blockers(Metoprolol), Digoxin
>
> Rhythm control: Amiodarone, Propafenone, Flecainide (15)

In a trial determining efficacy of magnesium sulfate for rate control (LOMAGHI) Low dose intravenous $MgSo_4$ (4.5g in 100mL of NS) showed a synergistic effect when combined with other AV nodal blockers resulting in improved rate control.(16)

<u>Approach</u>

Atrial fibrillation diagnosis

> Hemodynamically unstable: DC cardioversion
>
> Hemodynamically stable: Calculate CHA2DS2VASc score to detect the risk of thrombosis. If score $\geq$2 give anticoagulation
>
>> Duration of symptoms <48 hrs: Either Pharmacological or Electrical cardioversion with initial anticoagulation
>>
>> Duration of symptoms >48 hrs: TEE to look for clots, either Pharmacological or Electrical cardioversion with initial anticoagulation (15)

Multiple trials have been conducted till date to compare electrical vs pharmacological cardioversion strategies. Recently RAFF2 trial has had shown that both the strategies were equivalent to each other in reverting acute AF of <48hr duration.(17)

<u>Anticoagulation in AF</u>

Anticoagulation options in AF are: Vit K antagonist i.e. warfarin and Novel-oral anticoagulant drugs.

Multiple trials in recent times have shown the efficacy of NOACs over warfarin.

In the ROCKET AF trial, the oral direct Factor Xa inhibitor, rivaroxaban, at dosage of 20mg OD in patients with normal renal function, was equally efficacious as warfarin in prevention of stroke or systemic embolism and resulted in significantly fewer fatal bleeding events and hemorrhagic stroke. (18)

Dabigatran, was compared with warfarin in the RE-LY trial of 18,113 patients with AF at risk for stroke and was found to be quite efficacious with lesser events of major bleeding at a dosage of 150 mg or 110 mg per day in patients with creatinine clearance of >30.(19)

Based on the results of the ARISTOTLE (apixaban vs warfarin) and AVERROES (apixaban vs aspirin) trials, apixaban has been approved for prevention of VTE in patients undergoing major surgery and for stroke prevention in patients with AF at dose of 5mg twice daily, except in <80yrs, >60kg and <1.5mg/dl sr. creatinine individual. Dosage to be given half in these individuals. (20,21)

ENGAGE- TIMI 48 and ELDERCARE-AF compared edoxaban with warfarin in prevention of stroke and systemic embolization, and was found equally efficacious. However, edoxaban is particularly useful in patients with CrCl <95 and older population >80 yrs of age. A dose of 15mg/day was used in the later.(22,23)

AHA regularly updates the ACLS algorithm according to the latest evidence. Two new algorithms namely the opioid associated emergency algorithm and cardiac arrest in pregnancy were the new highlights of AHA 2020 ACLS guidelines. Role of calcium in cardiac arrest was debated for years. The recent ACLS guidelines do not recommend the use of calcium unless specifically indicated. Congruently recent COCA (Calcium in out of hospital cardiac arrest) trial has added another evidence that calcium does not have any role in out of hospital cardiac arrest setting, unless specifically indicated like in hyperkalemia, rather the trial was stopped because of its deleterious effects. (24) The use of Sodium Bicarbonate in cardiac arrest was not associated with improvements in the rates of ROSC or Survival to Discharge.

Vasopressin vs. Epinephrine- Vasopressin may be considered in a cardiac arrest but offers no advantage as a substitute for epinephrine in cardiac arrest (Class 2b; Level of Evidence C-LD). With respect to timing of epinephrine administration during cardiac arrest in a non-shockable rhythm, it is reasonable to give epinephrine as soon as possible.With respect to epinephrine for shockable rhythms, it is reasonable to give epinephrine after initial defibrillation has failed.

POCUS in cardiac arrest needs training for about 6 months to first identify the best cardiac window during an ongoing code. Pre-pause imaging has the potential to decrease time spent in pulse checks. CPR pause length time as close to 10 seconds has the potential to provide better care for our patients. ED physicians should continue to use POCUS to help diagnose, manage, and prognosticate patients presenting in cardiac arrest.

There was an addition of a new neuroprognostication and post cardiac arrest management timeline chart in the 2020 guidelines. Which according to the results of previous TTM1 trial recommends targeted temperature management to 32 to 36 degrees in patients with any level of altered sensorium. The succeeding TTM2 trial has shown no benefit of hypothermia (33 degree) over normothermia (37.5 degree with prevention of hyperthermia) in terms of neurological outcomes. (25)

2021 ERC guidelines currently suggest that emergent coronary angiography should be considered if there is high clinical suspicion of a coronary artery occlusion (e.g. haemodynamic compromise / electrical instability). This was based on the COACT trial.(26) TOMHAWK trial devised that in patients presenting with a suspected cardiac cause of OHCA who are hemodynamically stable, there appears to be no benefit from immediate angiography.(27)

Among patients with refractory out-of-hospital cardiac arrest, the bundle of early intra-arrest transport, ECPR, and invasive assessment and treatment did not significantly improve survival with neurologically favorable outcome at 180 days compared with standard resuscitation. ECPR may have promising results in future studies if the timing and appropriate patients are selected. It will likely require multiple system-wide factors such as a high rate of bystander CPR, a well-developed EMS system and a progressive multidisciplinary team of specialists providing intensive intra-arrest critical care at specialized cardiac centers.

Resuscitation with ECMO plus coronary angiography can improve survival compared to standard ACLS in OHCA with refractory VF or VT. ECMO achieves three goals pertinent to survival of OHCA: reliable normalization of perfusion, provides cardiopulmonary support to facilitate identification and treatment of the most common cause of refractory arrest (severe coronary artery disease with chronic or acute occlusion), becomes a bridge to recovery in ICU when multiorgan injury is sustained during long resuscitation.

Early ECMO-facilitated resuscitation for patients with OHCA and refractory ventricular fibrillation significantly improved survival to hospital discharge and functional status compared with patients receiving standard ACLS resuscitation.(ARREST trial)

In a wide complex tachycardia algorithm for adults, ALS recommends Amiodarone and procainamide as initial antiarrhythmic agents. PROCAMIO trial found an improved safety profile and efficacy of 10 mg/kg IV procainamide over 20 mins when compared with 5mg/kg IV amiodarone over 20 mins in tolerated wide complex tachycardia.0(28)

Among ED cardiac arrest patients, femoral artery Doppler ultrasound was more accurate than manual palpation for detecting any pulse. When using a PSV ≥ 20 cm/s, Doppler ultrasound was also more accurate for detecting a SBP ≥ 60 mmHg.

Hypertensive Urgency and Emergency

Hypertension is a significant modifiable risk factor for cardiovascular disease, stroke, renal disease, and death. Severe asymptomatic hypertension is defined as severely elevated blood pressure (180 mm Hg or more systolic, or 110 mm Hg or more diastolic) without symptoms of acute target organ injury. The short-term risks of acute target organ injury and major adverse cardiovascular events are low in this population, whereas hypertensive emergencies manifest as acute target organ injury requiring immediate hospitalization. Individuals with severe asymptomatic hypertension often have preexisting poorly controlled hypertension and usually can be managed in the outpatient setting. Immediate diagnostic testing rarely alters short-term management, and blood pressure control is best achieved with initiation or adjustment of anti-hypertensive therapy. Aggressive lowering of blood pressure should be avoided, and the use of parenteral medications is not indicated.

Effect of acute blood pressure management on short term adverse effects:

Despite the lack of evidence of an immediate increase in risk of major adverse cardiovascular events, primary care physicians often are hesitant to send patients with severe blood pressure elevations home. As a result, it remains common practice to acutely lower blood pressure using short-acting antihypertensive. Patients with symptoms such as headache, lightheadedness, shortness of breath, epistaxis, or anxiety are more likely to benefit from these agents. When blood pressure improves, long-acting anti-hypertensive therapy should be initiated, restarted, or adjusted and attempts to lower blood pressure acutely may not be necessary. Discharging patients with antihypertensive medications is a reasonable and safe option. (39).

Who should be hospitalized?

Patients with sustained diastolic blood pressure of 130 mm Hg or more should be considered for treatment with short-acting antihypertensive followed by long acting agents. Symptomatic patients with persistent systolic blood pressure elevations exceeding 240 mm Hg or diastolic blood pressure greater than 130 mm Hg despite appropriate rest and treatment with short-acting antihypertensive may benefit from hospitalization (40).

Management of hospitalized patients:

Blood pressure elevations during hospitalization are often exacerbated by pain, anxiety, or acute illness. When these factors have been excluded and the patient remains hypertensive, it is best practice to reinitiate or adjust oral antihypertensive therapy in those with preexisting hypertension. Parenteral medication is not indicated and should be reserved for the management of hypertensive emergencies (43). In patients without previous hypertension, oral antihypertensive therapy can be initiated during the hospitalization with close outpatient follow-up. Although there is often reluctance to discharge patients with systolic blood pressure of more than 180 mm Hg or diastolic blood pressure of more than 100 mm Hg, these values in the ambulatory clinic are appropriately managed in the outpatient setting. A significant benefit for hospitalized patients is the opportunity to recognize severe blood pressure elevations and improve transitional care for the primary care physician (41).

Preferred short acting agents:

1. Alpha blocker: Prazosin 1-2 mg BD
2. ACE inhibitor: captopril 25 mg BD/TDS
3. Beta blocker: Labetolol 100 mg BD
4. CCB: Diltiazem 30 mg QID
5. Centrally acting alpha 2 agonist: clonidine 0.1-0.2mg BD

Preferred longer acting agents:

1. ACE inhibitor: Lisinoprl 10 mg OD or Ramipril 2.5-10 mg OD
2. ARB: Telmisartan 40 mgOD
3. Beta blocker: Atenolol 25-50 mg OD or Metoprolol succinate 25-100 mg OD
4. CCB: Amlodipine 2.5-5 mg OD or Nifedipine 30 mg OD
5. Diuretic: Hydrochlorothiazide 12.5-25 mg OD

In conclusion, current recommendations are to gradually reduce blood pressure over several days to weeks and patients with escalating blood pressure, manifestation of acute target organ injury, or lack of compliance with treatment should be considered for hospital admission.

References

1. Dr. Smith's ECG Blog: The OMI Manifesto [Internet]. [cited 2022 Apr 6]. Available from: http://hqmeded-ecg.blogspot.com/2018/04/the-omi-manifesto.html
2. Aslanger EK, Yıldırımtürk Ö, Şimşek B, Bozbeyoğlu E, Şimşek MA, Yücel Karabay C, et al. DIagnostic accuracy oF electrocardiogram for acute coronary OCClUsion resuLTing in myocardial infarction (DIFOCCULT Study). Int J Cardiol Heart Vasc. 2020 Oct;30:100603.
3. Aslanger E, Yıldırımtürk Ö, Şimşek B, Sungur A, Türer Cabbar A, Bozbeyoğlu E, et al. A new electrocardiographic pattern indicating inferior myocardial infarction. J Electrocardiol. 2020 Aug;61:41–6.

4. Meyers HP, Bracey A, Lee D, Lichtenheld A, Li WJ, Singer DD, et al. Comparison of the ST-Elevation Myocardial Infarction (STEMI) vs. NSTEMI and Occlusion MI (OMI) vs. NOMI Paradigms of Acute MI. J Emerg Med. 2021 Mar;60(3):273–84.

5. 2020 ESC Guidelines for the management of acute coronary syndromes in patients presenting without persistent ST-segment elevation | European Heart Journal | Oxford Academic [Internet]. [cited 2022 Apr 6]. Available from: https://academic.oup.com/eurheartj/article/42/14/1289/5898842

6. Schüpke S, Neumann F-J, Menichelli M, Mayer K, Bernlochner I, Wöhrle J, et al. Ticagrelor or Prasugrel in Patients with Acute Coronary Syndromes. N Engl J Med. 2019 Oct 17;381(16):1524–34.

7. Yancy CW, Harrington RA. The TREAT Trial—Moving ST-Elevation Myocardial Infarction Care Forward, With More to Do. JAMA Cardiol. 2018 May 1;3(5):399–400.

8. Mewton N, Roubille F, Bresson D, Prieur C, Bouleti C, Bochaton T, et al. Effect of Colchicine on Myocardial Injury in Acute Myocardial Infarction. Circulation. 2021 Sep 14;144(11):859–69.

9. Tardif J-C, Kouz S, Waters DD, Bertrand OF, Diaz R, Maggioni AP, et al. Efficacy and Safety of Low-Dose Colchicine after Myocardial Infarction. N Engl J Med. 2019 Dec 26;381(26):2497–505.

10. Ducrocq G, Gonzalez-Juanatey JR, Puymirat E, Lemesle G, Cachanado M, Durand-Zaleski I, et al. Effect of a Restrictive vs Liberal Blood Transfusion Strategy on Major Cardiovascular Events Among Patients With Acute Myocardial Infarction and Anemia: The REALITY Randomized Clinical Trial. JAMA. 2021 Feb 9;325(6):552–60.

11. MD JLC. Myocardial Ischemia and Transfusion [Internet]. clinicaltrials.gov; 2022 Jan [cited 2022 Apr 4]. Report No.: NCT02981407. Available from: https://clinicaltrials.gov/ct2/show/NCT02981407

12. Mathew R, Di Santo P, Jung RG, Marbach JA, Hutson J, Simard T, et al. Milrinone as Compared with Dobutamine in the Treatment of Cardiogenic Shock. N Engl J Med. 2021 Aug 5;385(6):516–25.

13. Differentiating Acute Versus Chronic Right Heart Failure with Bedside Echocardiography [Internet]. [cited 2022 Apr 6]. Available from: http://www.emra.org/emresident/article/bedside-echo/

14. McDonagh TA, Metra M, Adamo M, Gardner RS, Baumbach A, Böhm M, et al. 2021 ESC Guidelines for the diagnosis and treatment of acute and chronic heart failure: Developed by the Task Force for the diagnosis and treatment of acute and chronic heart failure of the European Society of Cardiology (ESC) With the special contribution of the Heart Failure Association (HFA) of the ESC. Eur Heart J. 2021 Sep 21;42(36):3599–726.

15. Hindricks G, Potpara T, Dagres N, Arbelo E, Bax JJ, Blomström-Lundqvist C, et al. 2020 ESC Guidelines for the diagnosis and management of atrial fibrillation developed in collaboration with the European Association for Cardio-Thoracic Surgery (EACTS): The Task Force for the diagnosis and management of atrial fibrillation of the European Society of Cardiology (ESC) Developed with the special contribution of the European Heart Rhythm Association (EHRA) of the ESC. Eur Heart J. 2021 Feb 1;42(5):373–498.

16. Bouida W, Beltaief K, Msolli MA, Azaiez N, Ben Soltane H, Sekma A, et al. Low-dose Magnesium Sulfate Versus High Dose in the Early Management of Rapid Atrial Fibrillation: Randomized Controlled Double-blind Study (LOMAGHI Study). Acad Emerg Med Off J Soc Acad Emerg Med. 2019 Feb;26(2):183–91.

17. Stiell IG, Sivilotti MLA, Taljaard M, Birnie D, Vadeboncoeur A, Hohl CM, et al. Electrical versus pharmacological cardioversion for emergency department patients with acute atrial fibrillation (RAFF2): a partial factorial randomised trial. The Lancet. 2020 Feb 1;395(10221):339–49.

18. Patel MR, Mahaffey KW, Garg J, Pan G, Singer DE, Hacke W, et al. Rivaroxaban versus Warfarin in Nonvalvular Atrial Fibrillation. N Engl J Med. 2011 Sep 8;365(10):883–91.

19. Connolly SJ, Ezekowitz MD, Yusuf S, Eikelboom J, Oldgren J, Parekh A, et al. Dabigatran versus Warfarin in Patients with Atrial Fibrillation. N Engl J Med. 2009 Sep 17;361(12):1139–51.

20. Connolly SJ, Eikelboom J, Joyner C, Diener H-C, Hart R, Golitsyn S, et al. Apixaban in Patients with Atrial Fibrillation. N Engl J Med. 2011 Mar 3;364(9):806–17.

21. Granger CB, Alexander JH, McMurray JJV, Lopes RD, Hylek EM, Hanna M, et al. Apixaban versus Warfarin in Patients with Atrial Fibrillation. N Engl J Med. 2011 Sep 15;365(11):981–92.

22. Giugliano RP, Ruff CT, Braunwald E, Murphy SA, Wiviott SD, Halperin JL, et al. Edoxaban versus Warfarin in Patients with Atrial Fibrillation. N Engl J Med. 2013 Nov 28;369(22):2093–104.

23. Okumura K, Akao M, Yoshida T, Kawata M, Okazaki O, Akashi S, et al. Low-Dose Edoxaban in Very Elderly Patients with Atrial Fibrillation. N Engl J Med. 2020 Oct 29;383(18):1735–45.

24. Vallentin MF, Granfeldt A, Meilandt C, Povlsen AL, Sindberg B, Holmberg MJ, et al. Effect of Intravenous or Intraosseous Calcium vs Saline on Return of Spontaneous Circulation in Adults With Out-of-Hospital Cardiac Arrest: A Randomized Clinical Trial. JAMA. 2021 Dec 14;326(22):2268–76.

25. Dankiewicz J, Cronberg T, Lilja G, Jakobsen JC, Levin H, Ullén S, et al. Hypothermia versus Normothermia after Out-of-Hospital Cardiac Arrest. N Engl J Med. 2021 Jun 17;384(24):2283–94.

26. Olasveengen TM, Semeraro F, Ristagno G, Castren M, Handley A, Kuzovlev A, et al. European Resuscitation Council Guidelines 2021: Basic Life Support. Resuscitation. 2021 Apr;161:98–114.

27. Desch S, Freund A, Akin I, Behnes M, Preusch MR, Zelniker TA, et al. Angiography after Out-of-Hospital Cardiac Arrest without ST-Segment Elevation. N Engl J Med. 2021 Dec 30;385(27):2544–53.

28. Ortiz M, Martín A, Arribas F, Coll-Vinent B, Del Arco C, Peinado R, et al. Randomized comparison of intravenous procainamide vs. intravenous amiodarone for the acute treatment of tolerated wide QRS tachycardia: the PROCAMIO study. Eur Heart J. 2017 May 1;38(17):1329–35.

29. Rock W, Zbidat K, Schwartz N, et al. Pattern of blood pressure response in patients with severe asymptomatic hypertension treated in the emergency department. J Clin Hypertens (Greenwich). 2016; 18(8): 796-800.

30. Effects of treatment on morbidity in hypertension. Results in patients with diastolic blood pressures aver-aging 115 through 129 mm Hg. JAMA. 1967; 202(11): 1028-1034.

31. Axon RN, Garrell R, Pfahl K, et al. Attitudes and practices of resident physicians regarding hypertension in the inpatient setting. J Clin Hypertens (Greenwich). 2010; 12(9): 698-705.

32. Nakprasert P, Musikatavorn K, Rojanasarntikul D, Narajeenron K, Puttaphaisan P, Lumlertgul S. Effect of pre-discharge blood pressure on follow-up outcomes in patients with severe hypertension in the ED. Am J Emerg Med. 2016;34(5):834–839.

33. Adebayo O, Rogers RL. Hypertensive emergencies in the emergency department. Emerg Med Clin North Am. 2015; 33(3):539–551.

Syncope

A symptom that presents with an abrupt, transient, complete loss of consciousness, associated with inability to maintain postural tone, with rapid and spontaneous recovery. The presumed mechanism is cerebral hypoperfusion (1).

Presyncope (near-syncope)

The symptoms before syncope. These symptoms could include extreme lightheadedness; visual sensations, such as "tunnel vision" or "graying out"; and variable degrees of altered consciousness without complete loss of consciousness.

Presyncope could progress to syncope, or it could abort without syncope.

Orthostatic hypotension (OH)

A drop in systolic BP of $\geq$ 20 mm Hg or diastolic BP of $\geq$ 10 mm Hg with assumption of an upright posture (2).

Types of orthostatic hypotension (2,3)

1. Initial (immediate) OH A transient BP decrease within 15 s after standing, with presyncope or syncope.

2. Classic OH A sustained reduction of systolic BP of $\geq$ 20 mm Hg or diastolic BP of $\geq$ 10 mm Hg within 3 min of assuming upright posture.

3. Delayed OH A sustained reduction of systolic BP of $\geq$ 20 mm Hg (or 30 mm Hg in patients with supine hypertension) or diastolic BPof $\geq$ 10 mmHg that takes >3 min of upright posture to develop. The fall in BP is usually gradual until reaching the threshold.

4. Neurogenic OH A subtype of OH that is due to dysfunction of the autonomic nervous system and not solely due to environmental triggers(e.g., dehydration or drugs). Neurogenic OH is due to lesions involving the central or peripheral autonomic nerves.

Cardiac (cardiovascular) syncope (4)

Syncope caused by bradycardia, tachycardia, or hypotension due to low cardiac index, blood flow obstruction, vasodilatation, or acute vascular dissection.

Reflex (neurally mediated) syncope

Syncope due to a reflex that causes vasodilation, bradycardia, or both.

Types of reflex syncope:- (1-4)

A. Vasovagal syncope (VVS) The most common form of reflex syncope mediated by the vasovagal reflex.

1. May occur with upright posture(standing or seated or with exposure to emotional stress, pain, or medical settings;
2. Typically is characterized by diaphoresis, warmth, nausea, and pallor;
3. Is associated with vasodepressor hypotension and/or inappropriate bradycardia; and
4. Is often followed by fatigue. Typical features may be absent in older patients.

VVS is often preceded by identifiable triggers and/or by a characteristic prodrome. The diagnosis is made primarily on the basis of a thorough history, physical examination, and eyewitness observation, if available.

B. Carotid sinus syndrome Reflex syncope associated with carotid sinus hypersensitivity. Carotid sinus hypersensitivity is present when apause ≥3 s and/or a decrease of systolic pressure ≥50 mm Hg occurs upon stimulation of the carotid sinus. It occurs more frequently in older patients. Carotid sinus hypersensitivity can be associated with varying degrees of symptoms.

Carotid sinus syndrome is defined when syncope occurs in the presence of carotid sinus hypersensitivity.

C. Situational syncope Reflex syncope associated with a specific action, such as coughing, laughing, swallowing, micturition, or defecation. These Syncope events are closely associated with specific physical functions.

Postural (orthostatic) tachycardia syndrome (POTS)? (5)

A clinical syndrome usually characterized by all of the following: 1) frequent symptoms that occur with standing (e.g., lightheadedness, palpitations, tremulousness, generalized weakness, blurred vision, exercise intolerance, and fatigue);and 2) an increase in heart rate of ≥30 bpm during a positional change from supine to standing (or ≥40 bpm in those 12–19 y of age); and 3) the absence of OH (>20 mm Hg reduction in systolic BP).

Symptoms associated with POTSinclude those that occur with standing (e.g., lightheadedness, palpitations); those not associated with particular postures (e.g., bloating, nausea, diarrhea, abdominal pain); and those that are systemic (e.g., fatigue, sleep disturbance, migraine headaches). The standing heart rate is often >120 bpm.

Psychogenic pseudosyncope A syndrome of apparent but not true loss of consciousness that may occur in the absence of identifiable cardiac, reflex, neurological, or metabolic causes.

Epidemiology Syncope has many causes and clinical presentations; the incidence depends on the population being evaluated. Studies of syncope report prevalence rates as high as41%, with recurrent syncope occurring in 13.5%. The incidence follows a trimodal distribution in both sexes, with the first episode common around 20, 60, or 80 years of age and the third peak occurring 5 to 7 years earlier in males (6).

The prevalence of syncope as a presenting symptom to the ED ranged from 0.8% to 2.4% in multiple studies in both academic and community settings (7).

Initial Evaluation of Patients with Syncope

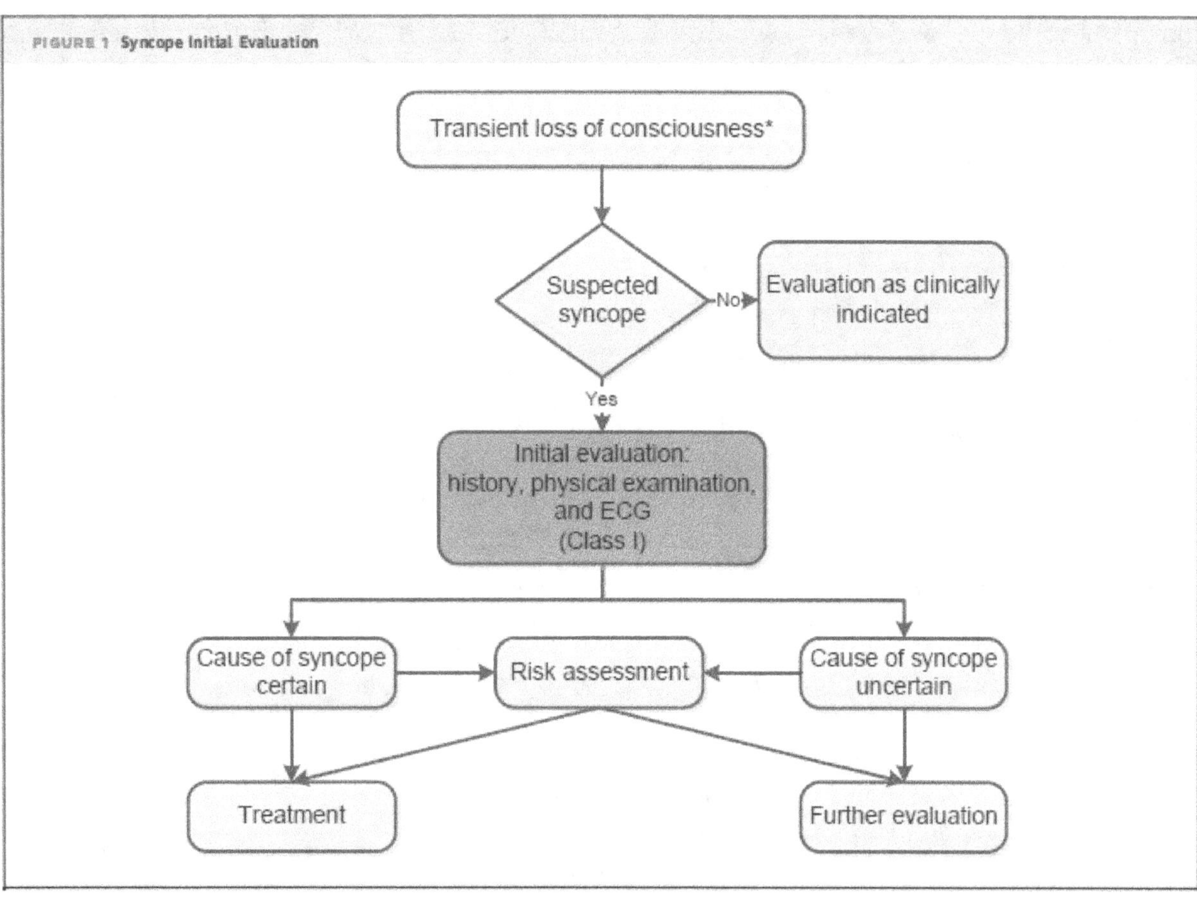

A detailed history and physical examination should be performed in patients with syncope (8). The history should aim to identify the prognosis, diagnosis, reversible or ameliorable factors, comorbidities, medication use, and patient and family needs. Cardiac syncope carries a significantly worse prognosis than does neurally mediated syncope.

The diagnostic history focuses on the situations in which syncope occurs, prodromal symptoms that provide physiological insight, patient's self-report, bystander observations of the event and vital signs, and post-event symptoms. Video recordings are helpful when available. Time relationship to meals and physical activities and duration of the prodrome are helpful in differentiating neurally mediated syncope from cardiac syncope. Comorbidities and medication use are particularly important factors in older patients. A history of past medical conditions should be obtained, particularly with regard to the existence of preexisting cardiovascular disease(8). A family history should be obtained, with particular emphasis on histories of syncope or sudden unexplained death (or drowning).

The physical examination should include determination of orthostatic blood pressure and heart rate changes in lying and sitting positions, on immediate standing, and after 3 minutes of upright posture. Careful attention should be paid to heart rate and rhythm, as well the presence of murmurs, gallops, or rubs that would indicate the presence of structural heart disease. A basic neurological examination should be performed, looking for focal defects or other abnormalities that would suggest need for further neurological evaluation or referral.

More Often Associated With Cardiac Causes of Syncope

- Older age (>60 y)
- Male sex
- Presence of known ischemic heart disease, structural heart disease, previous arrhythmias, or reduced ventricular function
- Brief prodrome, such as palpitations, or sudden loss of consciousness without prodrome
- Syncope during exertion
- Syncope in the supine position
- Low number of syncope episodes (1 or 2)
- Abnormal cardiac examination
- Family history of inheritable conditions or premature SCD (<50 y of age)
- Presence of known congenital heart disease

More Often Associated With Noncardiac Causes of Syncope

- Younger age
- No known cardiac disease
- Syncope only in the standing position
- Positional change from supine or sitting to standing
- Presence of prodrome: nausea, vomiting, feeling warmth
- Presence of specific triggers: dehydration, pain, distressful stimulus, medical environment
- Situational triggers: cough, laugh, micturition, defecation, deglutition
- Frequent recurrence and prolonged history of syncope with similar characteristics

SCD indicates sudden cardiac death.

Role of ECG:-

ECG is widely available and inexpensive and can provide information about the potential and specific cause of the syncopal episode (e.g., bradyarrhythmia with sinus pauses or high-grade conduction block; ventricular tachyarrhythmia). It may demonstrate an underlying arrhythmogenic substrate for syncope or SCD. Subsets of patients with Wolff-Parkinson-White syndrome, Brugada syndrome, long-QT syndrome (LQTS), hypertrophic cardiomyopathy (HCM), or arrhythmogenic right ventricular cardiomyopathy (ARVC) have characteristic ECGfeatures, which can prompt the decision to pursue further evaluation.

Patient disposition after initial evaluation for syncope

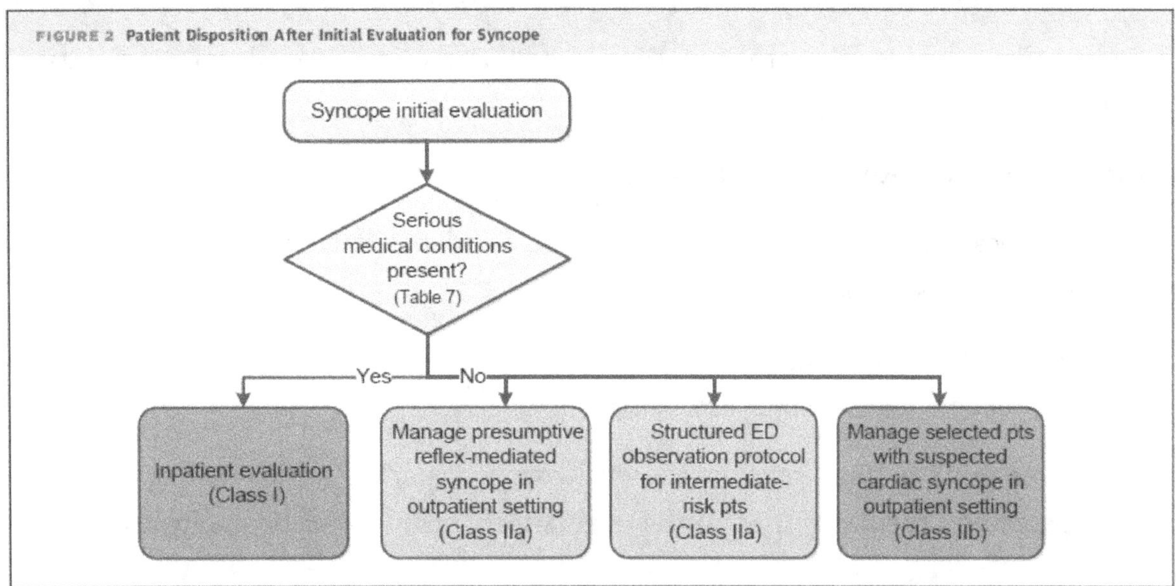

Additional evaluation and diagnosis for syncope

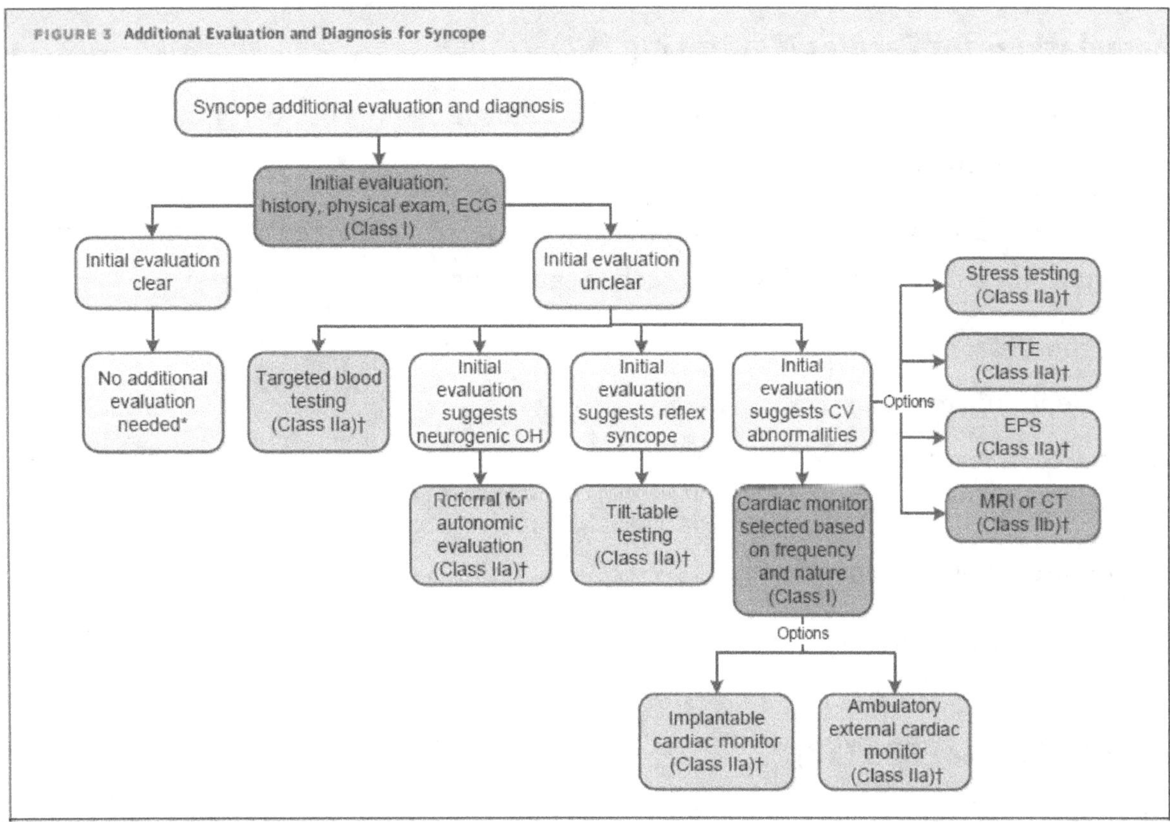

Blood Testing: Recommendations

Targeted blood tests are reasonable in the evaluation of selected patients with syncope identified on the basis of clinical assessment from history, physical examination, and ECG.

Usefulness of brain natriuretic peptide and high-sensitivity troponin measurement is uncertain in patients for whom a cardiac cause of syncope is suspected (9).

Routine and comprehensive laboratory testing is not useful in the evaluation of patients with syncope.(10).

Cardiovascular Testing: Recommendations

Transthoracic echocardiography can be useful in selected patients presenting with syncope if structural heart disease is suspected.

Computed tomography (CT) or magnetic resonance imaging (MRI) may be useful in selected patients presenting with syncope of suspected cardiac etiology.

Routine cardiac imaging is not useful in the evaluation of patients with syncope unless cardiac etiology is suspected on the basis of an initial evaluation, including history, physical examination, or ECG.

Exercise stress testing can be useful to establish the cause of syncope in selected patients who experience syncope or presyncope during exertion (11).

Recommendations for Cardiac Monitoring (12)

The choice of a specific cardiac monitor should be determined on the basis of the frequency and nature of syncope events.

To evaluate selected ambulatory patients with syncope of suspected arrhythmic etiology, the following external cardiac monitoring approaches can be useful:

1. Holter monitor
2. Transtelephonic monitor
3. External loop recorder
4. Patch recorder
5. Mobile cardiac outpatient telemetry

To evaluate selected ambulatory patients with syncope of suspected arrhythmic etiology, an ICM can be useful

Recommendations for EPS (13)

EPS can be useful for evaluation of selected patients with syncope of suspected arrhythmic etiology.

EPS is not recommended for syncope evaluation in patients with a normal ECG and normal cardiac structure and function, unless an arrhythmic etiology is suspected.

Recommendations for Tilt-Table Testing

If the diagnosis is unclear after initial evaluation, tilt-table testing can be useful for patients with suspected VVS. Tilt-table testing can be useful for patients with syncope and suspected delayed OH when initial evaluation is not diagnostic. Tilt-table testing is reasonable to distinguish convulsive syncope from epilepsy in selected patients. Tilt-table testing is reasonable to establish a diagnosis of pseudosyncope.

Neurological Testing: Recommendations (15)

Simultaneous monitoring of an EEG and hemodynamic parameters during tilt-table testing can be useful to distinguish among syncope, pseudosyncope, and epilepsy.

MRI and CT of the head are not recommended in the routine evaluation of patients with syncope in the absence of focal neurological findings or head injury that support further evaluation.

Carotid artery imaging is not recommended in the routine evaluation of patients with syncope in the absence of focal neurological findings that support further evaluation.

Routine recording of an EEG is not recommended in the evaluation of patients with syncope in the absence of specific neurological features suggestive of a seizure.

MANAGEMENT OF CARDIOVASCULAR CONDITIONS (16)

Arrhythmic Conditions:-

In patients with syncope and Bradycardia/ atrial fibrillation/ Supraventricular tachycardia and Ventricular Arrhythmias, Guideline Directed Medical Therapy (GDMT) is recommended.

Structural Conditions:-

In patients with syncope associated with ischemic and nonischemic cardiomyopathy, valvular heart disease and hypertrophic cardiomyopathy, GDMT is recommended.

ICD implantation is recommended in patients with ARVC who present with syncope and have a documented sustained VA.

Channelopathies (17)

ICD implantation is reasonable in patients with Brugada ECG pattern and syncope of suspected arrhythmic etiology.

Invasive EPS may be considered in patients with Brugada ECG pattern and syncope of suspected arrhythmia etiology

ICD implantation is not recommended in patients with Brugada ECG pattern and reflex-mediated syncope in the absence of other risk factors.

ICD implantation may be considered in patients with short-QT pattern and syncope of suspected arrhythmic etiology.

Beta-blocker therapy, in the absence of contraindications, is indicated as a first-line therapy in patients with LQTSand suspected arrhythmic syncope.

ICD implantation is reasonable in patients with LQTS and suspected arrhythmic syncope who are on beta-blocker therapy or are intolerant to beta-blocker therapy.

Left cardiac sympathetic denervation (LCSD) is reasonable in patients with LQTS and recurrent syncope of suspected arrhythmia mechanism who are intolerant to beta-blocker therapy or for whom beta-blocker therapy has failed.

REFLEX CONDITIONS: RECOMMENDATIONS

Vasovagal Syncope: Recommendations (18)

Patient education on the diagnosis and prognosis of VVS is recommended.

Patients with a syncope prodrome should be instructed to assume a supine position to prevent a faint and minimize possible injury. In patients with a sufficiently long prodrome, physical counter-maneuvers (e.g., leg crossing, limband/or abdominal contraction, squatting) are a core management strategy. In a randomized, parallel, open-label trial, leg crossing with conventional therapy (i.e., fluid, salt intake, counseling, and avoidance) was superior to conventional therapy in preventing syncope recurrence.

Midodrine is reasonable in patients with recurrent VVS with no history of hypertension, HF, or urinary retention.

Fludrocortisone might be reasonable for patients with recurrent VVS and inadequate response to salt and fluid intake, unless contraindicated.

Beta blockers might be reasonable in patients 42 years of age or older with recurrent VVS.

Encouraging increased salt and fluid intake may be reasonable in selected patients with VVS, unless contraindicated.

In selected patients with VVS, it may be reasonable to reduce or withdraw medications that cause hypotension when appropriate.

In patients with recurrent VVS, a selective serotonin reuptake inhibitor might be considered.

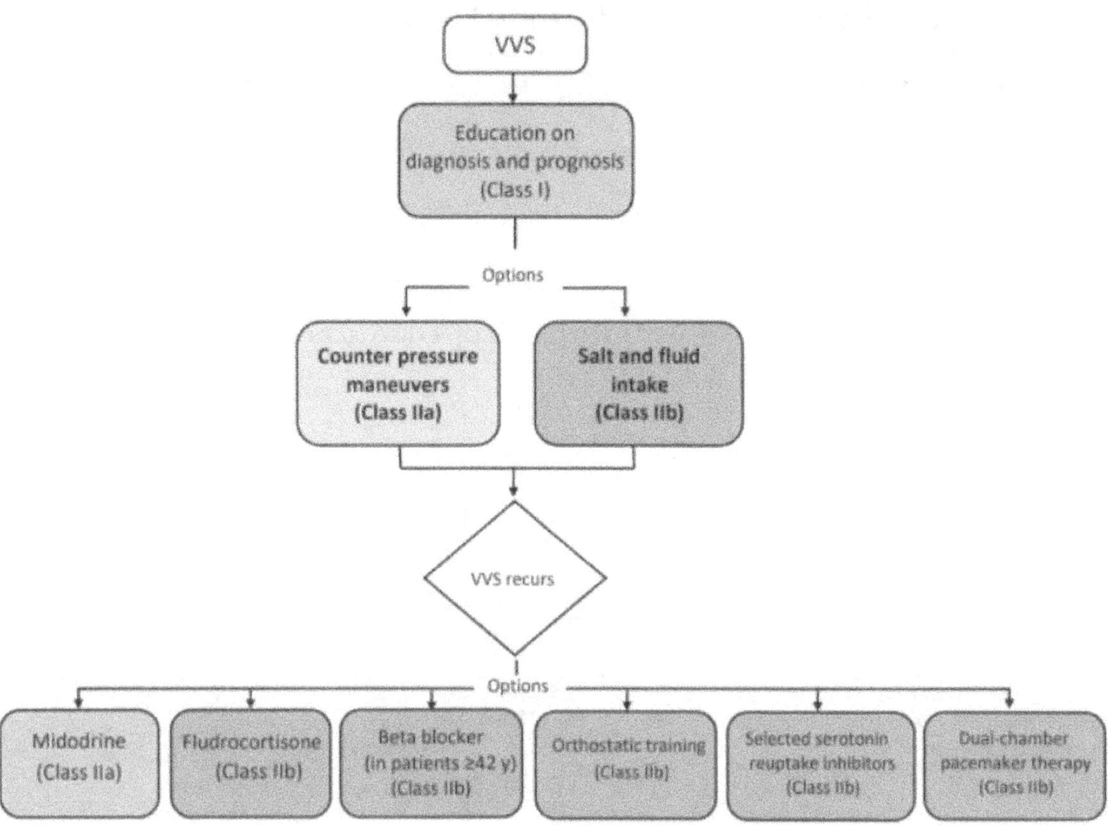

Dual-chamber pacing might be reasonable in a select population of patients 40 years of age or older with recurrent VVS and prolonged spontaneous pauses.

Permanent cardiac pacing is reasonable in patients with carotid sinus syndrome that is cardioinhibitory or mixed.

It may be reasonable to implant a dual chamber pacemaker in patients with carotid sinus syndrome who require permanent pacing.

ORTHOSTATIC HYPOTENSION: RECOMMENDATIONS (19)

Acute water ingestion is recommended in patients with syncope caused by neurogenic OH for occasional, temporary relief.

Physical counter-pressure maneuvers can be beneficial in patients with neurogenic OH with syncope Isometric contraction, such as by leg crossing, lower body muscle tensing, and maximal force handgrip, can increase blood pressure, with the largest effect occurring with squatting versus other counter-pressure maneuvers. Leg crossing increases cardiac output in patients with neurogenic hypotension. Similar or larger benefits would be expected with squatting and other isometric contraction. The benefit is limited to patients with sufficient prodrome and the ability to perform these maneuvers adequately and safely.

Compression garments can be beneficial in patients with syncope and OH.

Midodrine can be beneficial in patients with syncope due to neurogenic OH.

Droxidopa can be beneficial in patients with syncope due to neurogenic OH.

Fludrocortisone can be beneficial in patients with syncope due to neurogenic OH.

Encouraging increased salt and fluid intake may be reasonable in selected patients with neurogenic OH.(20).

Pyridostigmine may be beneficial in patients with syncope due to neurogenic OH who are refractory to other treatments.

Octreotide may be beneficial in patients with syncope and refractory recurrent postprandial or neurogenicOH.

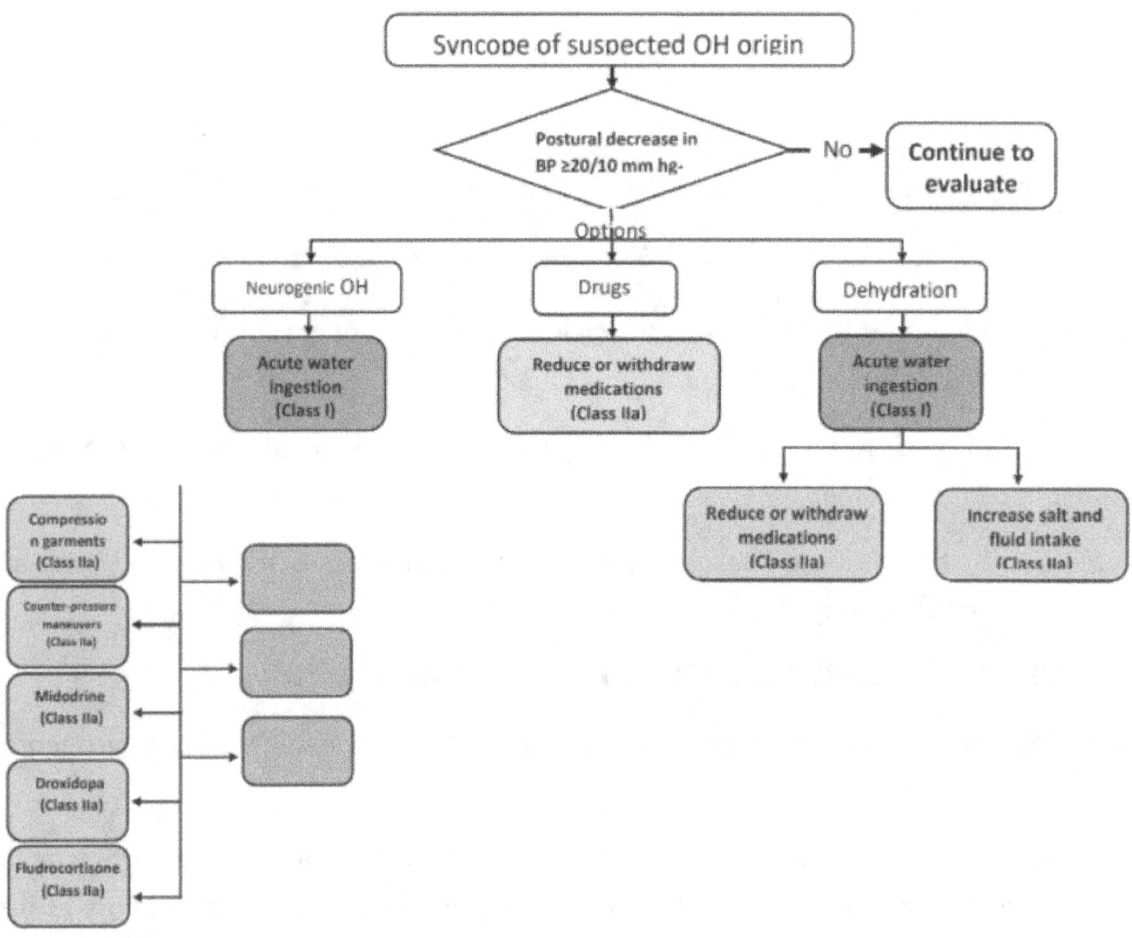

Recommendations for Dehydration and Drugs (21)

Fluid resuscitation via oral or intravenous bolus is recommended in patients with syncope due to acute dehydration.Reducing or withdrawing medications that may cause hypotension can be beneficial in selected patients with syncope. In selected patients with syncope due to dehydration, it is reasonable to encourage increased salt and fluid intake.

Recommendations for the Treatment of Pseudosyncope (22)

In patients with suspected pseudosyncope, a candid discussion with the patient about the diagnosis may be reasonable.Cognitive behavioral therapy may be beneficial in patients with pseudosyncope.

Classifying non cardiogenic syncope

Recent advances in the understanding of the pathophysiology of syncope have set the stage for a new classification, which can also be helpful in the identification of the most suitable strategies for recurrence prevention. Non-cardiac syncope can be classified into different phenotypes according to the predominant underlying hemodynamic mechanism, i.e., hypotension (vasodepression) or bradycardia, corresponding to hypotensive and bradycardic phenotypes.

NON CARDIAC SYNCOPE	
HYPOTENSIVE PHENOTYPE	BRADYCARDIC PHENOTYPE
Vasodepressor or mixed reflex syncope during table tilt	Cardioinhibitory response to table tilt
Vasodepressor or mixed carotid sinus syndrome	Cardioinhibitory carotid sinus syndrome
BP falls detected on 24h ambulatory monitoring	Syncopal reflex asystole (>3 sec) or non syncopal reflex asystole (>6 sec) detected by implantable loop detector
	Low adenosine syncope

Mechanism-based approach to syncope diagnosis

Identifying the syncope phenotype represents the first step towards effective syncope prevention. The syncope phenotype reveals which hemodynamic mechanism should be addressed by customized therapeutic interventions. Thus, a mechanism-based approach is required, aimed at documenting the correlation of syncope with hypotension and/or bradycardia.

The hypotensive phenotype

Hypotensive susceptibility leading to hypotensive phenotype syncope typically presents in patients with persistent or episodic hypotension, including orthostatic and postprandial hypotension.

Diagnosis of persistent hypotension — be it constitutional or drug-related — may be achieved using repeated office BPs or ABPM.

The bradycardic phenotype

Non-cardiac syncope with bradycardia phenotype is diagnosed if asystole >3 seconds is documented during syncope, thus indicating cardioinhibitory reflex susceptibility.

Asystole is most commonly a sinus arrest or atrioventricular(AV) block which is not related to cardiac conduction disorders but is reflex(30, 31). Diagnosis may be achieved using CSM, TT, and prolonged ECG monitoring.

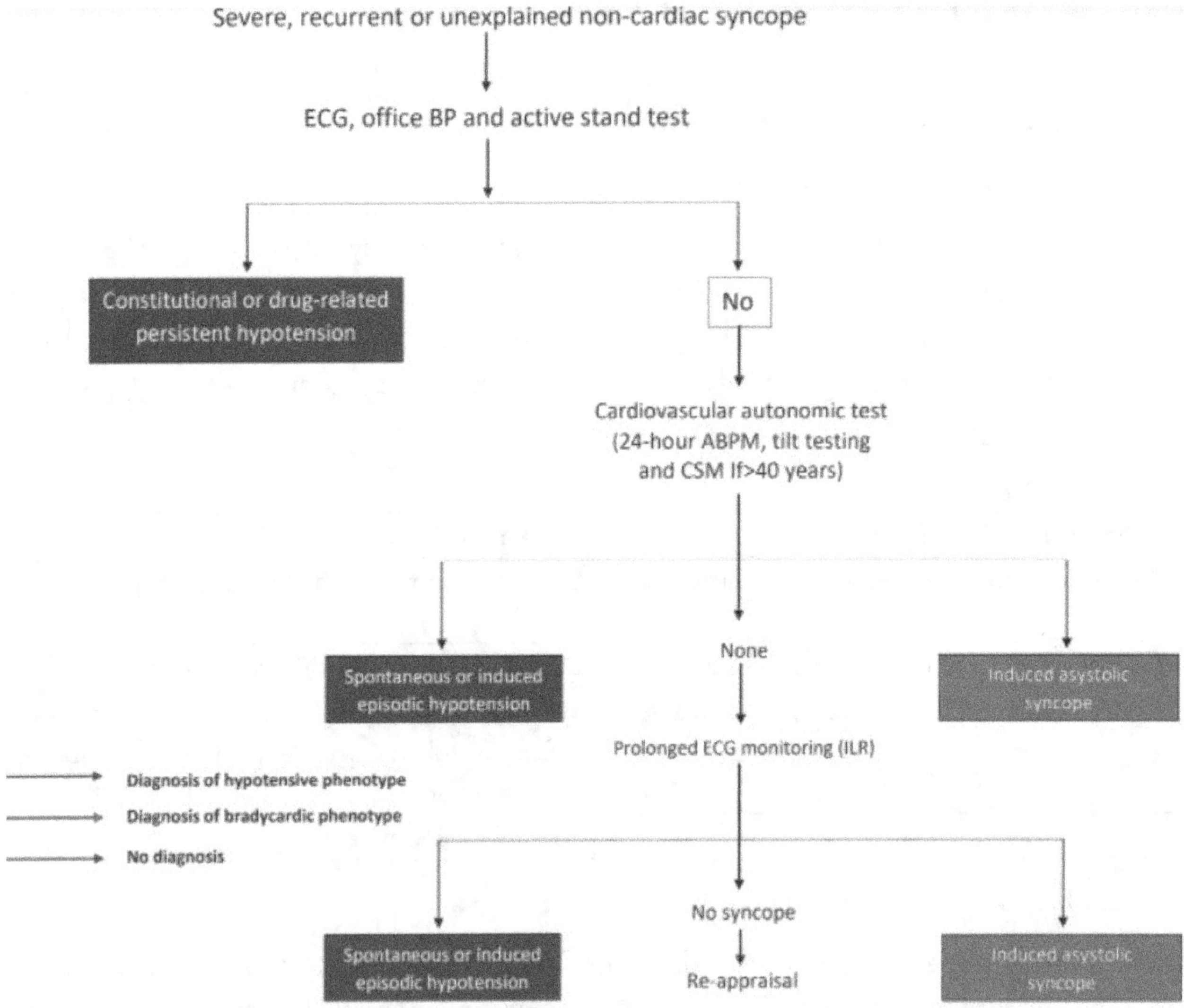

Existing and new strategies for syncope treatment

Alongside lifestyle measures aimed to counteract hypotensive susceptibility, a medication review and optimization should be carried out in all patients with syncope with the hypotensive phenotype.

Recent studies have provided data on the association between BP and hypotension-mediated adverse events, which may guide BP management in hypotensive susceptibility. From this evidence, systolic BP targets of 130–140 mm Hg can be recommended in hypertensive patients with hypotensive susceptibility, as more intensive treatment is expected to substantially increase the hypotensive syncope ris. Systolic BPs up to 160 mm Hg can be tolerated in older adults with severe frailty or disability – a vulnerable population in which fall risk is extremely high and the benefits of BP reduction remain doubtful.

Pharmacological therapies (23)

The α1-agonist midodrine is one available option in patients with the hypotensive phenotype. Midodrine increases BP in patients with constitutional hypotension and has demonstrated positive effects on symptoms due to neurogenic orthostatic hypotension and recurrent reflex syncope. The recent Prevention of Syncope Trial (POST) 4 re-emphasizes the value of midodrine in reflex syncope. The trial involved patients with severely symptomatic reflex syncope and showed a 40% relative risk reduction of recurrence using 10 mg 3/day compared with placebo; adverse events were modest and balanced in the two study groups.

Recent research has provided promising data on atomoxetine, a selective norepinephrine transporter (NET) inhibitor. Atomoxetine potentiates adrenergic drive to the heart, which may help to increase the heart rate, maintain cardiac output and BP during orthostatic stress. Moreover, in a recent double-blind placebo-controlled trial, atomoxetine significantly reduced the risk of (pre)syncope and prolonged presyncope-free survival in vasovagal syncope with greater benefit in participants with systolic BP <110 mm Hg.

Cardiac pacing (24)

Over the last decades, randomized controlled trials have provided evidence for the effectiveness of cardiac pacing in patients with predominant cardio inhibition documented by TT, CSM, or ILR, showing a significantly lower risk of syncope recurrence with pacing. The results of the multicentre randomized placebo-controlled BIOSync trial have shown a significantly lower risk of (pre) syncope recurrence in patients with documented cardioinhibition, receiving dual-chamber pacing with closedloop stimulation compared with pacing-off (a 77% and 46% relative and absolute risk reduction at 2 years, respectively) (36). Based on this evidence, the guidelines of the European Society of Cardiology (ESC) have upgraded the indication for pacing in reflex syncope from IIb to I (37). It must be understood that cardiac pacing is not always necessary but only indicated in patients aged >40-years affected by severe, recurrent, unpredictable syncope (i.e., often without prodrome) associated with a high risk of injuries (37). At present, there is no evidence to support pacing in patients <40-years presenting even with severe symptoms (37).

Theophylline

Recent studies advocate theophylline as a promising treatment in patients with low adenosine syncope, raising a potential alternative to cardiac pacing. Theophylline is a non-selective adenosine receptor antagonist, which competes with adenosine for receptor binding. In patients with low adenosine syncope, theophylline may prevent A1 receptor activation with subsequent bradycardia when plasma adenosine increases. Moreover, theophylline antagonizes adenosine A2 receptors mediating vasodilation, offering opposition to reflex vasodepression.

In a small study of low-adenosine syncope patients, a significant reduction of syncope and asystole burden during theophylline therapy compared with no treatment was observed. The therapeutic role of theophylline has yet to be defined.

References

1. Sheldon RS, Grubb BP, Olshansky B, et al. 2015 Heart Rhythm Society expert consensus statement on the diagnosis and treatment of postural tachycardia syndrome, inappropriate sinus tachycardia, and vasovagal syncope. Heart Rhythm. 2015;12:e41–63.

2. Freeman R, Wieling W, Axelrod FB, et al. Consensus statement on the definition of orthostatic hypotension, neurally mediated syncope and the postural tachycardia syndrome. Clin Auton Res. 2011;21:69–72.

3. Metzler M, Duerr S, Granata R, et al. Neurogenic orthostatic hypotension: pathophysiology, evaluation, and management. J Neurol. 2013;260:2212–9.

4. Soteriades ES, Evans JC, Larson MG, et al. Incidence and prognosis of syncope. N Engl J Med. 2002; 347:878–85.

5. Low PA, Sandroni P, Joyner M, et al. Postural tachycardia syndrome (POTS). J Cardiovasc Electrophysiol. 2009;20:352–8.

6. Schondorf R, Low PA. Idiopathic postural orthostatic tachycardia syndrome: an attenuated form of acute pandysautonomia? Neurology. 1993;43:132–7.

7. Morichetti A, Astorino G. [Epidemiological and clinical findings in 697 syncope events]. Minerva Med. 1998;89:211–20.

8. Alboni P, Brignole M, Menozzi C, et al. Diagnostic value of history in patients with syncope with or without heart disease. J Am Coll Cardiol. 2001;37: 1921–8.

9. Chiu DT, Shapiro NI, Sun BC, et al. Are echocardiography, telemetry, ambulatory electrocardiography monitoring, and cardiac enzymes in emergency department patients presenting with syncope useful tests? A preliminary investigation. J Emerg Med. 2014; 47:113–8.

10. Pfister R, Diedrichs H, Larbig R, et al. NT-pro-BNP for differential diagnosis in patients with syncope. Int J Cardiol. 2009;133:51–4.

11. Woelfel AK, Simpson RJ Jr., Gettes LS, et al. Exercise-induced distal atrioventricular block. J Am Coll Cardiol. 1983;2:578–81.

12. Sivakumaran S, Krahn AD, Klein GJ, et al. A prospective randomized comparison of loop recorders versus Holter monitors in patients with syncope or presyncope. Am J Med. 2003;115:1–5.

13. Gulamhusein S, Naccarelli GV, Ko PT, et al. Value and limitations of clinical electrophysiologic study in assessment of patients with unexplained syncope. Am J Med. 1982;73:700–5.

14. Gibbons CH, Freeman R. Clinical implications of delayed orthostatic hypotension: a 10-year follow-up study. Neurology. 2015;85:1362–7.

15. Van Dijk JG, Thijs RD, van Zwet E, et al. The semiology of tilt-induced reflex syncope in relation to electroencephalographic changes. Brain. 2014;137: 576–85.

16. Link MS, Laidlaw D, Polonsky B, et al. Ventricular arrhythmias in the North American multidisciplinary study of ARVC: predictors, characteristics, and treatment. J Am Coll Cardiol. 2014;64:119–25.

17. Gehi AK, Duong TD, Metz LD, et al. Risk stratification of individuals with the Brugada electrocardiogram: a meta-analysis. J Cardiovasc Electrophysiol. 2006;17:577–83.

18. Morley CA, Perrins EJ, Grant P, et al. Carotid sinus syncope treated by pacing. Analysis of persistent symptoms and role of atrioventricular sequential pacing. Br Heart J. 1982;47:411–8.

19. Tutaj M, Marthol H, Berlin D, et al. Effect of physical countermaneuvers on orthostatic hypotension in familial dysautonomia. J Neurol. 2006;253:65–72.

20. Young TM, Mathias CJ. The effects of water ingestion on orthostatic hypotension in two groups of chronic autonomic failure: multiple system atrophy and pure autonomic failure. J Neurol Neurosurg Psychiatry. 2004;75:1737–41.

21. Kenefick RW, O'Moore KM, Mahood NV, et al. Rapid IV versus oral rehydration: responses to subsequent exercise heat stress. Med Sci Sports Exerc. 2006;38:2125–31.

22. Goldstein LH, Chalder T, Chigwedere C, et al. Cognitive-behavioral therapy for psychogenic nonepileptic seizures: a pilot RCT. Neurology. 2010;74: 1986–94.

23. Sheldon R, Faris P, Tang A, et al. Midodrine for the prevention of vasovagal syncope: a randomized clinical trial. Ann Intern Med. 2021 [Epub ahead of print], doi: 10.7326/M20-5415, indexed in Pubmed: 34339231.

24. Glikson M, Nielsen JC, Kronborg MB, et al. 2021 ESC Guidelines on cardiac pacing and cardiac resynchronization therapy. Eur Heart J. 2021; 42(35): 3427–3520, doi: 10.1093/eurheartj/ehab364.

Abdominal Emergencies

Contributors

1. Dr. Chandni R,
2. Dr. Kavitha KP
3. Dr. Akhil SL
4. Dr. Austin Joju Mangal

Chapters

1. Abdominal Pain
2. Medical GI emergencies
3. Surgical GI emergencies

Approach to abdominal pain

Introduction and epidemiology

Abdominal pain is one of the commonest complaints that bring a patient to the ED and accounts for 5 to 10 percent of ED visits. Differential diagnosis in the ED is wide from life-threatening conditions to simple self-limiting conditions. Abdominal pain can also be a manifestation of extra-abdominal causes as well and the presentations can be atypical in extremes of age and in immunosuppression.

Pathophysiology

Abdominal pain can be broadly classified into visceral, parietal and referred.

Visceral pain

Unmyelinated fibres innervate the walls or capsules of organs. Due to obstruction, ischemic or inflammation, there will be stretching of these nerves and will cause visceral pain described as crampy, dull, or achy, type of pain. It can be either steady pain or intermittent pain

The visceral afferent follows segmental distribution and the pain can be localised by spinal cord level determined by the embryological origin of the involved organ from the foregut, midgut or hindgut.

The location of visceral pain and the possible involved organs are given in the table.

Location of visceral pain	Possible involved organs
Epigastric area	Stomach, first/second parts of duodenum, liver, gall bladder, pancreas
Periumbilical area	Third/Fourth parts of duodenum, jejunum, ileum, caecum, appendix, ascending colon, first $2/3^{rds}$ of transverse colon
Suprapubic area	Distal $1/3^{rd}$ of transverse colon, descending colon, sigmoid, rectum, intraperitoneal genitourinary organs.

As intraperitoneal structures are bilaterally innervated, stimuli will be sent to both sides of the spinal cord. This results in the pain that is felt at the midline independent of the left or right anatomical origin of the organ involved. For example, stimuli from the visceral fibres of the appendix enter the spinal cord at about T10 causing pain in the periumbilical region.

Parietal pain

Caused by irritation of myelinated fibres that cover the parietal peritoneum and pain can be localised superficial to the site of a painful stimulus. As the disease process evolves, the visceral pain gives way to parietal pain due to the localised peritonitis causing guarding and tenderness.

<u>Referred pain</u>

Pain felt at a distant place than the diseased organ. It also depends on the embryological origin of the organs. Referred pain is usually felt on the same side of the involved organ.

<u>Clinical Features</u>

We need to elicit a proper history specifically of the pain.

Pain- onset, duration, precipitating and relieving factors, quality, radiation, associated symptoms, timing, and what the treatment patient has taken for the pain.

In the examination, should look for abdominal distension, mass, scars, ecchymosis, stigmata of liver disease, tenderness, guarding, liver span, shifting dullness or fluid thrill. Voluntary guarding can be diminished by flexing the knees and distracting the patient by conversation while examining. Auscultation, look for decreased bowel sounds as in ileus, mesenteric infarction, narcotic use, or peritonitis; or increased bowel sounds as in small bowel obstruction.

Evaluate for abdominal aorta especially in patients with age more than 50 years.

In females, must include the examination of the pelvis along with an abdominal examination, to assess for vaginal infections and ectopic pregnancy.

In males, look for hernias, testicular and prostate examinations are also to be done.

Per rectal examination and to see for colour for bloody, maroon or tarry stools.

<u>Differential diagnosis</u>

Conventionally site of pain (diffuse pain, right, left upper and lower quadrants helps to narrow down the differentials in diagnosis.

Immediate life-threatening gastrointestinal emergencies include Perforation of the gastrointestinal tract (including peptic ulcer, bowel, oesophagus, or appendix), Acute bowel obstruction, Volvulus, Mesenteric ischemia, Splenic rupture (eg, secondary to Epstein-Barr virus [EBV], leukaemia, trauma)

Other important differentials include Myocardial infarction, Pulmonary embolism, ruptured/ leaking Abdominal aortic aneurysm, Ectopic pregnancy and Placental abruption.

Initial assessment and stabilization, bedside investigations, continued evaluation, and relevant advanced or specific investigations to be incorporated. Initial bedside assessment includes point of care ultrasound in the assessment of acute undifferentiated abdominal pain, life-threatening conditions like aortic aneurysm, assessment of shock and restricting more advanced studies like CT abdomen.

<u>Disposition</u>

The decision is based upon age, co-morbidities, initial and continued assessment, diagnosis, relief of symptoms and social support system.

For Further Reading:

1. Mattu A. Abdominal and Gastrointestinal Emergencies. Emerg Med Clin North Am. 2021 Nov;39(4):xiii-xiv. doi: 10.1016/j.emc.2021.08.006. PMID: 34600643.

2. Manning S, McCoin N. Gastrointestinal Emergencies. Emerg Med Clin North Am. 2021 Nov;39(4):xv-xvi. doi: 10.1016/j.emc.2021.08.003. PMID: 34600644.

3. Natesan S, Werley EB. Laboratory Tests in the Patient with Abdominal Pain. Emerg Med Clin North Am. 2021 Nov;39(4):733-744. doi: 10.1016/j.emc.2021.08.001. Epub 2021 Sep 9. PMID: 34600634.

4. Brenner DS, Fong TC. Approach to Abdominal Imaging in 2022. Emerg Med Clin North Am. 2021 Nov;39(4):745-767. doi: 10.1016/j.emc.2021.07.007. PMID: 34600635.

5. Murali N, El Hayek SM. Abdominal Pain Mimics. Emerg Med Clin North Am. 2021 Nov;39(4):839-850. doi: 10.1016/j.emc.2021.07.003. Epub 2021 Sep 10. PMID: 34600641; PMCID: PMC8430370.

6. Cullison KM, Franck N. Clinical Decision Rules in the Evaluation and Management of Adult Gastrointestinal Emergencies. Emerg Med Clin North Am. 2021 Nov;39(4):719-732. doi: 10.1016/j.emc.2021.07.001. Epub 2021 Sep 10. PMID: 34600633.

Medical Gastrointestinal Emergencies

Gastrointestinal emergencies are coming under common ED presentations. It could be abdominal pain, upper or lower GI bleed, jaundice, altered sensorium, giddiness and fall or ascites. ED presentation may be related or unrelated to common complaints listed and needs a high index of suspicion to include or exclude. The common medical gastrointestinal emergencies are included in this chapter.

1. Upper GI Bleed

Introduction

Gastrointestinal bleeding originating proximal to the ligament of Treitz is included as the upper GI bleed. Commonly presents with hematemesis (vomiting of blood of coffee-ground-like) and melena (black, tarry stools). Mortality varies between 3.5% to 10% in various studies. Factors associated with increased morbidity and mortality are advanced age, coexistent organ system disease, and recurrent haemorrhage.

Epidemiology

The most common causes of upper GI bleeding are peptic ulcer disease, which includes gastric, duodenal, oesophageal, and stomal ulcers.

Other causes are esophagogastric varices, portal hypertensive gastropathy, angiodysplasia, Mallory-Weiss syndrome, and Mass lesions (polyps/cancers). Usually, no lesion is identified in about 10 to 15 % of patients.

Approach in ED

Taking the appropriate history and physical examination help in identifying the potential sources of the upper GI bleed, assessing the severity, and thereby planning the subsequent management. To identify high-risk patients requiring emergency endoscopy various risk stratification schemes, including the Glasgow–Blatchford Score (GBS), Rockall score, and AIMS65, have been developed and validated.

There is an association between early nasogastric lavage with decreased time to endoscopy. This is because nasogastric tube placement and lavage aid in confirming the diagnosis of upper GI bleeding and correlate with the chance of high-risk lesions on endoscopy.

The aim of hemodynamic resuscitation is to maintain adequate tissue perfusion by restoring the intravascular volume and preventing end-organ damage. Initial management is stabilization. Patients in hemorrhagic shock require emergent resuscitation, including two large-bore IVs, typed and cross-matched blood with the consideration of massive transfusion protocols, and in selected cases, early airway management.

Treatment includes-

a. Blood transfusion – If Hb <= 7 g/dL and in older patients or with co-morbidities <=9 g/dL

b. Correct coagulopathy if identified

c. Use of Omeprazole (80 mg IV bolus and then infusion of 8 mg/h), Octreotide (50 microgram bolus followed by infusion of 25 micrograms/hr

d. Specific management like in variceal bleed with hepatic encephalopathy

Recent Updates

- Use of a risk assessment tool to identify patients with ≤1% risk of transfusion, hemostatic intervention, or death who may be discharged with outpatient management should reduce hospitalizations and costs.

- A Glasgow-Blatchford bleeding score (GBS) = 0–1 should meet this requirement and allows more patients to be discharged than GBS = 0, which was the threshold suggested in the 2012 ACG Guidelines.

- Patients with GBS ≤ 1 are at very low risk of rebleeding, mortality within 30 days, or needing hospital-based intervention and can be safely managed as outpatients with outpatient endoscopy.

- A restrictive RBC transfusion policy in which patients are transfused when hemoglobin falls below 7 g/dL seems to reduce further bleeding and death, a conclusion unchanged from the 2012 ACG Guidelines.

- Hypotensive patients may be transfused at higher hemoglobin levels given equilibration that occurs with fluid resuscitation and a threshold of 8 g/dL is reasonable in patients with pre-existing cardiovascular disease.

Pre-endoscopic medical therapy

- Infusion of 250 mg of erythromycin 20–90 minutes before endoscopy may reduce the need for repeat endoscopy and length of hospitalization, although is not documented to improve clinical outcomes such as further bleeding [1] The 2012 ACG Guidelines indicated such an infusion "should be considered".

- It promotes gastric emptying based upon its ability to be an agonist of motilin receptors, thereby improving gastric visualization [2]

- Tranexamic acid, an antifibrinolytic agent is found to be not beneficial in patients with upper GI bleeding [3].

- Patients admitted or under observation in a hospital with overt UGIB, whether predicted to be at low risk or high risk of further bleeding and death, undergo upper endoscopy within 24 hours of presentation.
- High-dose PPI therapy should be given continuously or intermittently for 3 days after successful endoscopic hemostatic therapy of a bleeding ulcer [1].

Nasogastric tube insertion

- Currently, the routine use of nasogastric tube (NGT) placement in patients with suspected acute upper GI bleeding is not recommended [4, 5].
- NGT lavage was associated with a shorter time to endoscopy. But, there were no differences with regard to mortality, length of hospital stay, surgery, or transfusion requirement when comparing those who underwent NGT lavage and those who did not [2].

2. Peptic Ulcer Disease

Brief overview

It is a chronic illness manifested by recurrent ulcerations in the stomach and proximal duodenum. It is a defect in the gastric or duodenal mucosa that extends through the muscularis mucosa into the deeper layers of the wall. H. pylori infection, is one of the main risk factors identified for peptic ulcer disease. It is one of the most prevalent human infections in the world, affecting at least 50% of the world's population. Dyspepsia having no definite findings on endoscopy has "functional" dyspepsia, accounting for more than 70% of patients.

Uncomplicated peptic ulcer disease can be strongly suspected in the presence of a classic history, including epigastric burning pain; relief of pain with ingestion of food, or antacids; and nocturnal pain accompanied by normal physical examination findings, including vital signs with or without mild epigastric tenderness.

The gold standard for diagnosis of peptic ulcer disease is the visualization of an ulcer by upper GI endoscopy. Proton pump inhibitors are considered as first-line non-eradication therapy for peptic ulcers. Known H. pylori-positive dyspeptic patients are treated with antimicrobial and antisecretory therapy followed by endoscopic study only in those with persistent symptoms. The main complications and indications for an ED visit are Upper GI haemorrhage, perforation, and obstruction.

Recent Updates

All patients diagnosed with peptic ulcer disease should undergo testing for *H. pylori* infection. All ulcers with malignant features should be biopsied.

Endoscopic features that suggest that an ulcer may be malignant include:

1. An ulcerated mass protruding into the lumen

2. Folds surrounding the ulcer crater that are nodular, clubbed, fused, or stop short of the ulcer margin

3. Overhanging, irregular, or thickened ulcer margins

   - A routine biopsy of benign-appearing duodenal ulcers is not recommended
   - Treatment of with patients with haemorrhagic peptic ulcers

     - Suspend antiplatelet agents, except for in patients at high risk for thromboembolic events [6]. Aspirin is continued for those at high risk for thromboembolic events. In patients receiving dual antiplatelet agents, aspirin alone should be continued [7].
     - Stop warfarin, if necessary, in endoscopic haemostasis patients. heparin or resuming warfarin as soon as haemostasis is established.

   - In patients undergoing refractory endoscopic treatment for haemorrhagic peptic ulcers, interventional radiology (IVR) is suggested due to its safety and effectiveness [8].
   - While using DAPT, the combined use of PPIs to prevent upper gastrointestinal bleeding [9].
   - Vonoprazan with amoxicillin and clarithromycin is used as triple eradication therapy for first line *H. pylori* eradication therapy and having a high eradication rate compared with that of PPIs [10].

3. Lower Gastro-Intestinal (GI) Bleed

<u>Introduction</u>

Loss of blood from the GI tract distal to the ligament of Treitz, typically present with hematochezia, and melena. In 80 to 85 percent of patients, bleeding will stop spontaneously. Upper GI bleeds are the most common source of lower GI bleed as blood traverse through the upper GI tract down to the lower GI system.

Mortality rate is 2 to 4 % [11] and should be considered a potentially life-threatening condition until proven otherwise.

<u>Clinical Manifestations</u>

Typically presents with hematochezia and approximately 10% of hematochezia episodes may be associated with upper GI bleeding. Melena (dark or black coloured stools) usually represents bleeding from an upper GI source.

<u>Causes of Lower GI Bleeding</u>

The most common cause of lower GI bleed is Upper GI source followed by diverticular disease, colitis, haemorrhoids, and adenomatous polyps/malignancies.

Hemodynamic instability, orthostatic hypotension, and an elevated blood urea nitrogen (BUN)-to-creatinine ratio are the findings that are suggestive of an upper GI source.

Physical Examination

Watch for signs of shock like tachycardia, hypotension, delayed capillary filling time, and cold clammy peripheries as happens in massive bleeding.

In patients with lower GI bleeding, a lack of abdominal tenderness suggests bleeding from disorders involving the vasculature, such as diverticulosis or angiodysplasia.

Inflammatory bowel disorders with lower GI bleeding are associated with abdominal tenderness on examination. Anoscopy can be performed to look for haemorrhoids

Laboratory tests

Include a complete blood count, serum electrolytes, liver function tests, and coagulation studies, blood grouping and cross-matching. The initial Hb level should be monitored frequently, depending on the severity of the bleed.

Imaging

Once an upper gastrointestinal (GI) bleeding source is excluded, colonoscopy is the initial examination of choice for the diagnosis and treatment of acute lower GI bleeding.

Other investigations like angiography, scintigraphy, or endoscopy may be of use but depend on the resource ability and clinician's preference.

In patients with severe bleeding who cannot be stabilized for colonoscopy or with severe ongoing bleeding despite colonoscopy, CT angiography may be used to select patients with active bleeding for subsequent angiography or, less commonly, to localize the source prior to surgery. Scintigraphy is more sensitive than angiography and can localize the site of bleeding at as low a rate as 0.1 mL/min. It has better potential value over angiography if bleeding occurs intermittently but requires a minimum of 3 mL of blood to pool.

Treatment

Resuscitate the patients in shock with first priority [12] and place two large bore IV lines and replace the volume with crystalloids.

Correct coagulopathy including if international normalized ratio is >1.5 or platelets are <50,000/μL.

Blood transfusion should be based on the clinical findings and if hemoglobin falls below 7 g/dL [13].

If colonoscopy fails to determine the source of bleeding, upper GI endoscopy can be considered to evaluate for an upper GI source of bleeding.

Repeat colonoscopy should be performed with endoscopic hemostasis if indicated in patients with significant, recurrent lower gastrointestinal bleeding [14].

4. Hepatic Disease

Introduction

Liver disease can be categorized as acute, chronic, or fulminant. Acute hepatitis typically presents with nausea, vomiting, and right upper quadrant abdominal pain. The most common causes are viral infection and toxic ingestion. Alcohol and acetaminophen are the most common toxic causes. Patients with chronic hepatitis display evidence of long-standing hepatocellular damage and scarring. Treatment of acute hepatitis from toxic causes includes supportive care and attention to associated conditions such as hyponatremia, alcohol or narcotic intoxication or withdrawal, alcoholic ketoacidosis, and hypoglycaemia. Liver failure is the potential final common pathway for both acute and chronic liver disease.

Definition

Acute liver failure refers to the development of severe acute liver injury with encephalopathy and impaired synthetic function with coagulopathy (INR of $\geq$1.5) in a patient within 26 weeks of illness onset, without cirrhosis or pre-existing liver disease and results from acute and massive hepatocellular destruction [15].

Acute liver failure can be subcategorized based on how long the patient has been ill and various cut offs have been used. Acute liver failure is classified as hyperacute (<7 days), acute (7 to 21 days), or subacute (>21 days and <26 weeks). In patients with hyperacute or acute liver failure, cerebral oedema is common, whereas it is rare in subacute liver failure [16].

Acute-on-chronic liver failure is a syndrome that affects patients with pre-existing chronic liver disease; and is characterized by intense systemic inflammation, organ failure, and a poor prognosis; and frequently develops with some identifiable pre- precipitating events.

Pathophysiology

In acute on chronic liver failure, there is dysregulated heightened inflammation and oxidative stress associated with high short-term mortality. The two precipitants of systemic inflammation that are frequently associated with acute-on-chronic liver failure are bacterial infections and acute alcoholic hepatitis. Severe GI haemorrhage can cause ischemic hepatitis, and also confers a predisposition to the development of bacterial infections [17]. The consensus recommendations of the Asian Pacific Association for the Study of the Liver described that of the survivors among 1844 patients with acute-on-chronic liver failure, 70% had a complete recovery. This finding emphasises that early diagnosis with the initiation of treatment can improve the outcome [18].

Management

Role of liver biopsy in ALF:

1. When a specific treatment or conduct can be decided (steroids in Autoimmune Hepatitis, drug-induced liver failure (N Acetyl cysteine in Paracetamol intoxication, antivirals in viral infections, mushroom ingestions, Wilson's disease, malignancy)

2. if it is not clear whether the patient has ALF or chronic liver disease.

But in the most severe cases, liver biopsy has no role in the treatment and liver transplantation should be considered.

Pregnancy-related liver disease includes pre-eclampsia/eclampsia, HELLP syndrome (defined as haemolysis, elevated liver enzymes and a low platelet count), Acute Fatty liver of Pregnancy (AFLP). These are associated with high mortality and pregnancy termination is the treatment of choice in these conditions [19].

Identifying and treating the precipitating event particularly bacterial or Fungal Infection, Acute Variceal Hemorrhage, Alcoholic hepatitis, Hepatitis B Virus Reactivation

Supportive Management

In haemodynamically unstable patients with acute liver failure, Normal saline should be given for hypotension. Patients who are acidotic can be resuscitated with half-normal saline with 75 mEq/L sodium bicarbonate.

Dextrose should be added to crystalloid solutions in patients with hypoglycemia.

As is seen in patients with septic shock, patients with acute liver failure may develop adrenal insufficiency. Thus, if hypotension persists despite volume repletion and vasopressor support, a trial of hydrocortisone is reasonable [16, 20].

For bleeding prevention, Prophylactic administration of fresh frozen plasma is not recommended since it has not been shown to influence mortality [17, 21]

Use of viscoelastic tests

Viscoelastic tests (VET), such as TEG and thromboelastometry, evaluate the coagulation phenotype through the different steps in clot formation. VET have been successfully used for guiding the administration of haemo derivatives before invasive procedures (Liver biopsy & LT) [22].

Among the acid-base disorders, alkalosis is more common than acidosis in the early stages of acute liver failure and is frequently a mixed respiratory and metabolic abnormality.

Lactulose is commonly used in patients with hepatic encephalopathy due to chronic liver disease. But its use in acute liver failure is controversial [17]. No difference in the severity of encephalopathy or in overall outcomes was found.

Liver transplantation is the only definitive treatment for cerebral oedema, though uncontrolled ICP elevation is a contraindication to liver transplantation.

Liver transplantation and prognostic scores

1. The King's College Criteria (KCC)
2. The MELD score

The Model for End-Stage Liver Disease with the addition of the serum sodium level (MELD-Na) score, in addition to scores based on the number of failing organs, provides accurate prognostication for individual patients with acute-on-chronic liver failure.

3. The APACHE II score
4. he SOFA score

King's College Criteria for establishing a poor prognosis and the need for liver transplantation (Table 1)

Table 1: King's College Criteria for acute liver failure

Acetaminophen-induced ALF
Arterial pH < 7.3 after fluid resuscitation
Or all of the following variables
Prothrombin time > 100 s (INR > 6.5)
Serum creatinine > 3.4 mg/dl (>259 mol/L)
Grade III–IV hepatic encephalopathy
Non-acetaminophen-induced ALF
Prothrombin time > 100 s (INR > 6.5)
Or three of the following variables
Non-A, non-B viral hepatitis, drug-induced or indeterminate aetiology of ALF
Time from jaundice to hepatic encephalopathy > 7 days
Age < 10 or >40 years
Prothrombin time >50 s (INR > 3.5)
Serum bilirubin > 17.4 mg/dl (>297.6 μmol/L)

Patients with grade IV encephalopathy, high ammonia levels (>150 micromol/L), or acute renal failure, and patients who require vasopressor support are considered as high risk patients and these patients can be prophylactically managed with hypertonic saline (3 percent), with a goal serum sodium of 145 to 150 mEq/L [18].

Seizures in patients with acute liver failure should be treated promptly because seizure activity increases ICP and may cause cerebral hypoxia. Consensus recommendations suggest treatment with phenytoin, since patients with acute liver failure have a severely impaired ability to clear sedatives. Patients who are refractory to phenytoin should receive short acting benzodiazepines.

5. Inflammatory bowel disease (IBD)

The term refers to two major categories of chronic relapsing inflammatory intestinal disorders: Crohn's disease (CD) and ulcerative colitis (UC).

A] Ulcerative colitis (UC)

Introduction

Ulcerative colitis (UC) is an idiopathic, chronic inflammatory disorder of the colonic mucosa that commonly involves the rectum and may extend in a proximal and continuous fashion to involve other parts of the colon. The classical clinical symptoms are bloody diarrhoea and rectal urgency with tenesmus, marked by exacerbations and remissions, typically affects individuals in the second or third decade of life. The diagnosis of UC is based on the clinical presentation, findings on colonoscopy or sigmoidoscopy showing continuous colonic inflammation starting in the rectum and Pathologic findings of chronic colitis [24].

ED presentation and recent management updates

Severe and fulminant disease presents to the ED with abdominal pain, anemia, loose bloody stools, tenesmus, systemic toxicity manifested as fever, tachycardia, raised ESR and CRP. Sigmoidoscopy or colonoscopy will aid in confirming the diagnosis along with biopsy.

Systemic steroids are used for induction of remission followed by oral steroids with close follow up for complications and tapering according to the response.

the steroid-refractory disease should be considered and rescue therapy with other therapeutic entities – either infliximab or cyclosporine – should be initiated, If there is no meaningful response to the intravenous steroids in acute severe disease within 3–5 days as determined by the Oxford index [24].

B] Crohn's disease

Brief overview

CD is typically characterized by transmural inflammation of the intestine and could affect any part of the gastrointestinal tract from mouth to perianal area. Abdominal Computed tomography (CT) enterography is the most preferred first-line radiologic study used in the assessment of small bowel CD. The most common scoring systems used to measure clinical disease activity include Crohn's Disease Activity Index (CDAI), Harvey-Bradshaw index (HBI), short inflammatory bowel disease questionnaire (SIBDQ) and Lehmann score.

Therapeutic interventions are done to address symptomatic response and subsequent tolerance of the intervention.

Chronology of treatment includes induction therapy, followed by maintenance therapy.

The medications which are highly effective in inducing remission include steroids and Tumor Necrosis Factor (TNF) inhibitors.

Medications used to maintain remission include 5-aminosalicyclic acid products, immunomodulators (Azathioprine, 6-mercaptopurine, methotrexate) and TNF inhibitors (infliximab, adalimumab, certolizumab and golimumab).

Two thirds of Crohn's Disease patients may require Surgical interventions like bowel resection, stricturoplasty or drainage of abscess during their lifetime [25].

References

1. Barkun AN, Almadi M, Kuipers EJ, Laine L, Sung J, Tse F, Leontiadis GI, Abraham NS, Calvet X, Chan FKL, Douketis J, Enns R, Gralnek IM, Jairath V, Jensen D, Lau J, Lip GYH, Loffroy R, Maluf-Filho F, Meltzer AC, Reddy N, Saltzman JR, Marshall JK, Bardou M. Management of Nonvariceal Upper Gastrointestinal Bleeding: Guideline Recommendations From the International Consensus Group. Ann Intern Med. 2019 Dec 3;171(11):805-822. doi: 10.7326/M19-1795. Epub 2019 Oct 22. PMID: 31634917; PMCID: PMC7233308.

2. Frossard JL, Spahr L, Queneau PE, Giostra E, Burckhardt B, Ory G, De Saussure P, Armenian B, De Peyer R, Hadengue A. Erythromycin intravenous bolus infusion in acute upper gastrointestinal bleeding: a randomized, controlled, double-blind trial. Gastroenterology. 2002 Jul;123(1):17-23. doi: 10.1053/gast.2002.34230. Erratum in: Gastroenterology 2002 Dec;123(6):2162. PMID: 12105828.

3. Bennett C, Klingenberg SL, Langholz E, Gluud LL. Tranexamic acid for upper gastrointestinal bleeding. Cochrane Database Syst Rev. 2014 Nov 21;2014(11):CD006640. doi: 10.1002/14651858.CD006640.pub3. PMID: 25414987; PMCID: PMC6599825.

4. Gralnek IM, Stanley AJ, Morris AJ, Camus M, Lau J, Lanas A, Laursen SB, Radaelli F, Papanikolaou IS, Cúrdia Gonçalves T, Dinis-Ribeiro M, Awadie H, Braun G, de Groot N, Udd M, Sanchez-Yague A, Neeman Z, van Hooft JE. Endoscopic diagnosis and management of nonvariceal upper gastrointestinal hemorrhage (NVUGIH): European Society of Gastrointestinal Endoscopy (ESGE) Guideline - Update 2021. Endoscopy. 2021 Mar;53(3):300-332. doi: 10.1055/a-1369-5274. Epub 2021 Feb 10. PMID: 33567467.

5. Rockey DC, Ahn C, de Melo SW Jr. Randomized pragmatic trial of nasogastric tube placement in patients with upper gastrointestinal tract bleeding. J Investig Med. 2017 Apr;65(4):759-764. doi: 10.1136/jim-2016-000375. Epub 2017 Jan 9. PMID: 28069629.

6. Kamada T, Satoh K, Itoh T, Ito M, Iwamoto J, Okimoto T, Kanno T, Sugimoto M, Chiba T, Nomura S, Mieda M, Hiraishi H, Yoshino J, Takagi A, Watanabe S, Koike K. Evidence-based clinical practice guidelines for peptic ulcer disease 2020. J Gastroenterol. 2021 Apr;56(4):303-322. doi: 10.1007/s00535-021-01769-0. Epub 2021 Feb 23. PMID: 33620586; PMCID: PMC8005399.

7. Sung JJ, Lau JY, Ching JY, et al. Continuation of low-dose aspirin therapy in peptic ulcer bleeding: a randomized trial. Ann Intern Med. 2010;152:1–9

8. Tarasconi A, Baiocchi GL, Pattonieri V, et al. Transcatheter arterial embolization versus surgery for refractory non-variceal upper gastrointestinal bleeding: a meta-analysis. World J Emerg Surg. 2019;14:3.

9. algimigli M, Bueno H, Byrne RA, ESC Scientific Document Group; ESC Committee for Practice Guidelines (CPG); ESC National Cardiac Societies et al. 2017 ESC focused update on dual antiplatelet therapy in coronary artery disease developed in collaboration with EACTS: The Task Force for dual antiplatelet therapy in coronary artery disease of the European Society of Cardiology (ESC) and of the European Association for Cardio-Thoracic Surgery (EACTS) Eur Heart J. 2018;39:213–260.

10. Sue S, Kuwashima H, Iwata Y, Oka H, Arima I, Fukuchi T, Sanga K, Inokuchi Y, Ishii Y, Kanno M, Terada M, Amano H, Naito M, Iwase S, Okazaki H, Komatsu K, Kokawa A, Kawana I, Morimoto M, Saito T, Kunishi Y, Ikeda A, Takahashi D, Miwa H, Sasaki T, Tamura T, Kondo M, Shibata W, Maeda S. The Superiority of Vonoprazan-based First-line Triple Therapy with Clarithromycin: A Prospective Multi-center Cohort Study on Helicobacter pylori Eradication. Intern Med. 2017;56(11):1277-1285. DOI: 10.2169/internalmedicine.56.7833. Epub 2017 Jun 1. PMID: 28566587; PMCID: PMC5498188.

11. Farrell JJ, Friedman LS. Review article: the management of lower gastrointestinal bleeding. Aliment Pharmacol Ther. 2005 Jun 1;21(11):1281-98. doi: 10.1111/j.1365-2036.2005.02485.x. PMID: 15932359.

12. Baradarian R, Ramdhaney S, Chapalamadugu R, Skoczylas L, Wang K, Rivilis S, Remus K, Mayer I, Iswara K, Tenner S. Early intensive resuscitation of patients with upper gastrointestinal bleeding decreases mortality. Am J Gastroenterol. 2004 Apr;99(4):619-22. doi: 10.1111/j.1572-0241.2004.04073.x. PMID: 15089891.

13. Triantafyllou K, Gkolfakis P, Gralnek IM, Oakland K, Manes G, Radaelli F, Awadie H, Camus Duboc M, Christodoulou D, Fedorov E, Guy RJ, Hollenbach M, Ibrahim M, Neeman Z, Regge D, Rodriguez de Santiago E, Tham TC, Thelin-Schmidt P, van Hooft JE. Diagnosis and management of acute lower gastrointestinal bleeding: European Society of Gastrointestinal Endoscopy (ESGE) Guideline. Endoscopy. 2021 Aug;53(8):850-868. doi: 10.1055/a-1496-8969. Epub 2021 Jun 1. Erratum in: Endoscopy. 2021 Jun 17;: PMID: 34062566.

14. Strate LL, Gralnek IM. ACG Clinical Guideline: Management of Patients With Acute Lower Gastrointestinal Bleeding. Am J Gastroenterol. 2016 Apr;111(4):459-74. doi: 10.1038/ajg.2016.41. Epub 2016 Mar 1. Erratum in: Am J Gastroenterol. 2016 May;111(5):755. PMID: 26925883; PMCID: PMC5099081.

15. Lee WM, Stravitz RT, Larson AM. Introduction to the revised American Association for the Study of Liver Diseases Position Paper on acute liver failure 2011. Hepatology. 2012 Mar;55(3):965-7. doi: 10.1002/hep.25551. PMID: 22213561; PMCID: PMC3378702.

16. Fyfe B, Zaldana F, Liu C. The pathology of acute liver failure. Clin Liver Dis 2018;22:257–68.

17. Bajaj JS, Kamath PS, Reddy KR. The evolving challenge of infections in cirrhosis. N Engl J Med 2021;384:2317-2330.

18. Sarin SK, Choudhury A, Sharma MK, et al. Acute-on-chronic liver failure: consensus recommendations of the Asian Pacific Association for the Study of the Liver (APASL): an update. Hepatol Int 2019;13:353-390.

19. M. Rovegno et al. / Annals of Hepatology 18 (2019) 543–552

20. Harry R, Auzinger G, Wendon J. The effects of supraphysiological doses of corticosteroids in hypotensive liver failure. Liver Int. 2003 Apr;23(2):71-7. doi: 10.1034/j.1600-0676.2003.00813.x. PMID: 12654129.

21. Alba L, Hay JE, Lee WM. Lactulose therapy in acute liver failure. J Hepatol 2002; 36:33A.

22. Rockey DC, Caldwell SH, Goodman ZD, Nelson RC, Smith AD. Ameri- can Association for the Study of Liver Diseases Liver biopsy. Hepatology 2009;49:1017–44.

23. European Association for the Study of the Liver. Electronic address: easloffice@easloffice.eu; Clinical practice guidelines panel, Wendon, J; Panel members, Cordoba J, Dhawan A, Larsen FS, Manns M, Samuel D, Simpson KJ, Yaron I; EASL Governing Board representative, Bernardi M. EASL Clinical Practical Guidelines on the management of acute (fulminant) liver failure. J Hepatol. 2017 May;66(5):1047-1081. doi: 10.1016/j.jhep.2016.12.003. PMID: 28417882.

24. Tripathi K, Feuerstein JD. Drugs in Context 2019; 8: 212572. DOI: 10.7573/dic.212572. ISSN: 1740-4398

25. M. Gajendran, P. Loganathan, A.P. Catinella, J.G. Hashash A comprehensive review and update on Crohn's disease Dis. Mon., 64 (2) (2018), pp. 20-57, 10.1016/j.disamonth.2017.07.001

Surgical Gastrointestinal Emergencies

Introduction

Surgical gastrointestinal emergencies are an important presentation to ED and we need to focus on identifying life-threatening problems. Patients usually come with common presentations of common problems. Unusual and rare presentations may need prompt intervention for stabilization and early diagnosis and management.

The following conditions are included in this chapter.

1. Acute Bowel Obstruction
2. Diverticulitis
3. Acute appendicitis
4. Acute Cholecystitis
5. Acute Pancreatitis
6. Perforated and bleeding peptic ulcer
7. Anorectal emergencies
8. Anorectal abscess
9. Perineal necrotizing fasciitis (Fournier's gangrene)

1. Acute Bowel Obstruction

What we already know:

- Bowel obstruction requires early identification of the cause and definitive intervention in a relatively short period of time to minimize morbidity and mortality.
- Adynamic ileus is usually self-limiting and does not require surgical intervention.
- Mechanical obstruction almost always requires surgical treatment.
- Differentiating small bowel from large bowel obstruction is important as the treatment varies.
- Adhesions remain the most common cause of small intestinal obstruction followed by incarcerated hernias.
- Neoplasms are the most common cause of large intestinal obstruction.

Recent Updates:

- The revised Bologna guidelines(2017) for the management of adhesive small bowel obstruction recommend that non-operative treatment should always be tried for a case of adhesive small bowel obstruction A(ASBO) unless there are signs of peritonitis, strangulation or bowel ischemia. (1)

- The cornerstone of non-operative management is nil per oral and decompression using a nasogastric tube or long intestinal tube. Non-operative management is effective in approximately 70–90% of patients with adhesive small bowel obstruction. (1)

- Non-operative management can be tried safely for 72 hours, during which time the imaging of choice would be CT with oral water-soluble contrast with a repeat X-ray in 24 hours. In the X-ray, if the contrast has reached the large bowel, the obstruction has resolved. (1)

- There is a higher rate of recurrence in patients who are treated nonoperatively because the cause of obstruction (adhesive disease) is not addressed. (2)

- In select patients with adhesive or partial SBO, oral administration of hypertonic water-soluble contrast media may have therapeutic effects and assist in resolution. Although the risk of vomiting and aspiration should be considered, a systematic review and meta-analysis of 14 prospective trials demonstrated a significant reduction in the need for surgery and shortened hospital stays in patients who received water-soluble contrast media. (2)

2. Diverticulitis

What we already know:

- The natural history of diverticulitis is usually benign and most cases can be managed medically, even with recurrent episodes.

- Observational treatment without antibiotics is appropriate for CT confirmed, uncomplicated acute diverticulitis in immunocompetent patients with mild symptoms.

- The 2015 American Gastroenterology Association guidelines recommended that antibiotics should be used selectively rather than routinely in patients with acute uncomplicated diverticulitis

- Complicated diverticulitis requires admission and in addition to bowel rest and antibiotics, may require surgery also.

Recent updates:

- The World Society of Emergency Surgery had published guidelines for the management of acute colonic diverticulitis in 2016 which were revised in 2020.

- Previously the Hinchey classification was used to classify diverticulitis with multiple modifications to it being suggested over time. The present WSES guidelines have proposed a new system of classification although they do not recommend any system to be superior.

- The WSES classification divides acute diverticulitis into 2 groups: uncomplicated and complicated. (3)

In the event of uncomplicated acute diverticulitis, the infection only involves the colon and does not extend to the peritoneum. In the event of complicated acute diverticulitis, the infectious process proceeds beyond the colon. Complicated acute diverticulitis is divided into 4 stages, based on the extension of the infectious process:

Uncomplicated diverticula: thickening of the wall, increased density of the pericolic fat

Complicated:

1a) Pericolic air bubbles or a small amount of pericolic fluid without abscess (within 5 cm from inflamed bowel segment)

1b) Abscess ≤ 4 cm

2a) Abscess > 4 cm

2b) Distant gas (> 5 cm from inflamed bowel segment)

3) Diffuse fluid without distant free gas

4) Diffuse fluid with distant free gas

- CECT abdomen is recommended as the imaging of the first choice. (3) (4)
- Image-guided percutaneous drainage is usually recommended for stable patients with abscesses >3 cm in size. (5)
- Tobacco cessation, reduced meat intake, physical activity and weight loss are recommended interventions to potentially reduce the risk of diverticulitis and therefore are useful discharge advice the emergency physician can give. (5)
- There is no evidence to support dietary restrictions during the acute stage. An unrestricted diet (when tolerated) is preferable. (4)
- Any evidence regarding bed rest is lacking and, since imposed physical inactivity may impair the patients' general condition, bed rest is not recommended. (4)
- Although a high-fibre diet may be recommendable for general health purposes, there is little evidence that it can prevent recurrent episodes or persistent symptoms in patients with acute diverticulitis. (4)
- It seems fairly safe to observe immunocompetent hemodynamically stable patients even if there are radiological signs of extraluminal air. Immediate surgery should be considered in hemodynamically unstable or septic patients. (4)

3. Acute appendicitis

What we already know:

- It is the most frequent cause of atraumatic abdominal pain in children and the most common non-obstetric surgical emergency in pregnancy.

- It must be considered in any patient with atraumatic right-sided abdominal, periumbilical or flank pain who has not previously undergone an appendicectomy.
- Ultrasound is the initial imaging modality of choice
- If USG is inconclusive, non-contrast CT is considered an acceptable modality.
- Alvarado score helps in the diagnosis and stratification of patients.
- The treatment is appendicectomy. While an antibiotics-only approach may be feasible and safe in select, uncomplicated patients, surgical management remains the accepted standard of care.

Recent updates:

- In July 2015, the World Society of Emergency Surgery (WSES) organized in Jerusalem the first consensus conference on the diagnosis and treatment of acute appendicitis (AA) in adult patients with the intention of producing evidence-based guidelines. An updated consensus conference took place in Nijemegen in June 2019 and the guidelines have now been updated in order to provide evidence-based statements and recommendations in keeping with varying clinical practice.
- Alvarado score is not recommended to positively confirm the clinical suspicion of acute appendicitis in adults.(6)
- The AIR (Appendicitis Inflammatory Response) score and the AAS (Acute Appendicitis Score) seem to be the best performing clinical prediction scores currently and have the highest discriminating power in adults with suspected acute appendicitis. The AIR and AAS scores decrease negative appendicectomy rates in low-risk groups and reduce the need for imaging studies and hospital admissions in both low- and intermediate-risk groups and hence are recommended as clinical predictors of acute appendicitis. (6)
- Although the Alvarado score is not sufficiently specific in diagnosing AA, a cutoff score of < 5 is sufficiently sensitive to exclude AA (sensitivity of 99%). The Alvarado score could, therefore, be used to reduce emergency department length of stay and radiation exposure in patients with suspected AA.(6)
- In paediatric appendicitis the two most used score were Alvarado score and Samuel's Pediatric Appendicitis Score (PAS). However, in a systematic review by Kulik et al. both scores failed to meet the performance benchmarks of CRP (C-reactive protein). On average, the PAS would over-diagnose AA by 35%, and the Alvarado score would do so by 32%.(6)
- A study by Macco et al. showed that the AIR had the highest discriminating power and outperformed the other two scores in predicting AA in children.(6)
- Recently, the new Pediatric Appendicitis Laboratory Score (PALabS) including clinical signs, leucocyte and neutrophil counts, CRP, and calprotectin levels has been shown to accurately

predict which children are at low risk of AA and could be safely managed with close observation. A PALabS ≤ 6 has a sensitivity of 99.2%, a negative predictive value of 97.6%, and a negative likelihood ratio of 0.03.(6)

- Contrast enhanced CT is now considered the imaging modality of choice in cases of diagnostic uncertainty over non-contrast CT and low dose contrast CT is said to be non-inferior to standard dose contrast CT.(6)

- Short, in-hospital surgical delay up to 24 h is safe in uncomplicated acute appendicitis and does not increase complications and/or perforation rate in adults. (6)

4. Acute Cholecystitis

What we already know:

- Gallstones are the cause of cholecystitis. Acalculous cholecystitis is a rare entity seen in critically ill patients.

- Abdominal ultrasound is the initial imaging modality of choice and contrast enhanced CT is recommended for confirmation and diagnosis of complications.

- Treatment is cholecystectomy.

Recent updates:

- Hepatobiliary iminodiacetic acid (HIDA) scan has the highest sensitivity and specificity for the diagnosis of ACC as compared to other imaging modalities.(7)

- Non-operative management is only recommended for patients refusing surgery or not suitable for surgery.(7)

- Antimicrobial regimens recommended for acute cholecystitis.

Good penetration efficiency Antibiotics Bile/serum (>=5)	Low penetration efficiency Antibiotics Bile/serum (<1)
Piperacillin/tazobactum	Cefotaxime
Tigecycline	Meropenem
Amoxicillin/clavulanate	Ceftazidime
Ciprofloxacin	Vancomycin
Ampicillin/Sulbactum	Amikacin
Ceftriaxone	Gentamicin
Levofloxacin	Cefepime
Penicillin G	Imipenem

Adopted from (7)

Classification system of the American Society of Gastrointestinal Endoscopy may be used to identify the risk of having associated common bile duct stones.(7)

5. Acute Pancreatitis

What we already know:

- Most cases are caused by gallstones or alcohol

- Most cases involve only mild inflammation and resolve with supportive care.

- Diagnosis is based on clinical findings, a serum lipase value elevated more than 3 times above the upper limit of normal and imaging findings.

- Treatment is supportive with aggressive hydration and control of pain and nausea.

- Prolonged bowel rest is not advisable.

Recent updates:

- Revised Atlanta Classification (RAC) and determinant-based classification (DBC) are 2 classification systems which are comparable in their efficacy maybe used interchangeably for classifying the severity of acute pancreatitis.(8)

- All patients with severe acute pancreatitis need to be assessed with contrast-enhanced computed tomography (CE-CT) or magnetic resonance imaging (MRI). Optimal timing for first the CE-CT assessment is 72–96 h after onset of symptoms.(8)

- C-reactive Protein level ≥ 150 mg/l at third day can be used as a prognostic factor for severe acute pancreatitis (2A).(8)

- Hematocrit > 44% represents an independent risk factor of pancreatic necrosis.(8)

- In the absence of gallstones or significant history of alcohol use, serum triglyceride and calcium levels should be measured. Serum triglyceride levels over 11.3 mmol/l (1000 mg/dl) indicate it as the etiology.(8)

- In idiopathic pancreatitis, biliary etiology should be ruled out with two ultrasound examinations, and if needed MRCP and/or endoscopic ultrasound EUS, to prevent recurrent pancreatitis(8)

- There are no "gold standard" prognostic score for predicting severe acute pancreatitis. Probably the bedside index of severity of acute pancreatitis (BISAP) score is one of the most accurate and applicable in everyday clinical practice because of the simplicity and the capability to predict severity, death, and organ failure as well as the APACHE-II (very complex) and other scores.(8)

- Recent evidences have shown that prophylactic antibiotics in patients with acute pancreatitis are not associated with a significant decrease in mortality or morbidity. Thus, routine prophylactic antibiotics are no longer recommended for all patients with acute pancreatitis (8)

- Procalcitonin is the most sensitive laboratory test for detection of pancreatic infection, and low serum values appear to be strong negative predictors of infected necrosis. Antibiotics are always recommended to treat infected severe acute pancreatitis. In patients with infected necrosis, the spectrum of empirical antibiotic regimen should include both aerobic and anaerobic Gram-negative and Gram-positive microorganisms. (8)

- Enteral nutrition is recommended to prevent gut failure and infectious complications. Total parenteral nutrition (TPN) should be avoided but partial parenteral nutrition integration should be considered to reach caloric and protein requirements if the enteral route is not completely tolerated(8)

6. Perforated and bleeding peptic ulcer:

In spite of various preventive strategies for use in peptic ulcer disease, complications like perforation and bleeding are not unusual.

In any emergency situation, a rapid ABC (airway, breathing, and circulation) evaluation should be done. Adopting scoring systems (SOFA, qSOFA) to evaluate and assess the severity of the disease in patients with perforated peptic ulcer (Weak recommendation based on low-quality evidences, 2 C) is suggested. The appropriate targets for resuscitation (the same used for sepsis and septic shock need to be considered. [9]

In general, the most important are:

- Mean arterial pressure (MAP) ≥ 65 mmHg
- Urine output ≥ 0.5 ml/kg/h
- Lactate normalization

7. Anorectal emergencies

This includes anorectal pain and bleeding, requiring emergency care.

This is a very common condition and may be life-threatening in some that require correct diagnosis and prompt management.

Patients delay reporting due to the embarrassment related to the affected anatomical region and present late and many times lack a timely proper clinical examination.

WSES-AAST guidelines (10) is an evidence-based international consensus statement on the management of anorectal emergencies in adult patients with suspected anorectal emergencies from the collaboration of a panel of experts. This has incorporated 7 main conditions namely retained anorectal bodies, perineal necrotizing fasciitis, complicated haemorrhoids, acute anal fissure, anorectal abscess, bleeding anorectal varices, complicated anorectal prolapse.

8. Anorectal abscess

This is characterized by an infection in the soft tissue around the anus and in about third of patients is associated with anal fistulas.

In patients with anorectal abscess and an obvious fistula, we suggest to perform a fistulotomy at the time of abscess drainage only in cases of low fistula not involving sphincter muscle (i.e., subcutaneous fistula) (weak recommendation based on low-quality evidence, 2C).

In patients with anorectal abscess and an obvious fistula involving any sphincter muscle, we suggest to place a loose draining seton (weak recommendation based on low-quality evidence, 2C).

In patients with anorectal abscess and no obvious fistula, we suggest against probing to search for a possible fistula, to avoid iatrogenic complications (weak recommendation based on low-quality evidence, 2C).

9. Perineal necrotizing fasciitis (Fournier's gangrene)

This is a rare but potentially life-threatening necrotizing infection involving the fascia and subcutaneous tissues of the external genitalia or perineum and may present or progress to septic shock and multiple organ failure. An impaired host resistance from reduced cellular immunity are associated with increased risk of Fournier's gangrene (i.e., diabetes, alcoholism, HIV, leukemia). Though idiopathic, the infection is typically polymicrobial. The predominant symptoms include perineal and/or scrotal pain, swelling, and erythema, along with fever, tachycardia, purulent discharge, crepitus progressing to florid gangrene. Testis is usually spared. It is a time sensitive disease and prompt recognition and treatment is of utmost importance.

In patients with suspected Fournier's gangrene, WSES-AAST guidelines suggested to use Laboratory Risk Indicator for Necrotising Fasciitis (LRINEC) score for an early diagnosis and Fournier's Gangrene Severity Index (FGSI) for prognosis and risk stratification (weak recommendation based on moderate quality evidence, 2B).

In patients with Fournier's gangrene, imaging should not delay surgical intervention (strong recommendation based on moderate quality evidence, 1B), along with prompt and aggressive antimicrobial therapy.

Summary:

All the common and some of the uncommon or unusual presentations of gastrointestinal emergencies and the recent updates are covered in the chapter. Time sensitive emergencies require recognition and proper interventions in the ED.

References

1. Broek RPG, Krielen P, Di Saverio S, Coccolini F, Biffl WL, Ansaloni L, et al. Bologna guidelines for diagnosis and management of adhesive small bowel obstruction (ASBO): 2017 update of the evidence-based guidelines from the world society of emergency surgery ASBO working group. World Journal of Emergency Surgery. 2018 Jun 19;13(1):24.

2. Jackson P, Cruz MV. Intestinal Obstruction: Evaluation and Management. AFP. 2018 Sep 15;98(6):362–7.

3. Sartelli M, Weber DG, Kluger Y, Ansaloni L, Coccolini F, Abu-Zidan F, et al. 2020 update of the WSES guidelines for the management of acute colonic diverticulitis in the emergency setting. World Journal of Emergency Surgery. 2020 May 7;15(1):32.

4. Schultz JK, Azhar N, Binda GA, Barbara G, Biondo S, Boermeester MA, et al. European Society of Coloproctology: guidelines for the management of diverticular disease of the colon. Colorectal Disease. 2020;22(S2):5–28.

5. Hall J, Hardiman K, Lee S, Lightner A, Stocchi L, Paquette IM, et al. The American Society of Colon and Rectal Surgeons Clinical Practice Guidelines for the Treatment of Left-Sided Colonic Diverticulitis. Diseases of the Colon & Rectum. 2020 Jun;63(6):728–47.

6. Di Saverio S, Podda M, De Simone B, Ceresoli M, Augustin G, Gori A, et al. Diagnosis and treatment of acute appendicitis: 2020 update of the WSES Jerusalem guidelines. World Journal of Emergency Surgery. 2020 Apr 15;15(1):27.

7. Pisano M, Allievi N, Gurusamy K, Borzellino G, Cimbanassi S, Boerna D, et al. 2020 World Society of Emergency Surgery updated guidelines for the diagnosis and treatment of acute calculus cholecystitis. World Journal of Emergency Surgery. 2020 Nov 5;15(1):61.

8. Leppäniemi A, Tolonen M, Tarasconi A, Segovia-Lohse H, Gamberini E, Kirkpatrick AW, et al. 2019 WSES guidelines for the management of severe acute pancreatitis. World Journal of Emergency Surgery. 2019 Jun 13;14(1):27.

9. Tarasconi A, Coccolini F, Biffl WL, Tomasoni M, Ansaloni L, Picetti E, Molfino S, Shelat V, Cimbanassi S, Weber DG, Abu-Zidan FM, Campanile FC, Di Saverio S, Baiocchi GL, Casella C, Kelly MD, Kirkpatrick AW, Leppaniemi A, Moore EE, Peitzman A, Fraga GP, Ceresoli M, Maier RV, Wani I, Pattonieri V, Perrone G, Velmahos G, Sugrue M, Sartelli M, Kluger Y, Catena F. Perforated and bleeding peptic ulcer: WSES guidelines. World J Emerg Surg. 2020 Jan 7;15:3. doi: 10.1186/s13017-019-0283-9. PMID: 31921329; PMCID: PMC6947898.

10. Tarasconi A, Perrone G, Davies J, Coimbra R, Moore E, Azzaroli F, Abongwa H, De Simone B, Gallo G, Rossi G, Abu-Zidan F, Agnoletti V, de'Angelis G, de'Angelis N, Ansaloni L, Baiocchi GL, Carcoforo P, Ceresoli M, Chichom-Mefire A, Di Saverio S, Gaiani F, Giuffrida M, Hecker A, Inaba K, Kelly M, Kirkpatrick A, Kluger Y, Leppäniemi A, Litvin A, Ordoñez C, Pattonieri V, Peitzman A, Pikoulis M, Sakakushev B, Sartelli M, Shelat V, Tan E, Testini M, Velmahos G, Wani I, Weber D, Biffl W, Coccolini F, Catena F. Anorectal emergencies: WSES-AAST guidelines. World J Emerg Surg. 2021 Sep 16;16(1):48. doi: 10.1186/s13017-021-00384-x. PMID: 34530908; PMCID: PMC8447593.

Obstetric Emergencies

Contributors

1. Dr. Ruby Bhatia
2. Dr. Rohan Bhatia

Chapters

1. Preeclampsia
2. Eclampsia

Preeclampsia

<u>PREVENTION AND MANAGEMENT OF ECLAMPSIA</u>

An eclamptic fit usually preceded by pre monitoring symptoms and signs of pre-eclampsia headache, epigastric pain, blurring of vision and sudden rise of blood pressure and increase reflexes. Rarely it may occur without warning sign in woman who appear to be imperfect health.

There is an unmet need in recognizing and managing hypertensive disorder of pregnancy in developing countries [Hypertensive disorders form a deadly triad along with hemorrhage and infection as a direct cause of near miss and maternal mortality accounting for sixteen percent in developed world, one forth or twenty six percent in Arabian and Latin America and nine percent of all maternal deaths in Asia and Africa.[2,3]

- Hypertensive disorders affect ten percent of all pregnancies globally. Of these preeclampsia and eclampsia occur in two to eight percent and is most ominous. Eclampsia occurs in 1.9 percent of all pregnancies with maternal deaths as high as four to six percent in India as reported by national eclampsia registry[4].

Hypertensive disorder in pregnancy may be classified into:

- Gestational hypertension
- Pre-eclampsia/ Eclampsia syndrome
  - Early onset pre-eclampsia <34 weeks
  - Late onset pre-eclampsia >34 weeks
- Chronic Hypertension
- Pre-eclampsia superimposed on chronic hypertension (ACOG2013B, reaffirmed 2019)[5].

  Preeclampsia & eclampsia syndrome are clinical **spectrum** of worsening disease with attenuated manifestation to cataclysmic deterioration associated with multiorgan dysfunction life threatening for both mother and fetus.

- **Preeclampsia is defined as Systolic blood pressure ≥140 mmHg and diastolic blood pressure ≥90 mmHg on at least 2 occasions at least four hours apart after 20 weeks of gestation in a previously normotensive patient and the new onset of one or more of the following:**

  Proteinuria ≥0.3 g in a 24-hour urine specimen or protein/creatinine ratio ≥0.3 (mg/mg) (30 mg/mmol) in a random urine specimen or dipstick ≥2+ if a quantitative measurement is unavailable

- Platelet count less than one lakh micromole/L
- >1.1 mg/dL (97.2 micromole/L) or doubling of the creatinine concentration in the absence of other renal disease
- Liver transaminases at least twice the upper limit of the normal concentrations for the local laboratory
- Pulmonary edema
- New-onset and persistent headache not accounted for by alternative diagnoses and not responding to usual doses of analgesics
- Visual symptoms (e.g., blurred vision, flashing lights or sparks, scotomata)

Preeclampsia is considered superimposed when it occurs in a woman with chronic hypertension. It is characterized by worsening or resistant hypertension (especially acutely), the new onset of proteinuria or a sudden increase in proteinuria, and/or significant new end-organ dysfunction after 20 weeks of gestation in a woman with chronic hypertension.

If systolic blood pressure is ≥160 mmHg or diastolic blood pressure is ≥110 mmHg, confirmation within minutes is sufficient. Response to analgesia does not exclude the possibility of preeclampsia. Adapted from: American College of Obstetricians and Gynecologists (ACOG) Practice Bulletin No. 222[6]: Gestational Hypertension and Preeclampsia. Obstet Gynecol 2020; 135:e237[7]

Indicators of severity of gestational hypertension/preeclampsia[8]

ABNORMALITY	NON SEVERE	SEVERE
Diastolic BP	<110 mm Hg	>=110 mm Hg
Systolic BP	<160 mm Hg	>=160 mm Hg
Proteinuria	None to positive	None to positive
New onset Headache	Absent	Present
Visual disturbances	Absent	Present
Upper abdominal pain	Absent	Present
Oliguria	Absent	Present
Convulsions (eclampsia)	Absent	Present
Serum creatinine	Normal	Elevated
Thrombocytopenia	Absent	Present
Serum transaminase elevation	Absent	Present
Fetal growth restriction	Absent	Present
Pulmonary edema	Absent	Present

Presence of one or more of the following indicates a diagnosis of "preeclampsia with severe features"

A. **Severe blood pressure elevation:** Systolic blood pressure ≥160 mmHg or diastolic blood pressure ≥110 mmHg on 2 occasions at least 4 hours apart while the patient is on bedrest; however, antihypertensive therapy generally should be initiated upon confirmation of severe hypertension, in which case criteria for severe blood pressure elevation can be satisfied without waiting until 4 hours have elapsed.

B. **Symptoms of central nervous system dysfunction:** New-onset cerebral or visual disturbance, such as: Photophobia, scotomata, cortical blindness, retinal vasospasm Severe headache (ie, incapacitating, "the worst headache I've ever had") or headache that persists and progresses despite analgesic therapy and not accounted for by alternative diagnoses

C. **Hepatic abnormality:** Impaired liver function not accounted for by another diagnosis and characterized by serum transaminase concentration >2 times the upper limit of the normal range or severe persistent right upper quadrant or epigastric pain unresponsive to medication and not accounted for by an alternative diagnosis

D. **Thrombocytopenia:** <1lakh/micromole/l

E. **Serum creatinine** concentration >1.1 mg/dl [97.2 micromole/L] or the doubling creatinine concentration in the absence of other renal disease)

F. **Pulmonary edema ACOG 2020 practice bulletin**[6]

Etiopathogenesis of preeclampsia:

Endovascular defective trophoblastic remodeling of spiral arterioles by extra villous trophoblast-small caliber vessel with high resistance to flow leading to endothelial cell activation and inflammation which further causing endothelial cell injury and atherosis with system wise micro coagulation and increased capillary permeability leading to thrombocytopenia, proteinuria and edema.

Endothelin's ET1, sFLT-1 & soluble endoglins increase while VEGF & PGF decreases Combination of uteroplacental ischemia with increased anti angiogenic factors with angiogenic imbalance triggers clinical spectrum of pre-eclampsia there is Intense vasospasm and Increase sensitivity to vasopressor substances Angiotensin -2 and Proteinuria is an objective marker reflecting system wide endothelial leak that characterizes Pre-eclampsia syndrome.

Eclampsia

- Eclampsia is defined by new onset focal or multifocal tonic clonic seizures or coma in a woman with preeclampsia (including HELLP syndrome or gestational hypertension) in the absence of other causative conditions as epilepsy, cerebral arterial ischemia- infarction, intracranial hemorrhage or drug use.

- Eclampsia is a clinical diagnosis and most ominous Incidence of eclampsia -1.5-10/10,000 deliveries (developed countries), 19.6-142/10,000 deliveries in developing countries, 2-3% in severe pre-eclampsia 0-0.6% - when anti-seizure prophylaxis not taken, Recurrence rate of eclampsia is one in every five pregnancies. ACOG practice bulletin June 2020[6]

- Eclampsia may occur in antepartum (38-53%), intrapartum (15-20%), post-partum (11-44%) and is most common in the third trimester. RISING TRENDS in postpartum eclampsia are observed

- Convulsions occurring < 20 wks. pregnancy or 48hrs postpartum is atypical eclampsia

- In fifty percent eclampsia occurs pre-term while in 20-30% it occurs between 20-30 weeks of gestation. With perinatal mortality as high as fifty percent in eclampsia, prematurity rather than eclampsia is the culprit.

Pathogenesis in Eclampsia

Hypertension - Breakdown of auto regulatory system in cerebral circulation – Hyper perfusion – endothelial dysfunction- Vasogenic/ cytotoxic edema. OR Hypertension – activation of auto regulatory system- Vasoconstriction of cerebral vessels – leading to hypoperfusion- ischemia- endothelial dysfunction – vasogenic/cytotoxic edema. Med Hypothesis 2014; 82:619, PLoS One 2014; 9: e 113670[9]. **Hemoconcentration is hallmark of eclampsia,** Normal hypervolemia of pregnancy is absent, Aggressive fluid therapy must be avoided in all cases of pre-eclampsia syndrome to prevent pulmonary edema, Do not use volume expansion, Limit maintenance fluid to 80ml/hr unless ongoing fluid losses.

Prevention of Eclampsia

1. Preconception counseling
2. Early detection of high-risk factors for prediction of pre-eclampsia to implement preventive measures before 16weeks of gestation.
3. Early diagnosis & treatment of pre-eclampsia non severe and gestational hypertension

4. Early diagnosis & treatment of preeclampsia with severe features
5. Preconception counseling for early detection of high-risk factor of pre-eclampsia remains cornerstone for prevention of eclampsia

High risk factors: Incidence 8% or more.

- Previous pregnancy with pre-eclampsia, especially early onset with adverse outcome.
- Multi fetal gestation.
- Chronic hypertension.
- Type 1 or 2 Diabetes mellitus.
- Chronic kidney disease
- Autoimmune disease (APLA, SLE).

Moderate risk factors:

- Nulliparity
- OBESITY-4.3% with BMI < 20 Kg/m2,13.3% with BMI >35 Kg/m2
- Family history of preeclampsia in mother or sister.
- Age >= 35 years.
- Sociodemographic characteristics. (African, American race, low socioeconomic level).
- Personal risk factors – previous pregnancy with LBW/ FGR/ stillbirth/ interval > 10 years between pregnancies.

Multiple moderate risk factors = High risk (UPSTF recommendation statement. Ann Intern Med 2014, 161:819)[10], **Most risk factors for pre-eclampsia are not modifiable-**Obesity and excessive gestational weight gain are modifiable risk factors, Smoking- reduces risk for hypertension during pregnancy, as it upregulates placental adrenomedullin expression & volume homeostasis, Women with any 1 high risk or 2 moderate risks should receive 81mg / day low dose aspirin between 12-28 weeks (<16 weeks) until delivery. (ACOG 2020)[6]. Genetic predisposition may also be etiological factors for pre-eclampsia and eclampsia 20-40% daughters of preeclampsia mothers, 11-37% sisters of preeclamptic women,22-47% twin sisters, 60% of monozygotic female twins may have preeclampsia

FOGSI-GESTOSIS-ICOG GCPR 2019 has listed following as high-risk factors for preeclampsia and eclampsia[1]

RISK FACTOR	SCORE
Age older than 35 years	1
Age younger than 19 years	1
Maternal anaemia	1
Obesity (BMI>30)	1
Primigravida	1
Short duration of sperm exposure (cohabitation)	1
Woman born as small for gestational age	1
Family history of cardiovascular disease	1
Polycystic ovary syndrome	1
Inter pregnancy interval more than 7 years	1
Conceived with Assisted Reproductive (IVF/ICSI) Treatment	1
MAP >85 mmHg	1
Chronic vascular disease (Dyslipidemia)	1
Excessive weight gain during pregnancy	1
Maternal hypothyroidism	2
Family history of preeclampsia	2
Gestational diabetes mellitus	2
Obesity (BMI>35kg/M^2)	2
Multifetal pregnancy	2
Hypertensive disease during previous pregnancy	2
Pregestational diabetes mellitus	3
Chronic hypertension	3
Mental disorders	3
Inherited / Acquired Thrombophilia	3
Maternal chronic kidney disease	3
Autoimmune disease (SLE/APLAS/RA)	3
Pregnancy with Assisted Reproductive (OD/ Surrogacy) Treatment	3

Preventive measures

- Low dose aspirin 81mg daily at bedtime w.e.f. from 12- 28weeks preferably before 16wks. discontinued ecosprin 5- 10 days before delivery 100- 150[6,10] mgs/day, Low dose acetyl salicylic acid (75mg/day) in high-risk women, started before 16 wks. of pregnancy[11], Low dose Aspirin 75-150mg /day in high-risk women before 12 weeks[1,12]. With good compliance > 90% in high-risk women leads to more than 10% reduction in incidence of pre-eclampsia, FGR and preterm birth.

- High dose Calcium supplementation 1.5-2.0gm daily. Dietary manipulation - ample amount of protein, no salt restriction, pre pregnancy weight loss in over weight and obese women, Advice for rest, exercise and work to all women with gestational hypertension, pre-eclampsia and chronic hypertension should be same as for normal pregnant woman, Role of metformin, sildenafil, statin - for prevention of pre-eclampsia investigation, not to be recommended outside clinical trials[1,6,11,12].

STANDARD PRENATAL CARE WITH CLOSE FOLLOW UP OF HIGH-RISK WOMEN FROM MID GESTATION IS ADVISED IN FOLLOWING CONDITION

- Women without overt hypertension with suspicion of early developing eclampsia
- New onset DBP>80
- Sudden abnormal wt gain > 2 pounds /wk
- A sudden rise in MAP (DELTA HYPERTENSION)
- Rise in 30 mm hg SBP or 15 mm of hg DBP
- Close observation for eclampsia & HELLP syndrome while still normotensive

OUTPATIENT SURVEILLANCE AT 7 DAY INTERVAL TILL OVERT HYPERTENSION & FEATURES OF PREECLAMPSIA SUPERVENES

An increased MAP >85 or >90mmhg predicts transient hypertension and a small risk of developing preeclampsia, MAP is a better predictor for preeclampsia than systolic, diastolic BP or increased blood pressure

Early diagnosis & treatment OF GESTATIONAL HYPERTENSION/ non-severe pre-eclampsia prevents eclampsia,- Women with gestational hypertension/non severe preeclampsia with no indication for delivery at <37 wks. Expectant management with maternal & fetal monitoring is suggested, Women with gestational hypertension or non-severe pre-eclampsia at or beyond 37 weeks, delivery rather than continued observation is suggested[1,6,12.]

Strict bed rest or rest at home is not recommended in women at risk. Diet rich in calories with ample proteins/no salt restrictions, Sodium and fluid intake should not be limited or forced. Goal is to keep B.P. 130/85 mmHg- **Antihypertensives**, Tab. Labetalol 100-200mg bd/ tds till max. 2400mg/day or Tab Nifedipine 10 mg bd/tds, max. 90 mg/day or Tab Methyldopa 500mg 6-8 hrly, max 2gm/day for control of blood pressure is recommended.

Antihypertensives are recommended for treatment at BP > 140 mm systolic or > 90 mm Hg diastolic or both[1,12]

ACOG 2019/2020[6] do not recommend antihypertensives if blood pressure is less than 160/100mmhg.

Women with gestational hypertension/non severe preeclampsia may be discharged after 72 hours with follow up after 2 weeks,6-8 weeks and 12 weeks[1,6,11,12]

Instruct to report immediately- symptoms of impending eclampsia are headache not accounted for by alternative diagnosis and not responding to usual dose of analgesics, blurring of vision, flashing lights, sparks, scotoma, epigastric pain, photophobia[1,6,12]

Progression to severe preeclampsia could happen within days in non-severe preeclampsia. Progression to severe preeclampsia in mild gestational hypertension could develop within 1 to 3 wks. Best practice indicates hospitalization in level II or III in all cases of severe/ imminent/ impending eclampsia. Termination of pregnancy is the only cure for preeclampsia. Never allow pregnancy to be postdated[1,6,12]

- Magnesium sulphate not to be administered universally for prevention of eclampsia in women with BP< 160/110 mm of Hg and with no symptoms of imminent eclampsia[1,12] However ACOG 2020[6] keeps IT OPTIONAL as per clinician choice.

Symptoms and Signs of Imminent/ impending Eclampsia:

Severe headache, Drowsiness, Mental confusion, Visual disturbances (e.g., blurred vision, flashes of light, double vision, photophobia), Epigastric pain/right upper quadrant pain, Nausea, vomiting, Shortness of breath, Decreased urinary output. Rarely prodormal symptoms MAY BE ABSENT. A sharp rise in the BP, Increased proteinuria, Exaggerated knee jerk may be reported before eclampsia.

ALL Cases of SEVERE PREECLAMPSIA/ IMPENDING/IMMINENT ECLAMPSIA to be treated as eclampsia hospitalization in level 2 or 3 -mandatory. GOAL is to forestall convulsions, prevent Intracranial hemorrhage, Prevent serious damage to vital organs, Safety of mother, Delivery of a healthy newborn

CLINICAL MANAGEMENT ALGORITHM FOR SUSPECTED SEVERE PREECLAMPSIA AT <34 WEEKS[8]

SEVERE PRE-ECLAMPSIA

- Admit
- Maternal & fetal assessment
- Consider Mgso4
- Treat dangerous hypertension

CONTRAINDICATIONS TO CONSERVATIVE MANAGEMENT

Uncontrolled severe hypertension

Eclampsia, Pulmonary edema,

Persistent headache refractory to treatment,

HELLP syndrome, Epigastric pain

Visual disturbances, Altered sensorium,

Significant renal dysfunction, Coagulopathy

Stroke, MI, Abruption

Previable fetus, Fetal compromise, persistent reverse end diastolic flow- Umbilical artery

Fetal death

INDICATIONS FOR DELIVERY IN severe preeclampsia <34 Weeks GESTATION

Corticosteroid therapy for lung maturation and immediate delivery after maternal stabilization (initial dose only, don't delay delivery)

A. **MATERNAL INDICATION-** Uncontrolled severe hypertension, Eclampsia, Pulmonary oedema, Placental abruption, DIC, non-reassuring fetal status, Fetal demise

B. **FETAL INDICATION-** Severe FGR, Persistent oligohydramnios, BPP 4/10 or less on two occasions 6 hrs apart, Reversed End diastolic flow in umbilical A doppler, Recurrent variable late decelerations in NST, Fetal death

Delivery decision should not be based on amount of proteinuria, Severe preeclampsia before fetal viability delivery after maternal stabilization should be planned as expectant management not recommended.

- **MANAGEMENT OF ECLAMPSIA:** New onset generalized tonic clonic seizures/convulsions or coma in women with preeclampsia not attributed to other causes, Hypertension>=160/110, proteinuria, multiorgan dysfunction and convulsions

  Status Eclampticus is defined as convulsions or eclamptic fits that continue incessantly one after the other Dangerous for both mother and fetus with High maternal and fetal mortality.

  Stages of an Eclamptic fit- 1. Premonitory stage: 10-20 seconds, eyes roll or stare, muscles of the face and hand(s) twitch, loss of consciousness.

  2. Tonic stage: 10-20 second, muscles go stiff or rigid, diaphragm in spasm, breathing stops, cyanosis occurs, back may be arched, teeth are clenched; eyes bulge.

  3. Clonic stage: 1-2 minutes, violent contraction and relaxation of the muscle, increased salivation causing "frothing", deep, noisy breathing, inhalation of mucus or saliva, face congested and swollen, tongue may be bitten by violent clenching of the teeth and jaws.

  4. Coma Stage (Post Ictal phase): several minutes or hours/days, stage of deep unconsciousness, breathing is noisy and rapid, cyanosis fades, face congested and swollen, further fits may occur before the woman, regains consciousness

FETAL RESPONSE TO ECLAMPSIA: Fetal bradycardia for at least three to five minutes is common after the seizure, Resolution of maternal seizure activity is associated with loss of variability, fetal tachycardia and transient decelerations, FHS improves with maternal and fetal therapeutic interventions, A non-reassuring FHS with frequent recurrent decelerations for > 10-15mins despite maternal/fetal resuscitative interventions suggests occult abruption.

RECOMMENDED LEVEL OF CRITICAL CARE FOR MANAGEMENT

LEVEL I- Preeclampsia with hypertension

LEVEL II- Severe preeclampsia with: Eclampsia, HELLP Syndrome, Hemorrhage, Hyperkalemia, Severe oliguria, Coagulation support, IV Antihypertensive treatment, Initial stabilization of severe hypertension, Evidence of cardiac failure, Abnormal neurology

LEVEL III- Severe preeclampsia and eclampsia needing assisted ventilatory support.

Patients should be managed In Eclampsia room in HDU Obstetrics, with Multidisciplinary approach, Inform consultant obstetrician/anesthetist/HDU team/ pediatrician and 1:1 nursing care, Eclampsia Tray should always be ready, Never leave the patient alone

STEPS OF MANAGEMENT-

1. Prevention of maternal hypoxia and trauma
2. Prevention of recurrent seizures.
3. Treatment of severe hypertension
4. Controlling the fluid balance
5. Evaluation for prompt delivery.
6. Care after delivery
7. Postpartum follow up

MAINTAIN AIRWAY PATENCY AND PREVENT ASPIRATION.

Place the woman on her left side, use a bed with padded railing, in a dark room, Clean the mouth and nostrils by gentle suction, Give oxygen 8-10L/min and continue for five minutes after each fit, or longer if cyanosis persists. **Make sure that:** airway remains clear, injury, especially tongue bite, is prevented during the clonic stage of convulsions, by placing padded tongue blades between her teeth; however do NOT attempt this during a convulsion.

Control the fits: Magnesium sulphate (MgSO47H2OUSP) drug of choice worldwide.

- Reduces recurrent seizures by ½ to 2/3 and maternal death by 1/3.
- Low cost
- Ease of administration.
- Cardiac monitoring is unnecessary.
- Lack of sedation.
- Reduces risk of cerebral palsy & severe motor dysfunction in fetus born prematurely.

Following regimens for control of fits in eclampsia are used worldwide:

(A) Continuous intravenous infusion- Zuspan Regimen

4-6g loading dose diluted in 100ml IV fluid administered over 15-20min

Begin 2g/hr or 1g/hr in 100ml of IV maintenance infusion

Assess deep tendon reflexes periodically

Maintain Serum magnesium levels between 4-7 mEq/l

Measure magnesium level if serum creatinine >1 mg/dl

Discontinue 24hrs after delivery

For settings where it's not possible to administer the full magnesium sulphate regimen, the use of magnesium sulphate loading dose followed by immediate transfer to a higher-level health care facility is recommended for women with severe preeclampsia & eclampsia

A lower dose maintenance regimen 2.5gm intramuscular every four hours may also be effective as well as cost effective in low resource area.[6,11]

(B) Intermittent intramuscular injection- Pritchard's Regimen

Loading dose: Inj. Magnesium sulphate 4-6 g (20 ml of 20% solution), slow IV, at the rate of 1 ml every minute. Thereafter administer Inj. Magnesium sulphate 5 g (10 ml of 50% solution), deep IM, with 1 ml of 2% Lignocaine in the same syringe in each gluteus. Every 4hr thereafter 5 g of 50% magnesium sulphate deep in upper outer quadrants alternate buttocks, only after ensuring:

- patellar reflex present
- Respiratory rate >12/min
- Urine output>100ml in previous 4hrs
- SPO_2 >92% at room air

Discontinue magnesium sulphate 24- 48hr after delivery or last fit whichever is later

MAGNESIUM SULPHATE TOXICITY

- Deep tendon reflexes are lost at serum magnesium levels of 7meq/l, Respiratory depression at 10 meq/l and Cardiac arrest at 25 meq/l
- Reduce maintenance dose by half if serum creatinine is 1 to 1.5mg/dl. Withhold magnesium sulphate maintenance dose if serum creatinine >1.5mg/dl or urinary output < 20ml/hour.

Contraindication to magnesium sulphate: Myasthenia Gravis, Hypocalcemia, Moderate to severe renal failure, Cardiac ischemia / heart block / myocarditis

Precautions: Do NOT give 50% Magnesium sulphate solution intravenously without diluting it20%.

- Do NOT give a rapid IV infusion, as it can cause respiratory failure or death.
- If respiratory depression occurs (RR <16 breaths/minute) after giving Magnesium sulphate, discontinue the drug. Give the antidote; Calcium gluconate 10 mg IV (10 ml of 10% solution) over a period of 10 minutes[6,11,9]
- Women who require LSCS should continue magnesium sulphate infusion during delivery, Magnesium sulphate prolongs duration of nondepolarizing muscle relaxants with a half-life of 5 hrs, discontinuing iv magnesium sulphate infusion before cesarean delivery minimally reduces Magnesium concentration & increases the risk of seizures

Failure of Magnesium Sulphate: woman has convulsions despite magnesium sulphate:

1. One convulsion within 30min – No further treatment
2. More than one convulsion within 30 minute or convulsion after 30 minute– Additional 2g 20% Magnesium sulphate @ 1g/ min which may be given twice if required at interval of 15 mins.

If fits still not controlled:

- **Na Amobarbital** 250mg IV in 3 minutes
- **Thiopental / Phenytoin** 4mg/ml in NS (1g in 250ml NS) @ 25mg/min)- 1250mg IV Patient should be on Cardiac monitor.
- Endotracheal intubation & assisted ventilators in ICU
- **Diazepam** 10mgIV slowly over 2 minutes. Can repeat the loading dose after 10 mins. Maximum 30mg. Maintenance dose Diazepam 40 mg in 500ml NS/RL titrated to keep women sedated but able to be roused.
- **Lorazepam** 4 mg IV over 2 minutes
- **Midazolam** 1-2mg IV @ 2 mg/min. Repeat every 5 mins until seizures stop. Max dose 2mg/kg body weight.

Controlling the blood pressure emergency therapy (ACOG Practice Bulletin 2020)[6]

- In severe pre-eclampsia and eclampsia injectable anti-hypertensives are recommended if BP $\geq$ 160/110mmhg. Goal: keep the diastolic pressure between 90 and 105 mmHg / systolic 140 to 155 mmHg to prevent cerebral hemorrhage.
- **Labetalol** Alpha1 beta blocker, 20mg IV over 2 mins followed by double dose at 10min interval up to 80mg with a total of 300mg (20-40-80-80 mg), 200mg orally 12 hourly up to 2400mg,

B.P. uncontrolled- Change Anti-hypertensive. Contraindication: Myocardial disease, Asthma, Decompensated cardiac failure.

- **Hydralazine** 5 mg slow IV in 3-4 min followed by 5-10mg at 15-20 min until diastolic BP b/w 90-110, Total dose-20mg/treatment cycle, Onset of action 10min, sudden hypotension. Side effects: tachycardia, nausea and vomiting, headache, muscle tremors, fetal distress; a sudden fall in BP-reduced uteroplacental perfusion

- **Nifedipine** Calcium channel blocker, 10 mg orally, repeat in 30mins up to maximum of 90 mg in 24hrs, never give sublingual nifedipine, Nifedipine extended release 30mg orally.

USE WITH CAUTION: Concomitant use of nifedipine and parenteral Magnesium sulphate may cause profound hypotension, Theoretical concern exists that the combined use of nifedipine and Magnesium sulphate can result in excessive hypotension and neuromuscular blockade[6,9,11]

- **Nicardipine** parenteral 3-9mg/hour IV infusion with programmed infusion pump.

- **Nitroglycerine:** 50mg NTG in 500ml isotonic saline, drug concentration of 100mcg/ml, Start @5mcg/min and increase by 5mcg/min every 5 minutes to max up to 200mcg/min, Infusion rate @5mcg/min corresponds to 3ml/hr and for every increment by 5mcg/min, increase rate by 3ml/hr.

LABETALOL AND HYDRALAZINE ARE THE DRUG OF CHOICE FOR MANAGEMENT OF HYPERTENISVE CRISIS IN ECLAMPSIA

Fluid balance: Restrict fluid intake, sodium lactate or 5% dextrose @ 80 ml (maximum) per hour unless there is an unusual fluid loss from vomiting, diarrhea, or excessive blood loss at delivery. Catheterise after stabilization (1hr), Record the urine output every 4 hours, urine output <100 ml per 4 hours, Suspect renal failure

Delivery of the baby: Eclampsia per se isn't an indication for cesarean section. Mode of delivery determined by: Gestational age, fetal presentation, Bishop score, Maternal fetal condition. Steps to affect vaginal delivery are to be used initially. Wait for 15-20mins until the mother and fetus show signs of recovery (control of seizures, mother oriented to Time, Place, Person fetal heat reassuring) before proceeding for cesarean if possible.

Cesarean section rate increases with decreasing gestational age at 28WKS -93-97%, 28-32WKS- 53-65% and 32-34 WKS-31-38%

Fetus benefits from in utero resuscitation before delivery.

Observation and Monitoring: Vitals, SPO_2, Reflexes and Urinary output- hourly, Temperature- 4 hourly, Transcutaneous pulse oximetry, Arterial blood gas analysis if $SpO_2 \leq 92\%$. Cut short the second stage of labor with ventouse or outlet forceps. Active management of third stage of labor:

Close watch for PPH as they are much less tolerant of even normal blood loss as normal hypervolemia of pregnancy is absent in Eclampsia. Avoid injection methergine after delivery.

- **Indications for Anesthesia Referral:** Deranged ABG, Unconscious Patient, Recurrent Convulsions, Suspected Aspiration and LSCS, **Administration of neuraxial anesthesia (spinal/epidural) is recommended for cesarean delivery or analgesia in labor with stable platelet count >70,000/mm3 with no coagulopathy and patient not on anticoagulant therapy.**[6]

- **For pain relief – systemic opioids/epidural analgesia may be considered.**

- **Thromboprophylaxis** with anti-embolic stockings & LMWH recommended till the patient is fully mobile extended thromboprophylaxis if multiple risk factors present

- **Role of Neuroimaging MRI/CT: Consider alternatives diagnosis in women with convulsions occuring more than 48 hours postpartum, focal neurological deficits, prolonged coma, Atypical eclampsia**

Indications of Invasive Hemodynamic Monitoring: Severe Cardiac disease, Acute kidney injury, Refractory hypertension, Oliguria, Pulmonary edema

Maternal and Fetal complications of Eclampsia:

A. Maternal: Immediate: Aspiration of vomitus, pulmonary oedema, bronchopneumonia, asphyxia, RDS, Abruptio placentae, PPH, HELLP syndrome (haemolysis, elevated liver enzymes, low platelet count), DIC, Acute kidney injury, Cerebral haemorrhage, thrombosis, oedema, Blindness (Amaurosis), Liver necrosis, Thromboembolic events, Persistent postpartum hypertension, Postpartum psychosis, Maternal death

   LONG TERM: There is a twofold rise in incidence of: hypertension, ischemic heart disease, stroke, chronic renal failure.

B. Fetus: Prematurity, FGR, LBW, Physical handicap, Cerebral palsy, Mental retardation, Stillbirth

   - **Follow up:** Close observation in immediate postpartum period for 48-72hrs.

   - Don't discharge before 72hrs

   - Repeat Postnatal visit 2 wks, 6-8 wks & 12wks after delivery

   - Fits may occur for the first time postpartum

   - Discharge instructions to include-information about signs & symptoms of imminent eclampsia & prompt reporting

   - Parenteral Magnesium sulphate is suggested with new onset hypertension with headache or blurred vision or preeclampsia

   - Persistent postpartum hypertension needs continued antihypertensive treatment. Prefer once daily antihypertensives – Enalapril, Amlodipine, Nifedipine

- Avoid diuretics, methyldopa and ARBs in postpartum period
- Safe use of NSAIDs is in for pain relief over opioids.[6,11]

Summary: All pregnant women with convulsions should be considered and managed as ECLAMPSIA unless proved otherwise at secondary or tertiary care level.

Early prediction of pre-eclampsia, low dose aspirin (81mg daily), from 12 wks until delivery, standard prenatal care, close follow up of high risk pregnancies may prevent eclampsia.

- Early diagnosis with appropriate management of pre-eclampsia may prevent eclampsia.
- Women with gestational hypertension, pre-eclampsia non severe delivery rather than expectant management is recommended at – 37 0/7 weeks
- Preeclampsia with severe features/ impending/ imminent eclampsia should be treated with magnesium sulphate in dose similar to as in eclampsia with mandatory admission at level II/ III health care facility.

Eclampsia is not preventable in physician error, lack of prenatal care, abrupt onset, magnesium sulphate failure, early onset (<21 weeks) or late post-partum onset. No matter where a woman delivers, giving birth should be a moment of joy, not a sentence to death

PPROMT Trial – "Immediate delivery compared with expectant management after preterm pre-labour rupture of the membranes close to term"

Background

Preterm pre-labour ruptured membranes close to term is associated with increased risk of neonatal infection, but immediate delivery is associated with risks of prematurity.

Aim of trial is to establish whether immediate birth in singleton pregnancies with ruptured membranes close to term reduces neonatal

infection without increasing other morbidity.

Methods

The PPROMT trial was a multicentre randomised controlled trial done at 65 centres across 11 countries

Inclusion – Women aged over 16 years with singleton pregnancies and ruptured membranes before the onset of labour between 34 weeks and 36 weeks and 6 days weeks who had no signs of infection were included.

Outcomes

Primary outcome – incidence of neonatal sepsis.

Secondary infant outcomes

1. Sepsis
2. Mechanical ventilation

   ≥24 h
3. Stillbirth
4. Neonatal death
5. Respiratory distress syndrome
6. Any mechanical ventilation duration of stay in a neonatal intensive or special care unit.

Secondary maternal outcomes

1. Antepartum or intrapartum haemorrhage
2. Intrapartum fever, postpartum treatment with antibiotics
3. Mode of delivery

Conclusion

In the absence of overt signs of infection or fetal compromise, a policy of expectant management with appropriate surveillance of maternal and fetal wellbeing should be followed in pregnant women who present with ruptured membranes close to term

References

1. FOGSI-GESTOSIS-ICOG Hypertensive Disorders in Pregnancy (HDP) Good Clinical Practice Recommendations 2019

2. Khan KS, Wojdyla D, Say L, et al: WHO analysis of causes of maternal death: a systematic review, Lancet 367: 1066, 2006 f

3. ACOG Practice Bulletin No. 202: Gestational Hypertension and Preeclampsia Obstetrics & Gynecology: June 2020 - Volume 135 - Issue 6 - p e237-e260PMID: 32443079

4. NATIONAL ECLAMPSIA REGISTRY- FOGSI ICOG 2013. www.ner-fogsi.in

5. American College of Obstetricians and Gynecologists; Task Force on Hypertension in Pregnancy Hypertension in pregnancy. Report of the American College of Obstetricians and Gynecologists' Task Force on Hypertension in Pregnancy. Obstet Gynecol. 2013;122(5):1122–31. doi: 10.1097/01.AOG.0000437382.03963.88. [PubMed] 5A- ACOG 2013B5B-REAFFIRMED 2019

6. Gestational Hypertension and Preeclampsia: ACOG Practice Bulletin, Number 222 Obstetrics & Gynecology: June 2020 - Volume 135 - Issue 6 - p e237-e260PMID: 32443079. DOI: 10.1097/AOG.0000000000003891

7. GESTATIONAL HYPERTENSION AND PRE-ECLAMPSIA. OBSTETGYNECOL 2020: 135; E237

8. Hypertensive disorders: Cunningham, F. grey, Kenneth J. Leveno, Steven L. Bloom, Catherine Y. Spong, Jodi S. Dashe, Barbara L. Hoffman, Brian M. Casey, Williams Obstetrics 25th edition. New York: McGraw- Hill Education: 2018

9. A Marra et al. posterior reversible encephalopathy syndrome: the endothelial hypotheses MED HYPOTHESIS 2014; 82:619, PLOS ONE 2014; 9: E 113670.

10. Screening for Hypertension in Adults: UPSTF recommendation statement. Ann Intern Med 2014, 161:819

11. WHO Recommendation for Prevention And Treatment of Pre-Eclampsia And Eclampsia 2017(http://whqlibdoc.who.int/hq/2011/WHO_RHR_11.25_eng.pdf)

12. Hypertension in pregnancy: diagnosis and management *NICE guideline Published: 25 June 2019 www.nice.org.uk/guidance/ng133*

Renal Emergencies

Contributors-

1. Dr. Ashima Sharma
2. Dr. Nidhi Kaeley
3. Dr. M Rahul Rohan
4. Dr. Sukhdeep Somal

Chapters-

1. AKI
2. Acute urinary retention
3. Urinary tract stones
4. UTI
5. Hematuria

AKI (Acute Kidney Injury)

Acute Kidney Injury (AKI) is one of the common presentations in the Emergency Department. It presents a wide spectrum of diseases. The epidemiology of AKI has not been clearly defined.

<u>Definition</u>

According to the kidney Disease Improving global outcomes (KDIGO) group, 2012, AKI is defined as increase in serum creatinine greater than equal to 0.3mg/dl within 48 hours or an increase in serum creatinine greater than 1.5 times baseline within seven days or decrease in urine out output for 6 hours. Multiple other classifications have been proposed such as RIFLE (Risk Injury Failure Loss End-stage) and AKIN (Acute Kidney Injury Network). KDIGO covers the parameters of both AKIN and RIFLE. AKI is characterized as acute reduction of renal function associated with fall in glomerular filtration rate presenting as increase in serum creatinine and reduced urine output.

AKI is categorized into three types

    a. Pre-renal

    b. Intrarenal

    c. Post-renal

KDIGO (Kidney Disease: Improving Global Outcomes Guidelines) (1)

AKI Stage	Serum Creatinine	Urine Output
1st	1.5-1.9 times baseline or 7/0.3mg/dl increase	<0.5ml/kg/h for 6-12 hours
2nd	2-2.9 times baseline	<0.5ml/kg/h For 7-12 hours
3rd	3 times the baseline or serum creatinine increase 4 mg/dl or initiation of renal replacement therapy	<0.3ml/kg/h For 7-24 hour or...... 12 hours

Intramural AKI is further classified as glomeruli, vasculature or interstitial.

<u>Etiology</u>

1. Pre-renal AKI caused by acute volume depletion (vomiting, diarrhea, bleeding, renal losses as diuretics, skin and respiratory losses).

2. Intra renal causes include glomerular, tubular (ischemia, infection, nephrotoxins, vascular)

3. Post renal causes include bladder obstruction (Prostate enlargement, urinary retention, malignancy), nephrolithiasis

(1) Detailed history to be taken in all the patients such as that of vomiting, diarrhea, bleeding on sepsis). Identify the underlying, contrast induced)

(2) Evaluation

Physical Examination can give clearance towards the diagnosis such as

1. Signs of dehydration suggest pre-renal cause of AKI.
2. Long rash suggests acute interstitial nephritis.
3. Underlying heart failure may suggest cardio-renal syndrome.
4. Underlying chronic liver disease with portal hypertension may suggest hepatorenal syndrome.

Urine analysis can be done by urine routine/microscopy, 24-hrs urinary protein or albumin, spot urine protein to creatinine ratio or albumin to creatinine ratio.

Quantitative Measurement- The gold stand technique is 24-hours urinary protein measurement. However, multiple shortcuts have been divided such as urinary protein creatinine ratio (or urinary albumin creatinine ratio). The shortcomings of UPCR ratio are observed in patients with large muscle mass and higher creatinine excretion, wherein proteinuria is underestimated. Also, in patients with small muscle mass and creatinine excretion less than 1000mg/day, UPCR is overestimated.

In (39) NEPTUNE (Nephrotic Syndrome Study Network), proteinuria was measured at baseline and during subsequent visits. No significant variation was observed between spot sample and 24-hours urinary protein values among various kinds of glomerular diseases.

Measurement of total urinary protein excretion

1. Urinary dipstick method- It mainly detects albumin and is insensitive to non-albumin proteins. False positive urinary dipstick results are seen in post-use of iodinated radiocontrast agents for at least 24 hours, alkaline urine, gross hematuria and usage of antiseptic such as chlorhexidine.
2. Sulfosalicylic acid test- It detects not only albumin but all kinds of proteins. Both urinary dipstick and sulfosalicylic acid tests can detect urinary lysozyme in patients with hypovolemic shock.

Following are the subtypes of proteinuria

a. Isolated proteinuria – Proteinuria without underlying abnormalities of urinary sediments such as hematuria, hypertension and diabetes or reduce glomerular filtration rates.
b. Glomerular Proteinuria- It occurs as a result of increased filtration of macromolecules such as albumin through the glomerular capillary wall. For example in diabetic nephropathy, other glomerular diseases, orthostatic or exercise induced proteinuria.

c. Tubular Proteinuria-The lower molecular weight proteins such as beta 2-microglobulin, immunoglobulin, light chains, retinol binding protein can easily filter along the glomerular capillary membrane. They then get completely reabsorbed in the proximal Tubule. Tubulo interstitial disease can result in excretion of these lower molecular weight proteins. Tubular proteinuria is not diagnosed clinically by dipstick method as it can detect only albumins.

d. Overflow Proteinuria - This occurs because of excessive production of a particular protein leading to increased glomerular filtration and excretion. For example in multiple myeloma, acute myelomonocytic, intra vascular hemolysis.

e. Post renal proteinuria- It is caused by inflammation of the urinary tract such as in patients with urinary tract infection, nephrolithiasis and tumors.

Other Tests:-

a. Urine-analysis- it can be done by urine dipstick and microscopic examination. They detect urine pH, protein (albumin), glucose, hemoglobin (myoglobin), leukocyte esterase (pyuria) and specific gravity.

b. Urinary sodium excretion can be detected by calculating fractional urine excretion (FeNA) to distinguish between pre-renal and ATN.

c. Measurement of urinary volume oliguria is urine volume less than 500ml/day.

d. Serological markers and kidney biopsy.

Crush –related acute kidney injury

Crush injury induced systemic manifestations are called crush syndrome. (2)

Renal manifestations of crush injury include.

a. Acute Kidney Injury- It can be further classified as-

   i. Pre-renal AKI- It occurs as a consequence of vascular injury leading to with acute macrocytic and myelocytic leukemia.

   ii. Intrarenal AKI- It occurs because of rhabdomyolysis. The patient can have dark red, brown and black urine. Microscopic examination may reveal pigmented granular east.

   iii. Post-renal AKI- It occurs above do to traumatic injury or urinary outflow tract obstruction,

Biochemical abnormalities include rhabdomyolysis associated hyperkalemia hyperphosphatemia, hypercalcaemia high creatinine kinase and lower fractional execution of sodium, hardly higher levels of myoglobin are detected.

Prevention

In order to prevent rhabdomyolysis induced AKI due to crush injury, easily aggressive fluid replacement is of paramount importance. Continuous monitoring of the patient for six hours after initiation of the fluids. As per renal disaster relief task force (RDRTF) of the International society of Nephrology (ISN), isotonic alkaline solution can be used to achieve forced alkaline diuresis. Heme-protein precipitation with Tamm-Horsfall protein, intratubular pigment cast formation and uric acid precipitation can be prevented by raising the urinary PH more than 6.5.

Alkalinization can aid in limiting the release of free iron from the myoglobin and formation of F2 isoprotanes, which increase renal vasoconstriction.Potential risk of alkalization include hypocalcemia.

The two proposed regimens of bicarbonate administration are

a. One Litre of isotonic saline alternating with 1 Litre of half isotonic saline plus 50 mEq of sodium bicarbonate.

   or

b. Isotonic saline for the first two hours followed by half isotonic saline plus 150mEq of sodium bicarbonate.

Use of mannitol: There is no consensus regarding the use of mannitol in crush injury patients. However, some experts advice if urinary output is adequate defined as more than 20ml/hour, 50ml of 20% mannitol may be added to each Litre of fluid. If desired urine output is not achieved discontinue mannitol.

Other treatment modalities include treatment of hypokalemia hypocalcemia, fluid overload and dialysis whenever indicated.

Hepatorenal syndrome (3)

It is one of the important causes of acute kidney injury in patients with chronic liver disease.

<u>Pathophysiology</u>

Arterial vasodilation in the splanchnic circulation plays a key role in the pathogenesis. As the liver disease advances there is continuous rise in cardiac output and drop in systemic vascular resistance hypotension induces activation of renin angiotensin and sympathetic nervous system. Both fall in total vascular resistance and bacterial translocation into the mesenteric lymph nodes play a key role in pathogenesis of hepatorenal syndrome.

Hepatorenal syndrome is characterized by-

a. A progressive decline in serum creatinine.
b. Usually normal urinary sediment.
c. Minimal protein urine.
d. Very low sodium excretion less than 10 mEq/l
e. urea or oliguria

Hepatorenal syndrome are of two types

A. Type 1 Hepatorenal syndrome is a more catastrophic forms characterized by two fold increase of serum creatinine with in a period less than two weeks.

B. Type 2 Hepatorenal syndrome is a less serious variant. The differentiating feature is ascites resistant to diuretics.

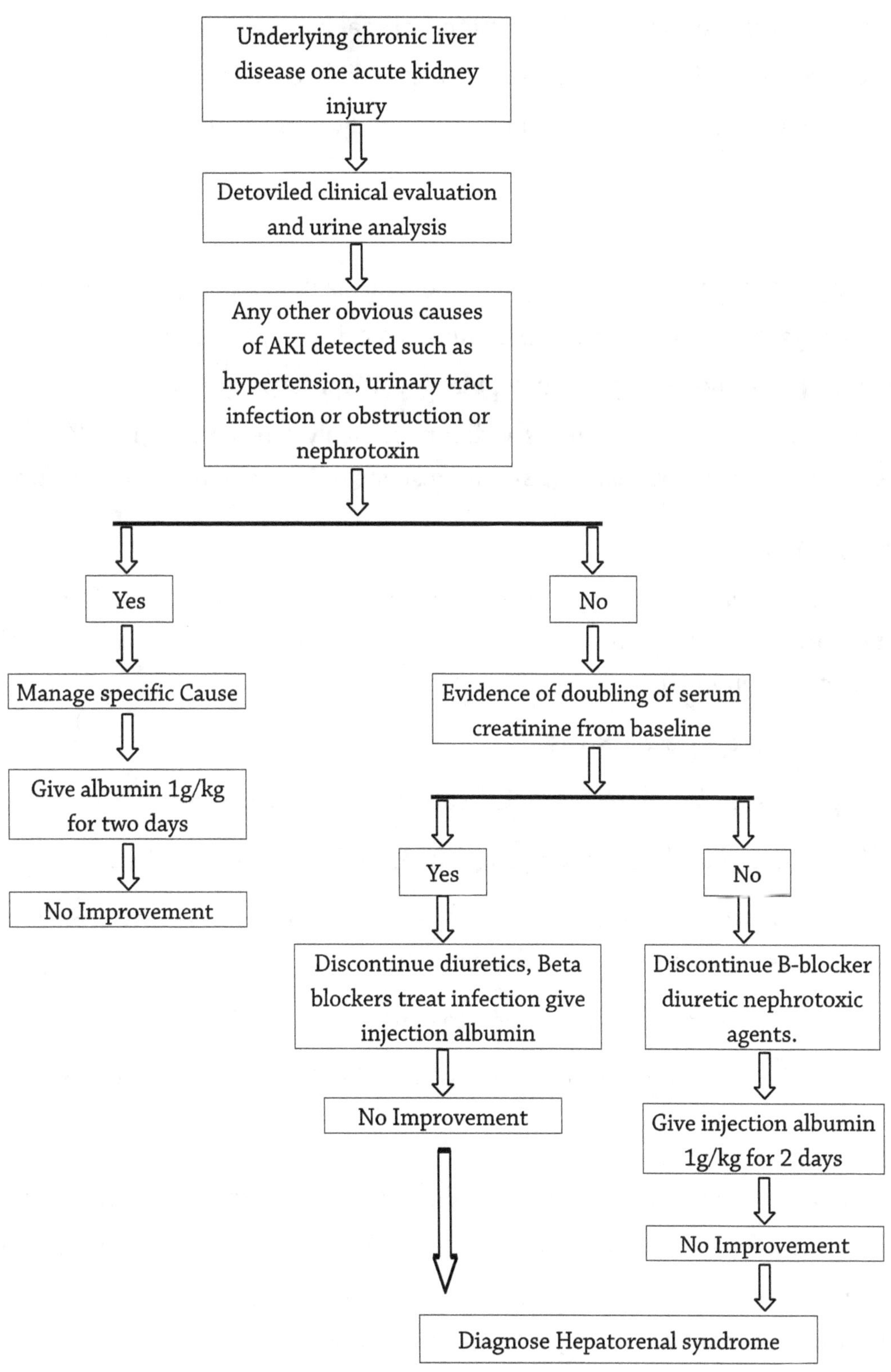

According to the American association for the study of liver disease (AASLD) and international club of ascites (ICA) following are criteria of hepatorenal syndrome.

I. Chronic liver disease or acute liver disease with portal hypertension.

II. Acute kidney injury which is defined as per KDIGO criteria.

III. Absence of any other apparent cause of AKI including shock, nephrotoxic drugs, ultrasonographic features of urinary obstruction or renal parenchymal disease.

IV. Urinary red cell excretion less than 50 cells per high fever field.

V. No improvement after giving albumin (1g/kg body weight) for two days and withdrawing diuretics.

<u>Treatment</u>

I. Terlipressin as intravenous (1 to 2 mg every four to six hours along with albumin for two days)

II. If terlipressin is unavailable, midodrine plus octreotide can be given.

III. Patients who fail above therapy transjugular intrahepatic portosystemic shunt can be tried.

IV. Renal replacement therapy in patients with continuously deteriorating renal function especially they are waiting for liver transplant and with scope of improvement of liver function.

Cardio Renal Syndrome

As per 2004 report of National Heart, Lung and Blood Institute CRS is defined as a condition in which therapy to relieve symptoms of heart failure is limited by a decline in renal function as manifested by a reduction in GFR.

Ronco and colleagues categorized CRS as

Type I (acute)- Acute heart failure resulting in acute kidney injury.

Type 2 CRS – Chronic cardiac dysfunction progressive to chronic kidney disease.

Type 3- Abrupt onset of worsening of kidney dysfunction leading to renal ischaemia or glomerulonephritis which is manifested as heart failure.

Type 4- Primary chronic kidney disease leading to cardiac dysfunction.

Type5 (secondary) - Acute or chronic systemic disorders leading to cardiac and renal dysfunction.

<u>Diagnosis</u>

- The most common test to document reduction in glomerular function test is serum creatinine.
- Blood urea nitrogen to creatinine ratio (BUN/Cr) helps to distinguish pre renal and intrinsic renal disease.
- Urinary sodium concentration may also aid in diagnosis.

<u>Pathophysiology-</u>

Variety of factors have been associated with worsening renal function.

1. Reduction in systolic blood pressure ESCAPE trial (Evaluation study of congestine heart failure and pulmonary catheterization concluded that coarsening renal function was significantly associated with mortality in patients with reduced systolic blood pressure.

2. Neurohumoral adaptations such as stimulating sympathetic nervous system and serum angiotensin-aldosterone system leading to increase in vasopressin and endothelin-I, This cause salt and water retention.

3. Reduced renal perfusion.

4. Increased renal venous pressure increase in intra abdominal and central venous pressure leads to increase in renal venous pressure.

5. Right ventricular dilatation and dysfunction. the result increase in central venous pressure can further reduce the GFR. Right ventricular dilation leads to reduction in left ventricular filling and forward cardiac output.

<u>Management-</u>

1. Improvement in cardiac function- INTER MAC registry demonstrated that early improvement in eGFR with left ventricular Assist Device was transient and persisted only for weeks to months.

   MIRACLE trial demonstrated cardiac resynchronization therapy improved the LV ejection fraction and eGFR in few patients with heart failure. (4, 5)

2. Diuretic therapy should not be deferred in patients with fluid overload in heart failure.

   CARRESS-HF trial- compared the effect of ultra filtration with that of stepwise pharmacological therapy renal function. (6)

3. Renin-angiotensin- system antagonists (7)

   Angiotensin connection enzyme (ACE) inhibitor, angiotensin receptor neprilysin inhibitor (ARNI), angiotensin II receptor blocker (ARB) is a known therapy in patients with heart failure with reduced ejection fraction.

   According to SOLVD trials, no difference was observed in chronic eGFR decline over a period of three years in patients with heart failure with reduced ejection fraction between enalapril and placebo group.

PARADIGM-HF- As per this trial, a decrease in eGFR during follow up was lesser in patients on ARNI therapy compared to ACE inhibitors. It was found that sacubitril /valsartan were associated with slower decline in eGFR compared to enalapril. (8)

4. Vasodilators-

    According to the acutely decompensated heart failure National registry (ADHERE) the rate of worsening of renal function was more in patients with intravenous diuretics along with nitroglycerin and nitropruesside as compared to intravenous diuretics only.(9)

5. Clinical and safety profile of dopamine has not been established. As per DAD-HF trial similar urine output was observed in patients on combination of dopamine and low dose furosemide as compared only furosemide.(10)

6. The renal optimization strategies evaluation (ROSE) trial did not find any benefit of low dose dopamine in enhancing decongestion and improvement of renal function patients with heart failure.(11)

7. Ultrafiltration – Three important trials UNLOAD, RAPID-CHF and CARESS-HF compared ultrafiltration with diuretic therapy in patients with heart failure.

    Ultrafiltration therapy is associated with rise in serum creatinine and increased rates in adverse events.(12)

8. Tolvaptan – As per EVEREST outcome trial, tolvaptan was found to have no effect on mortality in patients with heart failure.(13)

9. Adenosine acts on adenosine – I receptor. As per PROTECT trial, no benefit was observed in cardiovascular outcome and persistent of renal function in patients with heart failure.(14)

Biomarkers in AKI

Diagnostic Biomarkers (15,16)

a. Urinary tubular enzymes proximal renal tubular epithelial antigen (HRTE –I), alpha glutathione s- transferase (alpha GST) pi-glutathione S- transferase (pi GST), gamma-glutamyl-transpeptidase (gamma-GT), Alanine aminopeptidase (AAP), lactate dehydrogenase, N-acetyl-beta glucosaminidase (NAG) alkaline phosphatase.

b. Urinary low molecular weight proteins – alpha I – microglobulin, beta 2 microglobulin, retinol binding protein, adenosine deaminase binding protein and urinary cystatin C.

c. Neutrophil gelatinase associated lipocalin (NGAL)

d. Urinary kidney injury molecule.

e. Urinary interleukin 18.

f. Urinary liver type fatty acid binding protein in acute kidney injury.

g. soluble urokinase plasminogen activator receptor (suPAR)

h. Furosemide stress test.

Prognostic Biomarkers

1. Urinary renin and angiotensinogen

2. Plasma NGAL

3. Urinary insulin like growth factor protein 7 (IGFBP7) and tissue inhibitor of metalloproteinase-2 (TIMP2)

NAGL is expressed in the kidney after renal ischemia. If functions as anti-apoptosis by stimulating proliferation of renal tubular cells. It upregulates home oxygenase- I, thus protecting the kidney tubular cells. It has been found to be a significant biomarker of ATN. NGAL is helpful in differentiating between pre-renal AKI and ATN.

Recent updates in AKI

1. **STARRT-AKI Trial** [17]- In this trial, the need for accelerated or standard renal replacement therapy resulting in lower risk of death from any cause at 90 days in critically ill patients with acute kidney injury was studied. Before discussing this trial, it is important to know that the previous trials were ELAIN, IDEAL and AKIKI. The ELAIN trial was the only one of the three to show reduced 90-day mortality with early vs delayed initiation of RRT and was the smallest in sample size. The two strategies which were compared were *Accelerated Strategy: Clinicians were to start RRT as soon as possible and within 12 hours after patients had met full eligibility criteria.*

   Standard Strategy: Clinicians were discouraged to start RRT unless development of one or more of the following:

   - *Serum Potassium Level > 6.0 mmol or more per Litre*

   - *pH of 7.20 or less*

   - *Bicarbonate level of 12 mmol per Litre or less*

   - *Evidence of severe respiratory failure based on $PaO_2:FiO_2$ < 200 or less AND clinical perception of volume overload*

   - *Persistent AKI for least 72 hours after randomization*

     Outcomes studied were -

     Primary

   - Death from any cause at 90 days after randomization

     Secondary

   - Major Adverse Kidney Event (MAKE) = Death, dependence on RRT or a sustained reduction in kidney function (estimated GFR < 75% of baseline value)

   - Death in the ICU at 28 days or during hospitalization

- Number of days free of RRT at 90 days
- Number of ventilator and vasoactive-free days at 28 days
- Length of hospitalization
- Hospitalization free at 90 days
- Hospital related quality of life assessed using EQ-5D-5L questionnaire

Authors concluded that among critically ill patients with acute kidney injury, an accelerated renal-replacement strategy was not associated with a lower risk of death at 90 days than a standard strategy.

2. **Post Contrast Acute Kidney Injury (PC-AKI)** [18]- This was the single center retrospective observational study performed in Korea to estimate if the level of estimated glomerular filtration rate (eGFR) observed in the emergency department (ED) is significantly associated with the occurrence of postcontrast acute kidney injury (PC-AKI) in patients undergoing CTPA. **Outcomes of the study were-**

   Primary: PC-AKI (Defined as increase in serum creatinine concentration ≥0.3mg/dL or a ≥1.5 – 1.9 fold increase from baseline within 48 – 72hrs after contrast)

   Secondary: Multivariate logistic regression analysis was used to confirm the effect of eGFR in the ED on the occurrence of PC-AKI after adjustment for confounding variables.

   This current study shows that the last eGFR prior to CTPA in patients with suspected acute pulmonary embolism in the ED was not associated with occurrence of PC-AKI, even if the eGFR was <30mL/min/1.73m2, but there was certainly a trend toward increased AKI in this patient population. What we need now is not another retrospective observational study, and although a randomized clinical trial would be great, it is unlikely to ever happen.

3. **The Kompas Trial** [19]: Sodium Bicarbonate Prehydration in Adults with CKD Prior to Contrast-Enhanced CT- In this trial, they studied the effect of omission prophylactic prehydration with sodium bicarbonate prior to iodine-based contrast media administration in patients with stage 3 CKD. Patients were randomized to receive:No prehydration vs Prehydration with 250mL of 1.4% sodium bicarbonate administered in a 1hr infusion. The **Outcomes studies included-Primary:** Mean relative increase (percentage) in serum creatinine level 2 to 5 days after contrast administration compared with baseline (noninferiority margin <10% increase in serum creatinine level)

   Secondary-

1. Incidence of PC-AKI 2 to 5 days after contrast administration (Defined as an increase in creatinine level greater than 25% or greater than 0.5mg/dL) [To convert to micromoles/L, multiply by 88.4]

2. Mean relative increase in creatinine level 7 to 14 days after contrast administration

3. Recovery of renal function in patients with PC-AKI after 2 months

4. Incidence of acute heart failure

5. Incidence of renal failure requiring dialysis

6. Health care costs

They concluded that among patients with stage 3 CKD undergoing contrast-enhanced computed tomography, withholding prehydration did not compromise patient safety. The findings of this study support the option of not giving prehydration a safe and cost-efficient measure.

4. **ELAIN FOLLOW UP Trial** [20]- long term outcomes after early initiation of RRT in critically ill patients with AKI was studied. In this, early initiation of RRT was compared with delayed RRT in reducing composite end points of MAKE 365, consisting of death, RRT and persistent renal dysfunction at one year. Authors concluded that in the cohort of critically ill patients with AKI, early initiation of RRT as compared to delayed RRT continues to have benefit in improving composite end points such as mortality, dialysis dependence and renal function.

References

1. 1KIDGO Clinical Practice Guideline for Acute Kidney Injury. Kidney Int Suppl 2012; 2:8).

2. Odeh M. The role of reperfusion-induced injury in the pathogenesis of the crush syndrome. N Engl Med 1991; 324:1417.

3. Gines P, Guevara M, Arroyo V, Rodes J. Hepatorenal Syndrome. Lancet 2003; 362:1819.

4. Brisco MA, Kimmel SE, Coca SG, et al. Prevalence and prognostic importance of changes in renal function after mechanical circulatory support. Circ Heart Fail 2014; 7:68.

5. Adelstein EC, Shalaby A, Saba S. Response to cardiac resynchronization therapy in patients with heart failure and renal insufficiency. Pacing Clin Electrophysiol 2010; 33:850.

6. Grodin JL, Stevens SR, de Las Fuentes L, et al. Intensification of Medication Therapy for Cardiorenal Syndrome in Acute Decompensated Heart Failure. J Card Fail 2016; 22:26.

7. McCallum W, Tighiouart H, Ku E, et al. Trends in Kidney Function Outcomes Following RAAS Inhibition in Patients With Heart Failure With Reduced Ejection Fraction. Am J Kidney Dis 2020; 75:21.

8. Damman K, Gori M, Claggett B, et al. Renal Effects and Associated Outcomes During Angiotensin-Neprilysin Inhibition in Heart Failure. JACC Heart Fail 2018; 6:489.

9. Costanzo MR, Johannes RS, Pine M, et al. The safety of intravenous diuretics alone versus diuretics plus parenteral vasoactive therapies in hospitalized patients with acutely

decompensated heart failure: a propensity score and instrumental variable analysis using the Acutely Decompensated Heart Failure National Registry (ADHERE) database. Am Heart J 2007; 154:267.

10. Giamouzis G, Butler J, Starling RC, et al. Impact of dopamine infusion on renal function in hospitalized heart failure patients: results of the Dopamine in Acute Decompensated Heart Failure (DAD-HF) Trial. J Card Fail 2010; 16:922.

11. Chen HH, Anstrom KJ, Givertz MM, et al. Low-dose dopamine or low-dose nesiritide in acute heart failure with renal dysfunction: the ROSE acute heart failure randomized trial. JAMA 2013; 310:2533.

12. Yancy CW, Jessup M, Bozkurt B, et al. 2013 ACCF/AHA guideline for the management of heart failure: executive summary: a report of the American College of Cardiology Foundation/American Heart Association Task Force on practice guidelines. Circulation 2013; 128:1810.

13. Konstam MA, Gheorghiade M, Burnett JC Jr, et al. Effects of oral tolvaptan in patients hospitalized for worsening heart failure: the EVEREST Outcome Trial. JAMA 2007; 297:1319.

14. Dohadwala MM, Givertz MM. Role of adenosine antagonism in the cardiorenal syndrome. Cardiovasc Ther 2008; 26:276.

15. Morioka S, Maueröder C, Ravichandran KS. Living on the Edge: Efferocytosis at the Interface of Homeostasis and Pathology. Immunity 2019; 50:1149.

16. Wagener G, Gubitosa G, Wang S, et al. Urinary neutrophil gelatinase-associated lipocalin and acute kidney injury after cardiac surgery. Am J Kidney Dis 2008; 52:425.

17. STARRT-AKI Investigators; Canadian Critical Care Trials Group; Australian and New Zealand Intensive Care Society Clinical Trials Group; United Kingdom Critical Care Research Group; Canadian Nephrology Trials Network; Irish Critical Care Trials Group, Bagshaw SM, Wald R, Adhikari NKJ, Bellomo R, da Costa BR, Dreyfuss D, Du B, Gallagher MP, Gaudry S, Hoste EA, Lamontagne F, Joannidis M, Landoni G, Liu KD, McAuley DF, McGuinness SP, Neyra JA, Nichol AD, Ostermann M, Palevsky PM, Pettilä V, Quenot JP, Qiu H, Rochwerg B, Schneider AG, Smith OM, Thomé F, Thorpe KE, Vaara S, Weir M, Wang AY, Young P, Zarbock A. Timing of Initiation of Renal-Replacement Therapy in Acute Kidney Injury. N Engl J Med. 2020 Jul 16;383(3):240-251. doi: 10.1056/NEJMoa2000741. Erratum in: N Engl J Med. 2020 Jul 15;: PMID: 32668114.

18. Cheng W, Wu X, Liu Q, Wang HS, Zhang NY, Xiao YQ, Yan P, Li XW, Duan XJ, Peng JC, Feng S, Duan SB. Post-contrast acute kidney injury in a hospitalized population: short-, mid-, and long-term outcome and risk factors for adverse events. Eur Radiol. 2020 Jun;30(6):3516-3527. doi: 10.1007/s00330-020-06690-3. Epub 2020 Feb 21. PMID: 32080754; PMCID: PMC7248019.

19. Timal RJ, Kooiman J, Sijpkens YWJ, et al. Effect of No Prehydration vs Sodium Bicarbonate Prehydration Prior to Contrast-Enhanced Computed Tomography in the Prevention of Postcontrast Acute Kidney Injury in Adults With Chronic Kidney Disease: The Kompas Randomized Clinical Trial. *JAMA Intern Med.* 2020;180(4):533–541. doi:10.1001/jamainternmed.2019.7428

20. Meersch M, Küllmar M, Schmidt C, Gerss J, Weinhage T, Margraf A, Ermert T, Kellum JA, Zarbock A. Long-Term Clinical Outcomes after Early Initiation of RRT in Critically Ill Patients with AKI. J Am Soc Nephrol. 2018 Mar;29(3):1011-1019. doi: 10.1681/ASN.2017060694. Epub 2017 Dec 1. PMID: 29196304; PMCID: PMC5827600.

Acute Urinary Retention

Acute urinary retention (AUR) is a common problem presenting to ED mostly seen in elderly males. It is more dangerous if the patient is young, female, febrile or postprostatectomy.

The common causes of AUR are:-

Intestine	Severe constipation- compression of bladder neck against hardened stool in colon
Bladder	Neurogenic- diabetic cystopathy, multiple sclerosis, Parkinson's disease, stroke, cord compression due to lesion, and cord disruption due to trauma. Calculi Stones Malignancy
Prostrate	BPH Prostatitis Trauma/avulsion Malignancy
Urethra	Urethral strictures Urethral inflammation Urethral foreign body
Penile	Meatal stenosis Phimosis Trauma Paraphimosis

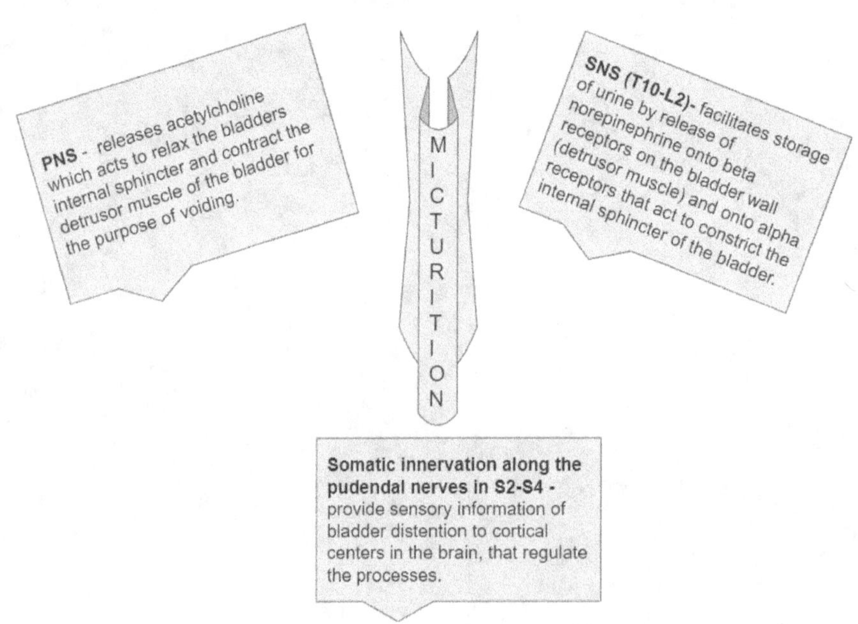

Act of micturition-

The salient points in history taking and examination are listed below.

Medications	Recreational drugs, Anticholinergic Agents Calcium Channel Blockers, NSAIDS, alpha-adrenergic Agonist, beta-adrenergic Agonist, Opioids, Sedative-Hypnotics, Antipsychotics, Antiparkinsonian Agents, Anesthetics
Pain	Location and duration
Weight loss	malignancy
Presence of fever	infection
Previous gynaec or urologic procedures	trauma
Presence of incontinence, nocturia, and urinary frequency	
Direct rectal exam	Decreased anal tone, saddle anesthesia- Neurogenic bladder
	Tender prostate - Prostatitis
Bimanual examination in females	Uterine Prolapse
Per abdomen palpation	Bladder for masses Flank tenderness- obstructive lesions proximal to the bladder Scrotal tenderness- obstructive lesions distal to the bladder

Investigations for AUR-

Urine examination	infectious cells, hematuria or gross blood with clots, large amounts of glucose that may point to poorly controlled diabetes
Renal ultrasound	obstructive process has led to hydronephrosis
CT of the renal collecting system	to assess for tumor, metastasis, stranding to indicate infection, presence of prolapse, or other gynecologic pathology.
Labs	Basic Metabolic panel to evaluate renal function through BUN: Creatinine ratio and electrolyte abnormalities that may be associated with drug use or cancers
	CBC - for infection and in cases where hemorrhagic cystitis or other causes of bleeding are suspected

Formulas for ED calculation-

Estimated Bladder Capacity in Ounces	Age in years + 2 (for children with AUR). Fluid Ounce = ~ 30 mL
Normal post-void residual (PVR) < 50 ml (may be up to 100 ml in patients > 65 years)	PVR = 0.5 X AP diameter X lateral diameter X sagittal diameter of the bladder

<u>ED management-</u>

Placement of foley catheter to drain the bladder with slow injection of a good amount of lidocaine jelly in urethral meatus. Sometimes a short acting opioid analgesic like fentanyl may be required. A 16 F catheter is invariably used which should be 18F in prostate hypertrophy is suspected as a thicker catheter will not get entrapped in the many crevices of prostate gland. The size should be decreased if there is a stricture. If the patient has a history of radical prostatectomy and if the catheter is not passing, think bladder neck obstruction and consult urology. Suprapubic catheters are considered after unsuccessful attempts with urethral catheters usually in the setting of severe urethral strictures or complex prostatic disease. Another indication for suprapubic catheter is urethral disruption due to trauma. Contraindications to placing a suprapubic catheter include empty or unidentifiable bladder and bowel anterior to the bladder wall.

- Few patients may develop post obstructive diuresis defined as urinary output > 200 mL for at least 2 hours after urethral catheter insertion, or > 3L in 24hrs. This is after the initial volume of urine has come out. These patients should be observed for at least 4 hours following urethral catheter insertion and if urinary output is > 200ml/hr, they should be admitted with a consultation to general medicine for electrolyte disturbances.

- Foley catheters can remain in the bladder for 7-10 days. Antibiotic prophylaxis is *not* recommended unless there is an underlying infection present. In patients with benign prostatic hypertrophy as a cause of retention, an alpha-blocker such as tamsulosin 0.4mg daily has been shown to decrease the likelihood of re-catheterization after a trial of void.

- In men who report unprotected sexual activity, therapy should be targeted toward gonorrhea and chlamydia.

- In the case of diabetic cystopathy and other non-reversible causes of retention that are secondary to chronic disease, treatment options include: scheduled voiding, cholinergic receptor agonist therapy (Bethanechol improves contractility of bladder smooth muscle and is prescribed in doses of 10-50mg TID or QID), and intermittent self-catheterization.

Studies:

1. <u>Boettcher S et al</u> conducted a prospective RCT in 294 male patients with urinary obstruction who were randomized to: Rapid Decompression (RD) vs Gradual Decompression (GD)(17). GD meant that After every 200mL of urine drained the catheter clamped for 5 min until bladder was completely empty and RD was to completely drain the bladder by placing the foley bag to gravity. The patients were observed for vital signs, hematuria and symptoms over the next 30 minutes. An assumed complication of RD is circulatory collapse due to viscerovascular reflexes In which the overdistended bladder leads to hypertension from increased arterial wall tonus and vasoconstriction throughout the sympathetic nerve mediated vesicovascular reflex. Also pain from the urinary retention raises

their blood pressure. When the painful stimulus is removed, blood pressure decreases. The authors concluded that Rapid drainage of the bladder in urinary retention does not cause more hematuria requiring intervention, renal failure, or hemodynamic collapse compared to gradual drainage of the bladder.

2. <u>Karavitakis M et al</u> identified 2074 citations and only Twenty-one studies were included in the systematic review.(18) The evidence for managing patients with UR/BPO with pharmacological or nonpharmacological treatments is limited.Pooled results indicated that α1-blockers provided significantly higher rates of successful trial without catheter compared with placebo [alfuzosin: 322/540 (60%) vs 156/400 (39%); participants=940; studies=7; low CoE); tamsulosin: 75/158 (47%) vs 40/139 (29%); participants=297; studies=3; low CoE)] with rare adverse events. Nonpharmacological treatments have been evaluated in RCTs/prospective comparative studies only sporadically. The meta analysis concluded that there is some evidence that alfuzosin and tamsulosin may increase the rates of successful trials without catheter, but little or no evidence on various nonpharmacological treatment options for managing patients with urinary retention secondary to benign prostatic obstruction.

3. <u>Salem Mohamed SH et al</u> enrolled 60 men with BPH and AUR and they were randomly allocated to receive 0.4 mg tamsulosin hydrochloride for 3 days or 7 days, after that the catheter was removed and the ability to void unaided was assessed.(19) Eighteen men taking tamsulosin for 3 days and 21 patients taking tamsulosin for 7 days did not require recatheterization on the day of the TWOC (60% and 70%, respectively, P = 0.417). Complication as urinary tract infection, urine leakage, hematuria, or catheter obstruction occurred in five (16.7%) men who received tamsulosin for 3 days and 13 (43.3%) men who received tamsulosin for 7 days (P = 0.024). The study concluded that Men catheterized for AUR can void successfully after catheter removal if treated with alpha-1 blockade, and success rate of TWOC is controversial regarding the duration of catheterization. However, the complications increased with the period of catheterization.

AUR should not be taken lightly even if BPH is a strong suspicion. Drainage of urine with catheterization under aseptic conditions is necessary. The catheterizations which are difficult require an ED consult with a urologist who can perform cystoscopy under local anesthesia and place the foley catheter. It is important to connect the patient for an early urology referral in other cases.. The septic patient, oliguric or anuric patient and conditions like priapism causing AUR should be early identified.

References

1. Salim Rezaie, "Urinary Retention: Rapid Drainage or Gradual Drainage to Avoid Complications?", REBEL EM blog, April 4, 2017 on Boettcher S et al. Urinary Retention: Benefit of Gradual Bladder Decompression – Myth or Truth? A Randomized Controlled Trial. Urol Int 2013

2. Karavitakis M, Kyriazis I, Omar MI, Gravas S, Cornu JN, Drake MJ, Gacci M, Gratzke C, Herrmann TRW, Madersbacher S, Rieken M, Speakman MJ, Tikkinen KAO, Yuan Y, Mamoulakis C. Management of Urinary Retention in Patients with Benign Prostatic Obstruction: A Systematic Review and Meta-analysis. Eur Urol. 2019 May;75(5):788-798. doi: 10.1016/j.eururo.2019.01.046. Epub 2019 Feb 14. PMID: 30773327.

3. Salem Mohamed SH, El Ebiary MF, Badr MM. Early versus late trail of catheter removal in patients with urinary retention secondary to benign prostatic hyperplasia under tamsulosin treatment. Urol Sci 2018;29:288-92

Urinary Tract Stones

The true incidence of urolithiasis in India is still not known. It is commonly seen in western states, hypothetically, attributable to high salinity of water.

<u>Renal stones Investigations:- (1)</u>

USG KUB	If the patient has a solitary kidney, history of fever, the diagnosis of stone is in doubt
Excretory urography	Gold standard in the work up for urolithiasis
Non contrast computerized tomography(NCCT) scan	Quick and safe, contrast free alternative to excretory urography. Contrast media should not be given or should be avoided when there is a elevated creatinine level, pregnancy or lactation
Analysis of stone composition	Stone analysis is desirable in recurrent stone formers- X ray crystallography. Infrared spectroscopy, Radiographic characteristics of the stone, Microscopic examination of the urinary sediments to detect crystals. Urine Ph (alkaline in infection stones and acidic in uric acid stones
Special Investigations	Urine culture, renal scintigraphy, antegrade, retrograde contrast study.

<u>The indications for stone removal are:-</u>

When the stone diameter is more than 7 mm (because of low rate of spontaneous passage)
When adequate pain relief is not achieved.
When there is stone obstruction associated with infection
Obstruction in single kidney
Bilateral obstruction

<u>Treatment options:-</u>

Extracorporeal shock wave lithotripsy (ESWL)	The contraindications for ESWL for renal stones include pregnancy, bleeding disorders, uncontrolled urinary tract infections, morbid obesity, aortic aneurysms
	Routine use of stents is not recommended for ESWL for renal stones
	The stone clearance is lower for stones in the lower calyx as compared to anywhere else in the kidney.
	20 mm should be considered the upper limit for stones in the lower calyx to be recommended for ESWL.
	Cystine stones are harder to fragment, hence cystine stones larger than 15mm should not be treated with ESWL
	The measurement of stone density with NCCT helps in predicting success rates of ESWL. Stones with greater than 1000 Hounsfield units (HU) show poor results with ESWL.

Percutaneous Nephrolithotomy	Indications for PCNL are larger than 20mm2, staghorn, partial staghorn calculi and stones in patients with chronic kidney disease
Flexible ureterorenoscopy	For calculi less than 20mm in size. The procedure wherein flexible ureteroscopy is used in the kidney is called retrograde intrarenal surgery (RIRS). It has been demonstrated as an effective way of treating stones which are refractory to ESWL.
Open surgery	recommended only if the stones are not expected to be removed in a reasonable number of stages.

Pain management:- (2)

NSAID by any route	as first-line treatment for adults, children and young people with suspected renal colic
Intravenous paracetamol	to adults, children and young people with suspected renal colic if NSAIDs are contraindicated or are not giving sufficient pain relief
Opioids	for adults, children and young people with suspected renal colic if both NSAIDs and intravenous paracetamol are contraindicated or are not giving sufficient pain relief
Antispasmodics	Do not offer to adults, children and young people with suspected renal colic
Medical expulsive therapy	alpha blockers for adults, children and young people with distal ureteric stones less than 10 mm. This is a new information after the SUSPEND trial (Pickard et al. 2015), the largest RCT on this subject which had, concluded that there was no benefit in using alpha blockers

Treatment options based on stone size, position and symptoms:-

	ADULTS	CHILDREN AND YOUNG PEOPLE
Asymptomatic renal stones	Watchful waiting for stones less than 5 mm, but may also apply to larger stones.	
Ureteric stones, less than 10 mm	ESWL- First choice URS - alternative choice if, - stone clearance is not possible within 4 weeks with SWL, - there are contraindications to SWL, - the stone is not targetable, or - a course of SWL has previously failed (because patients tend to form the same type of stones)	Either ESWL or URS - both equally recommended

Ureteric stones, 10 to 20 mm	URS- First choice ESWL- alternative choice if local facilities allow stone clearance within 4 weeks. PCNL- for larger impacted stones, particularly in the proximal ureter	Children have a higher incidence of spontaneous passage of larger stones than adults. Either ESWL or URS - both equally recommended
Ureteric stones, greater than 20 mm	No recommendation	No recommendation
Renal stones, less than 10 mm	ESWL- First choice URS- alternative choice PCNL- when both SWL and URS have failed or are not an option	Either ESWL or URS - both equally recommended PCNL- when other treatment has failed.
Renal stones, 10 to 20 mm	Both ESWL and URS are equally effective based on the clinician's decision. PCNL- again depends on clinical judgment	Clinical judgment should be used when deciding which treatment to use (URS, ESWL or PCNL).
Adults, renal stones, larger than 20 mm	PCNL- First choice URS- for people with high comorbidity, anesthetic risks or anatomical considerations	Either URS or PCNL could be considered, and ESWL should not be ruled out.
Adult, renal stones, staghorn	PCNL	PCNL

Surgical treatment should be offered within 48 hours of diagnosis or readmission, to people presenting with ureteric stones and renal colic, if the pain is ongoing and not tolerated or the stone is unlikely to pass. Although the evidence was from people with stones less than 20 mm, the committee agreed that ureteric stones of all sizes should be treated within this timeframe.

Studies:

3. Hollingsworth JM et al searched 443 articles and finally included 55 studies in their systematic review and meta-analysis on the utility and outcome of alpha blockers.(22) The results suggested that alpha blockers had no benefit in stone passage if the size is < 5mm with a RR = 1.19 but showed modest benefit for stones larger than 6 mm. (RR = 1.57). The other findings were a shorter time to passage with alpha blockers of 3.79 days, lower risk of surgical intervention and lower risk of admission to hospital. These results support current guideline recommendations advocating a role for alpha blockers in patients with ureteric stones

4. Meltzer AC et al recruited 512 adult patients presenting to the ED with a symptomatic urinary stone determined by CT to be < 9 m in diameter and located in the ureter. 267 patients received Tamsulosin 0.4 mgOD whereas 245 were enrolled in placebo arm.(23) 49.6% patients on tamsulosin

reported passage of stone versus 47.3% in placebo group.(No statistically significant difference). There was more dizziness amongst patients receiving tamsulosinAmongst males, there was a significantly higher rate of abnormalities with ejaculation in the tamsulosin arm (18.2% vs 7.4%). Tamsulosin did not significantly increase the stone passage rate compared with placebo. The findings do not support the use of tamsulosin for symptomatic urinary stones smaller than 9 mm. Guidelines for medical expulsive therapy for urinary stones may need to be revised.

Lidocaine is known to possess analgesic and anti-inflammatory properties with a short half life of 1-2 hours and predictable adverse effects. Oliveira L et al(5) performed a systematic review of RCTs and observational studies using lidocaine for pain management in the ED(24). Intotal, 8 RCTs, 1 observational study and 1 case series were included. 6 RCTs were on renal colic. One trial on renal colic compared lidocaine infusion with morphine and showed lidocaine as a superior analgesic. The most common side effect was dizziness. One patient who had received 400 mg lidocaine had seizure, bradycardia and cardiac arrest. The patient could be resuscitated with complete neurological recovery. The authors advised caution in the use of IV lidocaine in patients over the age of 65 years and those with structural heart disease as there is no strong evidence to support its effectiveness, with the known potential harms. The usual dose of lidocaine is 2mg/kg of IV lidocaine and typically given as an infusion over several minutes as opposed to IV push. The review concluded that there is limited current evidence to define the role of intravenous lidocaine as an analgesic for patients with acute renal colic in the ED.

<u>Summary-</u> The red flags of renal stones is obstructive uropathy with renal failure, localized or systemic infections and pain refractory to regular analgesics. These should be recognized and treated. Patients may require HD for preoperative stabilization. Syndromes with recurrent urinary stones should be investigated for parathyroidism and also referred for endocrinologist opinion.

References

1. Urolithiasis And Ureteric Colic-Standard Treatment Guidelines By Supriya Kashyap Kashyap Published On 13 Apr 2017 9:59 AM | Updated On 13 Apr 2017 9:59 AM

2. NICE Releases 2019 Guidelines For Management Of Renal And Ureteric Stones By Hina Zahid Published On 12 Jan 2019 7:00 PM | Updated On 12 Jan 2019 7:00 PM

3. Hollingsworth JM et al. Alpha blockers for treatment of ureteric stones: systematic review and meta-analysis. BMJ 2016.

4. Meltzer, AC et al. Effect of Tamsulosin on Passage of Symptomatic Ureteral Stones: A Randomized Clinical Trial. JAMA Intern Med 2018

5. Oliveira L et al. Safety and Efficacy of Intravenous Lidocaine for Pain Management in the Emergency Department: A Systematic Review. Ann Emerg Med 2018.

Studies and Guidelines

Common pathogens: E. coli is responsible for about 80-90% of UTI in the community. This is followed by Proteus sp., Klebsiella sp., Staphylococcus aureus, etc. Staphylococcus saprophyticus causes infection in young women in many countries but this is rare in India.(1) In hospital acquired UTIs or in the presence of devices, Pseudomonas aeruginosa, Acinetobacter sp, Enterococci etc., are causative agents depending on the setting. In patients on long term catheters and antibiotic therapy, Candida sp is also implicated.

Investigation from ED should be a Urine Specimen Clean catch midstream. Suprapubic aspiration is performed in cases of small children where voided urine is difficult to collect or in adults in case diagnosis is not getting confirmed by voided specimen. The specimen must be transported as early as possible. For up to 4 hours delay, the urine should be refrigerated. 0.8% boric acid as a preservative can be used to store urine for up to 24 hours if transported from distance. The urine sample is studied for 1. Direct Microscopy- Pus cells, RBC, Casts etc. 2. Rapid- Presence of pus cells by leukocyte esterase/nitrate reduction tests. 3. Culture- Semiquantitative culture for determining significant counts.

The diagnosis is based on the presence of "significant bacterial" counts in the urine specimen. Urine is otherwise a sterile fluid in the bladder but during the passage through the urethra can get contaminated with perineal flora colonizing the lower urethra. A count of 10^5 bacteria/ml of urine in a clean catch midstream specimen is "Significant bacteriuria" in a person with symptoms of the lower urinary tract like dysuria, frequency, suprapubic pain and hematuria.

On a urine microscopy, pus cells > 10,000/ml along with positivity for nitrite or leukocyte esterase in symptomatic individuals indicate probable UTI. In children commonly, one bacteria per oil immersion field in an uncentrifuged urine sample is considered a possible indication of a UTI. Rarely due to the inflammation red blood cells may be present and thus falsely increase the number of pus cells. Even if urine microscopy or urine cultures are not indicative of a UTI, caution should be exercised in case of obstructive uropathy, patient on antibiotics, hematogenous route of infection, in suprapubic aspirate specimen if the patient is clearly symptomatic. In children suprapubic aspirate may be needed due to the problem in collecting an appropriate specimen. Any count in this sample is considered significant. Recurrent UTIs may suggest an underlying anatomic abnormality and a urological evaluation with contrast imaging may be required for delineation of the same.

E. coli and other members of family Enterobacteriaceae remain the most common cause of UTI, however antimicrobial resistance is very high to the commonly prescribed antibiotics in various

Indian studies and the ICMR AMR network data. Most Enterobacteriaceae isolates are ESBL or extended spectrum beta lactamase producing curbing the utility of 3rd and 4th generation cephalosporins and most beta lactam antibiotics. Most often we have to resort to Carbapenems.

Table 1: General treatment of UTI

Clinical Condition	Common Pathogens	Empiric AMA	Alternate AMA	Comments
Acute Cystitis (in absence of cultures)	E.coli, Proteus sp Klebsiella sp.	• Nitrofurantoin 100 mg BD for 7 days • Cotrimoxazole 500/125 mg BD for 3-5 days • Ciprofloxacin 500 mg BD for 3-5 days	• Cefuroxime 250 mg BD for 3-5 days • Cefixime 400mg BD for 5 days	Staphylococcus saprophyticus (in sexually active young women) but is not common in India. In pregnancy the duration of treatment is longer
Acute Pyelonephritis (individualized based on data from each center) If blood culture is positive, a carbapenem is preferred.	E.coli, Klebsiella sp Proteus sp S. aureus	• Piperacillin tazobactam 4.5 gm IV 6 hourly for 10 days • Ertapenem 1 g IV OD for 7 days	• Imipenem 500 mg IV 8 hourly for 10 days or • Inj Amikacin 5mg/kg IV once daily x 10 days	Urine and blood culture should be done before the start of treatment. Amikacin 1gm OD IV or Gentamicin 7 mg/kg as prescribed doses. Close monitor on renal parameters is needed and watch out for relapse
Acute prostatitis	Enterobacteriaceae (E. coli, Klebsiella sp.)	• Doxycycline 100 mg BD for 2-3 wks • Co-trimoxazole 960 mg BD for 2-3 wks Ciprofloxacin 500 mg BD for 2-3 wks	• Piperacillin tazobactam 4.5 gm IV 6 hourly • Cefoperazone sulbactam 3 gm IV 12 hourly • Ertapenem 1 gm IV OD or Imipenem 1 gm IV 8 hourly or Meropenem 1 gm IV 8 hourly	Get urine and prostatic massage cultures before antibiotics. Treatment may be needed for longer duration
All these regimens need to be tailored according to susceptibility patterns at individual centers				

Recurrent urinary tract infection (UTI) in adults is defined as repeated UTI with a frequency of 2 or more UTIs in the last 6 months or 3 or more UTIs in the last 12 months (European Association of Urology [EAU] guidelines on urological infections [2017]).(2)

Recurrent UTI is diagnosed in children and young people under 16 years if they have: 2 or more episodes of UTI with acute pyelonephritis/upper UTI or 1 episode of UTI with acute pyelonephritis plus 1 or more episode of UTI with cystitis/lower UTI or 3 or more episodes of UTI with cystitis/lower UTI.

Recurrent UTI may be due to relapse (with the same strain of organism) or reinfection (with a different strain or species of organism) and is particularly common in women. Consider the lowest effective dose of vaginal oestrogen (for example, estriol cream) for postmenopausal women with recurrent UTI if behavioural and personal hygiene measures alone are not effective or not appropriate.

Some women with recurrent UTI may wish to try D-mannose if they are not pregnant, some women with recurrent UTI may wish to try cranberry products if they are not pregnant (evidence of benefit is uncertain and there is no evidence of benefit for older women), some children and young people under 16 years with recurrent UTI may wish to try cranberry products with the advice of a pediatric specialist (evidence of benefit is uncertain). Evidence is inconclusive about whether probiotics (lactobacillus) reduce the risk of UTI in people with recurrent UTI.

Table 2: People aged 16 years and over

Antibiotic prophylaxis	Dosage
First choice	Trimethoprim200 mg single dose when exposed to a trigger or 100 mg at night
	Nitrofurantoin – if eGFR ≥45 ml/minute 100 mg single dose when exposed to a trigger or 50 to 100 mg at night
Second choice	Amoxicillin 500 mg single dose when exposed to a trigger or 250 mg at night
	Cefalexin 500 mg single dose when exposed to a trigger or 125 mg at night

Table 3: Children and young people under 16 years

Antibiotic prophylaxis	Dosage
Children under 3 months	Refer to paediatric specialist
Children aged 3 months and over (specialist advice only)	
First choice	

Trimethoprim	3 to 5 months, 2 mg/kg at night (maximum 100 mg per dose) or 12.5 mg at night
	6 months to 5 years, 2 mg/kg at night (maximum 100 mg per dose) or 25 mg at night
	6 to 11 years, 2 mg/kg at night (maximum 100 mg per dose) or 50 mg at night
	12 to 15 years, 100 mg at night
Nitrofurantoin – if eGFR ≥45 ml/minute	3 months to 11 years, 1 mg/kg at night
	12 to 15 years, 50 to 100 mg at night
Second choice	
Cefalexin	3 months to 15 years, 12.5 mg/kg at night (maximum 125 mg per dose)
Amoxicillin	3 to 11 months, 62.5 mg at night
	1 to 4 years, 125 mg at night
	5 to 15 years, 250 mg at night

A catheter-associated urinary tract infection (CAUTI) is an asymptomatic infection of the bladder or kidneys in a person with a urinary catheter. (3) After 1 month of catheterization, nearly all people have bacteriuria but antibiotic treatment is not routinely needed for asymptomatic patients. The catheter should be changed if it has been in place for more than 7 days in the presence of CAUTI. A urine sample should be obtained from the catheter before replacing and also before antibiotics are given. When urine culture and susceptibility results are available, change the antibiotic according to susceptibility results if the bacteria are resistant, using narrow-spectrum antibiotics wherever possible. The Symptoms should start improving in 48 hours and if it does not happen, consider sepsis. An urgent specialist referral is needed for critically ill CAUTI patients, are pregnant, have a known or suspected structural or functional abnormality of the genitourinary tract, or are diabetics or immunosuppressed or have recurrent CAUTI or have bacteria that are resistant to oral antibiotics.

Table 4: Antibiotics for non-pregnant women and men aged 16 years and over

Antibiotic	Dosage and course length
First-choice oral antibiotic if no upper UTI symptoms	
Nitrofurantoin – if eGFR ≥45 ml/minute	100 mg modified-release twice a day for 7 days
Trimethoprim – if a low risk of resistance	200 mg twice a day for 7 days
Amoxicillin (only if culture results available and susceptible)	500 mg three times a day for 7 days
Second-choice oral antibiotic if no upper UTI symptoms (when first-choice not suitable)	
Pivmecillinam (a penicillin)	400 mg initial dose, then 200 mg three times a day for a total of 7 days

First-choice oral antibiotic if upper UTI symptoms	
Cefalexin	500 mg twice or three times a day (up to 1 to 1.5 g three or four times a day for severe infections) for 7 to 10 days
Co-amoxiclav (only if culture results available and susceptible)	500/125 mg three times a day for 7 to 10 days
Trimethoprim (only if culture results available and susceptible)	200 mg twice a day for 14 days
Ciprofloxacin (consider safety issues)	500 mg twice a day for 7 days
First-choice intravenous antibiotic (if vomiting, unable to take oral antibiotics or severely unwell). Antibiotics may be combined if susceptibility or sepsis a concern	
Co-amoxiclav (only in combination, unless culture results confirm susceptibility)	1.2 g three times a day
Cefuroxime	750 mg to 1.5 g three or four times a day
Ceftriaxone	1 to 2 g once a day
Ciprofloxacin (consider safety issues)	400 mg twice or three times a day
Gentamicin	Initially 5 to 7 mg/kg once a day, subsequent doses adjusted according to serum gentamicin concentration
Amikacin	Initially 15 mg/kg once a day (maximum per dose 1.5 g once a day), subsequent doses adjusted according to serum amikacin concentration (maximum 15 g per course)
Second-choice intravenous antibiotic	Consult local microbiologist

Table 5: Antibiotics for pregnant women aged 12 years and over

Antibiotic	Dose and course length
First-choice oral antibiotic	
Cefalexin	500 mg twice or three times a day (up to 1 to 1.5 g three or four times a day for severe infections) for 7 to 10 days
First-choice intravenous antibiotic (if vomiting, unable to take oral antibiotics, or severely unwell)	
Cefuroxime	750 mg to 1.5 g three or four times a day
Second-choice antibiotics or combining antibiotics if susceptibility or sepsis a concern	
Consult local microbiologist	

Table 6: Antibiotics for children and young people under 16 years

Antibiotic	Dosage and course length
Children under 3 months	Refer to pediatric specialist and treatment with intravenous antibiotics in line with the NICE guideline on fever in under 5
Children aged 3 months and over	
First-choice oral antibiotics	
Trimethoprim – if the low risk of resistance	3 to 5 months, 4 mg/kg (maximum 200 mg per dose) or 25 mg twice a day for 7 to 10 days 6 months to 5 years, 4 mg/kg (maximum 200 mg per dose) or 50 mg twice a day for 7 to 10 days 6 to 11 years, 4 mg/kg (maximum 200 mg per dose) or 100 mg twice a day for 7 to 10 days 12 to 15 years, 200 mg twice a day for 7 to 10 days
Amoxicillin (only if culture results available and susceptible)	3 to 11 months, 125 mg three times a day for 7 to 10 days 1 to 4 years, 250 mg three times a day for 7 to 10 days 5 to 15 years, 500 mg three times a day for 7 to 10 days
Cefalexin	3 to 11 months, 12.5 mg/kg or 125 mg twice a day for 7 to 10 days (25 mg/kg two to four times a day [maximum 1 g per dose four times a day] for severe infections) 1 to 4 years, 12.5 mg/kg twice a day or 125 mg three times a day for 7 to 10 days (25 mg/kg two to four times a day [maximum 1 g per dose four times a day] for severe infections) 5 to 11 years, 12.5 mg/kg twice a day or 250 mg three times a day for 7 to 10 days (25 mg/kg two to four times a day [maximum 1 g per dose four times a day] for severe infections) 12 to 15 years, 500 mg twice or three times a day (up to 1 to 1.5 g three or four times a day for severe infections) for 7 to 10 days
Co-amoxiclav (only if culture results available and susceptible)	3 to 11 months, 0.25 ml/kg of 125/31 suspension three times a day for 7 to 10 days (dose doubled in severe infection) 1 to 5 years, 0.25 ml/kg of 125/31 suspension or 5 ml of 125/31 suspension three times a day for 7 to 10 days (dose doubled in severe infection) 6 to 11 years, 0.15 ml/kg of 250/62 suspension or 5 ml of 250/62 suspension three times a day for 7 to 10 days (dose doubled in severe infection) 12 to 15 years, 250/125 mg or 500/125 mg three times a day for 7 to 10 days

First-choice intravenous antibiotics (if vomiting, unable to take oral antibiotics or severely unwell). Antibiotics may be combined if susceptibility or sepsis a concern	
Co-amoxiclav (only in combination unless culture results confirm susceptibility)	3 months to 15 years, 30 mg/kg three times a day (maximum 1.2 g three times a day)
Cefuroxime	3 months to 15 years, 20 mg/kg three times a day (maximum 750 mg per dose); (50 to 60 mg/kg three or four times a day [maximum 1.5 g per dose] for severe infections)
Ceftriaxone	3 months to 11 years (up to 50 kg), 50 to 80 mg/kg once a day (maximum 4 g per day) 9 to 11 years (50 kg and above), 1 to 2 g once a day 12 to 15 years, 1 to 2 g once a day
Gentamicin	Initially 7 mg/kg once a day, subsequent doses adjusted according to serum gentamicin concentration
Amikacin	Initially 15 mg/kg once a day, subsequent doses adjusted according to serum amikacin concentration
Second-choice intravenous antibiotic	
Consult local microbiologist	
Do not routinely offer antibiotic prophylaxis to prevent catheter-associated UTIs in people with a short-term or a long-term (indwelling or intermittent) catheter. Give advice about seeking medical help if symptoms of an acute UTI develop.	

Lower urinary tract infection (UTI) is an infection of the bladder usually caused by bacteria from the gastrointestinal tract entering the urethra and traveling up to the bladder.(4)

Table 7: Antibiotics for non-pregnant women aged 16 years and over

Antibiotic	Dosage and course length
First choice	
Nitrofurantoin – if eGFR ≥45 ml/minute	100 mg modified-release twice a day for 3 days
Trimethoprim – if low risk of resistance	200 mg twice a day for 3 days
Second-choice (no improvement in lower UTI symptoms on first-choice taken for at least 48 hours, or when first-choice not suitable)	
Nitrofurantoin – if eGFR ≥45 ml/minute4 and not used as first-choice	100 mg modified-release twice a day for 3 days

Pivmecillinam (a penicillin)	400 mg initial dose, then 200 mg three times a day for a total of 3 days
Fosfomycin	3 g single dose sachet

Table 8: Antibiotics for pregnant women aged 12 years and over

Antibiotic	Dosage and course length
Treatment of lower UTI-First choice	
Nitrofurantoin (avoid at term) – if eGFR ≥45 ml/minute	100 mg modified-release twice a day for 7 days
Second-choice (no improvement in lower UTI symptoms on first-choice taken for at least 48 hours or when first-choice not suitable)	
Amoxicillin (only if culture results available and susceptible)	500 mg three times a day for 7 days
Cefalexin	500 mg twice a day for 7 days
Alternative second-choices	
Consult local microbiologist, choose antibiotics based on culture and susceptibility results	
Treatment of asymptomatic bacteriuria Choose from nitrofurantoin, amoxicillin or cefalexin based on recent culture and susceptibility results	

Table 9: Antibiotics for men aged 16 years and over

Antibiotic	Dosage and course length
First choice	
Trimethoprim	200 mg twice a day for 7 days
Nitrofurantoin – if eGFR ≥45 ml/minute	100 mg modified-release twice a day for 7 days
Second-choice (no improvement in UTI symptoms on first-choice taken for at least 48 hours or when first-choice not suitable)	
Consider alternative diagnoses and follow recommendations in the NICE guidelines on pyelonephritis (acute): antimicrobial prescribing or prostatitis (acute): antimicrobial prescribing, basing the antibiotic choice on recent culture and susceptibility results.	

Table 10: Antibiotics for children and young people under 16 years

Antibiotic	Dosage and course length
Children under 3 months	Refer to pediatric specialists and treat with intravenous antibiotics in line with the NICE guideline on fever in under 5s.
Children aged 3 months and over	
First choice	

Trimethoprim – if low risk of resistance	3 to 5 months, 4 mg/kg (maximum 200 mg per dose) or 25 mg twice a day for 3 days
	6 months to 5 years, 4 mg/kg (maximum 200 mg per dose) or 50 mg twice a day for 3 days
	6 to 11 years, 4 mg/kg (maximum 200 mg per dose) or 100 mg twice a day for 3 days
	12 to 15 years, 200 mg twice a day for 3 days
Nitrofurantoin – if eGFR ≥45 ml/minute	3 months to 11 years, 750 micrograms/kg four times a day for 3 days
	12 to 15 years, 50 mg four times a day or 100 mg modified-release twice a day for 3 days
Second-choice (no improvement in lower UTI symptoms on first-choice taken for at least 48 hours or when first-choice not suitable)	
Nitrofurantoin – if eGFR ≥45 ml/minute6and not used as first-choice	3 months to 11 years, 750 micrograms/kg four times a day for 3 days
	12 to 15 years, 50 mg four times a day or 100 mg modified-release twice a day for 3 days
Amoxicillin (only if culture results available and susceptible)	1 to 11 months, 125 mg three times a day for 3 days
	1 to 4 years, 250 mg three times a day for 3 days
	5 to 15 years, 500 mg three times a day for 3 days
Cefalexin	3 to 11 months, 12.5 mg/kg or 125 mg twice a day for 3 days
	1 to 4 years, 12.5 mg/kg twice a day or 125 mg three times a day for 3 days
	5 to 11 years, 12.5 mg/kg twice a day or 250 mg three times a day for 3 days
	12 to 15 years, 500 mg twice a day for 3 days

Trials

5. <u>Kjölvmark, Charlott, et al.</u> compared cohorts of asymptomatic elderly nursing home residents and patients living in the community or at nursing homes with symptomatic UTI. Urinary IL-6 and Urinary heparin-binding protein (HBP) were compared to distinguish between patients with cystitis or asymptomatic bacteriuria. There was a statistically significant rise in urinary IL-6 levels in patients with cystitis (5)

6. <u>ProACT and subsequent Trials-</u> Serum levels of Procalcitonin have been used to decide the presence of true bacteremia in patients and initiate or stop antibiotics. The ProACT Trial where patients with LRTI were screened, did not produce convincing results. Procalcitonin failed miserably in limiting unnecessary antibiotic utilization. Consequent to it, Levine et al performed a retrospective analysis of UTIs and found a negative predictive value of 91% for a low procalcitonin, arguing strongly for its use as an adjunct in the non-initiation of empiric antibiotics. Procalcitonin

is presently considered as a reliable and objective diagnostic waypoint to limit costly, harmful, and unnecessary antibiotics.

7. <u>Chris H et al</u> from the United Kingdom recruited 240 adult women who had at least three UTI episodes in the previous 12 months from urology and urogynecology centers. The participants were randomly assigned 1:1 to receive either twice-daily oral doses of methenamine hippurate or daily doses of antibiotics (nitrofurantoin, trimethoprim, or cefalexin) for a year, with a 6-month follow-up period. The primary clinical outcome was the incidence of self-reported symptomatic, antibiotic-treated UTIs over the 12-month treatment period. Secondary outcomes included incidence of UTIs during the 6-month follow-up period, total antibiotic use, and antibiotic-resistance profiles in *Escherichia coli* isolated from urine and perineal swabs. The non-inferiority margin was a difference of one UTI episode per year. The results were as follows- (Table 10).

Treatment Period		Absolute difference
Incidence of symptomatic UTI	0.89 episodes per person year in the antibiotic arm	0.49
	1.38 episodes per person year (95% CI 1.05 to 1.72) in the methenamine hippurate arm	
6-month follow-up period	1.19 in the antibiotic arm	0.53
	1.72 in the methenamine hippurate arm	
Therapeutic antibiotics for UTI over the 12-month treatment period.	43% of participants in the antibiotic arm	Overall antibiotic use among women who received prophylactic methenamine hippurate was lower
	56% in the methenamine hippurate arm	
Resistance to at least one antibiotic in *E coli* isolated from perineal swabs	antibiotic arm (46 of 64, 72%)	Urine cultures showed higher rates of resistance in *E coli* to trimethoprim, co-trimethoxazole, and cephalosporins in antibiotics arm
	methenamine hippurate arm (39/70, 56%)	At month 18, multidrug resistance in *E coli* was higher in the methenamine group (20% vs 5%).

The results showed that while women who received prophylactic treatment with methenamine hippurate had a higher rate of UTI episodes than those treated with prophylactic antibiotics, the absolute difference has limited clinical significance. This new research increases the confidence with which methenamine hippurate can be offered as an option to women needing prophylaxis against recurrent urinary tract infection.

<u>Summary-</u> Keep a watchful eye on the symptoms of UTI which have a higher likelihood ratio for diagnosis rather than treating a lab / culture report. Always consider the local flora and antibiotic sensitivity and resistance report from your microbiologist. Look out for causes for severe UTI or nonresponsive to AMA especially structural causes like stone disease and immunosuppression like DM. Procedure like DJ stenting for pyelonephritis will help to clear the stagnation and promote efficacy of AMA. Use of CT scan KUB are also indicated in patients with obstructive or structural uropathy. Contrast scan is rarely required in such scenarios. Serious infections with raised serum creatinine should be referred to a nephrologist to consider a few sessions of Hemodialysis.

References

1. Antimicrobial Guidelines For Urinary Tract Infections- ICMR By Supriya Kashyap KashyapPublished On 5 Mar 2017 11:44 AM | Updated On 18 Aug 2021 5:28 PM

2. Antimicrobials In Recurrent UTI: NICE 2018 Guideline By Hina Zahid. Published On 2 Nov 2018 7:00 PM | Updated On 2 Nov 2018 7:00 PM

3. Antibiotic Use In Catheter-Associated UTI: NICE Guidelines By Vinay Singh Singh. Published On 5 Dec 2018 7:00 PM | Updated On 9 Aug 2021 5:01 PM

4. Antimicrobial Prescribing In Lower Urinary Tract Infection: NICE Guideline By Hina Zahid Published On 14 Mar 2019 7:00 PM | Updated On 14 Mar 2019 7:00 PM

5. Kjölvmark, Charlott, et al. "Distinguishing asymptomatic bacteriuria from urinary tract infection in the elderly–the use of urine levels of heparin-binding protein and interleukin-6." Diagnostic microbiology and infectious disease85.2 (2016): 243-248. PMID: 27039283

6. Levine, Alexander R., et al. "Utility of initial procalcitonin values to predict urinary tract infection." The American journal of emergency medicine (2018). PMID 29530360

7. Chris Harding et al. Alternative to prophylactic antibiotics for the treatment of recurrent urinary tract infections in women ALTAR trial: multicentre, open label, randomised, non-inferiority trial. BMJ 2022; 376..

Hematuria is a common presentation to the emergency department which can be traumatic, nontraumatic and incidental (in upto 40% of patients).

The causes of hematuria are tabulated in Table

Vascular	Kidney	Ureter	Bladder	Urethra
AV malformations	Benign tumors	Malignancy	Malignancy	BPH
Renal artery embolus, infarct, dissection, or aneurysm	Malignant tumors	Ureterolithiasis	Cystitis*	Urethritis, prostatitis
Renal vein thrombosis*	Glomerulonephritis (IgA nephropathy, streptococcal	Stricture	Radiation Cystitis	Prostate cancer*
AAA	Familial disease like alport syndrome			Recent procedures
	PCKD			Traumatic catheterization*
	Nephrolithiasis			Urethral diverticulum
	HSP	Causes in bold text have a higher incidence of life threatening hematuria. Starred *= most common causes of hematuria in our ED(unpublished report)		
	Hydronephrosis			
	Pyelonephritis*			
	Malignant Hypertension			
	Papillary necrosis			

Trials -

1. The article by Willis GC is very informative especially on the usefulness of urine dipstick test in ED to confirm hematuria.(33) Healthy individuals may have up to 7 RBCs/mL of urine. Urine dipstick is able to detect the presence of 10 RBCs/mL which makes it highly sensitive to detect physiologic abnormal hematuria. The pitfalls are-

1. Urine with high specific gravity and low pH can have false negative results. Same can happen after high consumption of vitamin C.
2. Myoglobin from rhabdomyolysis or by intravascular hemolysis releasing free hemoglobin can cause false positive results. All positive dipstick tests should be sent for microscopic analysis to determine true presence of red blood cells.

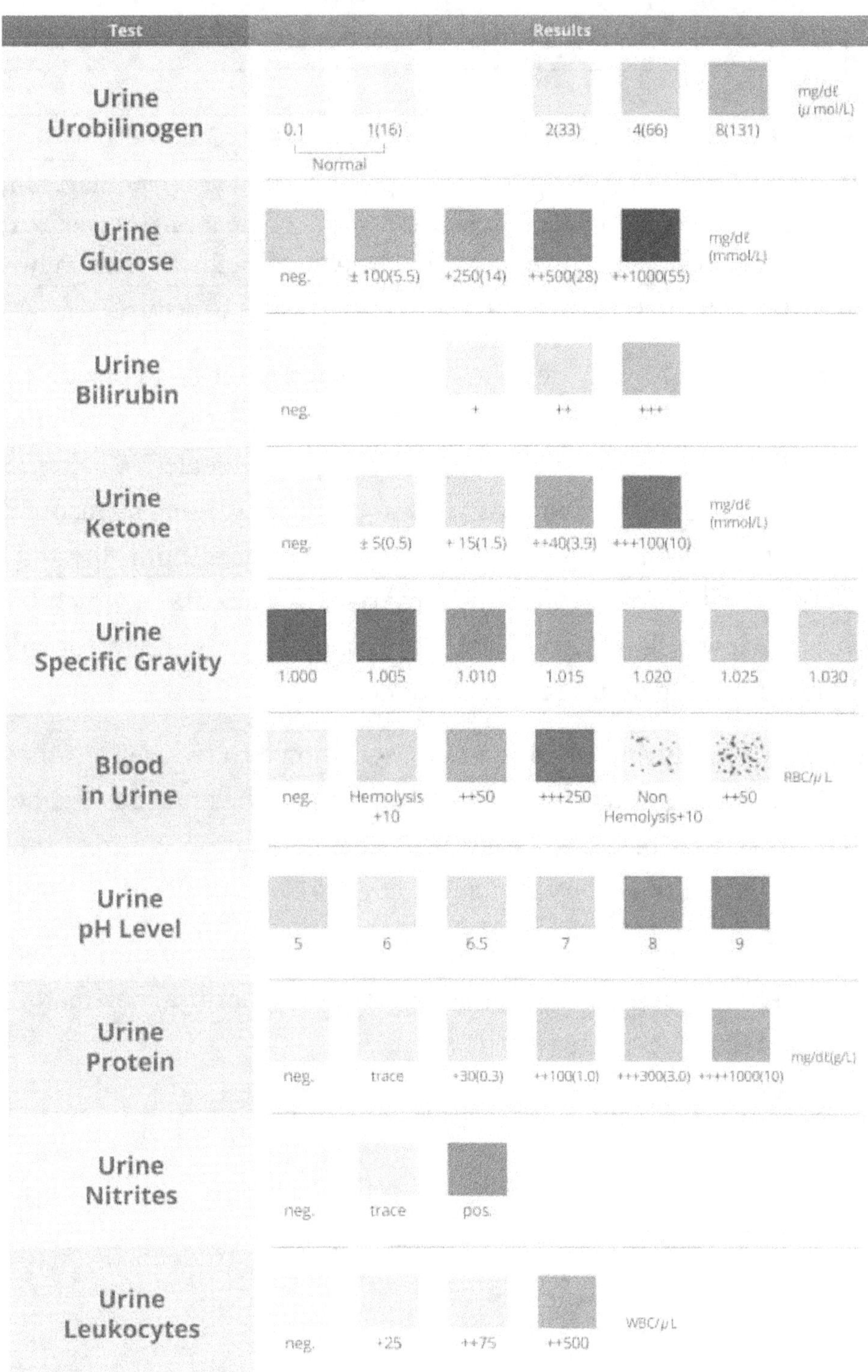

Microscopic hematuria is defined as ≥3-5 RBCs/hpf.(2) Asymptomatic microscopic hematuria is seen in young individuals after vigorous exercise, sexual intercourse or with febrile illness. Elevated INR may lead to microscopic hematuria, however this rarely occurs in the therapeutic range. The current American Urological Association (AUA) clinical practice guidelines recommend urological referral for all patients with microscopic hematuria in which a benign cause has been ruled out, and cystoscopy for all patients aged ≥35 or with current or past tobacco use or exposure to caustic chemicals.

An Algorithmic Approach Guiding Management. (3)

Risk level	Risk factors
Low	men<40, women<50, <10 pack year smoking, <10 RBC/hpf
Intermediate	Men 40-59, women 50-59, 11-25 rbc/hpf,10-30 pack year smoking, family history of urothelial cancer, prior microscopic hematuria, occupational exposure to benzenes, aromatic amines, chemotherapy with cyclophosphamide, chronic indwelling foleys
High	Age > 60, > 25rbc/hpf, >30 pack year smoking, gross hematuria

The AUA recommends referral for CT urogram and cystoscopy for any episode of hematuria that falls in the high risk category. CT has a near 100% sensitivity for detecting malignancy of the upper urinary tracts and with proper excretory phase a 95% negative predictive value for tumors of the bladder. However, in intermediate risk patients and in pregnancy, renal ultrasound is a reasonable initial imaging modality, which has 82% sensitivity for renal tumors, but is limited in its evaluation of more distal structures. MRI is a reasonable alternative for patients in which CT is unable to be performed, however with lower sensitivity than CT. While plain films and retrograde urethrography have minimal utility in detecting underlying malignancy.

Role of TXA- Infusion of TXA during irrigation has been shown to reduce the amount of irrigation needed and decrease hematuria detected by dipstick, however has not been shown to reduce the need for transfusion in serious bleeding.Reversal of anticoagulation is rarely indicated except in cases of life-threatening hemorrhage or vascular etiology.(4)

Workup of hematuria (5)-The figure outlines the workup of patients presenting with hematuria in ED by the authors. It takes into account the various causes of hematuria, risk factors for malignancy and involvement of specialist doctors as per the need.

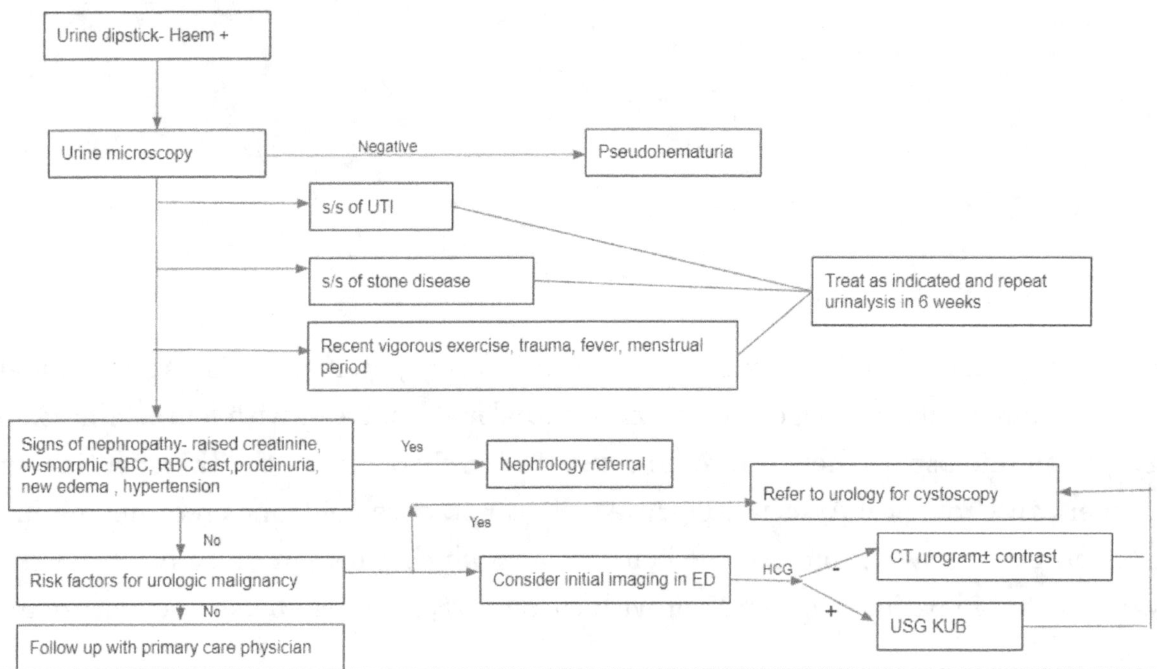

History, urine microscopy and ultrasound KUB are the most important parts of evaluation of hematuria. Special investigations like CT scan and urograms are indicated in patients where specialist referrals are not available or loss to followup is strongly suspected. Red flag like acute anemias, severe pain, urinary retention, acute renal dysfunction and further darkening of urine should be monitored, A three way foley's catheter for irrigation till the outflow is clear is helpful.

References

1. Willis GC, Tewelde SZ. The Approach to the Patient with Hematuria. Emerg Med Clin North Am. 2019;37(4):755-769. doi:10.1016/j.emc.2019.07.011

2. Barocas D, Boorjian S, Alvarez R, et al. Microhematuria AUA/SUFU Guideline. American Urologic Association, 2020.

3. Dulku G, Shivananda A, Chakera A, Mendelson R, Hayne D. Painless Visible Haematuria in Adults: An Algorithmic Approach Guiding Management. Cureus. 2019;11(11):e6140. Published 2019 Nov 13. doi:10.7759/cureus.6140

4. Moharamzadeh P, Ojaghihaghighi S, Amjadi M, Rahmani F, Farjamnia A. Effect of tranexamic acid on gross hematuria: A pilot randomized clinical trial study. Am J Emerg Med. 2017;35(12):1922-1925. doi:10.1016/j.ajem.2017.09.012

5. Kurz M, Feldman AS, Parezella, MA. Etiology and evaluation of hematuria in adults. In: UpToDate, Lam AQ (Ed), UpToDate, Waltham, MA, 2018

Infectious and Tropical Diseases

Contributors

1. Dr. Nidhi Kaeley
2. Dr. Hari Prasad
3. Dr. Vikram Jain
4. Dr. Monika Pathania

Chapters

1. Sepsis and Septic shock
2. Scrub Typhus
3. Infective endocarditis
4. Urosepsis
5. Dengue
6. Fungal infections
7. Viral infections
8. Mycobacterial infections
9. Parasitic infections
10. Tropical diseases
11. Vaccines
12. Leptospirosis

Sepsis and Septic Shock

Definition as per The Third International Consensus Definitions for Sepsis and Septic Shock (Sepsis-3)

Sepsis – It is defined as organ dysfunction caused by dysregulated host response to infection. It is estimated that it affects around 49 million people yearly with up to 19.7 % of mortality rate worldwide. Timely diagnosis and treatment can prevent significant mortality in patients with sepsis in the emergency department.(1)

Septic shock – is defined as a subset of sepsis in which underlying circulatory and metabolic abnormalities are profound enough to substantially increase mortality. Septic shock can be identified with a clinical construct of sepsis with persistent hypotension, requiring vasopressor therapy to elevate MAP more than or equal to 65 mm Hg and lactate less than 2 mmol/L despite adequate fluid resuscitation.

Pathophysiology There is a complex interplay of dysregulated inflammatory and anti-inflammatory markers. Multiple cytokines, inflammatory mediators and pathogen related molecules are released. The first step is activation of specific receptors on the surface of antigen presenting cells by the recognition of pathogen derived molecular patterns (PAMPs) such as endotoxins and exotoxins, lipids, DNA sequences and endogenous host derived danger signals (DAMPs). This leads to progressive inflammation and multi organ dysfunction. Also, in few patients, there is increased apoptosis of immune cells and T cell exhaustion, called immunoparalysis.

Sepsis induced coagulopathy-It is characterized by presence of organ dysfunction, decreased platelet count and increased PT INR.

Complement system in sepsis-Complement activated products (C3a, C5a, C4a) are activated. C5a attracts the neutrophils. After binding with C5a receptors the neutrophils change into migratory cells and develop the ability to enter the inflamed tissues and aid in removing the pathogen and debris. Both PAMPs and DAMPs stimulate the release of neutrophil extracellular trap, granular enzymes and reactive oxygen species. Thus, the prothrombotic state is activated and fibrinolysis is inhibited. This prothrombotic state leads to consumption coagulopathy, leading to overt DIC.

Sepsis induced immunosuppression and persistent inflammation catabolism syndrome-In the early stage, there is depletion of both B and T lymphocytes as a result of increased apoptosis rate of stromal cells and antigen presenting cells. In the beginning, B cells are stimulated by pathogen recognition receptors, which in turn activate the innate immune response. There is alteration in different peripheral B cell subgroups such as immature/ transitional B cells, naïve B cells, tissue like memory B cells. In later stages, there is sepsis induced lymphopenia, increased rate of antigen presenting cells and monocytes leading to reduction of cytotoxic and helper T cells.

Cellular, tissue and organ dysfunction-Hypoperfusion in sepsis occurs as a result of cardiovascular dysfunction. This leads to decreased oxygen delivery and utilization to the tissues.

Management

Surviving Sepsis Campaign changed recommends the 1-hour sepsis bundle which requires the physician to do the following all within 1 hour of ED triage. (1)

- measuring a lactate
- obtaining blood cultures
- starting antibiotics
- beginning 30 mL/kg crystalloid for hypotension or lactate >4 mmol/L
- initiating vasopressors without waiting for central venous access during or after fluid resuscitation to maintain a mean arterial pressure >65 mm Hg
- administration of iv hydrocortisone for ongoing shock

The approach to a patient with sepsis or septic shock in the emergency department is to start assessing the patient with primary survey and resuscitate simultaneously.

- Secure airway and breathing- supplemental oxygen to be started whenever indicated to maintain oxygen saturation between 90% and 96%. Mechanical ventilation to be initiated to reduce the work of breathing followed by intubation.

- Establish venous access - Peripheral venous access is sufficient for initial fluid resuscitation. Intravenous fluids (balanced crystalloids or normal saline) therapy to be started at 30 ml/kg in 1 hour and completed by 3 hours of presentation. The clinical and hemodynamic response and the presence or absence of pulmonary edema must be assessed before and after each bolus. Intravenous fluid challenges can be repeated until blood pressure and tissue perfusion are acceptable, pulmonary edema ensues, or fluid fails to augment perfusion. The insertion of a central line should not delay the administration of resuscitative fluids and antibiotics. A central venous catheter (CVC) can be used to infuse intravenous fluids, vasopressors, and blood products, as well as to draw blood for frequent laboratory studies. The role of CVP and $ScvO_2$ monitoring to determine the progress of sepsis is limited.

- Initial blood investigations include complete blood count, serum lactate levels, peripheral blood cultures(aerobic and anaerobic cultures from at least two different sites), urinalysis, and microbiologic cultures from suspected sources (eg, sputum, urine, intravascular catheter, wound or surgical site, body fluids) and an arterial blood gas analysis.

- <u>Imaging targeted at the suspected site of infection</u> is warranted (eg, chest radiography, computed tomography of chest and/or abdomen).

- <u>Vasopressors and inotropes</u> - In patients with shock, use of <u>norepinephrine</u> as a first line vasopressor therapy is recommended if not responsive to intravenous fluid therapy. Target a MAP (mean arterial pressure) of 65 mmHg. If target MAP is not achieved, vasopressin can be added as a second line or also as a first line agent in patients with significant tachycardia (eg, fast atrial fibrillation, sinus tachycardia >160/minute), agents that completely lack beta adrenergic effects. Similarly, dopamine may be acceptable in those with significant bradycardia; but low dose DA should **not** be used for the purposes of "renal protection." Phenylephrine is recommended as a first line in patients with atrial fibrillation with rapid ventricular rate. Epinephrine and dobutamine are effective inotropic agents.

- <u>Steroids</u> - In patients of septic shock on ongoing vasopressor therapy (dose of norepinephrine or epinephrine more than or equal to 0.25 microgram/kg/min for at least 4 hours after initiation to maintain target MAP) can be started on intravenous hydrocortisone at 200mg/day as 50 mg intravenously every 6 hourly or as continuous infusion.

- <u>Antibiotics</u> – should be started within the first hour of presentation. In patients with sepsis or septic shock at high risk of MRSA, starting antibiotics with MRSA coverage is recommended. It should not be initiated in patients with low risk of MRSA. In patients with sepsis or septic shock, at high risk of multi-drug resistant organism, should be initiated at two antimicrobials with gram negative coverage. Anti-fungal therapy should be added only in patients at risk of fungal infections. Source of infection should be actively looked for and drainage of abscess, empyema etc., is needed.Other examples include removing other infected implantable devices/hardware, when feasible, abscess drainage (including thoracic empyema and joint), percutaneous nephrostomy, soft tissue debridement or amputation, colectomy (eg, for fulminant *Clostridium difficile*-associated colitis), and cholecystostomy. The choice of antimicrobials should consider the patient's history (eg, recent antibiotics received, previous organisms), comorbidities (eg, diabetes, organ failures), immune defects (eg, HIV), clinical context (eg, community- or hospital-acquired), suspected site of infection, presence of invasive devices, Gram stain data, and local prevalence and resistance patterns making each prescription tailored to each individual. The patients with sepsis and septic shock have increased volume of distribution due to the administration of fluid and therefore higher clinical success rates have been reported in patients with higher peak concentrations of antimicrobials by giving high end dosing. Continuous infusions of antibiotics as compared with intermittent dosing regimens remains investigational.

- <u>Albumin</u> can be initiated in patients who have already received larger volumes of crystalloids. There is no role of hypertonic saline.

- <u>Levosimendan</u> – can be added in patients with septic shock and cardiac dysfunction with persistent hypotension despite adequate volume status and arterial blood pressure.

- In patients with septic shock, <u>invasive monitoring of arterial blood pressure</u> is recommended. Respiratory changes in the vena caval diameter, radial artery pulse pressure, aortic blood flow peak velocity, left ventricular outflow tract velocity-time integral, and brachial artery blood flow velocity are considered dynamic measures of fluid responsiveness. There is increasing evidence that dynamic measures are more accurate predictors of fluid responsiveness than static measures, as long as the patients are in sinus rhythm and passively ventilated with a sufficient tidal volume. For actively breathing patients or those with irregular cardiac rhythms, an increase in the cardiac output in response to a passive leg-raising maneuver (measured by echocardiography, arterial pulse waveform analysis, or pulmonary artery catheterization) also predicts fluid responsiveness.

- Recommendation is <u>AGAINST the use of qSOFA</u> compared with SIRS, NEWS or MEWS as a single tool for sepsis or septic shock.

- <u>Lactate level</u> more than 4 mmol/l indicate severity of the sepsis and need for therapeutic intervention. The lactate clearance is defined by the equation [(initial lactate – lactate >2 hours later)/initial lactate] x 100. The lactate clearance and interval change in lactate over the first 12 hours of resuscitation has been evaluated as a potential marker for effective resuscitation. Lactate is a poor marker of tissue perfusion after the restoration of perfusion. As a result, lactate values are generally unhelpful following restoration of perfusion, with one exception: a rising serum lactate level should prompt reevaluation of the adequacy of perfusion.

- <u>Diagnostic evidence of procalcitonin</u> is less clearly understood. Procalcitonin is mainly used to de-escalate or escalate antibiotic therapy. In few studies, it has shown mortality benefit but not an overall survival benefit to use procalcitonin guided antibiotic therapy.

Early Goal Directed Therapy for treating sepsis- Components were- 1.early administration of fluids and antibiotics (within one to six hours) using the following targets to measure the response: $ScvO_2$ ≥70 percent, CVP 8 to 12 mmHg, MAP ≥65 mmHg, and urine output ≥0.5 mL/kg/hour. Almost all trials did not show a mortality benefit to EGDT, it is thought that the lack of benefit was explained by an overall improved outcome in both control and treatment groups, and to improved clinical performance by trained clinicians in academic centers during an era that followed an aggressive sepsis education and management campaign. In support of this hypothesis is that central line placement was common (>50 percent) in control groups so it is likely that CVP and $ScvO_2$ were targeted in these patients.

Recent updates on sepsis

- **SAFE trial** (Saline versus Fluid administration) in 2004 showed that the use of 4 percent albumin or normal saline for fluid resuscitation results in similar outcomes in 28 days. (2)

- **VISEP study** (The efficacy of volume substitution and insulin therapy in severe sepsis) in 2008 placed critically ill patients with sepsis at increased risk for serious adverse events related to hypoglycemia. Hydroxy-ethyl pentastarch (10 percent) was harmful and its toxicity increased with accumulating doses. the trial was stopped prematurely. (3)

- **ProMise trial** (2014) showed that early administration of intravenous antibiotics and 6 hour base resuscitation as per EGDT (early goal-directed therapy) protocol in patients with septic shock did not lead to an improvement in outcome. (4)

- **ProCESS trial (2014)** showed that protocol based resuscitation of patients in whom septic shock was diagnosed in the emergency department did not show significant difference in 90-day mortality, 1-year mortality, or need for organ support. (5)

- **ARISE trial (2014)** did not show significant difference in survival time, in-hospital mortality, duration of organ support, or length of hospital stay in patients with early septic shock who were given protocol-based resuscitation. (6)

- **FABLED study (2019)** studied the outcome of blood culture sensitivity when drawing blood before and after antimicrobial administration in patients with severe manifestations of sepsis. They included adults with severe manifestations of sepsis, including systolic blood pressure less than 90 mm Hg or a serum lactate level of 4 mmol/L or more. The study concluded that drawing blood cultures after antimicrobial therapy in patients with severe sepsis significantly reduces the sensitivity of the blood culture. Positive blood cultures occur more likely if cultures are drawn prior to antibiotic therapy. (7)

- **CORTICUS trial** (2008) was an RCT (randomized control trial) done for patients with septic shock where 50 mg of intravenous hydrocortisone was given 6th hourly for 5 days in one arm and placebo in the other arm. There was no improvement in survival or the reversal of shock. (8)

- **ADRENAL trial** (2013) explored the efficacy of corticosteroids in critically ill patients with septic shock and did not result in lower 90-day mortality. (9)

- **Antibiotic Delays and Feasibility (2020)-** Four factors were independently associated with both definitions of antibiotic delay: vague (ie, non explicitly infectious) presenting symptoms, triage location to non acute areas, care before the quality improvement intervention, and lower Sequential [Sepsis-related]Organ Failure Assessment scores. The quality improvement intervention significantly reduced antibiotic delays, yet most septic patients did not receive antibiotics within 1 hour of triage. Compliance with the 2018 Surviving Sepsis Campaign would require a wholesale alteration in the management of ED patients with either vague symptoms or absence of triage hypotension. (10)

Scrub Typhus

Scrub typhus (Chigger borne typhus, Tsutsugamushi fever) is caused by Orientia tsutsugamushi. Unlike other bacteria of the family Rickettsiaceae, it lacks lipopolysaccharide and peptidoglycan in cell wall and does not have an outer slime layer. It is endowed with a major surface protein (56kDa) and some minor surface protein (110, 80, 46, 43, 39, 35, 25 and 25kDa).

Demography

The disease was first observed in Japan and called tsutsugamushi (from tsutsuga meaning dangerous and mushi meaning insect or mite). This disease is found in various part of the world. In India, scrub typhus has been reported from Rajasthan, Jammu & Kashmir and Vellore.

Serological tests- Several serological tests are currently available for the diagnosis of rickettsial diseases like Weil-Felix Test (WFT), Indirect Immunoflourescence (IIF), Enzyme linked Immunosorbent assay (ELISA). ELISA techniques, particularly immunoglobulin M (IgM) capture assays, are probably the most sensitive tests available for rickettsial diagnosis, and the presence of IgM antibodies, indicate recent infection with rickettsial diseases.

Recent updates:

Identification of a Novel Antigen for Serological Diagnosis of Scrub Typhus

O. tsutsugamushi 56-kDa type-specific antigen (TSA) is commonly used for serological diagnosis of scrub typhus, the 56-kDa TSA shows variations among O. tsutsugamushi strains, which may lead to poor diagnostic results. O. tsutsugamushi 27 kDa antigen through an immunoinformatic approach and verified its diagnostic potential using patient samples. O. tsutsugamushi 27-kDa antigen shows potential as a novel serological diagnostic antigen for scrub typhus, providing higher diagnostic accuracy for O. tsutsugamushi than the 56-kDa antigen.

Infective Endocarditis

Definition- Infective endocarditis is defined as infection of the endothelium of the heart.

Epidemiology

The annual incidence is around 3-10/100,000 of the population with mortality of around 30% at 30 days. The most common causative organism is Staphylococcus aureus followed by streptococcus viridans (18.7%), other streptococci (17.5%), and enterococci (10.5%).

Clinical features

The clinical features of infective endocarditis are divided as acute, subacute, and chronic. Most of the patients present with fever, night sweats, fatigue, weight, and appetite loss. Up to one-fourth of patients present with embolic phenomenon. The predisposing factors of infective endocarditis encompass cardiac conditions such as bicuspid aortic valve, mitral valve prolapse, rheumatic valve disease, congenital heart disease, history of prior infective endocarditis, implanted cardiac device, and prosthetic heart valve. Also, comorbidities such as intravenous drug use, chronic kidney disease, chronic liver disease, malignancy, advanced age, corticosteroids use, poorly controlled diabetes Mellitus, and immunocompromised status predispose the patients to infective endocarditis

Diagnosis

According to Modified Duke's criteria,

- **Definitive diagnosis** of infective endocarditis should include *two major* or *one major and three minor* or *five minor.*
- **Possible infective endocarditis** is defined as *one major and one minor* or *three minor criteria*
- **Rejected** infective endocarditis is when there is
  - a firm alternate diagnosis
  - Resolution of clinical manifestations occurs after ≤4 days of antibiotic therapy.
  - No pathological evidence of infective endocarditis is found at surgery or autopsy after antibiotic therapy for four days or less.
  - Clinical criteria for possible or definite infective endocarditis is not met

Table 1: Modified Dukes major and minor criteria

Major criteria
Positive blood culture for IE (any one of the following):
typical micro-organisms consistent with infective endocarditis from two separate blood cultures *staphylococcus aureus, viridans group streptococcus, streptococcus bovis group, HACEK group, or community acquired enterococci with absence of primary focus or organisms consistent with infective endocarditi,* **OR**
Persistent bacteremia ≥2 positive blood cultures drawn >12 hours apart; or all of three or a majority of ≥4 separate blood cultures (first and last samples ≥1 hour apart); **OR**
Single Positive serology for Coxiella or a phase IgG antibody titre >1:800
Evidence of endocardial involvement (any one of the following) -
Positive echocardiography
Vegetation (oscillating intracardiac mass on a valve or on supporting structures, in the path of regurgitant jets, or on implanted material, in the absence of an alternative anatomic explanation, **OR**
Abscess, **OR**
New partial dehiscence of prosthetic valve
New valvular regurgitation
Increase in or change in preexisting murmur not sufficient
Minor criteria
predisposing heart condition (prosthetic valves) or intravenous drug use
fever >38°C and 100.4°F
vascular phenomena (including those detected by imaging alone): arterial emboli, splenic infarction, mycotic aneurysms, intracranial haemorrhage and Janeway lesions
immunological phenomena: glomerulonephritis, Osler's nodes, Roth's spots and rheumatoid factor
microbiological evidence: positive blood cultures not meeting major criteria above or serological evidence of infection with organism consistent with IE

Management according to European Society of Cardiology guidelines 2015 (1)

Table 2: Proposed antibiotic regimens for initial empirical treatment of IE in acutely severely ill patients (before pathogen identification) –

Community-acquired native valves or late prosthetic valve endocarditis (≥12 months post surgery)
Ampicillin 12g/day IV in 4-6 doses **with** Flucloxicillin 12g/day IV in 4-6 doses **with** Gentamicin 3 mg/kg/day IV or IM in 1 dose
Early PVE (<12 monnths post surgery) or nosocomial and non nosocomial healthcare associated endocarditis
Vancomycin 30mg/kg/day with Gentamycin 3mg/kg/day IV or IM in one dose with Rifampin 900-1200 mg IV or orally in 2-3 divided doses

Table 3: Antibiotic regime for pathogen specific IE

For staphylococcus aureus (methicillin-sensitive)
• Native valve - Flucloxacillin 12 g IV in 4-6 doses
• Prosthetic valve - Flucloxacillin 12 g IV in 4-6 doses with Rifampicin 900-1200 mg IV or orally in 2-3 doses and Gentamycin 3mg/kg IV or IM in 1 or 2 doses
Staphylococcus aureus (methicillin-resistant)
• Native valve – Vancomycin 30-60mg/kg/day IV in 2-3 doses
• Prosthetic valve –Vancomycin 30-60mg/kg/day IV in 2-3 doses and rifampicin 900-1200 mg IV or orally in 2-3 doses and gentamycin 3mg/kg IV or IM in 1 or 2 doses
Viridans group streptococci and Streptococcus Bovis
• Native valve –   4 week regimens – Benzylpenicillin 12-18 MU/day IV in 4-6 doses or continuously; **or** Ceftriaxone 2 gm/day IV/IM in one dose   2 week regimens – Benzylpenicillin 12-18 MU/day IV in 4-6 doses or continuously **or** Ceftriaxone 2 g/day IV/IM in one dose **plus** Gentamicin 3 mg/kg IV/IM in one dose (Native valve)   • Prosthetic valve – Benzylpenicillin 1.2 gm fourth hourly; or Ceftriaxone 2 gm once a day
Enterococcus faecalis
• Native valve –   Amoxicillin 2gm fourth hourly and gentamycin 1mg/kg BD or ceftriaxone 2 gm BD   • Prosthetic valve –   Amoxicillin 2gm fourth hourly and gentamycin 1mg/kg BD or ceftriaxone 2 gm BD
Culture negative Endocarditis
It is endocarditis without etiology following inoculation of three blood samples in a standard blood culture system.   Following are the reasons for culture negative endocarditis   • Prior administration of antibiotics without sending blood cultures   • Inappropriate microbiological techniques   • Infection by fastidious or non-bacterial pathogens   • Coxiella burnetti and Bartonella species are common causes of culture negative endocarditis   *Coxiella burnetii* – Doxycycline 200mg/24h plus Cotrimoxazole (960 mg/24 h) plus rifampin (300-600/24 h) for ≥3-6 months orally   *Bartonella spp.* – Doxycycline100mg/12 h orally fro 4 weeks plus gentamicin (3mg/24 h) IV for 2 weeks

<u>Recent Updates</u>

Partial Oral Treatment of Endocarditis (POET) Trial was a step down therapy study (2019) with oral antibiotics in patients with left-sided endocarditis. The patients were randomly assigned to either continue IV antibiotics or to step down to oral antibiotics after atleast ten days of initial

IV antibiotics. The study was shown to be non inferior to continued intravenous antibiotics even after six months in terms of death from any cause, unplanned cardiac surgery, embolic events, and relapse of positive blood culture (primary outcome). There were no indications for longer term treatment failure among the patients who received step-down treatment with oral antibiotics. (2)

References

1. Habib G, Lancellotti P, Antunes MJ, Bongiorni MG, Casalta J-P, Del Zotti F, et al. 2015 ESC Guidelines for the management of infective endocarditis: The Task Force for the Management of Infective Endocarditis of the European Society of Cardiology (ESC)Endorsed by: European Association for Cardio-Thoracic Surgery (EACTS), the European Association of Nuclear Medicine (EANM). Eur Heart J [Internet]. 2015 Nov 21;36(44):3075–128. Available from: https://doi.org/10.1093/eurheartj/ehv319

2. Pries-Heje MM, Wiingaard C, Ihlemann N, Gill SU, Bruun NE, Elming H, et al. Five-Year Outcomes of the Partial Oral Treatment of Endocarditis (POET) Trial. N Engl J Med [Internet]. 2022 Feb 9;386(6):601–2.

Urosepsis

Urinary tract infection are one of the most common causes of sepsis among patients presenting to the hospital. Escherichia coli remains the most common causative organism.

The classification of Urinary tract infection (1) –

1. <u>Asymptomatic bacteriuria</u> -

More than 10^5 CFU/ml of a single pathogen in TWO successive clean catch urine sample in a woman without symptoms.

More than 10^5 CFU in ONE clean catch urine sample in an asymptomatic man

More than 100 CFU/ml of a single isolate in a patient who is catheterised without symptoms.

Treatment of asymptomatic bacteriuria is recommended only for pregnant females.

2. <u>Urethritis and cystitis (Lower urinary tract infection)</u>

Cystitis is the infection and inflammation of the urinary bladder. It starts when the pathogens from the GI (Gastrointestinal tract) colonise the urethra and ascends to the bladder. Clinically, they can be diagnosed with dysuria, increase in the frequency and hematuria.

Urethritis is commonly associated with sexually transmitted diseases. The have similar symptoms as cystitis but with added discharge, irritation and lesions on the external genitalia.

3. <u>Pyelonephritis (Upper urinary tract infection)</u> – infection of the renal parenchyma and pelvicalyceal system. The patient with present with flank pain or costovertebral tenderness, nausea and vomiting, with or without fever. There will be positive urine cultures of 10^5 CFU/ml. This can progress to urine bacterial nephritis, renal abscess and emphysematous pyelonephritis.

Uncomplicated pyelonephritis refers to the clinical syndrome of fever and flank pain or tenderness with or without vomiting in a woman with an anatomically normal urinary tract without comorbidities. However, the recommended treatment of women with uncomplicated pyelonephritis is similar to recommendations for patients with complicated UTI.

4. <u>Uncomplicated UTI</u> – A man or non-pregnant woman without any structural or functional abnormalities in the urinary tract or kidney parenchyma, without comorbidities (which places the patient at a risk for more severe infection) and not associated with any GU (genitourinary tract instrumentation). The diagnosis is a positive urine culture of more than 10^5 CFU/ml.

5. <u>Complicated UTI</u> – functional or anatomically abnormal urinary tract or infection in the presence of comorbidities that place the patient at risk for more serious adverse outcomes

6. <u>Recurrent UTI</u> – defined as two uncomplicated UTIs in 6 months or three or more uncomplicated UTIs in the preceding 12 months. It can be subdivided to –

Relapse of UTI is a recurrence of a UTI within 2 weeks of treatment completion caused by the same organism from a focus within the urinary system.

Reinfection is a recurrent UTI caused by a different bacterial isolate or by previously isolated bacteria after a negative intervening culture or a period of >2 weeks between infections.

7. <u>Catheter-associated UTI (CAUTI)</u> – refers to a UTI occurring in a person whose urinary tract is currently catheterized, or has been within the previous 48 hours. CAUTI is diagnosed when a patient has signs or symptoms compatible with a UTI with no other source identified and the presence of ≥10^3 CFU/mL of one or more bacterial species from a catheter urine specimen or midstream voided specimen if the catheter has been removed in the prior 48 hours.

IDSA (Infectious Diseases Society of America) guidelines for the treatment of UTI (2)

Table 1: Dosing of Antibiotics

Agent	Adult Dosage
Amikacin	Cystitis: 15 mg/kg/dose IV stat
	All other infections: 20 mg/kg/dose IV stat; subsequent doses and dosing interval based on pharmacokinetic evaluation
Amoxicillin-clavulanate	Cystitis: 875 mg (amoxicillin component) P.O. every 12 hours
Cefiderocol	2 g IV every 8 hours, infused over 3 hours
Ceftazidime-avibactam	2.5 g IV every 8 hours, infused over 3 hours
Ceftazidime-avibactam and aztreonam (infused together)	2.5 g IV every 8 hours, infused over 3 hours *plus* Aztreonam: 2 g IV every 8 hours, infused over 3 hours
Ceftolozane-tazobactam	Cystitis: 1.5 g IV every 8 hours, infused over 1 hour All other infections: 3 g IV every 8 hours, infused over 3 hours
Ciprofloxacin	400 mg IV every 8 hours
Colistin	Refer to international consensus guidelines on polymyxins
Eravacycline	1 mg/kg/dose IV every 12 hours
Ertapenem	1 g IV every 24 hours, infused over 30 minutes
Fosfomycin	Cystitis: 3 g PO stat
Gentamicin	Cystitis: 5 mg/kg/dose IV stat
	Other infections: 7 mg/kg/dose IV stat; subsequent doses and dosing interval based on pharmacokinetic evaluation

Imipenem-cilastatin	Cystitis (standard infusion): 500 mg IV every 6 hours, infused over 30 minutes
	All other infections (extended-infusion): 500 mg IV every 6 hours, infused over 3 hours
Imipenem-cilastatin-relebactam	1.25 g IV every 6 hours, infused over 30 minutes
Levofloxacin	750 mg IV/PO every 24 hours
Meropenem	Cystitis (standard infusion): 1 g IV every 8 hours
	All other infections (extended-infusion): 2 g IV every 8 hours, infused over 3 hours
Meropenem-vaborbactam	4 g IV every 8 hours, infused over 3 hours
Nitrofurantoin	Cystitis: macrocrystal/monohydrate (Macrobid®)100 mg P.O. every 12 hours
	Cystitis: Oral suspension: 50 mg every 6 hours
Plazomicin	Cystitis: 15 mg/kg IV × 1 dose
	All other infections: 15 mg/kg IV × one dose; subsequent doses and dosing interval based on pharmacokinetic evaluation
Polymyxin B	Refer to international consensus guidelines on polymyxins
Tigecycline	Uncomplicated intra-abdominal infections (standard dose): 100 mg IV × one dose, then 50 mg IV every 12 hours
	Complicated intra-abdominal infections (high dose): 200 mg IV × one dose, then 100 mg IV every 12 hours
Tobramycin	Cystitis: 7 mg/kg/dose IV × 1 dose
	All other infections: 7 mg/kg/dose IV × one dose; subsequent doses and dosing interval based on pharmacokinetic evaluation
Trimethoprim-sulfamethoxazole	Cystitis: 160 mg (trimethoprim component) IV/PO every 12 hours
	Other infections: 8–10 mg/kg/day (trimethoprim component) IV/PO divided every 8–12 hours; maximum dose 320 mg P.O. every 8 hours

Table 2: Recommended Antibiotic Treatment for Empiric or Confirmed Extended-spectrum β-Lactamase–Producing Enterobacteriaceae

Source of Infection	**Preferred Treatment**	**Alternative Treatment if First-line Options not Available or Tolerated**
Cystitis	Nitrofurantoin, trimethoprim-sulfamethoxazole	Amoxicillin-clavulanate, single-dose aminoglycosides, fosfomycin (*Escherichia coli* only)
		Ciprofloxacin, levofloxacin, ertapenem, meropenem, imipenem-cilastatin

Pyelonephritis or complicated urinary tract infection	Ertapenem, meropenem, imipenem-cilastatin, ciprofloxacin, levofloxacin, or trimethoprim-sulfamethoxazole	
Infections outside of the urinary tract	Meropenem, imipenem-cilastatin, ertapenem	
Oral step-down therapy to ciprofloxacin, levofloxacin, or trimethoprim-sulfamethoxazole should be considered		

Oral step-down therapy can be considered after susceptibility to the oral agent is demonstrated, patients are afebrile and hemodynamically stable, appropriate source control is achieved, and there are no issues with intestinal absorption.

Table 3: Recommended Antibiotic Treatment Options for Carbapenem-Resistant Enterobacteriaceae

Source of Infection	Preferred Treatment	Alternative Treatment if First- line Options not Available or Tolerated
Cystitis	Ciprofloxacin, levofloxacin, trimethoprim-sulfamethoxazole, nitrofurantoin, or a single dose of an aminoglycoside Meropenem (standard infusion): only if ertapenem-resistant, meropenem-susceptible, AND carbapenemase testing results are either not available or negative	Ceftazidime-avibactam, meropenem-vaborbactam, imipenem-cilastatin-relebactam, and cefiderocol Colistin (when no alternative options are available)
Pyelonephritis or complicated urinary tract infection	Ceftazidime-avibactam, meropenem-vaborbactam, imipenem-cilastatin-relebactam, and cefiderocol Meropenem (extended-infusion): only if ertapenem-resistant, meropenem- susceptible, AND carbapenemase testing results are either not available or negative	Once-daily aminoglycosides

Infections outside of the urinary tract - **Resistant to ertapenem, susceptible to meropenem, AND carbapenemase testing results are either not available or negative**	Meropenem (extended-infusion)	Ceftazidime-avibactam
Infections outside of the urinary tract - **Resistant to ertapenem, resistant to meropenem, AND carbapenemase testing results are either not available or negative** Ceftazidime-avibactam, meropenem- vaborbactam, and imipenem-cilastatin-relebactam Cefiderocol Tigecycline, eravacycline (generally limited to intra-abdominal infections)		
***Klebsiella pneumoniae* carbapenemases identified** (or carbapenemase positive but identified of carbapenemase unknown)	Ceftazidime-avibactam, meropenem-vaborbactam, imipenem-cilastatin-relebactam	Cefiderocol Tigecycline, eravacycline (generally limited to intra-abdominal infections)
Metallo-β-lactamase (ie, NDM, VIM, IMP) carbapenemase identified	Ceftazidime-avibactam + aztreonam, cefiderocol	Tigecycline, eravacycline (generally limited to intra-abdominal infections)
OXA-48-like carbapenemase identified	Ceftazidime-avibactam	Cefiderocol Tigecycline, eravacycline (generally limited to intra-abdominal infections)

Most infections caused by CRE are resistant to ertapenem but susceptible to meropenem are caused by organisms that do not produce carbapenemases.

The vast majority of carbapenemase-producing Enterobacterales infections in the United States are due to bacteria that produce Klebsiella pneumoniae carbapenemases (KPC). If a carbapenemase-producing Enterobacterales is causing the infection and the specific carbapenemase enzyme is unknown, it is acceptable to treat as if the strain is a KPC producer.

Table 4: Recommended Antibiotic Treatment Options for Difficult-to-Treat *Pseudomonas aeruginosa*, Assuming In Vitro Susceptibility to Agents in Table

Source of Infection	Preferred Treatment	Alternative Treatment if First-line Options not Available or Tolerated
Cystitis	Ceftolozane-tazobactam, ceftazidime-avibactam, imipenem-relebactam, cefiderocol, or a single dose of an aminoglycoside	Colistin
Pyelonephritis or complicated urinary tract infection	Ceftolozane-tazobactam, ceftazidime-avibactam, imipenem-cilastatin-relebactam, and cefiderocol	Once-daily aminoglycosides
Infections outside of the urinary tract	Ceftolozane-tazobactam, ceftazidime-avibactam, or imipenem-cilastatin-relebactam	Cefiderocol Aminoglycoside monotherapy: limited to uncomplicated bloodstream infections with complete source control

Intravesical bacteriophages for treating UTIs in patients undergoing TURP (3)

- A randomized, placebo-controlled clinical trial was done at the Alexander Tsulukidze National Centre of Urology, Tbilisi, Georgia.

- The study included men more than 18 years of age, who were scheduled for transurethral resection of the prostate (TURP), with complicated UTI or recurrent uncomplicated UTI but no signs of systemic infection.

- They were allocated to block randomization in a 1:1:1 ratio to receive intravesical Pyo bacteriophage (Pyophage; 20 mL) or intravesical placebo solution (20 mL) in a double-blind manner twice daily for seven days, or systemically applied antibiotics (according to sensitivities) as an open-label standard-of-care comparator.

- Urine culture was taken via a urinary catheter at the end of treatment (i.e., day 7) or after withdrawal from the trial.

- The primary outcome was microbiological treatment response after seven days, measured by urine culture; secondary outcomes included clinical and safety parameters during the treatment period.

- The study found intravesical bacteriophage therapy was non-inferior to standard-of-care antibiotic treatment but was not superior to placebo bladder irrigation in efficacy or safety in treating UTIs in patients undergoing TURP.

- Although bacteriophages are not yet a recognized or approved treatment option for UTIs, this trial provides new insight to optimize the design of further large-scale clinical studies to define the role of bacteriophages in UTI treatment.

Dengue

Demography:

The global burden of dengue is estimated to be 1.04 million cases as in 2017 and the incidence rate is 1371 per 1 lakh population. The overall seroprevalence of dengue infection in India is 48.7%.

Recent updates:

A pan-serotype dengue virus inhibitor targeting the NS3–NS4B interaction

Apart from symptomatic management we do not have specific antiviral therapy available against dengue. A highly potent dengue virus inhibitor (JNJ-A07) that exerts nanomolar to picomolar activity against a panel of 21 clinical isolates that represent the natural genetic diversity of known genotypes and serotypes has been developed.

A Dengue Virus Serotype 1 mRNA-LNP Vaccine Elicits Protective Immune Responses

a nucleotide-modified mRNA vaccine encoding the membrane and envelope structural proteins from DENV serotype 1 encapsulated in lipid nanoparticles (prM/E mRNA-LNP) is being developed. Vaccination of mice elicited robust antiviral immune responses comparable to viral infection, with high levels of neutralizing antibody titers and antiviral CD4+ and CD8+ T cells. Immunocompromised AG129 mice vaccinated with the prM/E mRNA-LNP vaccine were protected from a lethal DENV challenge. Both vaccine constructs demonstrated serotype-specific immunity with minimal serum cross-reactivity and reduced ADE in comparison to a live DENV1 viral infection.

Fungal Infections

<u>Candida infections</u>

Candidiasis is a fungal infection caused by a group of yeast organisms. The infections manifest by localizing to skin and mucous membranes and are rarely systemic. The most common organism among these is *Candida albicans*. They normally reside in the gastrointestinal tract. This infection is most commonly seen in patients who are immunocompromised like those with hematologic malignancies, recipients of solid organ malignancies, patients receiving chemotherapy for a variety of diseases and post transplant patient taking long term glucocorticoid therapy. The greatest number of such infections are seen in intensive care units especially in trauma and burns patients. Other risks factors –

- patients with abdominal surgeries (gastrointestinal perforations and anastomotic leaks)
- Acute kidney injury undergoing hemodialysis
- Central venous catheter in situ
- Patients receiving total parenteral nutrition
- Diabetes mellitus and HIV

Local mucocutaneous infections may present as white plaques on the tongue or buccal mucosa (eg. oral thrush); maceration, erythema, and fissures around oral commissures (eg. Perleche); onycholysis and paronychia around nails and intertriginous lesions in the form of satellite pustules on chronically wet and macerated skin. It can lead to balanitis and vulvovaginitis in males and females, respectively. Systemic lesions include esophageal candidiasis, hepatic candidiasis, disseminated candidiasis, or invasive candidiasis.

Diagnosis is by taking proper history and physical examination, KOH mounts, and cultures. Treatment of localized involvement includes removing the predisposing factors like chronic antibiotic therapy and chronic wet state of skin. Topical antifungals like miconazole, econazole, clotrimazole or clotrimazole are given. In case they do not respond, oral formulations of itaconazole, fluconazole, or nystatin can be started. Invasive candidiasis treatment includes caspofungin, fluconazole, and amphotericin B in non-neutropenic patients. Voriconazole can be used in neutropenic patients.

Micafungin is a semi-synthetic echinocandin which is derived from the fungus *Coleophama empedri*. The role of empirical micafungin in critically ill patients in the ICU with candida infections was studied in the *EMPIRICUS trial*. They included adult patients who were non neutropenic, non transplanted, critically ill patients with multiple organ failure exposed to broad spectrum antibiotics. This study showed that there was no statistical difference in patients alive and free from invasive fungal infection on day 28. The use of empirical micafungin decreased the rate of new invasive fungal infection. It was tolerated well with minimal adverse effects to the placebo. (1)

Candida auris

Candida auris is a fungus belonging to yeast and causes candidiasis in humans. It is an emerging multidrug-resistant yeast that can spread all over the world especially in long-term acute care hospitals. It requires unique identification methods. Clinical features are similar to *Candida albicans* but this is more common in diabetes mellitus, sepsis, and chronic kidney disease patients. The infection is primarily acquired in the hospital with a mortality rate of 30-60% in those with invasive candidiasis. Treatment is complex as it is multidrug-resistant. They are resistant to fluconazole, voriconazole, and amphotericin B. Echinocandins like caspofungin have shown susceptibility to *Candida auris*.

Public health authorities in southern California started proactive *C.auris* surveillance in September 2018 by detecting the species of *Candida* isolates in urine from patients in long-term acute care hospitals. The first *C. auris* case was identified in February 2019; subsequently, the point prevalence survey in 17 facilities identified 182 other cases. The gaps in hand hygiene, environmental cleaning, and transmission-based precautions were identified and addressed immediately; the outbreak was then contained to two facilities by October 2019. The findings demonstrated the importance of public health oversight and proper laboratory surveillance in reducing the risk *C. auris* transmission. (2)

Reference

1. Timsit J-F, Azoulay E, Schwebel C, Charles PE, Cornet M, Souweine B, et al. Empirical Micafungin Treatment and Survival Without Invasive Fungal Infection in Adults With ICU-Acquired Sepsis, Candida Colonization, and Multiple Organ Failure: The EMPIRICUS Randomized Clinical Trial. JAMA. 2016 Oct;316(15):1555–64.

2. Karmarkar EN, O'Donnell K, Prestel C, Forsberg K, Gade L, Jain S, et al. Rapid Assessment and Containment of Candida auris Transmission in Postacute Care Settings-Orange County, California, 2019. Ann Intern Med. 2021 Nov;174(11):1554–62.

Respiratory Syncytial Virus

Respiratory Syncytial Virus (RSV) is a common respiratory virus that usually causes mild, cold-like symptoms in all age groups. Infection most commonly occurs in winter. It is a significant cause of death in infants and children. Risk factors include infants less than six months of age, those with congenital heart disease, Down syndrome, any age group patient with persistent asthma, and elderly patients. RSV is a single-stranded RNA virus of the *Pneumoviridae* family.

RSV enters the nasopharynx, multiplies there, infects small bronchiolar epithelium except for basal cells, then spreads to type 1 and 2 pneumocytes. Lower respiratory tract infection occurs 1 to 3 days after that.

Clinical symptoms include cough, coryza, and rhinorrhea. It can also cause conjunctivitis, ear infections, sinusitis, pneumonia, bronchitis, acute exacerbation of asthma, or COPD.

Diagnosis is made based on clinical suspicion, especially in infants with respiratory symptoms who present during the winter season. Laboratory diagnosis requires analysis of respiratory secretions like a nasal wash, nasopharyngeal swab or mid-turbinate swab, tracheal aspirate, or bronchoalveolar lavage. The analysis is done by PCR-based assays; however, isolation of RSV in human epithelial type 2 (Hep-2) cells is the gold standard. Rapid antigen testing can also be performed with 80% sensitivity and 97% specificity.

Treatment is primarily supportive, which includes oxygen therapy, adequate fluids administration, and continuous monitoring of the clinical status. Inhaled bronchodilators, inhaled hypertonic saline, and corticosteroids are not routinely recommended. Ribavirin and RSV immunoglobulin have also been tried in immunocompromised patients. Palivizumab is a humanized monoclonal antibody used as prophylaxis in at-risk populations and as a part of treatment for hematopoietic cell transplant recipients with RSV infection.

EDP-938 is a nonfusion replication inhibitor of RSV, which modifies the viral nucleoprotein. In a two-part phase 2a, double-blind, randomized placebo-controlled challenge trial, participants inoculated with RSV-A Memphis 37b were assigned to receive either EDP-938 or placebo. Different doses of EDP-938 were analyzed. Nasal-wash samples were obtained from day 2 to day 12 for assessments. The participants were assessed clinically, and pharmacokinetic profiles were obtained. The primary endpoint taken was the area under the curve (AUC) for the RSV viral load, as measured by reverse-transcriptase–quantitative polymerase-chain-reaction assay. The key secondary endpoint was the AUC for the total symptom score. In part 1 of the trial, EDP-938 in a dose of 600 mg once daily or 300 mg twice daily after a loading dose of 500-mg or placebo. In part 2, EDP-938 in a dose of 300 mg once daily after a 600-mg loading dose or 200 mg twice daily after a loading dose of 400-mg or placebo. In both parts, mucus production was >70% lower in each EDP-938 group than in the placebo group. The four EDP-938 regimens had a safety profile similar to a placebo. All EDP-938 regimens were superior to placebo concerning lowering the viral load, total symptom scores, and mucus weight without apparent safety concerns. (1)

HIV Infections

HIV accounts for the highest number of deaths attributable to a single agent. It is estimated that 5.2 million people are infected with HIV in India. Opportunistic infections are a reason for increased morbidity and mortality.

Acute HIV syndrome occurs within 3-6 weeks after primary infection, but clinical severity varies, and it is attributed to the plasma viral load and re-trafficking of lymphocytes. Symptoms may persist for weeks and may present with opportunistic infections. The leading cause is a reversal of the CD4/CD8 ratio. Generalized weakness and lymphadenopathy are more common in the initial stage. Other features include fever, pharyngitis, lymphadenopathy, myalgia, headache, anorexia, nausea, vomiting, weight loss, or neurologic manifestations like meningitis, encephalitis, and peripheral neuropathy. This is followed by stages of clinical latency and symptomatic disease.

Diagnosis is with fourth-generation antigen/ antibody combination HIV-1/2 immunoassay with a confirmatory HIV -1/2 antibody differentiation immunoassay.

The first-line treatment is zidovudine + lamivudine + nevirapine for patients with hemoglobin more than 8g/dL. The second choice will include a combination of stavudine, lamivudine, and nevirapine.

Dolutegravir is a human immunodeficiency virus (HIV) integrase inhibitor which targets the viral integrase. There are limited options for effective antiretroviral treatment (ART) in children with human immunodeficiency virus type 1 (HIV-1) infection. An open-label, noninferiority randomized trial comparing three-drug ART based on the HIV integrase inhibitor dolutegravir and standard care therapy (non–dolutegravir-based ART) in children and adolescents starting first- or second-line ART. The primary endpoint taken was the proportion of participants with virologic or clinical treatment failure. Within 96 weeks, 47 participants in the dolutegravir group and 75 in the standard care group had treatment failure. Treatment effects were the same in groups with first- and second-line therapies. A total of 35 participants in the dolutegravir group and 40 in the standard care group experienced at least one profound adverse effect. And a total of 73 in the dolutegravir group and 86 in the standard care group had at least one adverse event of grade 3 or higher, respectively. At least one ART-modifying adverse event occurred in 5 participants in the dolutegravir group and 17 in the standard care group. This trial showerd that dolutegravir-based ART was superior to standard care. (2)

Prevention includes safe sex practices by using condoms, avoiding the sharing of IV syringes, and, if exposed, immediately started on postexposure prophylaxis. Cabotegravir extended-release suspension is a long-acting integrase inhibitor, approved by the U.S. Food and Drug Administration (FDA) on Dec 20, 2021 as the first injectable medication to prevent HIV. It is given as an IM injection every two months. It is given to adults and adolescents weighing more than 35 kilograms to reduce the risk of sexually acquired HIV. Two randomized clinical trials, first in May 2020, the *HPTN 083 trial* among men who have sex with men and transgender women, and in November 2020 among women in sub-Saharan Africa, demonstrated that the use of long-acting cabotegravir prevents HIV acquisition compared to the daily oral medications. The advantages of the medication were partly due to the high efficacy of the drug and other integrase inhibitors and, in part, due to better adherence to an injection compared to a once-daily pill regimen. It is hoped that the new tool for HIV prevention will accelerate progress toward reducing new infections. (3)

Rotavirus

This virus is a common cause of severe gastroenteritis in children less than five years of age. Severe infection occurs in immunologically naïve, unimmunized children between the age of six months and two years, immunocompromised individuals, and residents of long-term care facilities. Transmission is by the fecal-oral route, and infection can occur at any time of the year.

Clinical features include vomiting, watery, non-bloody diarrhea, fever, dehydration, and seizures. It can cause travelers diarrhea in adults. The pathophysiology includes the interplay between loss of brush border enzymes, the direct effect of rotavirus enterotoxin NSP4, and activation of the enteric nervous system.

Diagnosis is based on clinical grounds, and specific diagnosis includes detection of rotavirus in stool by immune-based assays like ELISA and nucleic acid testing like PCR. Stool cultures for viral isolation can also be used but not used routinely for diagnosis.

Treatment includes supportive care in the form of volume repletion and zinc supplementation. Antidiarrheals and antiemetics are not commonly recommended. Prevention is by proper hand washing, diaper changing, water, disinfection, contact isolation, and vaccination.

The oral rotavirus vaccine is included in the national immunization schedule at 6,10, and 14 weeks of age.

Two vaccines are licensed in the United States and demonstrated high effectiveness against moderate to severe diseases. A tr study utilized a test-negative case-control design and applied four distinct case definitions based on reverse transcription-quantitative real-time PCR (qRT-PCR) assay and enzyme immunoassay (EIA) test results. Vaccine effectiveness analysis population comprised of 842 children, 799 (95%) of whom had mild diseases requiring at most a clinic visit and 698 (83%) were fully vaccinated against rotavirus. Age-adjusted vaccine effectiveness was 70%

against disease defined solely by qRT-PCR results, 72% against disease as defined by qRT-PCR with a quantification cycle (*Cq*) value <27, 73% against a disease that was qRT-PCR positive but enzyme immuneassay (EIA) negative, and 62% against disease defined solely by EIA. Results were similar when restricting to disease resulting in an ambulatory clinic or emergency department visit. These results supported the rotavirus vaccination's effectiveness in protecting U.S. children from mild to moderate and severe diseases. (4)

References

1. Ahmad A, Eze K, Noulin N, Horvathova V, Murray B, Baillet M, et al. EDP-938, a Respiratory Syncytial Virus Inhibitor, in a Human Virus Challenge. N Engl J Med [Internet]. 2022 Feb 16;386(7):655–66. Available from: https://doi.org/10.1056/NEJMoa2108903

2. Turkova A, White E, Mujuru HA, Kekitiinwa AR, Kityo CM, Violari A, et al. Dolutegravir as First- or Second-Line Treatment for HIV-1 Infection in Children. N Engl J Med. 2021 Dec;385(27):2531–43.

3. Sharfstein JM, Killelea A, Dangerfield D. Long-Acting Cabotegravir for HIV Prevention: Issues of Access, Cost, and Equity. JAMA. 2022 Mar;327(10):921–2.

4. Burke RM, Groom HC, Naleway AL, Katz EM, Salas B, Mattison CP, et al. Rotavirus Vaccine Is Effective Against Rotavirus Gastroenteritis Resulting in Outpatient Care: Results From the Medically Attended Acute Gastroenteritis (MAAGE) Study. Clin Infect Dis an Off Publ Infect Dis Soc Am. 2021 Jun;72(11):2000–5.

Mycobacterial Infections

Recent updates

1. <u>WHO guidelines: treatment of MDR tuberculosis(TB)</u>

   The World Health Organization (WHO), in June 2021, published updated guidelines for the treatment of multidrug-resistant tuberculosis (MDR-TB). For nonpregnant patients who have uncomplicated MDR-TB, WHO supports treatment with a bedaquiline-containing regimen rather than a regimen including injectable agents. For six months, one preferred regimen in several T.B. programs is BPaL, an all-oral regimen of bedaquiline, pretomanid, and linezolid. In settings where pretomanid and linezolid cannot be used, a 9 to 12-month oral multidrug regimen which included bedaquiline for the first 4 to 6 months was started. Patients who do not meet the criteria for an abbreviated bedaquiline-containing regimen should be treated with a more extended, individualized regimen. (1)

2. <u>Bedaquiline-Resistant Tuberculosis Associated with Rv0678 Mutations</u>

   Bedaquiline is a diarylquinoline antimycobacterial drug used with other antituberculosis medications to treat multidrug-resistant tuberculosis. The addition of bedaquiline to antituberculosis drug regimens has been linked to an increased rate of transient serum liver test abnormalities during treatment and several instances of clinically apparent liver injury. Bedaquiline use began in South Africa in 2015 to treat drug-resistant tuberculosis. A non–target based mutation in the *mmpR* (*Rv0678*) gene encoding an efflux pump repressor has been identified in the majority of bedaquiline-resistant isolates over the past five years. (2)

3. <u>Biomarker-guided tuberculosis preventive therapy (CORTIS): a randomized controlled trial</u>

   Targeted preventive therapy for individuals at the highest risk of incident tuberculosis might impact the epidemic by interrupting transmission. A transcriptomic signature of tuberculosis (RISK11) and the efficacy of signature-guided preventive therapy were tested.

   - Adult volunteers were recruited to five geographically distinct communities in South Africa. Whole blood was sampled for RISK11 by quantitative RT-PCR assay from eligible volunteers without HIV, recent previous tuberculosis (i.e., <3 years before screening), or comorbidities at screening.

   - RISK11-positive participants were randomized to either once-weekly, directly-observed, open-label isoniazid and rifapentine for 12 weeks (3 HP) or no treatment.

- Prognostic discrimination of incident tuberculosis in the untreated RISK11-positive versus RISK11-negative groups and treatment efficacy in the 3HP-treated versus untreated RISK11-positive groups during active surveillance through 15 months were tested.

- The primary endpoint taken was microbiologically confirmed pulmonary tuberculosis. The primary outcome measures were risk ratio for tuberculosis of RISK11-positive to RISK11-negative participants and treatment efficacy.

- The RISK11 signature discriminated between individuals with prevalent tuberculosis or progression to incident tuberculosis and individuals who remained healthy, but the provision of 3HP to signature-positive individuals after exclusion of baseline disease did not lower progression to tuberculosis over 15 months. (3)

4. <u>Comparing the accuracy of lipoarabinomannan urine tests for diagnosis of pulmonary tuberculosis in children from four African countries</u>

- Urine-based lipoarabinomannan assays such as Fujifilm SILVAMP TB LAM (FujiLAM) and Alere Determine TB LAM Ag (AlereLAM) were assessed for diagnostic accuracy in childhood tuberculosis.

- A cross-sectional study tested urine samples from children younger than 15 years with presumed pulmonary tuberculosis using FujiLAM and AlereLAM assays. The researchers quantified diagnostic performance against a microbiological reference standard (confirmed tuberculosis) and a composite reference standard (confirmed and unconfirmed tuberculosis).

- 15% of children had confirmed tuberculosis, 27% had unconfirmed tuberculosis, and 58% were unlikely to have tuberculosis. Sixty-one children were HIV-positive, with a prevalence of 15%.

- Using the microbiological reference standard of confirmed tuberculosis, the sensitivity of FujiLAM was 64·9%, and the sensitivity of AlereLAM was 30·7%. The specificity of FujiLAM was 83·8%, and the specificity of AlereLAM was 87·8%.

- Against the composite reference standard of confirmed and unconfirmed tuberculosis, both assays had decreased sensitivity; the sensitivity of FujiLAM and AlereLAM was 32·9% and 20·2%, respectively. The specificity of FujiLAM and AlereLAM was 83·3% and 90·0%, respectively. By comparing AlereLAM with FujiLAM, the latter had higher sensitivity and similar specificity than the former. FujiLAM could add value to the rapid diagnosis of tuberculosis in children in the future. (4)

5. <u>Daratumumab (Anti-CD38) for Treatment of Disseminated Nontuberculous Mycobacteria in a Patient With Anti–Interferon-γ Autoantibodies</u>

- Despite aggressive antimicrobial treatment, patients with autoantibodies to interferon-γ (IFN-γ) develop severe and progressive infections with mycobacteria and other intracellular pathogens.

- Rituximab has been shown to improve symptoms, disease burden, and mycobacteremia and decrease anti–IFN-γ autoantibody titers.

- This was a case report where the use of daratumumab (an anti-CD38 monoclonal antibody targeting plasma cells approved for treating multiple myeloma [MM]) in a patient with autoantibodies to IFN-γ who had progressive mycobacterial infection despite multiple cycles of rituximab, resulting in clinical and radiographic improvement. (5)

6. <u>$CD38^+CD27^-TNF-\alpha^+$ on Mtb-specific $CD4^+$ T Cells Is a Robust Biomarker for Tuberculosis Diagnosis</u>

- *Mycobacterium tuberculosis* (*Mtb*)-specific CD4+ T cells have shown significant promise as alternative means of detecting and distinguishing active disease from latent infection.

- A study was done to see the diagnostic ability of phenotypic markers on *Mtb*-specific cytokine-producing immune cell subsets for identifying active T.B.

- Subjects recruited were pulmonary and extrapulmonary T.B., latent T.B., cured T.B., healthy controls, and sick controls.

- Polychromatic flow cytometry identified host immune biomarkers in an exploratory cohort comprising 56 subjects using peripheral blood mononuclear cells. The clinical performance of the identified biomarker was evaluated using whole blood in a blinded validation cohort comprising 165 individuals.

- Cytokine secreting frequencies of *Mtb*-specific clusters of differentiation 4-positive ($CD4^+$) T cells with $CD38^+CD27^-$ phenotype clearly distinguish infected individuals with active tuberculosis from those without the disease.

- Tumor necrosis factor-α (TNF-α) secretion from $CD38^+CD27^-CD4^+$ T cells upon stimulation with ESAT6/CFP10 peptides had the excellent diagnostic accuracy at a cutoff of 9.91% (exploratory: 96.67% specificity, 88.46% sensitivity; validation: 96.15% specificity, 90.16% sensitivity).

- Additionally, this subset differentiated treatment-naive patients with T.B. from individuals cured of T.B. following the completion of anti-TB therapy.

- Hence, *Mtb*-specific $CD38^+CD27^-TNF-\alpha^+CD4^+$ T-cell subset is a robust biomarker for diagnosing T.B. and assessing cure. (6)

7. <u>Plasma Kynurenine-to-Tryptophan Ratio - a Highly Sensitive Blood-Based Diagnostic Tool for Tuberculosis in Pregnant Women Living With Human Immunodeficiency Virus (HIV)</u>

- Plasma indoleamine 2,3-dioxygenase (IDO) activity measured using kynurenine-to-tryptophan (K/T) ratio has been suggested as a blood-based T.B. biomarker.

- A study was done to investigate whether a plasma K/T ratio could be used to diagnose active T.B. among pregnant women with HIV.

- Using enzyme-linked immunosorbent assay (ELISA), investigators measured K/T ratio in 72 pregnant women with an active T.B. and compared them to 117 pregnant women with HIV but without T.B., matched by age and gestational age.

- Pregnant women who received isoniazid preventive therapy (IPT) before enrollment had a lower plasma K/T ratio than those who did not get IPT (P =.0174).

- The Plasma K/T ratio was elevated in women with active T.B. at the time of diagnosis compared to those without T.B.

- The plasma K/T ratio gave a higher diagnostic sensitivity of 94% and specificity of 90%, positive predictive value (PPV) of 85%, and negative predictive value (NPV) of 98%. (7)

8. <u>Multidrug-Resistant Tuberculosis Treatment Regimens - Based on DNA Sequencing</u>

- The study determined whether next-generation sequencing (NGS) analysis of *Mycobacterium tuberculosis* complex isolates and genes responsible for drug resistance can guide the design of effective multidrug-resistant/rifampicin-resistant tuberculosis (MDR/RR-TB) treatment regimens.

- NGS-based genomic DST predictions of isolates of *M. tuberculosis* complex done in MDR/RR-TB patients admitted to a T.B. reference center in Germany between Jan 1, 2015, and Apr 30, 2019, were compared with phenotypic DST results in mycobacteria growth indicator tubes (MGIT).

- Standardized treatment algorithms were applied to design individualized therapies based on either genomic or phenotypic DST results, and disparities were further evaluated by determining minimal inhibitory drug concentrations (MICs) using Sensititre MYCOTBI and UKMYC microtiter plates.

- Among 70 patients with MDR/RR-TB, agreement among 1048 pairwise comparisons of genomic and phenotypic DST was 86.3%; 7.2% of results were discordant, and 6.5% could not be evaluated due to the presence of polymorphisms with yet unknown implications for drug resistance.

- Notably, 549 of 561 predictions of drug susceptibility were phenotypically confirmed in MGIT, and 27 of 64 false-positive results were linked to previously described mutations mediating a low or moderate MIC increase. Virtually all drugs (99.0%) used in combination therapies inferred from genomic DST were confirmed to be susceptible by phenotypic DST. NGS-based genomic DST can reliably guide the design of effective MDR/RR-TB treatment regimens. (8)

References

1. Mirzayev F, Viney K, Linh NN, Gonzalez-Angulo L, Gegia M, Jaramillo E, et al. World Health Organization recommendations on the treatment of drug-resistant tuberculosis, 2020 update. Eur Respir J. 2021 Jun;57(6).

2. Omar S V, Ismail F, Ndjeka N, Kaniga K, Ismail NA. Bedaquiline-Resistant Tuberculosis Associated with Rv0678 Mutations. Vol. 386, The New England journal of medicine. United States; 2022. p. 93–4.

3. Scriba TJ, Fiore-Gartland A, Penn-Nicholson A, Mulenga H, Kimbung Mbandi S, Borate B, et al. Biomarker-guided tuberculosis preventive therapy (CORTIS): a randomised controlled trial. Lancet Infect Dis. 2021 Mar;21(3):354–65.

4. Nkereuwem E, Togun T, Gomez MP, Székely R, Macé A, Jobe D, et al. Comparing accuracy of lipoarabinomannan urine tests for diagnosis of pulmonary tuberculosis in children from four African countries: a cross-sectional study. Lancet Infect Dis. 2021 Mar;21(3):376–84.

5. Ochoa S, Ding L, Kreuzburg S, Treat J, Holland SM, Zerbe CS. Daratumumab (Anti-CD38) for Treatment of Disseminated Nontuberculous Mycobacteria in a Patient With Anti-Interferon-γ Autoantibodies. Clin Infect Dis an Off Publ Infect Dis Soc Am. 2021 Jun;72(12):2206–8.

6. Acharya MP, Pradeep SP, Murthy VS, Chikkannaiah P, Kambar V, Narayanashetty S, et al. CD38+CD27-TNF-α+ on Mtb-specific CD4+ T Cells Is a Robust Biomarker for Tuberculosis Diagnosis. Clin Infect Dis an Off Publ Infect Dis Soc Am. 2021 Sep;73(5):793–801.

7. Adu-Gyamfi C, Savulescu D, Mikhathani L, Otwombe K, Salazar-Austin N, Chaisson R, et al. Plasma Kynurenine-to-Tryptophan Ratio, a Highly Sensitive Blood-Based Diagnostic Tool for Tuberculosis in Pregnant Women Living With Human Immunodeficiency Virus (HIV). Clin Infect Dis an Off Publ Infect Dis Soc Am. 2021 Sep;73(6):1027–36.

8. Grobbel H-P, Merker M, Köhler N, Andres S, Hoffmann H, Heyckendorf J, et al. Design of Multidrug-Resistant Tuberculosis Treatment Regimens Based on DNA Sequencing. Clin Infect Dis an Off Publ Infect Dis Soc Am. 2021 Oct;73(7):1194–202.

Malaria

Malaria is a life-threatening disease caused by parasites transmitted through the bites of infected female anopheles mosquitoes. It is endemic in tropical and subtropical regions. WHO reported 241 million cases and 627 thousand death from malaria in 2020 (227 million cases and 558 thousand deaths in 2019). The main species are Plasmodium vivax, P. falciparum, P. malariae, P.ovale, and P.knowlesi. The definitive malaria host is the female Anopheles mosquito, while the intermediate host is human. Malaria is transmitted by the bite of the female Anopheles mosquito through blood and transplacental. Main clinical features include flu symptoms, headaches, anorexia, nausea, vomiting, myalgia, diarrhea, and abdominal pain. Signs include abdominal tenderness, splenomegaly, and hepatomegaly. Tertian malaria is caused by P. vivax and P.ovale with fever every 48 hours. Quartan malaria is caused by P. malariae with fever every 72 hours. Investigations include a complete blood count with erythrocyte sedimentation rate, renal function tests, liver function tests, coagulation profile, urine analysis, random blood sugar, and CSF examination. Specific tests include thin smear microscopy, which helps identify species and needs more than 1000/mcL parasites. Thick smear microscopy has several layers of red cells and can identify the presence of parasites even at 40/mcL parasites. Other tests include quantitative buffy coat tests, rapid diagnostic tests, and polymerase chain reactions. Treatment of uncomplicated P. vivax and P. ovale, chloroquine-sensitive, includes chloroquine 25mg/kg body weight divided over three days. In the case of chloroquine resistance, artemisinin combined therapy is used except in the first trimester of pregnancy, where quinine is recommended. A 14-day course of primaquine 0.25mg/kg is given to prevent relapse. For G6PD deficiency, primaquine 0.75mg/kg once a week for eight weeks is recommended with close medical supervision for primaquine-induced hemolysis. For uncomplicated P. falciparum malaria, artemisinin combined therapy for three days is recommended. Seven days of quinine with clindamycin in pregnancy is recommended in first trimester infections. Indications for hospitalization in uncomplicated malaria include young children, immunocompromised patients, patients with no acquired immunity, and patients with hyperparasitemia. Complicated malaria includes the presence of P. falciparum parasitemia and one or more of the following- impaired consciousness, prostration, acidosis, jaundice, convulsions, shock, hyperparasitemia, hypoglycemia, pulmonary edema, severe anemia, bleeding, and renal impairment.

Treatment of complicated malaria includes oxygen, iv fluids, glucose, antipyretics, antiepileptics, blood transfusion, and antibiotics. Artesunate 2.4mg/kg iv for 0,8,24 hours and then daily for seven days is recommended by WHO. Other alternative is quinidine gluconate. Artemisinin is the cornerstone of current antimalarial treatments worldwide. The drug of choice for severe malaria is artesunate. Artemisinin combination therapies (ACT) are first-line treatments for uncomplicated falciparum malaria and serve as alternatives to chloroquine for the other malaria types. These highly effective and well-tolerated antimalarials have contributed to global reductions in malaria deaths and complications. Fifteen years ago in Western Cambodia, the first clear evidence of artemisinin resistance in Plasmodium falciparum parasites came.

Recent updates:

Tools for malaria prevention include vaccination and chemoprophylaxis; their combination improves protection in endemic areas. In a trial done in Burkina Faso and Mali, more than 6000 children (aged 5 to 17 months) were randomly assigned to receive vaccination (primary three-dose series of RTS, S/AS01and then two annual boosters), chemoprophylaxis done withfour monthly doses of sulfadoxine-pyrimethamine and amodiaquine annually, or both. Therewas a significant reduction in three-year incidences of uncomplicated malaria, severe malaria, and death from malaria among those who received both interventions (protective efficacy for each of those outcomes ranged from 60 to 75 percent than either intervention alone). These findings supported a combination approach to reduce seasonal malaria; delivery optimization to high-burden areas is needed.

Monoclonal antibodies may be a valuable tool for malaria prevention in the future. CIS43LS, an antibody targeting the P. falciparum circumsporozoite protein, is required for parasite motility and hepatocyte invasion. A phase 1 trial was done among 25 healthy adults with no prior history of malaria infection or vaccination; CIS43LS was administered iv at one of three doses. No adverse events were noted; a dose-dependent increase in serum antibody concentrations was seen with a half-life of 56 days. Among 15 adults who got controlled exposure to mosquitoes carrying P. falciparum sporozoites, parasitaemia was not observed in any nine participants who received CIS43LS and five of six controls. Available data will quickly translate into malaria prevention among travelers, seasonal malaria control, and elimination campaigns.

Oxidative Stress and Pathogenesis in Malaria-

The precise role and the mechanisms of oxidative stress in malaria pathogenesis are still not well defined. On one hand, there is abundant evidence of strong correlations between levels of oxidative stress in malaria patients and disease severity in general disease severity or specific complications. Together with multiple studies in mice treated with antioxidants, the data suggest that oxidative stress is a major contributor to malaria pathogenesis. On the other hand, despite multiple proposed mechanisms, there is no specific demonstrated causal link between oxidative stress and pathogenesis in human malaria.

Overall, maintaining oxidative balance in the host in the context of Plasmodium infection may be beneficial as it could prevent the development of pathologic complications. However, since the oxidative burst in phagocytes and anti-malarial treatments mechanism of action is mediated by inducing oxidative killing of the parasite, the possible interference of antioxidant treatments with parasite elimination must be carefully analyzed before treatment.

Diagnostic Methods for Non-Falciparum Malaria-

TABLE 1 | Summary of diagnostic methods for non-falciparum (nf) malaria.

Classification	Method	Sensitivity (a) Specificity for nf spp (b)	Advantages or Strengths	Disadvantages or Weaknesses
Field diagnosis	Microscopy (Section 2a)	a. LOD ~50-200 parasites/µL b. High in single infections	Gold-standard method for malaria diagnosis in field. Low cost PoC detection	Unable to detect sub-microscopic infections. Requires well-trained technicians. Eventual spp misidentification. Under-diagnosis of minority spp in mixed infections.
	RDTs (Section 2b)	a. Expected: 75% at 200 parasites/µL b. not specific for nf spp except Types 5-6 for Pv (see **Table 2**)	Rapid (~20 minutes) Low cost – independent of equipment Requires minimal training PoC detection	Unable to detect sub-microscopic infections. Unable to differentiate among nf spp. Low sensitivity for nf spp in field (frequently lower than expected).
Laboratory diagnosis	Immunological methods (Section 3a)	a. Commercial ELISA kits: 95% to detect clinical malaria. b. Commercial ELISA kits: not specific for nf spp.	Useful for epidemiological surveys seeking to study malaria prevalence. Promising results on detection of active infections could be useful to develop new RDTs or biosensors.	Requires trained personnel and laboratory equipment. In-house assays were validated in field using relatively low numbers of samples and require further validation to determine sensitivity and spp specificity.
	Detection of iRBCs (Section 3b)	–	Promising results that require further validation.	Requires trained personnel and laboratory equipment. High cost of required equipment.
	PCR (Section 3c)	a. LOD 0.2-5 parasites/µL (blood) b. High (~85-100%, compared to microscopy).	Gold-standard method for detecting sub-microscopic infections. Quantitative determination (qPCR). Most assays were able to differentiate among nf spp.	Requires trained personnel and laboratory equipment. High cost of reagents and equipment. Even though several assays were validated with samples from endemic areas, this method remains mostly used only for research purposes.
New potential PoC diagnosis	Biosensors (Section 4a)	a. Highly variable. b. Mostly specific for Pf and Pv determination.	Analytical performance well documented. Promising results that require further validation.	Currently requires trained personnel and laboratory equipment. These methods were not yet validated in field.
	"Lab-on-chip" or LAMP-based methods (Section 4b)	a. High, ~95-100% compared to PCR. b. High, ~85-100% depending on the assays and the comparator.	Requires less training and equipment than PCR, while obtaining similar results. Commercial kits with high sensitivity available. Potentially PoC.	Prone to contamination (requires high care in sample and reagents manipulation). Commercial kits currently available do not discriminate among nf spp.

*Source: Gimenez AM, Marques RF, Regiart M, Bargieri DY. Diagnostic Methods for Non-Falciparum Malaria. Front Cell Infect Microbiol. 2021 Jun 17;11:681063. doi: 10.3389/fcimb.2021.681063. PMID: 34222049; PMCID: PMC8248680.

New treatment regimens for Chagas disease

Chagas disease is caused by the protozoan parasite *Trypanosoma cruzi*. It is responsible for morbidity and mortality in countries of the Western hemisphere. It is transmitted by the bite of triatomine bugs through vertical transmission from mother to fetus, transfusion of infected blood components, transplantation of organ from infected donor, and ingestion of contaminated food or water.

Clinical features include nonspecific symptoms like malaise, fever, anorexia, and can even be asymptomatic. Chagomas are seen on the face or extremities. Romana's sign is a characteristic unilateral swelling of the upper and lower eyelid. In a small subset of patients, manifestations include acute myocarditis, pericardial effusion, or meningoencephalitis.

Acute Chagas disease should be suspected in individuals from endemic areas with typical clinical features. The acute phase lasts for 8 to 12 weeks. Circulating trypomastigotes can be identified by microscopy of fresh blood or buffy coat smears. The polymerase chain reaction is another sensitive diagnostic tool. Direct demonstration of parasites by hemoculture or xenodiagnosis indicates actual infection. Differential diagnoses include preseptal cellulitis, infectious mononucleosis, and acute HIV infection.

For more than five decades, the quest to find effective aetiological treatments for Chagas disease was continued. There has been some renewed interest in the past decade by the use of molecules such as azoles.

In the last 50 years, only two drugs were recommended to treat Chagas disease have been available which are benznidazole and nifurtimox. Benznidazole was launched in 1971 but was not approved by the U.S. FDA until 2017. Despite benznidazole being highly effective and capable of eradicating 100% of parasites, substantial limitations, including toxicity (peripheral neuropathy, granulocytopenia, and severe gastrointestinal symptoms) lead to the discontinuation of treatment. These have been reported in up to 25% of patients with Chagas disease.

Babesiosis

Babesiosis is an infection caused by protozoa *Babesia*, infecting and lyse red blood cells. It is transmitted by tick or blood transfusion and rarely organ transplantation and congenital transmission. The main species is *Babesia microti*.

Infection can range from asymptomatic to fatal. The incubation period lasts between 1 to 4 weeks. Most common features include chills, sweats, and myalgia. Other features include anorexia, headache, nausea, dry cough, arthralgia, shortness of breath, sore throat, vomiting, diarrhea, photophobia, weight loss, conjunctival injection, and abdominal pain. Splenomegaly, hepatomegaly, icterus, pharyngeal erythema, and retinopathy with splinter hemorrhages were examined.

Laboratory features include low hematocrit, hemoglobin, elevated lactate dehydrogenase, reticulocytosis, raised transaminitis, elevated alkaline phosphatase, elevated bilirubin, BUN and creatinine. A peripheral blood smear examination or polymerase chain reaction (PCR), rather than antibody testing should be used. For babesiosis patients with a positive *Babesia* antibody test, the recommendation is to confirm using peripheral blood smear or PCR before treatment.

Treatment of babesiosis includes a combination of atovaquone plus azithromycin or clindamycin plus quinine. Atovaquone plus azithromycin is the recommended antimicrobial combination for patients with babesiosis, while clindamycin plus quinine is the choice. The duration of therapy is 7 - 10 days in immunocompetent patients but is often extended when there is an immunocompromised patient.

Table 1. Infectious Diseases Society of America (IDSA) 2020 Guidelines on Diagnosis and Management of Babesiosis (1)

Patient Category	Treatment Regimen	
	Adult doses	**Pediatric doses**
Ambulatory patients: mild to moderate disease	**Preferred**	
	Atovaquone 750 mg orally (with a fatty meal) Q12h plus azithromycin 500 mg orally on day 1, then 250 mg Q 24h for 7 to 10 days.	Atovaquone 20 mg/kg per dose (up to 750 mg) Q12h orally plus azithromycin 10 mg/kg orally on the day of admission, then 5 mg/kg (up to 250 mg) Q24h for 7 to 10 days.
	Alternative	
	Clindamycin 600 mg orally Q8h plus quinine sulfate 542 mg base (which equals 650 mg salt) orally Q6h–8h for 7 to 10 days.	Clindamycin 7–10 mg/kg orally Q8h plus quinine sulfate 6 mg base/kg (which equals 8 mg salt/kg) (up to 542 mg base or 650 mg salt/ dose) orally Q6–8h for 7 to 10 days.

Hospitalized patients: acute severe disease	**Preferred**	
	Atovaquone 750 mg orally Q12h plus azithromycin 500–1000 mg IV Q24h until symptoms abate, then convert to all-oral therapy (see step-down therapy).	Atovaquone 20 mg/kg per dose (up to 750 mg) Q12h orally plus azithromycin 10 mg/kg (up to 500 mg) Q24h IV until symptoms abate, then convert to all-oral therapy (see step-down therapy).
	Alternative	**Alternative**
	Clindamycin 600 mg IV Q6h plus quinine sulfate 542 mg base (which equals 650 mg salt) orally Q6h–8h until symptoms abate, then convert to all-oral therapy (see step-down therapy).	Clindamycin 7–10 mg/kg IV plus quinine sulfate 6 mg base/kg (which equals 8 mg salt/kg) per dose (up to 542 mg base or 650 mg salt) Q6–8h orally until symptoms abate, then convert to all-oral therapy (see step-down therapy).
Hospitalized patients: step-down therapy (transition to oral therapy)	**Preferred**	
	Atovaquone 750 mg orally Q12h plus azithromycin 250–500 mg orally Q24h. Treatment of acute disease plus step-down therapy typically lasts 7–10 days in total. A high dose of azithromycin (500–1000 mg) should be considered for immunocompromised patients.	Atovaquone 20 mg/kg per dose (up to 750 mg) orally Q12h plus azithromycin 10 mg/kg (maximum dose 500 mg) orally Q24h. Treatment of acute disease and step-down therapy typically last 7–10 days in total.
	Alternative	
	Clindamycin 600 mg orally Q8h plus quinine sulfate 542 mg base (which equals 650 mg salt) orally Q6h–8h. Treatment of acute disease plus step-down therapy typically lasts 7–10 days.	Clindamycin 7–10 mg/kg orally (up to 600 mg/dose) orally Q8h plus quinine sulfate 6 mg base/kg (which equals 8 mg salt/kg) (up to 542 mg base or 650 mg salt/ dose) orally Q6–8h. Treatment of acute disease plus step-down therapy typically lasts 7–10 days.
Highly immunocompromised patients	Start with one of the regimens recommended for hospitalized patients: acute severe disease and follow with step-down therapies but treat for at least six consecutive weeks, including two final weeks during which parasites are no longer detected on the peripheral blood smear. A 500–1000 mg daily dose should be considered when oral azithromycin is used. If infection relapses, consider one of the regimens listed in Table 3.	

Exchange transfusion is considered for patients with high-grade parasitemia (>10%) or those with one or more of the following complications

- severe hemolytic anemia
- severe pulmonary, renal, or hepatic compromise.

Expert consultation with transfusion services physician or hematologist in conjunction with an infectious diseases specialist is strongly suggested.

For immunocompetent patients, a recommendation is to monitor *Babesia* parasitemia during the acute phase of therapy using peripheral blood smears but recommend strongly against testing for parasitemia once symptoms have resolved.

It is also recommended to monitor Babesia parasitemia using peripheral blood smears even after they become asymptomatic and until blood smears are negative for immunocompromised patients. PCR testing should be used if blood smears turn hostile.

References

1. Krause PJ, Auwaerter PG, Bannuru RR, Branda JA, Falck-Ytter YT, Lantos PM, et al. Clinical Practice Guidelines by the Infectious Diseases Society of America (IDSA): 2020 Guideline on Diagnosis and Management of Babesiosis. Clin Infect Dis an Off Publ Infect Dis Soc Am. 2021 Jan;72(2):e49–64.

Recent updates on Vaccines

Hepatitis B vaccine

Hepatitis B virus (HBV) is a global health issue, with 257 million carriers worldwide and 887,000 causing HBV-related liver disease in 2015. Chronic HBV prevalence among children less than five years of age is less than 1%. This reflects a global vaccination problem. HBV is transmitted by sexual route, through blood and transplacental route. WHO recommends screening with HBsAg and hepatitis B core antigen before blood transfusion in donors.

The HBV spectrum infection range from acute to chronic disease. The acute features include subclinical or anicteric hepatitis, icteric hepatitis, and finally, fulminant hepatitis. Chronic illnesses include an asymptomatic carrier state to chronic hepatitis, cirrhosis, and hepatocellular carcinoma. The incubation period lasts one to four months. Chronic HBV patients are asymptomatic and sometimes fatigued. Physical examination may be normal, or there can be stigmata of chronic liver disease. Jaundice, ascites, peripheral edema, splenomegaly, and encephalopathy are common in decompensated ones. Chronic HBV infection has 4 phases -

- immune tolerant
- HBeAg positive chronic hepatitis
- inactive carrier state, and
- reactivation HBeAg negative chronic hepatitis.

There can be coinfection with Hepatitis C, D virus, and sometimes HIV.

HBV should be tested in two populations –

- Those with signs and symptoms of acute or chronic hepatitis
- Asymptomatic patients who are at high risk for HBV exposure or at risk of severe adverse outcomes from undiagnosed infection.

For screening asymptomatic persons, HBsAg and anti-HBs are recommended. Anti HBc can be used to screen HIV patients, those with HCV infection on direct-acting antivirals, patients who require immunosuppressive therapy, and blood and organ donors. HBV DNA is also used with a cut-off of 10 to 20 IU/mL.

Acute hepatitis B treatment includes tenofovir or entecavir as monotherapy. Lamivudine or telbivudine can be used for short-duration therapy. Adefovir is usually avoided because of weak antiviral activity.

In a case of chronic hepatitis B, after history and physical examination, lab tests should include a complete blood count, liver function tests, coagulation profile, renal function tests, HBeAg, HBV DNA, and IgG hepatitis A. Also, evaluate for other causes of liver disease, HIV, and HCC screening. Antiviral therapy is based on the presence or absence of cirrhosis, ALT, and HBV DNA levels. Drugs include nucleoside analogs, pegylated interferon, and anti-CD-20.

HBV vaccines can be a single antigen recombinant, most commonly yeast-derived using S protein of the surface antigen (Recombivax HB and Engerix -B), which use aluminum adjuvant. They are given in three doses over six months period intramuscularly. In December 2021, the U.S. FDA approved a trivalent mammalian cell-derived recombinant vaccine that contains two pre-S epitopes apart from the S antigen. Compared to conventional hepatitis B vaccines, the new vaccine is more immunogenic in older adults. Despite this, its role remains uncertain since it causes more side effects than conventional hepatitis B vaccines, and more doses are required than the adjuvanted recombinant hepatitis B vaccine (HepB-CpG; three versus two doses). (1)

Human papillomavirus vaccination

Papillomaviruses are double-stranded DNA viruses belonging to the Papillomaviridae family. There are more than 200 types of HPV which infects only humans. They are subdivided into cutaneous or mucosal categories based on tissue tropism. It has two encapsulating structural proteins, L1 and L2. L1 protein assembles itself in the absence of a viral genome to form viral-like particles (VLP). This L1 VLP is an immunogen used in HPV vaccines.

HPV 9 valent vaccine, the two doses are given at 0 and 6 to 12 months between 9 to 15 years of age. Three doses of HPV vaccine should be given at 0, 1 to 2 and 6 months. Quadrivalent HPV and Bivalent HPV vaccines are also there.

Cutaneous HPV types include plantar and common warts, including types 1,2 and 4. Flat warts are caused by HPV types 3 and 10. The anogenital epithelium is affected by genital warts HPV 6 and 11 and squamous intraepithelial lesions by HPV 15 and 16.

Human papillomavirus (HPV) vaccination was shown to reduce the incidence of HPV infection and cervical intraepithelial neoplasia (CIN). 13.7 million follow-up females aged 20 to 30 years were included in a registry-based observational study. Females who received the bivalent HPV vaccine at a younger age were found to have a significant relative reduction in the incidence of cervical cancer and CIN3 (34% for vaccination at age 16 to 18 years, 62% at age 14 to 16 years, and 87% at age 12 to 13 years) compared with the unvaccinated cohort. This lends further support to vaccinating against HPV at a younger age. (2)

Herpes zoster vaccination

Varicella-zoster virus infection causes two clinically distinct diseases – varicella and shingles. During the initial phase of varicella, VZV infects nasopharyngeal lymphoid tissue through airborne infection. Risk factors include the elderly, immunocompromised patients, transplant patients, autoimmune diseases, and HIV.

Clinical features include rash, headache, fever, malaise, and fatigue. Common complications include postherpetic neuralgia and ocular, neurologic, and bacterial superinfection of the skin. Diagnosis is made clinically, and tests include polymerase chain reaction and direct fluorescent antibody testing.

Herpes zoster vaccination is indicated for those ≥50 years of age to reduce the risk of herpes zoster and postherpetic neuralgia. Two doses of vaccine is administered two to six months after the first dose and given intramuscularly. Adverse effects include injection site reactions, myalgia, fatigue, headache, shivering, and Guillain-Barre syndrome.

The U.S. FDA and the European Medicines Agency have now approved the recombinant zoster vaccine (RZV) for use in individuals ≥18 years old who are at increased risk of herpes zoster due to immunodeficiency or immunosuppression. RZV has been shown to reduce the incidence of herpes zoster in immunocompromised adults. Specific recommendations from the United States Advisory Committee on Immunization Practices regarding the use of RZV in those ≥18 years of age are pending. (3)

Vaccination with live virus vaccine is not recommended for transplant recipients or immunosuppressive treatment. It is given as one time subcutaneous injection. Adverse events include injection site reactions, acute retinal necrosis, and uveitis.

Ebola vaccine

Ebola virus comprises of six species, namely, Zaire, Sudan, Bundibugyo, Tai Forest, Reston, and Bombali, belonging to Filoviridae. It is a nonsegmented, negative-sense, single-stranded RNA virus. It is transmitted by contact with tissues or body fluids, airborne transmission, and nosocomial exposure to bats.

Clinical features include fever and chills, fatigue, headache, vomiting, diarrhea, rash, loss of appetite, altered level of consciousness, hyperreflexia, myopathy, stiff neck, gait instability, and seizures.

Laboratory features include leucopenia, thrombocytopenia, abnormal hematocrit, transaminitis, prolonged prothrombin and partial thromboplastin time, proteinuria, elevated blood urea nitrogen, and creatinine electrolyte abnormalities. RTPCR can be tested to identify viruses.

Effective Ebola virus disease treatment requires aggressive supportive care to correct volume losses, correct electrolyte abnormalities, and prevent shock as complications of vomiting and diarrhea.

After the re-emergence of Ebola virus disease in Guinea, it became the epicenter of the 2014–16 epidemic in West Africa five years after the initial wave that claimed more than 11 000 lives, and following it, successive outbreaks were reported in the Democratic Republic of the Congo, the need for safe and effective vaccines to prevent disease transmission remains urgent. In May 2020, the Janssen Vaccines & Prevention developed a heterologous primary and booster Ebola vaccine regimen. This included the adenovirus type-26 vector-based vaccine having Zaire Ebola virus glycoprotein (Ad26.ZEBOV). The modified vaccine Ankara vector-based vaccine, encoded glycoproteins from strains like Sudan virus, Zaire Ebola virus, Marburg virus, and nucleoprotein expressed on the Tai Forest virus (MVA-BN-Filo). They are administered eight weeks apart. European Commission granted authorization for marketing for the prevention of Ebola virus disease in adults and children aged one year or older.

Clinical development of the Ad26.ZEBOV and MVA-BN-Filo vaccine regimen included several phases 1 clinical trial done in concert at various sites in Uganda, which is an endemic country for Ebola virus and is at risk of an outbreak, with reported Ebola virus cases; in Tanzania and Kenya, which were also at risk of an outbreak but had no previously reported cases of the disease; and in the U.K. and the USA, that is only at risk of imported cases of the disease.

These trials helped in the collection of safety, tolerability, and immunogenicity data across various epidemiological settings. African participants include malaria-naive individuals from high-altitude settings of Nairobi, Kenya, and individuals with partial immunity to malaria from Mwanza, Tanzania, and Masaka, Uganda. This strategic approach has led to the generation of locally relevant data and provided a solid evidence base to inform the selection of Ad26.ZEBOV as a prime and MVA-BN-Filo to boost phase 2 clinical trial. (4)

CYD-TDV dengue vaccine (CYD65)

Dengue is the most rapidly spreading mosquito-borne viral disease, with a 30-fold increase in global incidence over the last five decades. Every year, thousands of cases of dengue fever occur all over the country, giving rise to a significant number of deaths and morbidity. The case fatality rate for dengue fever varies by region and age, and most fatal cases are among children and young adults— the WHO enlisted dengue fever as one of the threats to global health in 2019.

In India, Aedes aegypti is the primary vector in most urban areas. The climatic variations, temperature, and rainfall play a vital role in the life cycle, breeding, longevity of vectors, and transmission of the disease. Aedes is a daytime feeder and can fly up to a limited distance of 400m. There are four dengue virus serotypes designated DENV-1, DENV-2, DENV-3, and DENV-4. The dengue virus genome is composed of three structural protein genes encoding the nucleocapsid of core protein (C), a membrane-associated protein (M), an envelope protein(E), and seven nonstructural (NS) proteins - NS1, NS2A, NS2B, NS3, NS4A, NS4B, and NS5.

The onset of dengue fever is usually with a sudden rise in temperature, which may be biphasic, lasting 2-7 days. Headache, flushing, retro-orbital pain and rash, myalgia, maculopapular or rubelliform rash usually appears after the third or fourth day of fever and is commonly seen on the face, neck, and other parts of the body; it generally fades away in the latter half of febrile phase.

Mild dengue fever and body aches are best treated with paracetamol. Salicylates and other non-steroidal anti-inflammatory drugs (NSAIDs) should be avoided as these may predispose to mucosal bleeds. The patient should be encouraged to drink plenty of fluids. In moderate and severe dengue, these patients should be admitted to the hospital and given intravenous fluids. Crystalloids are the preferred fluids.

Three doses of the licensed tetravalent CYD-TDV (Dengvaxia, Sanofi Pasteur, Lyon, France) dengue vaccine are immunogenic and effective against symptomatic dengue individuals who are dengue seropositive. Previous trials have provided little evidence that antibody responses elicited after one or two doses of CYD-TDV would be similar to those elicited after three doses.

In a randomized, controlled, phase 2 non-inferiority study (CYD65), healthy individuals aged 9–50 years were recruited from the community in three sites in Colombia and three sites in the Philippines. Participants were assigned (1:1:1) randomly, to receive, at 6-month intervals (on day 0, month 6, and month 12), three doses of CYD-TDV (three-dose group); one dose of placebo (on day 0) and two doses of CYD-TDV (each at 6 and 12 months; two-dose group); or two doses of placebo (on day 0 and 6 months) and one dose of CYD-TDV (at 12 months; one-dose group). Each dose of 0·5 mL CYD-TDV was administered subcutaneously into the deltoid of the upper arm. The primary endpoints taken were geometric mean titers (GMTs) of neutralizing antibodies against each dengue virus serotype after 28 days and one year, after the final injection. After an amendment of protocol during the conduct of the study, the original primary objectives of non-inferiority of the one-dose and two-dose groups to the three-dose group were altered to include non-inferiority of a two-dose group to three-dose group only, which assessed individuals who were dengue seropositive at baseline. Safety was assessed among all participants who received at least one study drug injection, regardless of serostatus. At 28 days of the last injection, neutralizing antibody GMTs were 899 in the two-dose group versus 822 in the three-dose group against dengue serotype one versus 875 against serotype 2; 599 versus 610 against serotype 3; and 510 versus 531 against serotype 4. At one year, GMTs had decreased but remained above baseline for all serotypes: 504 in a two-dose group versus 490 in a three-dose group against serotype one versus 821 against serotype 2; 437 versus 477 against serotype 3; and 238 versus 270 against serotype 4. Most adverse events after injection were non-serious and systemic. A two-dose CYD-TDV regimen might be an alternative to the licensed three-dose regimen in dengue seropositive individuals at baseline and aged nine years and older. Vaccination with reduced doses could improve vaccine compliance and coverage, especially in low-resource settings. (5)

Leptospirosis

Leptospira organisms are obligate aerobic spirochetes which are tightly coiled and very thin having unique motility.

The genus is divided into two species leptospira interrogans end leptospira Biflexa. Humans are accidental host in whom the severity of disease ranges from subclinical infection to fatal infections. The primary host are wild and domestic animals In whom infection causes severe economic loss in dairy and meat industry.

Recent Updates:

Leptospira collagenase and LipL32 for antibody detection in leptospirosis

Leptospira whole-genome sequencing demonstrated that pathogenic Leptospira contained the nucleotide sequence (colA gene) coding for the collagenase. A study was done to demonstrate where cloned ColA protein, in comparison with LipL32 which is widely used in the leptospira study, was used as an antigen for antibody detection. Data suggested that sensitivity and specificity of ColA protein for Leptospira antibody detection were 100%. In addition, ColA protein showed higher specificity than LipL32.

Hematological Emergencies

Contributors

1. Dr. Dipali Rajpal
2. Dr. Nidhi Kaeley
3. Dr. Archana Bairwa

Chapters

1. Thrombocytopenia
2. Primary Immune thrombocytopenia
3. TTP
4. Transfusion reactions
5. Febrile neutropenia
6. SVC syndrome
7. Anticoagulation reversal
8. American Society of Hematology Guidelines
9. VITT
10. Pediatric oncological emergencies

Thrombocytopenia

The reported prevalence of idiopathic thrombocytopenia is 9.5 per 100,000 in adults with an incidence of 3.3 per 100,000 in a year. Thrombocytopenia is defined as platelet count less than 1.5 lakh/microlitre. The normal platelet count ranges from 1.5 to 4.5 lakhs/microlitre. Platelet count is higher in women as compared to men. It is relatively higher in younger population.

Diagnostic approach to the adult with unexplained thrombocytopenia

Bleeding is a definite concern in patients with thrombocytopenia. Following are the criteria of increased bleeding risks.

- The risk of surgical bleeding is higher in patients with platelet count less than 50,000/microlitre.
- The risk of spontaneous bleeding is high in patients with platelet count less than 20,000/microlitre.
- It has been observed that the bleeding risk is slightly lesser in ITP (idiopathic thrombocytopenia) as compared to other conditions for the same platelet count.

In addition, thrombocytopenia has another risk of thrombosis; the following are the conditions:

- Heparin-induced thrombocytopenia (HIT) was seen in less than 5% of patients exposed to heparin. Heparin-induced antibodies are formed against the platelet factor 4 (PFF-4) epitope. This leads to thrombocytopenia and further platelet activation, further causing catastrophic venous and arterial thrombosis.
- Vaccine-induced immune thrombotic thrombocytopenia (VITT) has been observed in patients after vaccination with COVID-19 adenoviral vector vaccines [AstraZeneca and Janssen (Johnson and Johnson)]. The presentation is similar to HIT.
- Antiphospholipid syndrome is commonly found in patients with SLE and other infections.
- Disseminated Intravascular coagulation.
- Thrombotic microangiopathy
- Paroxysmal Nocturnal Hemoglobinuria
- ITP with a concomitant thrombotic disorder.

Idiopathic thrombocytopenia is defined as a low platelet count of less than 100X10q/L. Thrombocytopenia can occur as a result of decreased production, increased immune-mediated destruction, or splenic sequestration of platelets.

Common Causes of thrombocytopenia

- Pregnancy
- Chronic liver disease or hypersplenism
- Immune thrombocytopenia
- Congenital platelet disorders
  - MYH-19 related disorders
  - Berner – surlier syndrome
  - Gray platelet syndrome
- infections
  - viral
  - Bacterial/sepsis
  - HIV
  - Intracellular parasites
- Drug-induced thrombocytopenia
  - antibiotics (sulfonamides, ampicillin, piperacillin, Vancomycin, rifampicin)
  - antiplatelet agents (Carbamazepine, phenytoin)
  - quinine
- HIT (Heparin-induced thrombocytopenia)
- Drug-induced thrombotic microangiopathy (DITMA) is seen with quinine, several cancer therapies, calcineurin inhibitors, and drugs of abuse.
- Alcohol
- Malignancy
- Nutritional (vitamin B_{12}, folate deficiency)
- Thrombotic microangiopathy
- Bone marrow disorders
  - Myelodysplastic syndrome
  - Aplastic Anemia
  - Acute Leukemia

Rheumatological Disorders

- SLE
- Antiphospholipid syndrome
- Secondary ITP

Other Causes –

- giant capillary hemangioma
- large aortic aneurysms
- Cardiopulmonary bypass
- Intra-aortic balloon pumps

Physical Examination (Examine for)

- Petechiae
- Purpura
- Ecchymoses
- Hepatosplenomegaly
- Lymphadenopathy

Laboratory Investigations

1. Repeat CBC
2. Peripheral blood smear
3. Rule out pseudo thrombocytopenia
4. RBC and WBC abnormalities

    a. Schistocytes are seen in microangiopathic process (DIC, TTP, HUS, DITMA)

    b. Nucleated RBCs and Howell-Jolly BB bodies are seen in post-splenectomy patients

    c. Leucoerythroblastic findings, teardrop cells, nucleated RBCs, immature granulocytes suggest an infiltrative process in bone marrow

    d. Leucocytosis with band cells in sepsis

    e. Immature WBCs dysplastic WBCs in leukemia myelodysplasia

    f. Multilobe/hyper segmented neutrophils in patients with vitamin B_{12} or folate deficiency

5. Bone Marrow Examination

Primary Immune Thrombocytopenia

It is an autoimmune disease characterized by lower platelet count. The symptoms and signs of primary immune thrombocytopenia can range from mild to catastrophic presentation in the form of overt bleeding. Autoimmune diseases are known to affect around 3-9% of the population. However, ITP still remains a disease of exclusion after ruling out secondary causes of thrombocytopenia.

Pathophysiology

Following defects play a pivotal role in the underlying pathogenesis of ITP.

a. Defects in Antigen Presenting Cells – The autoimmune response is triggered by T-helper cells, which recognize the cognate antigens along with major histocompatibility complexes (MHC) on antigen-presenting cells (APC). APC includes dendritic cells, macrophages as well as platelets, and megakaryocytes, as per recent studies. Dendritic cells have the ability to stimulate autoreactive T-cell proliferation. In the case of inflammatory states such as sepsis, MHC class II molecules are upregulated and increase the antigen capacity of the cells. The macrophage destroys not only autoantibody-opsonized platelets but also presents platelet autoantigen to autoreactive T-helper cells.

b. Soluble factors – Patients with ITP have multiple abnormalities in soluble immune mediators such as cytokines/chemokines. one study demonstrated the production of macrophage inhibition factor (MIF) by lymphocytes in patients with ITP. It has been reported that ITP is a manifestation of defects in the number and defective suppressive capacity of regulator T-cell (Treg) in patients with ITP versus controls and restored Treg numbers and regulatory function, especially in responders, following treatment with rituximab. (1)

c. Dysregulation of natural killer (NK) cells and T-lymphocytes – The natural killer cells have the ability to recognize and kill the abnormal cells. A study found that in ITP, the ability for NK cells to kill K562 erythroleukemic target cells was significantly suppressed. thus as NK cells inhibit B-cell differentiation, their suppression can lead to formation of autoantibodies production in ITP.

d. Various other myeloid and lymphoid abnormalities have been reported in patients with ITP.

Treatment

The primary goal of treatment of ITP is the prevention of bleeding by increasing the platelet count up to 20,000/ul.

First-line Treatment

Both dexamethasone and prednisolone have been found to stimulate B-Cell and dendritic cell activation, thus leading to the deactivation of immune-mediated platelet destruction.

Prednisolone is started at this dose of 1mg/kg/day. A study found that in patients with an initial platelet count of less than 20,000/ul, dexamethasone given at a dose of 40mg for four days increased the platelet count to 50,000/ul. Steroids can be safely initiated in pregnant patients. In steroid-resistant patients, intravenous immunoglobulins of RHO(D) IVIG can be initiated at a dose of 1g/kg/day infusion for a day or two. IVIG is indicated in patients with rapidly falling platelet counts and active bleeding with an urgent need to build up platelet count. It should be started in conjunction with steroid therapy.

<u>Second-line Treatment</u>

According to ASH (American society of hematology) 2011, splenectomy is recommended in patients who failed therapy with steroids, IVIG, and anti-RhD. Splenectomy can be performed either open or laparoscopically. Laparoscopic splenectomy leads to a shorter hospital stay.

Anti-CD-20, rituximab is another option for chronic and persistent ITP. The standard dose of rituximab in ITP is 375 mg/m^2/week intravenously for four doses. The toxicity of rituximab includes infusion reactions, serum sickness, and arrhythmias.

<u>Third Line Treatment</u>

- Azathioprine - 150mg/day in Chronic refractory ITP.
- Cyclophosphamide
- Cyclosporine
- Diazole
- Dapsone
- mycophenolate mofetil
- Vinblastine
- Vincristine
- Thrombopoietin receptor agonists (TPO-RA)
  - romiplostim is fc peptide fusion peptibody. It stimulates megakaryopoiesis.
  - Eltrombopag is naphthalenesulfonic acid which also stimulates platelet production.
  - Avatrombopag- JAK-STAT pathway.
- Fostamatinib- a syk inhibitor
- Efgartigimod - Anti-Fc-Rn. It is found to decrease the half-life of IgG.
- Rozanolixizumab - Anti-Fc-Rn
- Rilzabrutinib - BTKI
- Sutimlimab - Anti-c/s

Thrombotic Thrombocytopenic Purpura

<u>Pathogenesis</u>

It is caused by severe deficiency of ADAMTS 13 (A Disintegrin and metalloprotease with a thrombospondin type motif, member 13) protease. The deficiency is less than 10% ADAMTS-13 functions as von willebrand factor (VWF) cleaning protease. It leads to cleaning of ultra large molecules of VWF, thus preventing the accumulation of ultra large mustiness of VWF in areas of stress.

<u>Histopathology</u>

It is characterized by changes in the small vessel wall such as swollen endothelial cell and sub-endothelial space thickening of vessel wall and platelet microthrombi leading to small arteriole and capillary occlusion. It involves multiple systems in the body.

   a.   Kidney- It causes severe acute kidney injury.
   b.   Central nervous system - It causes neurological manifestations such as headache, tonic-clonic seizure, come, stroke.
   c.   Hematological manifestations occur in the form of microangiopathic hemolytic anemia.

Clinical Presentation

The mean age of presentation of TTP is 40 years. Females are more commonly affected than males. Pregnancy is a risk factor of immune TTP. The key finding of TTP-HUS registry showed that microangiopathic hemolytic anemia and thrombocytopenia was present in all the patients. Severe neurological manifestations were present in 53% of cases, whereas 27% heal minor neurological manifestations, 5% of patients developed acute kidney failure, and 47% had reduced renal function. Gastrointestinal symptoms in the form of abdominal pain, nausea, vomiting, and diarrhea may be present. Cardiac manifestations in the form of chest pain, arrhythmias, myocardial infarction, heart failure, and cardiogenic shock may be present.

Evaluation and Diagnosis

TTP should be suspected when a patient presents with microangiopathic hemolytic anemia with severe thrombocytopenia.

PLASMIC SCORE

The score gives one point to each of the following.

- Platelet count <30,000/microlitre
- Hemolysis (defined as reticulocyte count >2.5%, undebatable haptoglobin or indirect bilirubin >1mg/dl)

- No active cancer
- No solid organ or stem cell transplant
- MCV <90 ft.
- INR <1.5
- Creatinine <2.0 mg/dl

6 to 7 points - high probability TTP

5 points- intermediate probability TTP

0 to 4 points - how probability TTP

Hereditary TTP occurs as a consequence of TMA caused by *balletic ADAMTS 13 mutations.*

Important Terminology in Treatment

- <u>Clinical response:</u> Constant normalization of platelet count and LDH < 1.5 times the upper limit of normal with therapeutic plama exchange anti-VWF therapy (Caplacizumab), with no new or progressive manifestations of ischemic organ injury.
- <u>Clinical remission:</u> A sustained clinical response > 30 days after stopping TPE and emapalumab or attainment of partial or complete ADAMTS 13 remission.
- <u>ADAMTS-13 Remission</u> - ADAMTS 13 activity recovery to > 20% is a partial ADAMTS 13 remission, ADAMTS 13 activity recovery to the lower limit of normal for the assay or greater is a complete ADAMTS 13 remission.
- <u>Refractory disease</u> - No clinical response with rituximab and anti-VWF
- <u>Disease exacerbation</u> - thrombocytopenia referred within 30 days of stopping TPE or anti-VWF therapy.
- <u>Clinical Relapse</u> - Thrombocytopenia recurrence following a remission
- <u>ADAMTS 13 relapse</u> - ADAMTS 13 activity < 20% following AAMS 13 remission

Treatment Approach

1. Calculate PLASMIC SCORE
2. Detect ADAMTS 13 activity –

   less than 10% is suggestive ofsevere deficiency.

   If 13 to 20%, it may support the diagnosis of TTP.

   If ADAMTS 13 activity > 20%, TTP is unlikely to be the diagnosis

3. Plasma Exchange.
4. Medical therapies include

a. Glucocorticoids

b. Rituximab

c. Caplacizumab

All the high-risk cases should receive methylprednisolone 100 mg a single dose on the first day, followed by 125 mg two to four times a day. If the patient is clinically improving, switch to prednisolone 1mg/kg/day

Transfusion Reactions

Types of acute transfusion Reactions

- a. Transfusion-related acute lung injury
- b. Transfusion-associated circulatory overload.
- c. Acute hemolysis
- d. Anaphylaxis
- e. Sepsis
- f. allergic Transfusion reactions
- g. Febrile non-hemolytic transfusion reactions

Transfusion-related acute lung injury

It occurs when a patient develops rapid onset of acute lung injury and non-cardiogenic pulmonary edema as a consequence of activation of immune cells in the lung. In 2004 and 2005, according to the national heart lung and blood institute (NHLBI) working group and the Canadian consensus conference (CCC), TRALI was defined as an acute lung injury or acute respiratory distress syndrome developing during or within six hours of blood product transfusion.

However, in 2019, Revised Delphi panel definition, *TRALI type I* was defined as having no risk factors of ARDS, and all the following criteria are met, including acute onset, hypoxemia (pao_2/fio_2 ≤300 mmhg hg or spo_2 <90% on room air), and no clear evidence of left atrial hypertension. If left atrial hypertension is present, it is judged not to be the underlying cause of hypoxemia. During or within six hours of transfusion, there should be no history of temporal relationship to any other alternative risk factors for ARDS.

TRALI type II - It is defined as when risk factors of ARDS are present or mild ARDS is evident at baseline but with respiratory deterioration judged based on either one of the following:

Finding as suggestive of TRALI Type - I

Stable respiratory status in the 12 hours before transfusion.

TRALI CRITERIA

These criteria require the presence of **new** acute respiratory distress syndrome (ARDS) occurring during or within six hours after blood product administration, documented by hypoxemia and abnormal chest imaging. Hypoxemia is documented when oxygen saturation is ≤90 percent on room air or the PaO_2/FIO_2 ratio is <300 mmHg, although other signs of hypoxia can also satisfy this criterion. Chest imaging must demonstrate bilateral pulmonary infiltrates.

In patients when TRALI cannot be distinguished from TACO when clinical findings are similar, and there is a lack of data if left atrial hypertension is absent or present.

Transfusion - associated dyspnea (TAD) - is defined when shortness of breath occurs within 24 hours post-cessation of transfusion and there is suspicion of temporal association with transfusion.

Risk factors of TRALI

- Chronic alcohol abuse
- Shock
- High-risk airway pressure while being mechanically ventilated
- Currently smoker
- High IL-8 levels
- Positive Fluid be Loma

Pathogenesis of TRALI

- **Neutrophil Sequestration and Priming** - Recipient factors such as endothelial injury trigger neutrophil priming and sequestration in the lung microvasculature. Priming occurs due to cytokine release.

- **Neutrophil activation**

  Recipient neutrophils are activated by factors in the blood product which results in the release of cytokines, reactive oxygen species, oxidases, and proteases. This causes damage to pulmonary capillary endothelium leading to pulmonary edema.

Clinical features

- Hypoxemia
- Pulmonary infiltrates on chest imaging
- If previously intubated, the presence of frothy pink secretions suggests TRALI
- Fever is present in 33% of cases
- Hypotension is present in 32% of cases
- Cyanosis is seen in 25% of cases

Differential Diagnosis

- Transfusion – associated circulatory overload (TACO)
- ARDS

- Sepsis
- Severe allergic transfusion reactions
- Thermolytic transfusion reactions

Treatment

- Immediately discontinue blood transfusions
- Proper ventilation and oxygenation
- Steroids – There is very limited evidence of corticosteroids in patients with TRALI. Hence, the routine use of corticosteroids is not recommended, especially in cases that present late after 14 days of syndrome onset.
- Multiple TRALI treatment and preventive strategies have been proposed such as HMG COA reductase inhibitors (statins) aspirin, allogenic blood products alternatives, however, none of these therapies have sufficient evidence of routine use in patients with TRALI.

Transfusion-associated Circulatory overload (TACO)

- Patients develop pulmonary edema due to volume excess or fluid overload.
- *Definitive TACO* – is defined as new-onset or exacerbation of three or more of the following within 12 hours of the end of a transfusion without another explanation:
    a. Respiratory diseases (acute or worsening)
    b. Evidence of pulmonary edema on examination or radiographs.
    c. Elevated brain natriuretic protein (BNP) or N-terminal prohormone BNP (NT-Pro-BNP)
    d. Other unexplained cardiovascular changes elevated (central venous pressure)
- Probable TACO – Finding as above, with transfusion as a likely contributor but the individual received other fluids as well or has a history of cardiac disease that could explain the findings.
- Possible TACO – Finding as above but pre-existing cardiac disease is a more likely explanation.

Following are risk factors of TACO –

- Age ≥ 85years
- History of heart failure
- Female sex
- While race
- History of chronic pulmonary disease the risk of TACO correlates.

Clinical Presentation

The possibility of TACO should be considered in any patient who has new or worsening respiratory problems during or within 12 hours of completing transfusion. The typical presentation of TACO include dyspnea, orthopnea with a variable severity ranging from mild dyspnea to acute respiratory decompensation, headache and seizures have been reported.

Management

- Oxygen

- Fluid mobilization – It is done with diuretics

- Ventilatory support

- Resuming transfusion – As the underlying pathogenesis of TACO is fluid overload, resumption of transfusion can be considered in these patients in case further transfusion is indicated and pulmonary edema has completely resolved. Also, if there is sufficient time to finish the transfusion under the four-hours limit.

Febrile Neutropenia

According to the infection disease society of America guidelines, fever in neutropenic patients is defined as Single oral temperature≥ 38.3·e (101 degree F) or a temperature of more than equal to 38.oc (100.4· f) sustained over on – hours period.

Neutropenia is defined as an absolute neutrophil count of less than 1500 or 1000 cells/ul, severe neutropenia as an ANC < 500 cell/ul or an ANC that is expected to decrease to <500cells/microlitre over the next 48 hours, or profound neutropenia as an ANC less than 100 cells/microlitre.

Neutropenic fever syndromes – the international immune-compromised host society has classified initial neutropenic fever syndromes into three categories.

I. Microbiologically documented infection which is defined as neutropenic fever with clinical focus of infection and associated pathogen.

II. Clinically documented infection is defined as neutropenic fever with a clinical fours but without isolation of associated pathogen.

III. unexplained fever – neutropenic fever with neither a clinical focus nor an identified pathogen.

Approach to management

Primary Prophylaxis

<u>Antibacterial Prophylaxis</u>

Fluoroquinolones (levofloxacin – 500mg or 750 mg orally once daily) and ciprofloxacin (500mg or 750 mg orally twice daily) for high-risk neutropenic patients i.e., patients anticipated to have absolute neutrophil count of less than 500 cell/ul for more than seven days, who do not have a contraindication to give fluoroquinolones.

Patients with any one of the following are considered to be at high risk of serious complications and should be considered for antibiotic prophylaxis.

a. Receipt of cytotoxic therapy (ANC <500/ul) for > 7days.

b. MASCC risk score < 21

c. CISNE Score ≥ 3

d. Presence of active uncontrolled co-morbid medical problems

- Severe sepsis/ septic shock

- oral or gastrointestinal mucositis

- Gastrointestinal symptoms such as abdominal pain, nausea, vomiting

- Intravascular catheter infection expectantly catheter tunnel infection
- New pulmonary infiltrators hypoxemia.
- Underlying Chronic lung disease
- Complex infection at the time of presentation.

e. Alemtuzumab or CAR-T cell use within the last two months

f. Uncontrolled progressive comes

g. Evidence of hepatic or renal insufficiency

Antifungal Prophylaxis

Keeping in mind the 2018 American Society of clinical oncology Guidelines and the IDSA guideline, the following recommendations have been proposed.

I. Prophylaxis against Candida infection is advised in patients receiving initial induction or salvage induction Chemotherapy who may develop severe oral or gastrointestinal mucositis. Tablet fluconazole 400mg once daily dose is preferred. Other agents are itraconazole, voriconazole, Posaconazole, micafungin, caspofungin, and anidulafungin.

II. Prophylaxis is recommended against mold infections and candida spp with Posaconazole or voriconazole in patients with severe neutropenia due to intensive chemotherapy. Delayed-release parconazole (taken with food) is preferred with oral suspension, loading dose 300mg every 12th hour on the first day followed by 300mg once daily subsequently.

III. Antifungal prophylaxis is not preferred in patients with Anticipated duration of neutropenia $\leq$ 7days. Pneumocystis pneumonia prophylaxis is preferred in patients with selected antilogous HCT recipients and in some patients receiving induction chemotherapy in acute lymphocytic leukemia.

Antiviral Prophylaxis

1. Annual immunization with an inactivated influenza vaccine is recommended in all the patients with cancer.
2. Those who are HSV seropositive or undergoing allogenic HCT or induction Chemotherapy should receive antiviral prophylaxis (400mg or 800mg orally twice day)
3. CMV prophylaxis is not indicated

Treatment

1. Perform a detailed general physical and systemic examination
2. Complete blood count and differential count to be sent.
3. Kidney and liver function tests to be sent

4. Two sets of blood culture, one from peripheral and the other from central line.

5. Testfor COVID-19 infection

6. Imaging studies to be performed

7. Antibiotic therapy targeting germ-negative and gram-positive infections should be initiated within 60 minutes.

Low-risk patients who are not receiving fluoroquinolone prophylaxis and not known to be colonized by extended-spectrum beta-lactamase-producing gram-negative bacilli should receive a combination of ciprofloxacin 750mg twice daily along with amoxicillin eliminate (500mg/125mg) orally three times a day.

Alternatively, monotherapy with levofloxacin/moxifloxacin ones daily can be given.

For patients who are in severe sepsis or septic shock (hypotension, altered mental status, oliguria, respiratory depression) should receive either one of the following

- piperacillin – tazobactam
- Cefepime
- meropenem or imipenem

For patients with in septic shock or oliguria or severe respiratory depression, another gram-negative agent such as aminoglycoside or fluoroquinolone can be added and also an agent with MRSA cover (Vancomycin).

- For patients with skin and soft tissue infection, MRSA cover to be added.
- If Vancomycin resistance is suspected, add linezolid or daptomycin.
- If Clostridium difficile infection is suspected, add Vancomycin.

Superior Vena Cava Syndrome

Introduction

It was first described in 1757 by Hunter in a patient suffering from a large syphilitic aneurysm. Superior vena cava syndrome (SVCS) is a condition that occurs when there is a mechanical obstruction to the SVC caused by either external compression, neoplastic invasion of the vessel wall, or internal obstruction. While the role of infections as a cause of SVC syndrome has declined with the use of antibiotics, malignancy has become the most common cause.

Pathophysiology

SVC is a thin-walled, low-pressure vein that drains blood from the head, neck, upper extremities, and upper thorax. Due to its location in the right mediastinum, it can be easily compressed by associated structures like the trachea, right bronchus, aorta, pulmonary artery, or perihilar and paratracheal lymph nodes. Compression of SVC leads to impairment of blood flow which leads to venous engorgement proximal to the site of obstruction resulting in classical signs and symptoms. Over time, even the collateral systems get dilated due to collateral flow into the azygos venous system and inferior vena cava.

The most common cause of SVC syndrome is malignancy, accounting for 90% of the cases, with 75% occurring secondary to lung cancer and 15% secondary to Non-Hodgkin's lymphoma. Cancers of the breast, thyroid, esophagus, germ cell tumors, thymoma are also associated with SVC syndrome. Right-sided lung cancers are more likely to cause SVCS. Small cell carcinomas are the most common type of lung cancer implicated

SVCS is more common in men after the age of 50 years.

Benign causes for SVCS are intravascular devices causing thrombosis, cardiac causes, mediastinal fibrosis, benign mediastinal tumors, vascular disease and infections.

Clinical features

History: Dyspnoea is the most likely presentation (about 63%). Association with cough is suggestive of malignancy. It can present with facial, neck, and arm swelling. There are also symptoms of headache, lightheadedness, distorted vision, nasal stuffiness, hoarseness of voice, stridor, chest pain, and dysphagia. Symptoms depend on the speed of SVC obstruction; the more acute the onset more severe the symptoms.

Examination: Facial and neck edema is the most common finding. Swollen extremities, plethora, alterations in mental status, and papilledema can be present. Laryngeal, bronchial, and cerebral edema are rare but life-threatening.

Investigations:

- *Chest radiography* – limited in use but can reveal evidence of a mass, perihilar lymphadenopathy, and mediastinal disease.

- *Venography* – Rarely done in ED. It was earlier considered to be the gold standard as it can find the exact location of the obstruction.

- *Ultrasound* – SVC cannot be directly visualized. The venous waveform in the subclavian and brachiocephalic veins may show dampening and loss of venous pulsatility and minimal respiratory variation when the SVC is obstructed. It can provide information about the presence and extent of thrombus and point to obstruction

- *CT scan with IV contrast* – Investigation of choice in ED. It has high sensitivity (96%) in diagnosis as well as information about the cause of SVCS, which in turn helps with the treatment plan. It can determine if there is a thrombosis, external compression, or both.

- *MRI* – In patients allergic to IV contrast and in renal failure, MRI can be done.

Treatment

Symptomatic treatment with supplemental oxygen, head-end elevation of the bed, and a course of parental steroids are started in the emergency department. Anti-coagulation or thrombolytic therapy should be considered when thrombus is present.

SVCS rarely requires emergent treatment in ED as it can rarely cause airway obstruction secondary to laryngeal edema. SVCS is often an urgency and needs to be directed toward appropriate care.

- Radiation and chemotherapy – Radiation therapy is the mainstay of treatment in SVCS secondary to small cell carcinoma of the lung. Shrinking the size of the tumor provides relief to the obstruction. Chemotherapy in chemosensitive tumors.

- Endovascular Therapy – mounting evidence indicates this as the best treatment for SVCS secondary to a benign cause. This includes stenting, angioplasty, and intravascular thrombolysis. Stenting can be done in malignant SVCS to relieve symptoms, escpecially after radio-chemotherapy failure.

Disposition

Consider admitting patients requiring anticoagulation or thrombolysis. Those who are newly diagnosed with cancer with moderate to severe symptoms must also be admitted. Patients with mild symptoms can be discharged, referred for outpatient evaluation and followed up with an oncologist.

AntiCoagulation Reversal

Introduction

Anticoagulant therapy is indicated for prophylaxis and treatment of thromboembolic disorders. Today vitamin K antagonists, Heparin, low molecular weight heparin, direct thrombin inhibitors, and Factor Xa inhibitors are commonly used. With millions of individuals using these agents worldwide, clinicians should be equipped with clear protocols to manage complicated bleeding from these therapies.

Clotting cascade

For reversal of anticoagulation, we first need to have a good grasp of the clotting cascade and the complex physiologic process to maintain homeostasis between clot formation and degradation. Vascular endothelial injury leads to clot formation, beginning with primary Hemostasis. Platelets bind to the damaged endothelium by an interaction between glycoprotein (IIb IIIa) and the Von Willebrand factor. With platelet activation and degranulation, more platelets are recruited to the site of injury, finally forming a platelet plug. The efficacy of the platelet plugs depends on the efficacy of the platelet and may vary from patient to patient.

Secondary hemostasis begins with activation of the clotting cascade; activated Factor Xa catalyzes the conversion of prothrombin to thrombin (factor 2 A). Thrombin converts fibrinogen to fibrin. Fibrin is responsible for crosslinking and strengthening the platelet Plug. Secondary hemostasis depends on the quantity of functioning coagulation factors and their activation.

In terms of laboratory analysis for assessing primary hemostasis, platelet function tests and platelet aggregation assays may be used. But these tests are poorly standardized and time-Consuming. Secondary hemostasis is assessed using Prothrombin time (PT) and International normalized ratio (INR) for Exstrinsic and common pathways (factor II, VII, and X). Activated Thromboplastin time(aPTT) is measured for intrinsic and common pathways (all factors except factor VII).

Reversal of Warfarin

Warfarin is indicated for the treatment and prophylaxis of venous thromboembolism (VTE), pulmonary embolism (PE), thromboembolic complications associated with atrial fibrillation or cardiac valve replacement, and for reduction of secondary emboli post Myocardial infarction (MI) and cerebrovascular incidents (CVA). Warfarin acts as a vitamin K Antagonist inhibiting the hepatic enzyme vitamin K epoxide reductase and limiting the synthesis of factors II, VII, XI, X and the procoagulant Protein C and Protein S. Therapeutic doses decrease the vitamin k dependent factors by 30-50%. PT and INR are used to monitor its anticoagulant effects.

Reversal of warfarin occurs by immediate and sustained therapy. Immediate therapy includes Prothrombin complex concentrate (PCC) and fresh frozen plasma (FFP). Sustained reversal is by Vitamin K administration.

***Prothrombin complex concentrate* (PCC)** – Available as 3-factor and 4-factor preparations. 3-factor PCC due to low factor VII does not satisfactorily decrease the supratherapeutic INR'S. In 2013, The FDA approved K centra, a 4-Factor PCC for reversal of warfarin-related coagulopathy. K centra contain factors II, VII, IX, and X. In addition, it also contains protein C and protein S. Heparin and antithrombin are added to keep the factors in the un-activated form. IV administration is based on the patient's baseline INR, with an initial dose of 25-50 IU/kg for significant bleeds.

Activated PCC, also known as Factor VIII inhibitor bypassing activity (FEIBA), is indicated for bleeding episodes from factor VIII and IX deficiencies. FEIBA contains primarily Factor VII and smaller quantities of factor II, IX, and X (Considered when 4 factor PCC is not available).

PCCs are contraindicated in patients with a history of anaphylaxis to PCC, Previous episodes of PE, MI, and disseminated intravascular coagulation. FEIBA may lead to an increase in the incidence of thrombosis as per FDA Pharmacovigilance data (8.24 PER 100,000 infusions).

Fresh frozen plasma(FFP) – Contains all coagulation factors. Rh compatibility is not required. Risks of transfusion like infections and allergic reactions are present. Each unit of FFP corrects clotting factor by 2-3% in a 70 kg man. Initial administration of 2 units of FFP for intracranial bleeds and 4 units for extracranial bleeds are advised. A volume of 10- 15 ml/kg of FFP may be required in life-threatening hemorrhages. Its use in patients with atrial fibrillation, cardiac valvular disease, and ventricular dysfunction is limited due to the risk of decompensated heart failure or transfusion-associated lung injury. FFP use is also limited due to the need to keep it frozen as time taken (15 -20 mins) to thaw.

Vitamin K – Vitamin K is an essential cofactor in the synthesis of factors II, VII, IX, X, and proteins C & S. Available both in oral and IV forms. Subacutaneous and Intramuscular routes are no longer recommended due to unpredictable absorption and the potential for hematomas. The time to onset from the administration of oral vitamin K is about 6 – 10 hours which peaks in about 24 to 48 hours. Actively bleeding patients should receive an IV dose of 5 to 10mg by slow infusion over 20 minutes. The onset of action in 1-2 hours and peaks action in 12- 24 hours.

An anaphylactic reaction is seen in 3 of 10,000 doses of parenteral infusion secondary to the diluent from Vitamin K preparation. After vitamin K administration, therapeutic anticoagulation cannot be obtained for nearly two weeks.

Recombinant factor VIII a – Used for the treatment of bleeding episodes in patients with Hemophilia A (factor VIII deficiency), Hemophilia B (Factor IX deficiency), and congenital factor

VII deficiency. Due to an increased risk of thromboembolic events, it is no longer recommended for reversal of warfarin.

Table 1: Managing elevated INR or bleeding in patients on vitamin k antagonist therapy

Condition	Description
INR supratherapeutic but <5; absent significant bleeding	Lower or omit dose. Increase frequency of monitoring. Resume therapy at a lower dose if INR is more than minimally supratherapeutic
INR>5 but <10; absent significant bleeding	Omit 1-2 doses, Increase the frequency of monitoring, Resume therapy when INR therapeutic or omit dose, give 1-2.5 mg oral vitamin k. If the patient is at higher risk of bleeding or requires rapid reversal for a surgical procedure, give 2-4 mg oral vitamin k; the INR should decrease within 24 hours. If INR remains elevated additional vitamin k maybe(1-2g) given
INR.10; absent significant bleeding	Hold warfarin therapy. Give 5-10mg of vitamin k; The INR should decrease in 24-48 hours. Increase the frequency of monitoring. Administer additional vitamin K if necessary. Resume therapy when INR is therapeutic.
Serious or life-threatening bleeding	Hold warfarin therapy. Give 10mg of vitamin k by slow IV infusion in addition to PCC or FFP, Vitamin K may be given every 12 hours

Table 2: Reversal agents for warfarin

Agent	Dose	Notes
Vitamin K	1.25-10 mg oral or IV	No IM or subcutaneous
PCC (KCENTRA)	Strategy 1: INR & Weight based INR 2-4: 25IU/KG IV PUSH INR >4-6: 35U/KG IV PUSH INR>6:50IU/KG IV PUSH Strategy 2:INR based dosing INR <5: 500IU INR>5: 1000U Strategy 3: fixed dosing 1500 U	Any strategy may be used with KCENTRA
Apcc (FEIBA)	50-100 U/KG	Used only when PCC not available

Reversal of Heparin and Low Molecular Weight Heparin

Heparin and LMWH (Enoxaparin, Dalteparin and Fondaparinux) are approved for the prophylaxis and treatment of DVT and PE. Enoxaparin maybe used in ST elevation MI. Enoxaparin and dalteparin maybe used for ischemic complication of unstable angina and non Q wave MI.

Heparin and LMWH act by binding to antithrombin III which activates the antithromin III complex which inhibits the factor Xa and inhibitory effect on thrombin.

The aPTT is used to assess the anticoagulation effect of heparin and LMWH. The chromogenic anti-factor X a assay is the gold standard to assess LMWH anticoagulation.

If urgent or emergent heparin reversal is required, heparin should be discontinued and protamine sulphate initiated. Protamine dose calculated depending on time since heparin administration. If immediate 1 to 1.5 mg of protamine should be given for every 100U of heparin delivered. If 30 to 60 minutes have elapsed 0.5 to 0.75 U for every 100 U and if greater than 2 hours since administration 0.250 to 0.375 mg per 100 U of heparin.

Protamine is only about 60% effective in reversal of Enoxaparin and Dalteparin due to limited ability to address Factor Xa inhibition. 1mg of protamine for every mg of Enoxaparin or Dalteparin. If bleeding is not controlled, an additional 0.5mg per 1mg can be given. Maximum dose shouldn't exceed 50 mg. (Paradoxical anticoagulation may occur secondary to factor V activation). Infusion shouldn't exceed more than 20mg/min due to risk of anaphylaxis, hypotension and bradycardia. Fondaparinux is not neutralised by protamine sulphate.

Table 3: Reversal agents for heparin and LMWH.

Agent	Dose	
Protamine for heparin	Time elapsed since heparin dose: Immediate Administer 1-1.5 mg/100U heparin 30-60 min Administer 0.5-0.75 mg/100 U heparin >2hours Administer 0.25-0.375 mg /100 U heparin	Dose should not exceed 50 mg
Protamine for LMWH	**Dalteparin** 1 mg of protamine neutralizes 100 U of Dalteparin If bleeding persist or aPTT remains prolonged after 2-4 hours, repeat dose 0.5mg/100 U Dalteparin **Enoxaparin** If <8hours since dose, 1mg per 1mg of enoxaparin If 8-12 hours since dose, 0.5mg per 1 mg of enoxaparin If >12 hours since dose, No protamine If bleeding persist or aPTT remains prolonged, repeat dose, 0.5 mg per mg of enoxaparin.	Only partially effective Not effective for fondaparinux

Reversal of direct oral anticoagulants

Direct thrombin inhibitors(DTI)

Dabigatran is an oral DTI indicated for the reduction of incidence of stroke and embolism in nonvalvular atrial fibrillation, for treatment of DVT and PE, and for prophylaxis of DVT and PE. In patients who have undergone Hip arthroplasty, Dabigatran binds to the active site of free and clot-bound thrombin, inhibiting the conversion of fibrinogen to fibrin and feedback activation of factors VII, IX, and V.

In 2015, FDA approved Idarucizumab, a humanized monoclonal antibody fragment for the reversal of dabigatran in the setting of emergent/urgent surgical procedures and life-threatening and severe bleeding. The recommended dose is 5g, provided as two vials of 2.5g/50ml administered no more than 15 minutes apart. The line should be flushed before the administration, and no other infusion should be co-administered in the same line.

Hemodialysis can be performed if Idarucizumab as dabigatran is predominantly excreated by the kidneys. American society of hematology also recommends the administration of PCC or aPPC for life-threatening bleeds and is supported by poor-quality evidence and with thrombotic risk. Cryoprecipitate administration is advised in patients with fibrinogen levels below 200md/Dl.

Table 4: Reversal agents for direct thrombin inhibitors

Agent	Dose	Notes
Idarucizumab	5g 2vials containing 2.5g/50ml	No data regarding repeat dosing
PCC	50U/kg	
FEIBA	50-100kg	
Cryoprecipitate	2 pools	Administer when fibrinogen <200md/dL

Factor Xa Inhibitors

Factor Xa inhibitors include Rivaroxaban, Apixaban, Edoxaban and Betrixaban. They have been approved for the risk reduction of stroke and systemic embolism in patients with non-valvular atrial fibrillation. Rivaroxaban has also been indicated for DVT and PE prophylaxis in patients undergoing knee and hip arthroplasty.

Factor Xa inhibitors selectively block the active site on factor Xa when free or bound to the prothrombinase complex. Inhibiting Factor Xa inhibits platelet aggregation induced by thrombin.

Peak plasma levels are attained within 2 hours of administration of rivaroxaban, apixaban, and edoxaban; 4 hours in the case of betrixaban dosing. After oral administration in patients with normal renal function, elimination half-lives is less than 12 hours.

At Therapeutic levels, all Factor Xa inhibitors prolong PT, INR, and aPTT, but responses are variable and are not useful for monitoring anticoagulant effects.

Andexanet alfa designed as a reversal agent for all factor Xa inhibitors, is a recombinant, modified Factor Xa molecule which competes with native factor Xa. It shows promising results in various trials. The trials are still underway to identify the best reversal agent for the same. Four factors PCC and Factor VIII, may be used.

Table 5. Reversal agents for factor X a inhibitors

Agent	Dose	
Four factor PCC	25-50 U/KG	Repeat dose beyond 50u/kg not recommended. Max dose 5000 U
Factor VIII inhibitor bypassing activity	50-100 U/kg	Repeat dose after 6 hours if bleeding persists

Antifibrinolytic therapy

Antifibrinolytic therapy with agents like tranexamic acid and aminocaproic acid in direct oral anticoagulation-associated bleeding is unknown. Due to a favorable safety profile and relatively inexpensive cost, these agents may be considered in the setting of life threatening bleeds.

Table 6: Antifibrinolytic

Agent	Dose	
Tranexamic acid	1g IV	Dose adjustments for renal impairments
Aminocaproic acid	4-5g IV infusion during the first hour of treatment followed by 1g/h for 8hours or until bleeding controlled	Avoid rapid IV infusion may cause hypotension, bradycardia, and arrhythmia

Reversal of Anti-platelet therapy

Antiplatelet agents include Aspirin (an irreversible inhibitor of cyclooxygenase 1 and 2), Thienopyridines, Clopidogrel, Prasugrel, and Ticlopidine, which irreversibly inhibit the P2Y12 receptor for adenosine diphosphate on platelets. Ticagrelor and Cangrelol are adenosine di phosphate inhibitors. Dipyridamole is a reversible inhibitor of adenosine di phosphate. Antiplatelet therapy is used to prevent platelet aggregation and thrombosis in the setting of acute MI, Non-ST-elevation MI, and Unstable angina. Antiplatelet therapy is also indicated for the prevention of ischemic CVA and MI and death in patients who have experienced acute coronary syndrome and to prevent stent thrombosis after percutaneous therapy.

There are no clinical guidelines for the treatment of life-threatening bleeding in the setting of antiplatelet therapy. PATCH trial (Platelet transfusion versus standard care after acute stroke due to spontaneous cerebral hemorrhage associated with antiplatelet therapy) showed platelet transfusions being ineffective in the reduction of bleeding. However, further research is required before making a recommendation regarding platelet transfusions.

Desmospressin is a synthetic analog of antidiuretic hormone indicated for the treatment of Bleeding episodes in persons with type 1 von Willebrand disease and Hemophilia A patients with greater than 5% factor V activity. A recent meta-analysis of ten randomized control Studies revealed that treatment with desmopressin reduced red blood cell transfusion in such individuals and had less blood loss. Current guidelines from the neuro critical care society Of critical care medicine support the use of a 0.3 microgram/kg intravenous dose of Desmopressin in patients on antiplatelet therapy who experience intracranial hemorrhage.

Table 7: Reversal of antiplatelet

Agents	Dose	
Platelets	2-3 units of pooled platelets or apheresis units	Mortality or morbidity benefit yet to be proven
Desmopressin	0.4 microg/kg	Consider in addition to platelet infusion

SUMMARY

Among individuals of age 65 and older, warfarin, Dabigatran, Rivaroxaban, and Enoxaparin account for nearly 60% of drug-related emergency medicine visits. An increasing number of patients are being prescribed these anticoagulants. Having a clear protocol for managing their bleeding complication is essential for emergency medicine physicians.

Vaccine Induced Immune Thrombotic Thrombocytopenia

Introduction

First observed in February 2021 in people who received the ChadOx1 CoV -19 vaccine (AstraZeneca, University of Oxford and Serum Institute of India). As the name suggests, thrombosis is followed by thrombocytopenia in most cases. It was later observed in a small number of individuals who received the Ad26.COV2. S vaccine (Jansen, Johnson and Johnson). Vaccine Induced Immune Thrombocytic Thrombocytopenia (VITT) is a syndrome observed in individuals who have received a certain adeno viral vector vaccine.

Epidemiology

Implicated vaccines are the ChadOx1 CoV -19 vaccine (AstraZeneca, University of Oxford and Serum Institute of India) and Ad26.COV2.S vaccine (Jansen, Johnson and Johnson). Incidence appears to be very rare; however, due to the mass vaccination drive of millions of individuals, several hundred patients have developed this condition. Initial reports suggest a female predominance and a younger age group (<55-60 years)

Pathophysiology

VITT occurs secondary to adeno viral vectored corona disease 2019 vaccination. These vaccines appear to stimulate antibodies to platelet factor 4(PF4), which activate the platelets and coagulation pathways and cause thrombosis and thromboembolic complications. Similar to Autoimmune Heparin-induced thrombocytopenia.

Clinical Features

VITT mimics autoimmune heparin-induced thrombocytopenia. Syndrome begins in a narrow window about 5-10 days post-vaccination; however, identification of cases occurs between 5-30 days due to delay in recognizing symptoms. The main presentations are thrombosis, thrombocytopenia, DIC, bleeding, and flu-like syndrome in the same time period has also been described, which suggests an enhanced inflammatory response.

Thrombosis is the presenting complaint in most initially reported cases most common is cerebral venous sinus thrombosis (CVST), followed by splanchnic, adrenal and ophthalmic vein, PE, and DVT. Arterial thrombosis may lead to stroke, myocardial ischemia, acute limb ischemia. Sudden death can occur secondary to any of the above conditions.

Thrombocytopenia presents as petechial or mucosal bleeds with a typical platelet count of 10,000 to 100000/ micro L. DIC/Coagulation abnormalities are seen frequently with VITT Intracranial hemorrhage secondary to CVST is seen.

Evaluation-

Suspect VITT in individuals who present with symptoms of thrombosis and Thrombocytopenia during an appropriate time frame following one of the implicated vaccines.

History

History of implicated Vaccine taken, interval since vaccine taken (5-30 days). Symptoms of Thrombosis and symptoms of Thrombocytopenia should be asked for.

Laboratory Testing

CBC and peripheral blood smear to document the degree of thrombocytopenia.

Coagulation testing includes Prothrombin time (PT), activated partial thromboplastin time (ApTT), fibrinogen and D-dimer to assess for DIC. PF4 antibody testing by ELISA is confirmatory.

Imaging

Imaging depending on the suspected site of thrombosis as per standard guidelines.

Differential diagnosis

Other causes of thrombosis and thrombocytopenia, like immune thrombocytopenia, thrombotic thrombocytopenia, and Heparin-induced thrombocytopenia should be ruled out.

Management

Anticoagulation – Full dose anticoagulation even if there are no signs of thrombosis. Avoid using heparin, especially when HIT cannot be ruled out. Do not delay anticoagulation for confirmatory tests.

IVIG -1gm/kg for two days for all patients of VITT.

Plasma exchange is used in refractory cases and in individuals with severe life threatening symptoms.

Platelet transfusions are reserved for patients with critical bleeding (hemodynamic compromise, bleeding into the critical anatomic site)

Fibrinogen administration in patients with critical bleeding and hypofibrinogenemia.

American Society of Hematology 2021 Guidelines for Management of Venous Thromolism: Prevention and Treatment in Patients with Cancer

The Risk of Venous Thromboembolism is greater in patients with cancer. Hence, certain recommendations were developed using the Grading of Recommendations Assessment, Development, and Evaluation (GRADE) approach to assess the certainty of the evidence and formulate recommendations.

Pharmacologic choices for VTE treatment and avoidance incorporate unfractionated heparin (UFH), low-molecular-weight heparins (LMWHs), and fondaparinux (an indirect synthetic inhibitor of activated factor Xa), vitamin K antagonists (VKAs), and direct oral anticoagulants (including direct thrombin inhibitors and factor Xa inhibitors.

Recommendations for Primary prophylaxis for hospitalized medical patients with cancer

- For hospitalized medical patients with cancer without VTE, the American Society of Hematology (ASH) guideline panel *suggests* using thromboprophylaxis over no thromboprophylaxis (conditional recommendation, very low certainty in the evidence of effects

- For hospitalized medical patients with cancer without VTE, in which pharmacological thromboprophylaxis is used, the ASH guideline panel *suggests* using LMWH over UFH (conditional recommendation, low certainty in the evidence of effects

- For hospitalized medical patients with cancer without VTE, the ASH guideline panel *suggests* using pharmacological thromboprophylaxis over mechanical thromboprophylaxis (conditional recommendation, very low certainty in the evidence of effects

- For hospitalized medical patients with cancer without VTE, the ASH guideline panel *suggests* using pharmacological thromboprophylaxis over a combination of pharmacological and mechanical thromboprophylaxis (conditional recommendation, very low certainty in the evidence of effects

- For hospitalized medical patients with cancer, the ASH guideline panel *suggests* discontinuing thromboprophylaxis at the time of hospital discharge rather than continuing thromboprophylaxis beyond the discharge date (conditional recommendation, very low certainty in the evidence of effects

Recommendations for Primary prophylaxis for patients with cancer undergoing surgery.

- For patients with cancer without VTE undergoing a surgical procedure at lower bleeding risk, the ASH guideline panel *suggests* using pharmacological rather than mechanical thromboprophylaxis (conditional recommendation, low certainty in the evidence of effects

- For patients with cancer without VTE undergoing a surgical procedure at high bleeding risk, the ASH guideline panel *suggests* using mechanical rather than pharmacological thromboprophylaxis (conditional recommendation, low certainty in the evidence of effects

- For patients with cancer without VTE undergoing a surgical procedure at high risk for thrombosis, except in those at high risk of bleeding, the ASH guideline panel *suggests* using a combination of mechanical and pharmacologic thromboprophylaxis rather than mechanical prophylaxis alone (conditional recommendation based on low certainty in the evidence of effects) or pharmacologic thromboprophylaxis alone (conditional recommendation, very low certainty in the evidence of effects

- For patients with cancer undergoing a surgical procedure, the ASH guideline panel *suggests* using LMWH or fondaparinux for thromboprophylaxis rather than UFH (conditional recommendation, low certainty in the evidence of effects)

- For patients with cancer undergoing a surgical procedure, the ASH guideline panel makes no recommendation on the use of VKA or DOAC for thromboprophylaxis, because there were no studies available.

- For patients with cancer undergoing a surgical procedure, the ASH guideline panel *suggests* using postoperative thromboprophylaxis over preoperative thromboprophylaxis (conditional recommendation, low certainty in the evidence of effects

- For patients with cancer who had undergone a major abdominal/pelvic surgical procedure, the ASH guideline panel *suggests* continuing pharmacological thromboprophylaxis postdischarge rather than discontinuing at the time of hospital discharge (conditional recommendation, very low certainty in the evidence of effects

Primary prophylaxis in ambulatory patients with cancer receiving systemic therapy.

- For ambulatory patients with cancer at low risk for thrombosis receiving systemic therapy, we *recommend* no thromboprophylaxis over parenteral thromboprophylaxis (strong recommendation, moderate certainty in the evidence of effects

- For ambulatory patients with cancer at intermediate risk for thrombosis receiving systemic therapy, the ASH guideline panel *suggests* no prophylaxis over parenteral prophylaxis (conditional recommendation, moderate certainty in the evidence of effects

- For ambulatory patients with cancer at high risk for thrombosis receiving systemic therapy, the ASH guideline panel *suggests* parenteral thromboprophylaxis (LMWH) over no thromboprophylaxis (conditional recommendation, moderate certainty in the evidence of effects

- For ambulatory patients with cancer receiving systemic therapy, the ASH guideline panel *recommends* no thromboprophylaxis over oral thromboprophylaxis with VKA (strong recommendation, very low certainty in the evidence of benefits but high certainty about the harms

- For ambulatory patients with cancer at low risk for thrombosis receiving systemic therapy, the ASH guideline panel *suggests* no thromboprophylaxis over oral thromboprophylaxis with a DOAC (apixaban or rivaroxaban) (conditional recommendation, moderate certainty in the evidence of effects

- For ambulatory patients with cancer at intermediate risk for thrombosis receiving systemic therapy, the ASH guideline panel *suggests* thromboprophylaxis with a DOAC (apixaban or rivaroxaban) or no thromboprophylaxis (conditional recommendation, moderate certainty in the evidence of effects.

- For ambulatory patients with cancer at high risk for thrombosis receiving systemic therapy, the ASH guideline panel *suggests* thromboprophylaxis with a DOAC (apixaban or rivaroxaban) over no thromboprophylaxis (conditional recommendation, moderate certainty in the evidence of effects

- For multiple myeloma patients receiving lenalidomide, thalidomide, or pomalidomide-based regimens, the ASH guideline panel *suggests* using low-dose acetylsalicylic acid (ASA) or fixed low-dose VKA or LMWH (conditional recommendation, low certainty in the evidence of effects.

Primary prophylaxis for patients with cancer with central venous catheter.

- For patients with cancer and a central venous catheter (CVC), the ASH guideline panel *suggests* not using parenteral thromboprophylaxis (conditional recommendation, low certainty in the evidence of effects

- For patients with cancer and a CVC, the ASH guideline panel *suggests* not using oral thromboprophylaxis (conditional recommendation, low certainty in the evidence of effects

- For patients with cancer and VTE, the ASH guideline panel *suggests* DOAC (apixaban or rivaroxaban) or LMWH be used for initial treatment of VTE for patients with cancer (conditional recommendation, very low certainty in the evidence of effects

- For patients with cancer and VTE, we *recommend* LMWH over UFH for initial treatment of VTE for patients with cancer (strong recommendation, moderate certainty in the evidence of effects

- For patients with cancer and VTE, the ASH guideline panel *suggests* LMWH over fondaparinux for initial treatment of VTE for patients with cancer (conditional recommendation, very low certainty in the evidence of effects

Short-term treatment for patients with active cancer (initial 3-6 months)

- For the short-term treatment of VTE (3-6 months) for patients with active cancer, the ASH guideline panel *suggests* DOAC (apixaban, edoxaban, or rivaroxaban) over LMWH (conditional recommendation, low certainty in the evidence of effects

- For the short-term treatment of VTE (3-6 months) for patients with active cancer, the ASH guideline panel *suggests* DOAC (apixaban, edoxaban, or rivaroxaban) over VKA (conditional recommendation, very low certainty in the evidence of effects

- For the short-term treatment of VTE (3-6 months) for patients with active cancer, the ASH guideline panel *suggests* LMWH over VKA (conditional recommendation, moderate certainty in the evidence of effects

- For patients with cancer and incidental (unsuspected) pulmonary embolism (PE), the ASH guideline panel *suggests* short-term anticoagulation treatment rather than observation (conditional recommendation, very low certainty in the evidence of effects

- For patients with cancer and subsegmental PE (SSPE), the ASH guideline panel *suggests* short-term anticoagulation treatment rather than observation (conditional recommendation, very low certainty in the evidence of effects

- For patients with cancer and visceral/splanchnic vein thrombosis, the ASH guideline panel *suggests* treating with short-term anticoagulation or observing (conditional recommendation, very low certainty in the evidence of effects

- For patients with cancer with CVC-related VTE receiving anticoagulant treatment, the ASH guideline panel *suggests* keeping the CVC over removing the CVC (conditional recommendation, very low certainty in the evidence of effects

- For patients with cancer and recurrent VTE despite receiving therapeutic LMWH, the ASH guideline panel *suggests* increasing the LMWH dose to a supratherapeutic level or continuing with a therapeutic dose (conditional recommendation, very low certainty in the evidence of effects

- For patients with cancer and recurrent VTE despite anticoagulation treatment, the ASH guideline panel *suggests* not using an inferior vena cava (IVC) filter over using a filter (conditional recommendation, very low certainty in the evidence of effects

Long-term treatment (>6 months) for patients with active cancer and VTE

- For patients with active cancer and VTE, the ASH guideline panel *suggests* long-term anticoagulation for secondary prophylaxis (>6 months) rather than short-term treatment alone (3-6 months) (conditional recommendation, low certainty in the evidence of effects

- For patients with active cancer and VTE receiving long-term anticoagulation for secondary prophylaxis, the ASH guideline panel *suggests* continuing indefinite anticoagulation over stopping after completion of a definitive period of anticoagulation (conditional recommendation, very low certainty in the evidence of effects

- For patients with active cancer and VTE requiring long-term anticoagulation (>6 months), the ASH guideline panel *suggests* using DOACs or LMWH (conditional recommendation, very low certainty in the evidence of effects.

PADUA PREDICTION SCORE FOR VTE

Active cancer (metastasis and/or chemoradiotherapy in the previous 6 months) 3 points
Previous VTE (with the exclusion of superficial vein thrombosis) 3 points
Reduced mobility 3 points
Already known thrombophilic condition 3 points
Recent (<1 month) trauma and/or surgery 2 points
Elderly age (>70 years) 1 points
Heart and/or respiratory failure 1 points
Acute myocardial infarction or ischemic stroke 1 points
Acute infection and/or rheumatologic disorder 1 points
Obesity (BMI >30 kg/sq.metre) 1 points
Ongoing hormonal treatment 14 points

SCORE GREATER THAN 4 IS HIGH RISK FOR VTE

Pediatric Oncological Emergencies

Cancer remains one of the leading causes of death in children worldwide. Professional health care providers should be aware of serious syndromes encountered in the management of pediatric oncologic conditions to prevent their occurrence and avoid potentially severe consequences through driven interventions. With newer interventions in this field, the survival rate has drastically improved and is beneficial for the patients survival. On the other hand, longer survival comes at the expense of an increasing number of disease and treatment-associated complications, as modern *cancer treatments can have potentially life-threatening side effects.*[1] *Early recognition and proper treatment of these oncologic emergencies can considerably reduce the chances of potential complications and improve clinical outcomes.*

Children may present emergently with signs and symptoms concerning an undiagnosed underlying malignancy or may present with life- threatening conditions related to a known malignancy or its therapy.

Patients undergoing therapy for their cancer will have compromised immune systems and decreased function of vital organs from chemotherapeutic agent toxicity, sometimes resulting in diagnostic and therapeutic dilemmas and hastening their demise.

Common oncological emergencies are summarized in table 1.

Table 1: Common oncological emergencies.

System	Oncological emergencies
Metabolic	Tumour lysis syndrome Hypocalcemia Hypercalcaemia Hypoglycaemia Hyperkalaemia Hyperphosphataemia
Haematological	Anaemia Leukopenia Hyperleukocytosis
	Hyperviscosity syndrome Disseminated intravascular coagulation Hemophagocytic lymphohistiocytosis
Cardiovascular	Superior vena cava syndrome
	Pericardial effusion/pericardial tamponade
Respiratory	Superior mediastinal syndrome Acute respiratory distress syndrome Pulmonary embolism
Neurological	Raised intracranial pressure and brain herniation
	Posterior reversible encephalopathy syndrome Spinal cord compression
	Brain metastasis

Infection	Sepsis
	Febrile neutropenia
Haematopoietic cell transplantation related	Graft *versus* host disease Sinusoidal obstruction syndrome Thrombotic microangiopathy

Tumour lysis syndrome

Tumour lysis syndrome (TLS) is a life-threatening oncological emergency resulting from the rapid lysis of tumour cells and abrupt release of their intracellular content into circulation.

Tumour lysis is a metabolic and oncological emergency commonly encountered in clinical practice. Majority of the symptoms seen in patients with tumor lysis syndrome are related to the release of intracellular chemical substances that cause impairment in functions of target organs.

Clinically, the syndrome is a combination of the following things which include hyperuricemia, hyperkalemia, hyperphosphatemia, hypocalcemia, and acute kidney injury.

The prevalence of TLS varies amongst different malignancies and definitions and is estimated to be between 4% and 42%, whilst the related mortality is reported to be up to 21% in paediatric patients with haematological malignancies.

TLS is most common in patients with haematological malignancies, particularly acute lymphoblastic leukaemia and Burkitt lymphomas in children and usually occurs after cytotoxic therapy.

The occurrence of TLS in patients with solid tumours is less frequent. Following are other tumour related risk factors include high tumor load, high proliferative rates, high tumour chemosensitivity and increased lactate dehydrogenase levels. Cairo and Bishop is the most common classification system for TLS. TLS can also be classified into laboratory TLS and clinical TLS. Laboratory TLS is defined as the presence of two or more blood abnormalities (uric acid, potassium, phosphorus, calcium) within 3 days before or 7 days after the initiation of chemotherapy, whilst clinical TLS is defined as the presence of laboratory TLS with one or more of the following: cardiac arrhythmia or sudden death and seizure.

The timing of TLS presentation is usually 12–72 hours after the initiation of cytotoxic therapy. Spontaneous TLS without any obvious trigger is rare but has been increasingly documented in Burkitt's lymphoma. The clinical manifestations of TLS include nausea, vomiting, diarrhoea, muscle cramps, paraesthesia, oedema, congestive heart failure, cardiac dysrhythmias, seizure and sudden death. The release of intracellular metabolites can overwhelm the normal homeostatic mechanism and can cause hyperkalemia, hyperphosphatemia, hypocalcaemia, hyperuricemia and acute renal failure.

Pathophysiology

Rapid tumor cell turnover leads to release of intracellular contents into the circulation. This release can overload renal elimination and cellular buffering mechanisms, leading to numerous metabolic derangements.

Clinically significant tumor lysis syndrome can occur spontaneously, but it is most often seen 48-72 hours after initiation of cancer treatment.

Hyperkalemia is often the earliest laboratory manifestation. Hyperkalemia and hyperphosphatemia result directly from rapid cell lysis.

Hypocalcemia is a consequence of acute hyperphosphatemia with subsequent precipitation of calcium phosphate in soft tissues.

In acute kidney injury, decreased calcitriol levels also cause hypocalcemia.

Uric acid is the terminal catabolic product of purine metabolism in humans. Nucleic acid purines, which are released by cell breakdown, are ultimately metabolized to uric acid by hepatic xanthine oxidase. This conversion leads to hyperuricemia. Uric acid is a weak acid with a pKa of approximately 5.4. It is soluble in plasma and is freely filtered at the renal glomeruli. However, uric acid is less soluble in renal tubular and collecting duct fluid due to normally acidic media, thus increasing the possibility of uric acid crystal formation in cases of hyperuricemia.

The kidney is the primary organ involved in the clearance of uric acid, potassium, and phosphate. Preexisting volume depletion or renal dysfunction predisposes patients to worsening metabolic derangements and Acute kidney injury (AKI).

Uric acid nephropathy, is the major cause of AKI, is due to mechanical obstruction by uric acid crystals in the renal tubules and Acute nephrocalcinosis from calcium phosphate crystal precipitation. This develops in the presence of hyperphosphatemia.

Clinical manifestation of Tumor lysis syndrome are

- Nausea
- Vomiting
- Diarrhoea
- Hematuria
- Cardiac arrhythmias
- Seizures
- Muscle cramps
- Tetany, syncope, sudden death

As per the Cairo-Bishop definition of Tumor lysis syndrome (TLS)

1. Laboratory TLS is defined as two or more abnormal serum values present within three days before or seven days after instituting chemotherapy in the setting of adequate hydration (with or without alkalinization) and use of a hypouricemic agent.

   I.   Uric acid value ≥8mg/dl or 476 umol/l or 25 % increase from bax liver

   II. Potassium ≥2.1 mmol.l or 6.5 mg/dl in children or 7/.45 mmol/l & (4.5 mg/dl) in adults or 25% increase.

   III. Calcium ≤1.75 mmol or 7 mg/dl of 25% decrease

2. Clinical TLS is defined

   laboratory TLS plus one or more of the following that was not directly or probably attributable to a therapeutic agent: increased serum creatinine concentration (≥1.5 times the ULN), cardiac arrhythmia/sudden death, or a seizure.

Management

The management of TLS includes Early recognition and treatment of metabolic and renal complications with close monitoring and prophylactic strategies for at-risk patients.

The risk assessment of acute leukaemia is based on white blood cell counts and LDH levels, where high values ($≥100 × 10^9$/L and $≥2 ×$ upper limit of normal, respectively) are considered high risk for TLS. Burkitt lymphoma/leukaemia is always classified as high risk forTLS. The risk of TLS is also higher in patients with pre-existing renal impairment or disease involving the kidney at diagnosis.

For high risk cases, TLS parameters, including potassium, phosphate, uric acid, calcium, creatinine and LDH levels, should be monitored every 4–6 hours and patients with proved TLS should ideally be monitored in high dependency or intensive care settings. Monitoring of urine output is of utmost importance as it may lead to oliguria by obstructive uropathy and hyperhydration can lead to fluid overload inpatients at risk. Preventive measures include aggressive hydration (3 L/m^2/day), diuresis to maintain a urine output of ≥100 mL/m^2/hour (3 mL/kg/hour if ≤10 kg) and antihyperuricemic agents.

Commonly used antihyperuricemic agents are allopurinol and rasburicase. These agents act on the purine catabolism pathway to reduce the uric acid level in the blood. In patients with hyperuricemia, rasburicase, a recombinant urate oxidase, can be used with a suggested dose of 0.2 mg/kg/dose daily for up to 5 days. It is contraindicated in patients with glucose-6- phosphate dehydrogenase deficiency.

Mechanism of action of allopurinol - It is a hypoxanthine analog that competitively inhibits xanthine oxidase. It blocks the conversion of hypoxanthine and xanthine to uric acid, it decreases the uric acid formation. It does not decrease the pre-existing uric acid levels. Hence, rasburicase is advocated over allopurinol in patients with pre-existing higher uric acid level.

Rasburicase – It is preferred for the initial management of high risk cases of TLS in most pediatric and adult populations. It is efficacious in especially those with underlying renal and cardiac dysfunction. Rasburicase is a modified strain of saccharomyces cerevisiae. It promotes degradation of uric acid and is very well tolerated.

Febexostat – It is a selective xanthine oxidase inhibitor. It is not a purine analogue. It inhibits both reduced and oxidized forms of xanthine oxidase. There is no dose modification required in patients with mild to moderate level impairment. There are lesser known drug- drug interactions as compared with allopurinol.

Management can be done according to the Risk groups namely

Low Risk- Monitoring and Hydration

Intermediate – Start Allopurinol with hydration

If hyperuricemia – Start rasburicase

High risk- Hydration + Rasburicase therapy

1. Hyperkalemia is the most catastrophic complication of TLS leading to cardiac erythema glucose – insulin, beta agonists and calcium gluconate to be initiated in these patients.
2. Symptomatic hypocalcemia should be treated with calcium at lowest dose until associated hyperphosphatemia is corrected. If severe hypocalcemia is present calcium replacement can be done irrespective of phosphates level.
3. Hyperphosphatemia can lead to acute kidney injury and should be addressed.
4. Indication of Dialysis –

    a. Severe oliguria of anuria
    b. Intractable fluid overload
    c. Persistent hyperkalemia
    d. Hyperphosphatemia induced symptomatic hypocalcemia
    e. Calcium phosphate product $\geq 70mg2/dl2$

Prevention

1. Intravenous hydration

    A 2008 International expert panel on TLS has recommended that both children and adults should receive 2-3 L/m2 per day of IV fluid, Urine output should be measured. Diuretics are contraindicated in patients with hypovolemia or obstructive uropathy.

2. Urinary alkalinization

   There is no data supporting the role of urinary alkalinization in patients with TLS. It is believed that urinary alkalinization promotes calcium phosphate deposition in the kidney, heart and other organs of the system. Hence sodium bicarbonate is only indicated in patients with severe metabolic acidosis

3. Hyperuricemia drugs

   For patients with TLS, allopurinol may be used instead of rasburicase. Only if the pretreatment level of uric acid is not higher than 9mg/dl. However, single dose rasburicase is also a reasonable approach.

Dose of allopurinol – 100mg/m2 three times a day.

In patients with acute kidney injury reduce the dose to half.

As per EMA (European Medicine Agency) and FDA (Food and Drug Administration) dose of rasburicase in high risk patients with uric acid level ≥8mg/dl, is 6.2mg/kg once daily for 5 to 7 days. In patients with intermediate risk and uric acid level < 8 mg/dl, dose of rasburicase is 0.15mg/kg.

Risks –

1. Hemolysis with G6PD deficiency.
2. Anaphylaxis
3. Meth henigkibubinemia
4. Spuriously lower uric acid level
5. Teratogenicity

Hyperleukocytosis

Hyperleukocytosis is defined as a peripheral white blood cell count >100 × 10^9/L, and it is a medical emergency. Its associated with haematological malignancies, in particular T cell acute lymphoblastic leukaemia (ALL), infant ALL and acute myeloblastic leukaemia (AML). As the size of myeloblasts in AML is twice that of lymphoblasts in ALL, patients with AML and hyperleukocytosis have a high risk of early morbidity and mortality compared to patients with ALL.

It leads to an increased whole blood viscosity leading to aggregation of blast cells in the microvasculature, leukostasis and microvascular occlusion, coagulopathy.

Symptoms include headache, seizures, dural sinus thrombosis, visual field changes, cortical infarction, retinopathy, pneumonitis, respiratory distress, myocardial ischaemia, disseminated intravascular coagulopathy and multiorgan failure.

Management

The principle in the management of hyperleukocytosis includes hyperhydration to reduce whole blood viscosity, the prevention of tumour lysis syndrome, correcting metabolic abnormalities and early chemotherapy. Leukapheresis for leukoreduction in leukemic patients is controversial and there are no guidelines for paediatric patients. Blood transfusion should be avoided in hemodynamically stable patients as it increases blood viscosity.

Disseminated intravascular coagulation

Disseminated intravascular coagulation (DIC) is a syndrome characterized by systemic activation of blood coagulation, which generates intravascular fibrin and thrombin.

The clinical presentation of DIC can be classified into three distinct groups:

- subclinical, where the effect of thrombin and plasmin generated can only be reflected in the laboratory markers, more likely in solid tumours;
- hyperfibrinolysis, where the predominant clinical symptoms are bleeding, as the activation of the fibrinolytic system dominates, more likely in acute promyelocytic leukaemia; and (3) hypercoagulation, where thrombosis is the predominant clinical symptoms, caused by excess thrombin, more likely in pancreatic and lung adenocarcinoma. Common clinical presentations include mucocutaneous haemorrhage, gastrointestinal haemorrhage, melena and haematuria. Less common presentations include haemothorax, sinus thrombosis and pulmonary embolism.

The platelet count is usually low or there could be a sudden drop along with prolonged clotting times, the presence of fibrin- degradation products, and low plasma levels of coagulation inhibitors. DIC should be considered in case of a sudden deterioration of laboratory parameters and >30% drop in platelet count.

Management

Mainstay of treatment is to treat the cause. Acute promyelocytic leukaemia is a common cause of cancer in children, All-trans retinoic acid should be given as soon as acute promyelocytic leukaemia is suspected; it has been associated with decreased rates of early haemorrhagic deaths.

Use of blood products and platelets, fibrinogen and cryoprecipitate. Blood transfusion is indicated in active bleeding or in patients at risk of bleeding). Platelet count of $>50\times10^9$/L and fresh frozen plasma (FFP) can be given too. In suspected fluid overload, Prothrombin complex concentrate can be given instead of FFP.

Patients with low fibrinogen level (<1.5g/L)- cryoprecipitate or fibrinogen concentrate can be given.

Heparin is reserved for symptomatic thrombosis. Tranexamic acid may be considered in hyperfibrinolytic DIC.

Superior vena cava syndrome and superior mediastinal syndrome

SVC syndrome is the compression or obstruction on major vessels. Superior mediastinal syndrome is the compression or obstruction of the SVC and airways. In children, superior mediastinal mass syndrome is more common. Childrens have a smaller airway diameter are especially prone to airway obstruction, in which a >30% decrease in the luminal area represents a grave risk for total airway obstruction. Anterior mediastinum is said to have the majority of mediastinal masses. Clinical signs that we could appreciate are cyanosis, upper body oedema, engorgement of veins and pulsus paradoxical changes in blood pressure might indicate significant mass effects on surrounding anatomical structures.

Management

A chest X-ray, an echocardiogram and CT scan are also useful diagnostic tools to evaluate the degree of compression by the mediastinal mass on the surrounding structures.

Elevation of the head, lateral or prone position can be considered to reduce the mediastinal mass effect. Fluid status should be optimized to maintain sufficient venous return and cardiac output.

Steroid therapy and radiotherapy can be considered to decrease the size of the tumour according to the presentation history and imaging findings. Extracorporeal membrane oxygenation (ECMO) to support the patient hemodynamically.

Acute respiratory distress syndrome

ARDS is characterized by tachypnoea, dyspnoea and hypoxemia,

The major cause of ARDS patients being extrapulmonary infection and invasive aspergillosis and *Pneumocystis* pneumonia. Diagnostic bronchopulmonary alveolar lavage (BAL) can be used to guide treatment, The etiology includes lung injury following aspiration, pneumotaxic drugs, radiation toxicity and post-thoracic surgical changes, reduced baseline lung function post-chemotherapy (e.g. bleomycin reducing the diffusing capacity of the lung for carbon monoxide), diffuse alveolar haemorrhage, pulmonary leukostasis, transfusion-related acute lung injury, pancreatitis and sepsis.

Management

The mainstay of management is to treat the underlying cause and to avoid secondary lung injury and extrapulmonary complications.

According to the latest paediatric ARDS guideline, Early non-invasive positive pressure ventilation, lung-protective ventilation strategies (moderately elevated PEEP, patient-specific tidal volume and permissive hypercapnia), the consideration of neuromuscular blockade to achieve effective mechanical ventilation, conservative fluid management and adequate nutrition. The use of ECMO and Mesenchymal stem cell therapy might be beneficial for ARDS.

Posterior reversible encephalopathy syndrome

Posterior reversible encephalopathy syndrome (PRES), also known as reversible posterior leukoencephalopathy syndrome is a common neurological complication. Common causes include severe hypertension, renal dysfunction, severe infections, selected autoimmune diseases and certain medications(Steroids, immunosuppressive agents or cytotoxic agents) are common triggers for PRES.

Symptoms include headache, changes in vision, seizures, confusion and weakness of one or more limbs. The diagnosis is usually made by MRI of the brain (vasogenic oedema within the posterior arterial watershed region).

Management

Symptomatic management stays as a first line modality in PRES. Although PRES is reversible in most cases, it can cause permanent neurological damage if not treated. Causative drugs and trigger events should be discontinued. Other supportive management includes sufficient hydration, maintaining arterial oxygenation, correction of hypoglycemia, electrolyte disturbances, and coagulopathy. If hypertension, the elevated blood pressure should be reduced by 25- 50% with gradual reduction over 24-96 hours. Intravenous nicardipine and labetalol are considered first-line therapies for the management of hypertensive crises in children. Anticonvulsants might be required for seizure control.

Infection

Paediatric oncology patients are highly at the risk of sepsis because of the intensive treatment, chemotherapy and immunosuppression Febrile neutropenia develops at least once during the course of treatment. Most common bacterial pathogens are gram-positive bacteria (e.g. *Streptococcus viridians* and *Staphylococcus aureus*), followed by gram-negative bacteria (e.g. *Escherichia coli*, *Klebsiella pneumonia* and *Pseudomonas aeruginosa*) and viruses.

Acute myeloid leukaemia, high-risk acute lymphoblastic leukaemia, relapsed acute leukaemia, those undergoing allogeneic hematopoietic cell transplantation, those receiving high dose steroids and those with prolonged neutropenia are at a high risk of invasive fungal disease. Viruses to be considered are cytomegalovirus, Epstein–Barr virus, varicella-zoster virus, human herpesvirus-6, human herpesvirus-7 and polyomavirus (e.g. BK virus)

Management

Febrile neutropenia patients should be started on empirical antibiotic therapy with broad coverage to tackle serious or life-threatening sepsis.

The American Society of Clinical Oncology recommends the first-line treatment of either monotherapy with an antipseudomonal β-lactam, a fourth-generation cephalosporin or carbapenem. For patients who are hemodynamically unstable and are suspected of resistant infection, a second antimicrobial effective for the treatment of gram- negative bacteria or a glycopeptide should be added. With the emergence of antibiotic-resistant pathogens (e.g. vancomycin- resistant *Enterococcus*, methicillin-resistant *Staphylococcus aureus*, multidrug resistant gram- negative bacteria, carbapenem- resistant *Enterobacteriaceae*), advanced antibiotics to cover these organisms can be considered. Potential sources of infection need to be treated with appropriate antibiotics and blood culture and sensitivity. Suspicion should be high in Central line-associated bloodstream infections and it can be a reason for prolonged hospitalization, intensive care admissions and increased mortality in oncology patients. G-CSF can be considered in bacteremia, fungemia, invasive bacterial tissue infiltration or invasive fungal infection, unresponsive to appropriate antimicrobial therapy. In haematopoietic cell transplant patients appropriate use of prophylactic antimicrobials should be considered.

Surgical Emergencies Updates

Contributors

1. Dr. Vempalli Nagasubramanyam
2. Dr. Ashima Sharma
3. Dr. Konda Sireesha
4. Dr. Lubna Tarannum

Chapters

1. Cholecystitis and cholangitis
2. Appendicitis
3. Pancreatitis
4. Lower GI bleed
5. Burn injury

Cholecystitis and Acute Cholangitis

Cholecystitis is inflammation of the gallbladder, most commonly occurring due to a gallstone obstruction. a few cases can be acalculous. Obstruction leads to gallbladder distension, inflammation resulting in acute cholecystitis. it may be due to gallstones in 95% of the cases. They can be pigment stones and cholesterol stones, tumor, lymphadenopathy, fibrosis, parasites and kinking of the duct.

Risk Factors are use of oral contraceptives or estrogen replacement therapy (alters cholesterol and bile salt metabolism leading to gallstone formation and gallbladder hypomotility), diseases of the terminal ileum (e.g. Crohns; secondary to poor bile salt reabsorption), cirrhosis (decreased bile acid secretion), hemolytic diseases (pigmented gallstones), pregnancy, obesity, TPN

This long-held notion that gallbladder outlet obstruction is the inciting event in acute cholecystitis has been challenged. Bile cultures are positive in about half of patients with acute cholecystitis and are usually polymicrobial.

<u>Clinical Features</u>

History	Physical Examination	Investigations	Treatment
Pain in the right upper quadrant of abdomen.	Tenderness in right upper quadrant	WBC elevated-	Asymptomatic gallstones generally require no treatment
Pain due to biliary colic is more around midnight	Rigidity, rebound tenderness	CRP elevated but not specific	ED management is mainly in symptom control. Symptom management includes NPO, IV fluids, antiemetics, analgesics and appropriate antibiotics
Associated nausea and vomiting	Fever in one third of cases	Liver function tests are often normal. Transaminitis allows for evaluation of choledocolithiasis	In acute cholecystitis surgical consultation is sought for early laparoscopic cholecystectomy
	Murphy's sign (tenderness and an inspiratory pause elicited by palpation of the RUQ during a deep breath)	Ultrasound-Imaging method of choice to identify Sonographic Murphy's sign and presence of gallstones.Other nonspecific findings are Gallbladder wall thickening>3 mm and pericholecystic fluid. GB wall thickness increases with age; an upper limit of 8mm for patients > age 50 is commonly cited.	

Diabetes is a risk factor for emphysematous cholecystitis: initiate antibiotic therapy directed against Gram-negative rods and anaerobes, and consult surgery	Jaundice is rare in acute cholecystitis	CECT may reveal complications of cholecystitis	Antimicrobials: Mildly ill: ciprofloxacin 400 mg IV + metronidazole 500 mg IV Critically ill: vancomycin 20 mg/kg (up to 2 g) IV + piperacillin/tazobactam 4.5 g IV

Acute acalculous cholecystitis (AAC) is due to inflammation of the gallbladder without evidence of gallbladder calculi. AAC is commonly associated with critically ill patients in the ICU, i.e. polytrauma patients, massive burns, cardiac surgery, abdominal vascular surgery, immunosuppression, sepsis, prolonged TPN administration. Maintain a high index of suspicion in patients who present to the ED with right upper quadrant pain even in the absence of a history of cholelithiasis. Men > 60 years old with atherosclerotic cardiovascular disease are the most common outpatient population to develop AAC. Fever is an associated symptom along with RUQ pain and leucocytosis found in acalculous cholecystitis.

The sensitivity of ultrasound for acute acalculous cholecystitis is not well established. If there is a high clinical suspicion and a negative ultrasound, pursue further diagnostic imaging with HIDA scan +/- CT imaging, followed by admission for diagnostic laparoscopy if all noninvasive testing is negative.

Acute acalculous cholecystitis follows a more fulminant course than calculous cholecystitis. Broad spectrum antibiotics with gram-negative coverage and fluid resuscitation should be started immediately if the diagnosis is suspected, with an emergent consultation to general surgery.

Cholangitis is the presence of increased hepatic intraductal pressure with a concurrent infection of the obstructed bile. The migration of bacteria from the duodenum into the hepatopancreatic duct, which can then spread to the bloodstream can occur in cholangitis and hence it can quickly progress to septic shock.Mortality approaches 100% if untreated. Even with appropriate diagnosis and therapy in the current era, mortality remains high (2-30%). The most common causes are bile duct stones and previous manipulation of the biliary tree (biliary calculi, benign biliary stricture and malignancy, ERCP) and primary sclerosing cholangitis. The other causes are Lemmel syndrome due to extrinsic compression of the bile duct due to a duodenal periampullary diverticulum, inflammation due to pancreatitis, Mirizzi syndrome due to impacted stone in the cystic duct or neck of the gallbladder and intrinsic obstruction by thrombosis and parasitic infection.

History	Physical Examination	Investigations	Treatment
Bizarre presentation with altered mental status or sepsis with unknown source	Charcot's triad of fever, right upper quadrant pain, and jaundice has a specificity of 85% and sensitivity of 25%.	AST/ALT is typically elevated, but degree of elevation varies. GGT and alkaline phosphatase are elevated in close to 90%; bilirubin may be over 4 mg/dL	Broad spectrum antibiotics, resuscitation (fluids, vasopressors), symptomatic therapy (analgesics, antiemetics), and consultation.
Fever in 40-100%,	Reynold's pentad is Charcot's triad plus hypotension and altered mental status, which has a sensitivity of < 7%.	Elevated WBC in 80%. Neutrophil to lymphocyte ratio is often > 5.	Consult GI in all patients for decompression with ERCP. Surgery should also be consulted if the patient is toxic with end organ injury.
Abdominal pain in 60-100%, but these are not specific.		Blood cultures are positive in 70%.	Antibiotics should cover enteric streptococci, coliforms, and anaerobes. No solid evidence for using antibiotics with high biliary penetration, but still must be considered in cholangitis. Vancomycin is needed in very few patients with cholangitis.
Jaundice is present in 60-70%. systemic symptoms like rigors, chills		Several options of imaging are US, CT, ERCP, MRCP. US can identify dilated intrahepatic ducts, as well as a dilated common bile duct to indicate common bile duct stone or other distal obstruction.CBD > 7 mm is dilated, but in those with prior cholecystectomy the dilation can be up to 10 mm. CBD may be normal early in the disease course.	Not sick: Piperacillin/tazobactam or ertapenem OR metronidazole PLUS cefazolin or cefuroxime or ceftriaxone or cefotaxime or ciprofloxacin or levofloxacin. Sick: Piperacillin/tazobactam, meropenem, imipenem-cilastatin OR metronidazole PLUS cefepime or ceftazidime.
Complications from bacteremia (shock, hepatic abscess).		CT with IV contrast can identify dilated intrahepatic and common bile ducts and may also identify a nearby mass causing external compression on the biliary structures.	Healthcare associated: Add ampicillin or vancomycin.
		MRCP is used for high diagnostic suspicion but inconclusive or negative CT/US.	

<u>Tokyo guidelines</u> are widely used for diagnosis and severity grading of cholangitis-

TG18 Diagnostic Criteria for Acute Cholangitis.

Category	
A. Systemic inflammation	
Fever or shaking chills	Body temperature > 38 degree C
Laboratory evidence of inflammatory response	WBC <4000 or >10000 CRP>1
B. Cholestasis	
Jaundice	Bilirubin ≥ 2 mg/dl
Abnormal LFT	Alk Phos> 1.5 times upper normal limit GGT > 1.5 times upper normal limit AST > 1.5 times upper normal limit ALT > 1.5 times upper normal limit
C. Imaging	
Biliary dilatation	
Evidence of etiology on imaging	
Suspect Cholangitis- one item from A plus one item from B or C Confirmed Cholangitis- one item from A, B and C are present.	

TG18 Severity Criteria for Acute Cholangitis-

Grade III- **Severe** dysfunction in atleast one of the following systems	Criteria	Treatment- Immediate Decompression
CVS	Hypotension requiring dopamine ≥ 5ug/kg/min or any dose of norepinephrine.	
CNS	AMS	
Resp	PaO_2/FiO_2< 300	
Renal	Oliguria or serum creatinine > 2 mg/dl	
Hepatic	INR > 1.5	
Hematological	Platelet count < 100,000/ mm^3	
Grade II- **Moderate** dysfunction in any two of the following		early decompression
Abnormal WBC count	< 4000 or >12000	
High fever	more than 39 degree C	
Hyperbilirubinemia	Total bilirubin ≥ 5 mg/dl	

Hypoalbuminemia	< 70% of the normal lower limit	
Advanced age	≥ 75 years	
Grade I- Mild		Medical management and surgical planned intervention later.
Does not meet the criteria of severe or moderate at diagnosis		

Certain antibiotics have good penetration efficiency for biliary sepsis. These are- Tigecycline, Ciprofloxacin, Penicillin G, Piperacillin/Tazobactum, Ampicillin/Sulbactam, Cefipime, Amoxicillin-clavulanate, Levofloxacin and Imipenem.

For the emergency physician, the most important factors are suspecting the disease, resuscitating, providing antibiotics, and recognizing those patients who require emergent surgical or GI evaluation in order to improve outcome in moderate or severe disease.

Acute Appendicitis

Acute appendicitis is most common in the age group of 10 to 19 years. In children >1 year old, it remains the most frequent cause of atraumatic abdominal pain. Acute appendicitis is the most common non obstetric surgical emergency in pregnancy. In any patient with acute atraumatic abdominal pain without prior appendectomy, consider appendicitis. Inflammation occurs due to intraluminal obstruction and subsequent engorgement from mucosal secretion distal to the obstruction. Eventually, bacteria multiply behind the obstruction, invade the appendix mucosa, and cause tissue necrosis, organ infarction, and perforation.

The risk factors are white ethnicity, male gender and young age (69% of cases occur in patients <30 years). Luminal obstruction may be the underlying pathophysiological factor. Causes of obstruction are fecalith, lymphatic tissue, gallstone, tumours and parasites.

History	Physical Examination	Investigations
Typical findings are the exception and not the rule in diagnosis of acute appendicitis.	Tenderness at McBurney's point	WBC >10000 with a leftward shift
Fever	Abdominal guarding, Rebound tenderness	WBC >10000 with CRP>1
Migrating pain- from periumbilical region to right lower quadrant (McBurney's point)	Rovsing's sign - pain over McBurney's point on palpating the descending colon in the left lower quadrant	Serum Bilirubin > 1 mg/dl
Nausea/vomiting follow pain	Psoas sign - while the patient lies on the left side, passive extension of the right leg at the hip produces abdominal pain	CT imaging-dilated appendix >6 mm with a thickened wall, peri appendiceal inflammation, and potential visualization of an appendicolith or abscess
	Obturator test - passive internal and external rotation of the flexed right thigh at the hip produces abdominal pain	US-thickened, noncompressible appendix > 6 mm in diameter

The 2015 American College of Radiology Appropriateness Criteria for right lower quadrant pain state that although US is the preferred initial imaging modality in children, CT is overall the most accurate imaging modality for suspected appendicitis.

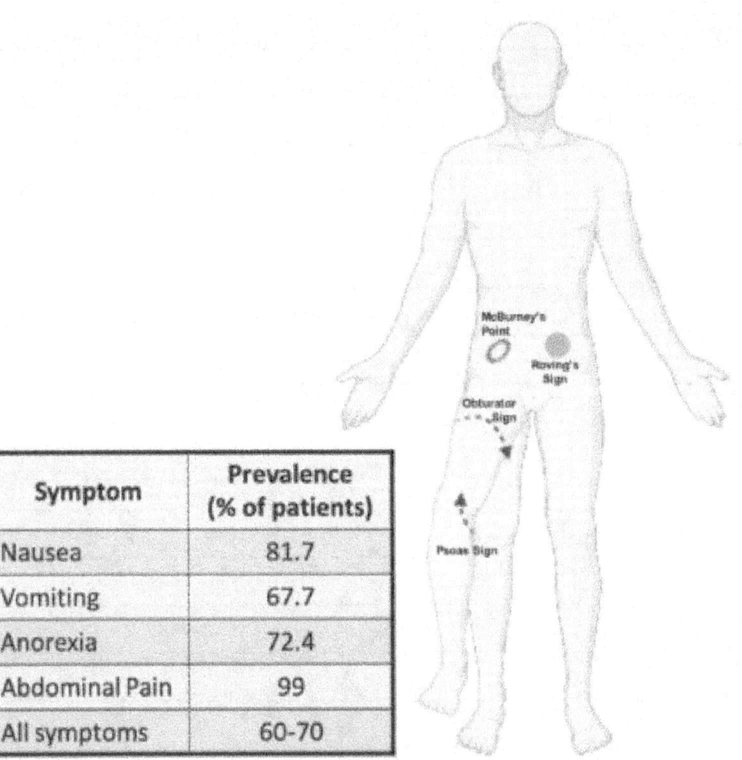

Symptom	Prevalence (% of patients)
Nausea	81.7
Vomiting	67.7
Anorexia	72.4
Abdominal Pain	99
All symptoms	60-70

Exam Findings	Sensitivity	Specificity
McBurney's Point Tenderness	50 – 94%	75 – 86%
Rovsing's Sign	22 – 66%	58 – 96%
Obturator Sign	8%	94%
Psoas Sign	13 – 42%	79 – 97%

Several risk scores are available to determine need for further evaluation, but each has limitations and biases.

Alvarado score	Points
Migratory pain	1
Anorexia	1
Nausea - vomiting	1
Rebound pain	1
Elevated temperature	1
Shift (left)	1
Tenderness in RLQ	2
Leukocytosis	2

Appendicitis Inflammatory Response (AIR) score	Points
Vomiting	1
RLQ pain	1
Rebound tenderness	
Light	1
Medium	2
Strong	3

Elevated temperature	1
PMN %	
70-84%	1
>85%	2
WBC (cells/uL)	
10-14.9	1
>14.9	2
CRP (g/L)	
10-49	1
>50	2

Pediatric Appendicitis Score	Points
Cough/ hopping/ percussion tenderness	2
Anorexia	1
Pyrexia	1
Nausea/emesis	1
Tenderness over RIF	2
Leukocytosis	1
PMNs elevation	1
Migration of pain	1

Scoring tool	Maximum Score	Low Risk	Intermediate Risk	High Risk
Alvarado	10	0-4 sens= 99%	5-6	7-10 Spec= 82%
AIR	12	0-4 sens= 96%	5-8	9-12 Spec= 99%
PAS	10	0-4 sens= 100%	-	5-10 Spec= 92%
Treatment		Discharge	Send for Imaging	Send to OT

Treatment-

1. Immediate surgical consultation is required.

2. Nil per oral (NPO)

3. IV fluids

4. Analgesics, antiemetics

5. Perioperative antibiotics

   – Antibiotic therapy has been proposed as an alternative to surgery for uncomplicated appendicitis. CODA trial (Comparison of Outcomes of Antibiotic drugs and Appendectomy,

2020) reported that 30-day general health status of patients treated with antibiotics was compared to the appendectomy group. 29% of medically treated patients required appendectomy by 90 days. Long term data from this trial now confirm high rates of subsequent appendectomy after initial medical therapy.40% at one year, 49% at two years, and 49% at 3 and 4 years. Due to high appendectomy rates in future, surgery is suggested for uncomplicated appendicitis and reserve medical therapy for those who are medically unfit for or decline surgery.(2)

— Similar experience noted in the COMMA trial documented 25 percent of recurrence rates at one year in patients initially treated with antibiotics. Quality of life scores are also better for immediate appendectomy groups.(3)

— For acute non perforated appendicitis appendectomy should be performed within 12 hours of diagnosis. Delaying appendectomy more than 48 hours associated with more surgical site infections and other complications. Single shot of prophylactic antibiotics should be given 60 minutes before the incision for appendectomy for preventing wound infection and intra-abdominal abscess development for patients proceeding directly from emergency room to operating room. For patients in whom immediate appendectomy is not possible, they should be admitted and started on intravenous antibiotics as soon as possible rather than waiting till just before surgery.(4)

Emergency Physicians should utilize prediction scoring tools: AIR score for high risk patients and Alvarado score for dischargeable patients. They should not hesitate to utilize CT imaging for intermediate risk patients, including pregnant women and children.

Acute Pancreatitis

Acute pancreatitis is one of the common causes of acute severe abdominal pain due to the inflammatory process. Incidence is increasing worldwide due to the increasing trend of obesity and gallstone disease.

Overall mortality rate of acute pancreatitis is 5%. Mortality rate of interstitial pancreatitis is 3% whereas necrotizing pancreatitis it is 17%. Mortality is mainly due to systemic inflammatory response syndrome and organ failure in the first 2-week period, but after 2 weeks it is due to sepsis and its complications.

<u>Etiology of pancreatitis-</u>

1. Gallstones (Most common - 40-70 %)
2. Alcohol (2nd most common - 20-35%)
3. Hypertriglyceridemia
4. Post ERCP
5. Genetic (PRSS1, SPINK, CTRC, CFTR gene mutation)
6. Drugs (6-Mercaptopurine, Azathioprine, Aminosalycilates, Diuretics, Valproic acid, Tetracycline, Steroids, Estrogen)
7. Hypercalcemia
8. Infections (Vital, Bacterial, Fungal, Parasites)
9. Anatomic abnormalities
10. Idiopathic

<u>Diagnosis requires at least two of three criteria.</u>

1. Clinical presentation consistent with acute pancreatitis.
2. Serum amylase or lipase significantly elevated above the upper limit of normal.
3. Imaging findings characteristic of acute pancreatitis (Transabdominal ultrasound, IV contrast enhanced CT, MRI)

<u>Classification is based on the Atlanta classification-</u>

1. Interstitial edematous acute pancreatitis- acute inflammation of the pancreatic parenchyma and peripancreatic tissues, but without recognizable tissue necrosis.
2. Necrotizing acute pancreatitis- inflammation associated with pancreatic parenchymal necrosis and/or peripancreatic necrosis.

<u>According to the severity, acute pancreatitis is divided into the following:</u>

- Mild acute pancreatitis- absence of organ failure and local or systemic complications
- Moderately severe acute pancreatitis- no organ failure or transient organ failure (<48 hours) and/or local complications.
- Severe acute pancreatitis- persistent organ failure (>48 hours) that may involve one or multiple organs

<u>Scoring Systems</u>

There are several scoring systems designed to predict mortality, necessity of intensive care, and pancreatitis severity.

Score	sensitivity	specificity	remarks
Ranson's	0-100%	14-97%	complete Ranson score cannot be calculated until 48 hours post-admission initial score >2 is often used as suggestive of admission
APACHE II	68-100%	21-96%	used in the ED to predict the necessity for an ICU admission.
BISAP			A score of 5 was found to suggest a mortality rate of 22%, and a score of 3 or more is suggestive of severe acute pancreatitis.
SIRS			presence of SIRS correlateD with a 25% mortality rate during the index admission vs 0% in patients who did not meet SIRS criteria
Balthazar CT severity score			Necrosis, local inflammation, and fluid collections are useful in predicting outcomes. mortality rates were 23% with any degree of necrosis and 0% without.

<u>Management-</u>

Initial management should focus on pain management, fluid resuscitation and nutritional support.

1. **Pain management**

   Appropriate pain management is mandatory to prevent hemodynamic instability. Adequate fluid management is one of the cornerstones in pain management as hypovolemia from vascular leak itself will lead to hemoconcentration and ischemic pain.

   – Opioids are the first line drugs for pain management. Intravenous opioids are preferred. Fentanyl or hydromorphone are used as bolus and constant infusion.

   – Fentanyl – 20-50 microgram bolus dose will be used typically.

   – Meperidine also will be considered over morphine in view of theoretical risk of increased sphincter of Oddi pressure due to morphine. But no clinical studies till now proved that morphine will aggravate or cause pancreatitis or cholecystitis.

- Ketamine infusions at 0.2-0.3 mg/kg have shown promise in patients with acute pancreatitis.

- Acetaminophen may be considered if available intravenously, although used cautiously if any significant hepatic dysfunction is present. NSAIDs, such as ketorolac, are less preferred due to the increased risk of kidney injury and gastrointestinal bleeding in patients already under significant systemic stress.

- Nausea should be treated with repeated doses of centrally-acting antiemetics such as ondansetron or metoclopramide. A baseline electrocardiogram may be useful to establish the QTc interval in the case that repeated doses of these medications become necessary.

2. **Fluid management**

   - In the initial stages (within the first 12 to 24 hours) of acute pancreatitis, fluid replacement has been associated with a reduction in morbidity and mortality. Inadequate hydration can lead to hypotension and acute tubular necrosis. Persistent hemoconcentration at 24 hours has been associated with development of necrotizing pancreatitis. Necrotizing pancreatitis results in vascular leak syndrome leading to increased third space fluid losses and worsening of pancreatic hypoperfusion. However, it is important to limit fluid resuscitation mainly to the first 24 to 48 hours after onset of the disease. Continued aggressive fluid resuscitation after 48 hours may not be advisable as overly-vigorous fluid resuscitation is associated with an increased need for intubation and increased risk of abdominal compartment syndrome.

     A practical solution advised is use of isotonic fluid (Normal saline or ringer lactate) to be used at a rate of 5-10 ml/Kg per hour to all patients with pancreatitis after ruling out fluid overload symptoms. In case of severe volume depletion rapid bolus infusion of 20 mg/kg followed by 3ml/kg/hour infusion for the next 12 hours.

   - Colloids should be avoided due no mortality benefit and risk of multi organ dysfunction.

   - Rate of fluid resuscitation can be adjusted by clinical monitoring (heart rate and mean arterial blood pressure and urine output) hematocrit and blood urea nitrogen levels.

   - Fluid resuscitation with ringer lactate can reduce the incidence of systemic inflammatory response syndrome as per limited conflicting evidence. Nineteen Patients receiving RL and 21 receiving NS were analyzed. The median number of SIRS criteria at 48 hours were 1 (1-2) for NS vs 1 (0-1) for RL, p = 0.060. CRP levels (mg/l) were as follows: at 48 hours NS 166 (78-281) vs RL 28 (3-124), p = 0.037; at 72 hours NS 217 (59-323) vs RL 25 (3-169), p = 0.043. In vitro, LR inhibited the induction of inflammatory phenotype of macrophages and NF-κB activation. This effect was not observed when using Ringer's solution without lactate, suggesting a direct anti-inflammatory effect of lactate.(5)

3. **Nutritional management**

   - In the absence of ileus, nausea or vomiting in mild acute pancreatitis oral feeding with low fat soft diet should be initiated within 24 hours as much as tolerated if pain and inflammatory markers are improving.
   - In patients with moderately severe to severe pancreatitis, where oral nutrition is not possible immediately, nasojejunal tube feeding can be initiated by day 5. In these patients parenteral nutrition should be initiated within 48-72 hours.
   - Early feeding (less than 48 hours after hospitalization) did not increase adverse effects and was associated with reduction in length of hospital stay.
   - A multicenter trial comparing enteral nutrition in the first 24 hours with enteral feeding after 72 hours in patients with predicted severe acute pancreatitis did not find any improved clinical outcomes with early enteral feeding.(6)

4. **Antibiotics**

   - Whenever infection is suspected antibiotics should be started. There is no role of prophylactic antibiotics irrespective of type or severity of disease.

5. **Other treatment**

   - Pentoxifylline

     Role of pentoxifylline studied in one randomized trial in severe acute pancreatitis within 72 hours of diagnosis revealed fewer admissions and longer hospital stay compared to placebo. (7)
   - Protease inhibitors – as per the evidence available till now protease inhibitors shown only marginal reduction of mortality in severe pancreatitis patients. (8)

6. **Catheter drainage in patients with infected pancreatic necrosis -** In a randomized trial of 104 such patients comparing immediate with delayed drainage (until necrotic collections were largely encapsulated but patients were clinically deteriorating or not improving), both approaches had similar complication and mortality rates; however, immediate drainage resulted in a higher number of interventions. Approximately one-third of patients improved with antibiotics without the need for intervention. These data support our approach to selectively perform nonsurgical drainage in patients with infected pancreatic necrosis who exhibit clinical deterioration or fail to improve with antibiotics, and delay drainage in clinically stable patients until the development of walled-off necrosis.(9)

Risky Discharges - The most significant risk factors were found to be:

- Gastrointestinal symptoms, specifically nausea, vomiting, or diarrhea

- A less than solid diet at discharge
- Moderate to severe alcohol use

The role of emergency physician is to establish the etiology of the pancreatitis. Imaging is not necessary but may be helpful in a particularly acute patient or in one with high levels of diagnostic uncertainty. Uncovering evidence of necrosis or localized complications will change the disposition.

POINTER Trial – Immediate versus Postponed Intervention for Infected Necrotizing Pancreatitis

Necrotizing pancreatitis – in 20-30% cases of acute pancreatitis. Current approach – IV antibiotics until the infected pancreatic and peripancreatic necrosis has become encapsulated – Then, catheter drainage.

Multicenter, randomized superiority trial to investigate whether immediate catheter drainage is superior to postponed catheter drainage in patients with infected necrotizing pancreatitis

DEFINITION OF INFECTED NECROSIS

- In 1ˢᵗ 14 days – positive Gram's stain or culture from a fine-needle aspiration or the presence of gas configurations within pancreatic and peripancreatic necrosis on contrast-enhanced computed tomography (CT)
- After the first 14 days after onset – Clinical signs of infection were considered diagnostic for infected necrosis, defined as persistent organ failure in patients admitted to the intensive care unit or the persistence of two inflammatory variables (temperature >38.5°C or elevated C-reactive protein levels or leukocyte counts) during 3 consecutive days in patients on regular hospital wards

PROCEDURE

- Patients were randomly assigned, in a 1:1 ratio, to immediate catheter drainage or postponed catheter drainage.
- Immediate catheter drainage included treatment with antibiotics and catheter drainage within 24 hours after randomization (which occurred as soon as infected necrosis was diagnosed).
- Postponed catheter drainage included treatment with antibiotics and supportive treatment aimed at postponing the drainage procedure until the stage of walled-off necrosis, when necrotic collections were largely or fully encapsulated

END POINTS

- Primary end point was the score on the Comprehensive Complication Index, including all complications that occurred between randomization and 6-month follow-up, graded according to the Clavien–Dindo classification

- Secondary End Point – death, new onset organ failure, number of patients with severe complications, total number of surgical, endoscopic, and radiologic interventions, total length of intensive care and hospital stay; and total inpatient hospital costs etc

<u>CONCLUSION</u>

104 patients were randomly assigned to immediate catheter drainage (55 patients) or postponed catheter drainage (49 patients)

No difference between the groups in the primary end point: the mean Comprehensive Complication Index score was 57 in the immediate-drainage group and 58 in the postponed drainage group (mean difference, –1; 95% CI, –12 to 10; P=0.90)

Mortality was 13% in the immediate-drainage group, as compared with 10% in the postponed-drainage group (relative risk, 1.25; 95% CI, 0.42 to 3.68)

No significant differences were found in the incidence of major complications.

This multicenter, randomized trial did not show the superiority of immediate catheter drainage over postponed catheter drainage in reducing complications in patients with infected necrotizing pancreatitis.

Lower Gastrointestinal (GI) Bleeding

It is the loss of blood from the GI tract distal to the ligament of Treitz. Blood from the upper GI tract also may mimic lower GI bleeding. About 80% of episodes of lower GI bleeding resolve spontaneously. Hematochezia is either bright red or maroon-colored rectal bleeding. Approximately 10% of hematochezia episodes may be associated with upper GI bleeding. Melena is dark or black colored stools and usually represents bleeding from an upper GI source.

Etiology-

- The most common cause is diverticular disease, followed by colitis, hemorrhoids, and adenomatous polyps/malignancies.

- Diverticulosis is identified by painless bleeding and right-sided diverticula are more likely to bleed.

- Vascular ectasia includes arteriovenous malformations and angiodysplasias of the colon. There is also a suggestion that valvular heart disease is a risk factor for developing bleeding vascular ectasias, although this is an area of debate.

- Ischemic Colitis is the most common cause of intestinal ischemia and is usually transient. Although most cases will resolve on their own, some patients require surgical intervention.

- Mesenteric ischemia can lead to bowel necrosis. Diagnosis is difficult and despite aggressive treatment, prognosis is poor, with a survival of 50% if diagnosed within 24 hours.

- Meckel's Diverticulum is a rare but important condition in younger age groups.

- Hemorrhoids is the most common source of anorectal bleeding but massive hemorrhage is unusual.

Diagnosis

History	Physical examination	Laboratory Testing
Hematochezia or melena	Visual inspection of the vomitus	Blood group and cross matching CBC, coagulation profile BUN, Creatinine Electrolyte, glucose Liver function tests
S/S of hypotension, tachycardia, angina, syncope, weakness, or altered mental status	hypotension and tachycardia, decreased pulse pressure or tachypnea are more subtle signs. If the patient is in shock-cool, clammy skin	Angiography -sometimes detects the site of bleeding.Provides therapeutic options such as transcatheter arterial embolization or the infusion of vasoconstrictive agents.

Weight loss and changes in bowel habits may suggest malignancy	Liver failure features	Scintigraphy localizes the site of bleeding.Can detect if bleeding occurs intermittently but requires a minimum of 3 mL of pooled blood.
Past history- prior history of GI bleeding, trauma, ingestion of foreign bodies, and recent colonoscopies	P/A--tenderness, masses, ascites, or organomegaly. A lack of abdominal tenderness suggests bleeding from disorders involving the vasculature, such as diverticulosis or angiodysplasia	CT angiography can be useful in unstable bleeds
Medication history- antiplatelets, NSAIDs and anticoagulants	P/R- laceration, masses, trauma, anal fissures, or external hemorrhoids	Sigmoidoscopy, Colonoscopy

Patients with acute lower GI bleed can be categorized as high or low risk based on the following features (10)

- Hemodynamic instability
- Persistent bleeding
- Comorbid illness
- Advanced age
- Prior history of bleeding from diverticulosis or angiodysplasia
- Current aspirin use
- Prolonged PT
- Anemia
- Elevated blood urea nitrogen
- Abnormal WBC

The British Society of Gastroenterology released guidelines for management of LGIB recently. these are-

1. Categorize the patient as stable versus unstable (defined as shock index > 1). Patients with an unstable bleed should be resuscitated and undergo CTA. Patients with stable bleeds and shock index < 1 are less likely to have severe, active bleeding.(11) These patients can be assessed with scoring systems, such as the Oakland score (weak recommendation, moderate quality evidence). It is used to determine safe discharge in patients with acute lower GI bleed. This score based on parameters such as age, sex, previous history of lower GI bleed, blood on per rectal examination, heart rate, systolic blood pressure and haemoglobin. Score of 8 or less can be considered for safe discharge. (12)

2. Glasgow-Blatchford score, typically used in UGIB, can also be utilized in LGIB.

3. Patients with minor, self-terminating bleeding with no other indications for admission can be discharged with urgent outpatient assessment (strong recommendation, moderate quality evidence). Colonoscopy is the recommended test, though endoscopy may be needed in higher risk patients.

4. Patients with major bleeding should be admitted for colonoscopy (strong recommendation, moderate quality evidence). Timing of colonoscopy is controversial, and patients with LGIB should "have an inpatient colonoscopy on the next available list."

5. If the patient is hemodynamically unstable or has a shock index > 1 after resuscitation or active bleeding is suspected, obtain CTA. This modality provides the fastest and most accurate means to finding the site of bleeding and allows for radiological intervention (strong recommendation, low quality evidence). CTA sensitivity and specificity range from 79-95% and 95-100%, respectively.

6. Upper endoscopy should be performed if CTA does not identify a source of bleeding, as LGIB with hemodynamic instability may be due to an UGIB source. Approximately 11-15% of patients thought to have a LGIB source actually have an UGIB source. NG placement for suspected UGIB is not recommended on a routine basis. Gastroscopy may be utilized if the patient stabilizes (strong recommendation, moderate evidence quality).

7. If CTA is positive, catheter angiography with embolization is recommended as soon as possible. In centers with 24/7 interventional radiology service, this should be completed within 1 hour for hemodynamically unstable patients (strong recommendation, low quality evidence).

8. Emergent laparotomy is the last line of therapy, which should be completed only after all other radiological and endoscopic modalities, except under exceptional circumstances (strong recommendation, low quality evidence).

9. Restrictive transfusion thresholds of 7 g/dL are recommended, with a Hb target of 7-9 g/dL after transfusion. In patients with cardiovascular disease, use a trigger of 8 g/dL and target of 10 g/dL (strong recommendation, low quality evidence). FFP and platelet transfusion is uncommon in these patients, with no randomized data for LGIB.

10. Interrupt warfarin therapy at presentation (weak recommendation, low quality evidence). If unstable LGIB, reverse anticoagulation with PCC and vitamin K (strong recommendation, moderate quality evidence).

11. For patients taking DOACs, stop therapy at presentation (strong recommendation, low quality evidence). Consider inhibitors such as idarucizumab or andexanet for life-threatening bleeding (strong recommendation, moderate quality evidence). Restart DOAC therapy at a maximum of 7 days after bleeding (weak recommendation, very low quality evidence).

12. TXA may benefit in acute GI bleeding, but the guidelines do not make any clear recommendations pending the HALT-IT trial.

13. The final recommendations state hospitals should have access to a GI bleeding lead and agreed pathways for management, colonoscopy access, and interventional radiology access (either on site or through transfer).

Burn Injury

Burn injury is one of the common emergencies seen in ED. A burn is defined as an injury to the skin or other organic tissue primarily caused by heat or due to radiation, radioactivity, electricity, friction or contact with chemicals. Heat burns occur when some or all of the different layers of cells in the skin are destroyed by a hot liquid (scald), a hot solid (contact burn) or a flame (flame burn). In India around 7 million people suffer from burn injuries each year with 1.4 lakh deaths and 2.4 lakh people suffer with disability.Care of burn patients has improved significantly over the last few decades.

<u>Pathophysiology</u>

LOCAL

The extent of injury depends on intensity of heat and duration of contact. Burn wounds are described by Jackson to be having three zones: zone of coagulation(necrosis), stasis(ischemia), hyperthermia (inflammation)(13).

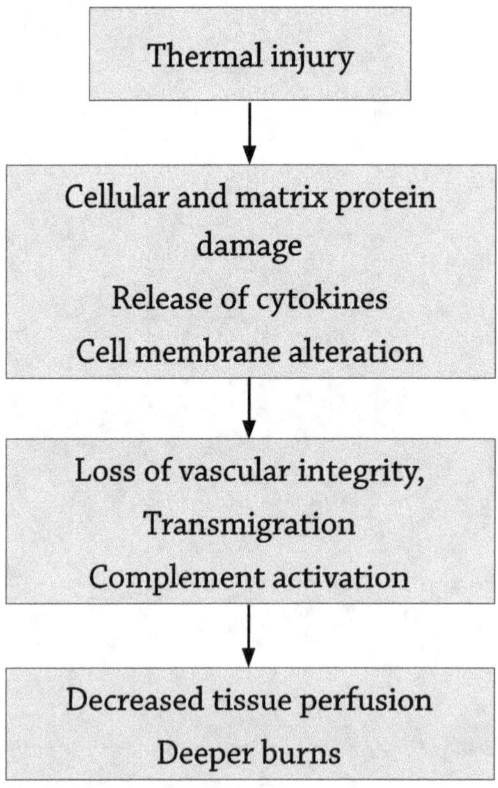

Resuscitation and local wound care can limit this reversible tissue loss.Maximal fluid shift occurs around 12 hours after burn and within 24 hours capillary integrity returns to near normal.

Burn shock may result from intravascular volume depletion, cardiac dysfunction and tissue hypoperfusion leading to multi organ dysfunction. Kidneys are particularly susceptible to damage from hypo perfusion leading to acute kidney injury.

PREHOSPITAL CARE

The risk of death from burns increases with large burn size, old age, female sex, presence of comorbidity and inhalation injury. Stop the burning process. Assess airway, breathing, circulation (ABC) and immobilize cervical spine if required. Remove any constricting materials like watches, rings and cover the patient in clean sheets to prevent hypothermia. Patients should be transported to appropriate facilities at the earliest.

TREATMENT

- Evaluation of patient

History from patient or bystanders, if patient is not able to communicate, about burn etiology, duration of burns, closed space burns	assess patient's ABC	If there is evidence of inhalation injury, intubate the patient.	Send routine laboratory tests, bedside chest Xray, ABG, ECG
AMPLE history	check for inhalation injury	If mechanical ventilation is needed, use low tidal volume ventilation to minimize airway pressures.	
	After the primary survey, do a secondary survey of head to toe examination, check for other traumatic injuries.	start resuscitation using large bore IV cannulas	
		Nasogastric tube is inserted to prevent ileus in burns >20% in adults, >10% in children and urinary catheter for monitoring urine output	
		Pain management with analgesics and prevent hypothermia.	
		Tetanus immunization should be updated	

Immediate referral to a burn specialist and continuous monitoring of patient vitals. In inhalation injury treatments that may be helpful inhaled nitric oxide to treat hypoxic vasoconstriction and aerosolized heparin and N-acetylcysteine (NAC) to remove bronchopulmonary casts.Prophylactic intravenous (IV) antibiotics are not needed.

Burns size

Burn injury size is determined by the percentage of body surface area (TBSA) involved. An accurate assessment of burn size is critical because triage and resuscitative efforts are based on the TBSA affected. Rule of Nine is simple and divides the body segments into multiples of 9%. Lund-Browder burn chart - accurate age adjusted burn size calculation. Palm method- patient's closed hand equals to approximately 1% TBSA.

Computer-based applications such as the SAGE diagram can give more precise assessments(10). Some mobile applications have also been validated.

Burn depth is determined mainly clinically. Though not being widely used yet, Ultrasound, laser Doppler, and fluorescein all have potential to assess perfusion of the burn wound and thus its depth(17). Based on depth burns are classified into:

1. Superficial burn (first degree burn)- involves only epidermis, have No blisters and are painful
2. Partial thickness burn
   a. Superficial partial thickness burn-involves epidermis and papillary dermis (second degree burn) -painful and blistered
   b. Deep partial thickness burn- in addition involves reticular dermis too (second degree burn) - variable degree of pain
   c. Full thickness burn- involves entire epidermis and dermis (third degree burn) - painless and leathery appearance
   d. Fourth degree burn - epidermis, dermis, fat, muscle, bone

Burn injuries that should be referred to a burn center include:

1. Partial thickness burns greater than 10% total body surface area (TBSA).
2. Burns that involve the face, hands, feet, genitalia, perineum, or major joints.
3. Third degree burns in any age group.
4. Electrical burns, including lightning injury.
5. Chemical burns.
6. Inhalation injury.

7. Burn injury in patients with preexisting medical disorders that could complicate management, prolong recovery, or affect mortality.

8. Any patient with burns and concomitant trauma (such as fractures) in which the burn injury poses the greatest risk of morbidity or mortality. In such cases, if the trauma poses the greater immediate risk, the patient may be initially stabilized in a trauma center before being transferred to a burn unit. Physician judgment will be necessary in such situations and should be in concert with the regional medical control plan and triage protocols.

9. Burned children in hospitals without qualified personnel or equipment for the care of children.

10. Burn injury in patients who will require special social, emotional, or rehabilitative intervention.

Resuscitation-

Resuscitation must proceed carefully because the consequences of both over or under resuscitation can be devastating.

The formulas used to calculate fluid for resuscitation are only a guide(14). Titration of fluid is recommended according to patients vitals, especially according to urine output. Fluid of choice is crystalloid like ringer lactate.

	Parkland formula	Modified Brooke formula or ABA consensus formula	Rule of Tens
ADULTS	4ml X Weight in kg X %BSA of burns for first 24 hrs — half of this is given in 8 hrs from time of burn — other half in following 16hrs — titrate to maintain UOP of 0.5ml/kg/hr and mean arterial pressure greater than 65 mm Hg	2 cc × weight [kg] × % TBSA	— Estimate TBSA of burns to the nearest 10 percent. — Multiply the %TBSA x 10 – The result gives the initial fluid rate in mL/hour for adults weighing 40 to 80 kg. — For patients who weigh > 80 kg, increase the rate by 100 mL/hour for every additional 10 kg of body weight.

CHILDREN	3ml X Weight in kg X %BSA of burns for first 24 hrs — half of this is given in 8 hrs from time of burn — other half in following 16hrs — add 5%dextrose as maintenance fluid in children weighing <20kg as they have lower glycogen reserves. — titrate to maintain UOP of 1ml/kg/hr		
		to prevent over resuscitation	

Tanaka et al. in 2000 found ascorbic acid at a dose of 66 mg/kg/h for 24 hours decreased overall volume requirements for resuscitation. The authors promote that vitamin C acts as an oxidative scavenger and may also limit tissue damage from the inflammatory process of the burn (15).

<u>Burn wound care</u>

1. After evaluation and initiating resuscitation focus on burn wound care. Do not apply any topical antibiotic dressing if a patient is being referred to a burn specialist. Use sterile moist dressing keeping in mind to avoid hypothermia. Check for circumferential burns or any constricting materials that may interfere with circulation.

2. Debridement of wounds should not delay the transfer of patients. Adequately sedate the patient before the procedure.

3. Escharotomy is indicated in circumferential burns leading to distal vascular compromise in limbs, circumferential burns of torso causing respiratory difficulty.

4. Fasciotomy- The incision is extended through the fascia exposing underlying muscles. This is done in circumferential burns with increased compartment pressure. In limbs incision is made along mid lateral line to the fat level avoiding incising fascia and major neurovascular structures. In chest, incision is made along the anterior axillary line from second to twelfth rib.

5. Newer dressings like collagen sheet or silver releasing dressings are available that can limit the frequency of multiple painful dressing changes

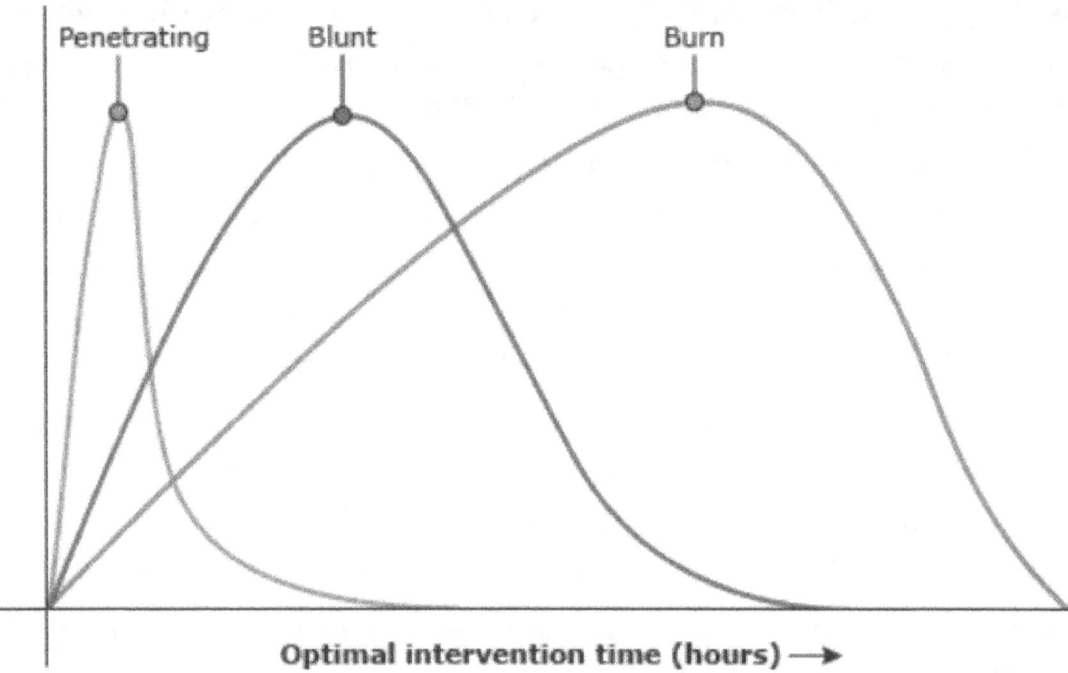

This figure depicts the optimal times for intervention in competing types of injury - penetrating, blunt, and burn. The priority of intervention changes over time (hours) and should be sequential. Penetrating injuries are best evaluated and addressed immediately. In the following minutes and/or hours, blunt injuries associated with thoracic or abdominal organs should be addressed. Cutaneous burns are the last priority and management can be initiated in the hours following stabilization and management of penetrating and blunt injuries.

Burn management requires an ABC approach with a special consideration to rapidly evolving, critical airways and pain management. CO and cyanide poisoning are treated if history, exam, or labs are suggestive. A burn patient can be MORE than just a burn with additional trauma, toxicologic etiologies, and blast injuries.

References

1. Gomi H, Solomkin JS, Schlossberg D, et al. Tokyo Guidelines 2018: antimicrobial therapy for acute cholangitis and cholecystitis. J Hepatobiliary Pancreat Sci 2018; 25:3.

2. CODA Collaborative, Flum DR, Davidson GH, et al. A Randomized Trial Comparing Antibiotics with Appendectomy for Appendicitis. N Engl J Med 2020; 383:1907.) (CODA Collaborative, Davidson GH, Flum DR, et al. Antibiotics versus Appendectomy for Acute Appendicitis - Longer-Term Outcomes. N Engl J Med 2021; 385:2395.

3. O'Leary DP, Walsh SM, Bolger J, et al. A Randomized Clinical Trial Evaluating the Efficacy and Quality of Life of Antibiotic-only Treatment of Acute Uncomplicated Appendicitis: Results of the COMMA Trial. Ann Surg 2021; 274:240.

4. United Kingdom National Surgical Research Collaborative, Bhangu A. Safety of short, in-hospital delays before surgery for acute appendicitis: multicentre cohort study, systematic review, and meta-analysis. Ann Surg 2014; 259:894

5. de-Madaria E etal.Fluid resuscitation with lactated Ringer's solution vs normal saline in acute pancreatitis: A triple-blind, randomized, controlled trial. United European Gastroenterol J. 2018;6(1):63. Epub 2017 Apr 27.

6. Ellery KM, Kumar S, Crandall W, Gariepy C. The Benefits of Early Oral Nutrition in Mild Acute Pancreatitis. *The Journal of pediatrics.* 2017;191:164-169.

7. Vege SS, Atwal T, Bi Y, et al. Pentoxifylline Treatment in Severe Acute Pancreatitis: A Pilot, Double-Blind, Placebo-Controlled, Randomized Trial. Gastroenterology 2015; 149:318.

8. Takeda K, Matsuno S, Sunamura M, Kakugawa Y. Continuous regional arterial infusion of protease inhibitor and antibiotics in acute necrotizing pancreatitis. Am J Surg 1996; 171:394.

9. Boxhoorn L, etal. Immediate versus Postponed Intervention for Infected Necrotizing Pancreatitis. Engl J Med. 2021;385(15):1372.

10. Aoki T, Nagata N, Shimbo T, et al. Development and Validation of a Risk Scoring System for Severe Acute Lower Gastrointestinal Bleeding. Clin Gastroenterol Hepatol 2016; 14:1562.

11. Oakland K, Chadwick G, East JE, et al. Diagnosis and management of acute lower gastrointestinal bleeding: guidelines from the British Society of Gastroenterology. Gut 2019; 68:776.

12. Oakland K, Jairath V, Uberoi R, et al. Derivation and validation of a novel risk score for safe discharge after acute lower gastrointestinal bleeding: a modeling study. Lancet Gastroenterol Hepatol 2017; 2:635.

13. Yin S. Chemical and common burns in children. Clinical Pediatrics (Phila). May 2017;56(5 Suppl):8S-12S

14. Satahoo SS, Palmieri TL Fluid resuscitation in burns: 2 cc, 3 cc, or 4 cc?.Curr Trauma Rep. 2019;5:99.

15. Tanaka, H, Matsuda, T, Miyagantani, Y, Yukioka, T, Matsuda, H, Shimazaki, S. Reduction of resuscitation fluid volumes in severely burned patients using ascorbic acid administration: a randomized, prospective study. Arch Surg. 2000;135(3):326-331

Endocrine Emergencies

Contributors:

1. Dr. Nidhi Kaeley
2. Dr. Rohan Bhatia
3. Dr. Salva Ameena M S
4. Dr. Silpa S

Chapters

1. Thyroid storm
2. Myxoedema coma
3. DKA/HHS
4. Adrenal insufficiency

Thyroid Storm

Thyroid storm is a rare life-threatening emergency. The patient presents with severe clinical manifestations of thyrotoxicosis.

Epidemiology and Risk factors [1]

- Long untreated hyperthyroidism
- Thyroidal or non-thyroidal surgery
- Trauma
- Infections/sepsis
- Acute iodine overload
- Pregnancy

Clinical features and signs [2-4]

- Tachycardia usually ≥140 beats per minute
- Congestive heart failure
- Hypotension
- Arrhythmias such as atrial fibrillation
- Hyperpyrexia- temperature ≥104 -106 degree F
- Agitation, delirium, psychosis, stupor, coma
- Physical examination may reveal Goiter, Graves disease ophthalmopathy, hand tremor, warm and moist skin
- Gastrointestinal symptoms – severe nausea, vomiting, diarrhea, abdominal pain, hepatic failure or jaundice

Laboratory investigations [5]

- In primary overt hyperthyroidism, there is low TSH, high FT4 and/or FT3 concentrations
- Mild hyperglycemia
- Mild hypercalcemia
- Abnormal liver tests
- Leukocytosis or leukopenia

Diagnostic criteria of thyroid storm

The Burch and Wartofsky's Scoring System uses precise clinical criteria for the identification of thyroid storm. Score of 45 or more highly suggests thyroid storm. A score of 25 to 44 is supportive of diagnosis and a score less than 25 makes the diagnosis unlikely.

Table 1. Burch and Wartofsky's Scoring System for thyroid storm [6]

Diagnostic Parameters	Scoring Points
1. Thermoregulatory dysfunction	
Temperature °C (°F)	
37.2–37.7 (99–99.9)	5
37.7–38.3 (100–100.9)	10
38.3–38.8 (101–101.9)	15
38.9–39.4 (102–102.9)	20
39.4–39.9 (103–103.9)	25
≥40 (≥104.0)	30
2. CNS effects	
Absent	0
Mild (agitation)	10
Moderate (delirium, psychosis, extreme lethargy)	20
Severe (seizures, coma)	30
3. GI-hepatic dysfunction	
Absent	0
Moderate (diarrhea, nausea/vomiting, abdominal pain)	10
Severe (unexplained jaundice)	20
4. CV dysfunction	
Tachycardia (beats/min)	
90–109	5
110–119	10
120–129	15
≥140	25
5. Congestive heart failure	
Absent	0
Mild (pedal edema)	5
Moderate (bibasilar rales)	10
Severe (pulmonary edema)	15
6. Atrial fibrillation	
Absent	0
Present	10

Treatment [5,7-15]

1. Beta blockers to control increased adrenergic tone signs and symptoms. Propranolol (60 to 80 mg) every 4-6 hours to be initiated.

2. Thionamide blocks synthesis of new hormones.

    - Propyl thiouracil (PTU)- 200 mg every 4 hours.
    - Methimazole- 20 mg every 4-6 hours.

3. Iodine solution blocks the new hormone release.

    - Potassium iodide- 5 drops orally every 6 hours.
    - Lugol's solution- 10 drops every 8 hours.
    - To be started after 1 hour of thioamide to prevent utilization of iodine as a substrate for new hormone synthesis.

4. Glucocorticoids

    - Hydrocortisone- 100 mg every 8th hourly.
    - Prevents the conversion of T4 to T3 and suppresses the autoimmune process.

5. Bile acid sequestrants in severe cases to reduce enterohepatic recycling of thyroid hormones.

Other therapies

- Plasmapheresis helps to remove cytokines, autoantibodies, and excessive thyroid hormones from the plasma. In a case series, free T4 was found to be reduced by 21% after each session of plasmapheresis in severe cases of thyroid storm. The American Society for Apheresis (ASFA) recommends that TPE be performed at a frequency of daily to every 2–3 days until clinical improvement is noted. Complications of TPE are seen in 5% of patients and include hypotension, hemolysis, allergic reactions, coagulopathy, vascular injury, and infection. [16, 17]

- Lithium has been found to block the release of thyroid hormones. However, it is associated with renal and neurological toxicities.

- Surgical Intervention- Following are the indications

    a. Failed medical therapy
    b. Severe reaction to antithyroid drugs
    c. Not a candidate for radio ablation therapy
    d. Persistent thyrotoxicosis despite maximum antithyroid drug/radio ablation therapy
    e. Underlying thyroid carcinoma
    f. Suspicious/malignant nodules on FNAC

References

1. Akamizu T, Satoh T, Isozaki O, et al. Diagnostic criteria, clinical features, and incidence of thyroid storm based on nationwide surveys. Thyroid 2012; 22:661.

2. Ngo SY, Chew HC. When the storm passes unnoticed--a case series of thyroid storm. Resuscitation 2007; 73:485.

3. Swee du S, Chng CL, Lim A. Clinical characteristics and outcome of thyroid storm: a case series and review of neuropsychiatric derangements in thyrotoxicosis. Endocr Pract 2015; 21:182.

4. Angell TE, Lechner MG, Nguyen CT, et al. Clinical features and hospital outcomes in thyroid storm: a retrospective cohort study. J Clin Endocrinol Metab 2015; 100:451.

5. B, Burman K. Thyrotoxicosis and thyroid storm. Endocrinol Metab Clin North Am 2006; 35:663.

6. Burch HB, Wartofsky L. Life-threatening thyrotoxicosis. Thyroid storm. Endocrinol Metab Clin North Am 1993; 22:263.

7. Chiha M, Samarasinghe S, Kabaker AS. Thyroid storm: an updated review. J Intensive Care Med 2015; 30:131.

8. Ross DS, Burch HB, Cooper DS, et al. 2016 American Thyroid Association Guidelines for Diagnosis and Management of Hyperthyroidism and Other Causes of Thyrotoxicosis. Thyroid 2016; 26:1343.

9. Cooper DS, Daniels GH, Ladenson PW, Ridgway EC. Hyperthyroxinemia in patients treated with high-dose propranolol. Am J Med 1982; 73:867.

10. A, Johnson EO, Kalogera CH, et al. The effect of thyrotoxicosis on adrenocortical reserve. Eur J Endocrinol 2000; 142:231.

11. Mazzaferri EL, Skillman TG. Thyroid storm. A review of 22 episodes with special emphasis on the use of guanethidine. Arch Intern Med 1969; 124:684.

12. Senda A, Endo A, Tachimori H, et al. Early administration of glucocorticoid for thyroid storm: analysis of a national administrative database. Crit Care 2020; 24:470.

13. Solomon BL, Wartofsky L, Burman KD. Adjunctive cholestyramine therapy for thyrotoxicosis. Clin Endocrinol (Oxf) 1993; 38:39.

14. Kaykhaei MA, Shams M, Sadegholvad A, et al. Low doses of cholestyramine in the treatment of hyperthyroidism. Endocrine 2008; 34:52.

15. Tsai WC, Pei D, Wang TF, et al. The effect of combination therapy with propylthiouracil and cholestyramine in the treatment of Graves' hyperthyroidism. Clin Endocrinol (Oxf) 2005; 62:521.

16. Muller C, Perrin P, Faller B, et al. Role of plasma exchange in the thyroid storm. Ther Apher Dial 2011; 15:522.

17. Tieken K, Paramasivan AM, Goldner W, et al. Therapeutic Plasma Exchange As A Bridge To Total Thyroidectomy In Patients With Severe Thyrotoxicosis. Aace Clin Case Rep 2020; 6:e14.

Myxedema Coma

Introduction and Epidemiology

It is defined as severe hypothyroidism characterized by hypothermia, altered mental state, and multi-organ dysfunction as a consequence of hypo functioning of organs. Hypothyroidism is four times more common in women than in men; 80 percent of cases of myxedema coma occur in females. Myxedema coma occurs almost exclusively in persons 60 years and older.

Risk factors [1]

- Severe long-standing hypothyroidism
- Infection
- Myocardial infarction
- Cold exposure
- Surgery
- Drugs such as amiodarone, anesthetic agents, narcotics, beta-blockers, lithium, diuretics, rifampicin, phenytoin, and phenothiazines

Clinical presentation [2-6]

1. Decreased mental state, lethargy, obtundation
2. Hypothermia
3. Hypotension
4. Bradycardia
5. Hyponatremia
6. Hypoglycemia
7. Hypoventilation
8. Puffiness of hands, face, thickened nose, swollen lips, enlarged tongue
9. Cardiovascular complications- congestive heart failure, decreased cardiac output

Following are the Organ Specific Manifestations of Hypothyroidism –

Cardiac Manifestations-

- Diastolic hypertension
- Hypotension, shock

- Arrhythmia and heart block
- Decreased myocardial contractility and reduced cardiac output
- EKG findings -Bradycardia, flattened T waves, low voltage, bundle branch blocks, and complete heart blocks
- Low voltage on EKG- pericardial effusion
- QT interval prolongations leading to "torsades de pointes,"

Neurological Manifestations

- Lethargy/coma
- Depression
- Disorientation
- Decreased deep tendon reflexes
- Psychosis, slow mentation, paranoia, and poor recall
- Status epilepticus

Respiratory Manifestations

- Hypoventilation
- Obstructive sleep apnea

Gastrointestinal Manifestations

- Abdominal pain, nausea, vomiting, ileus, anorexia, constipation, and ascites
- Ileus, megacolon
- Gastrointestinal bleeding

Renal and Electrolyte Manifestations

- Hyponatremia
- Decreased glomerular filtration rate
- Urinary retention

Hematologic Manifestations

Acquired von Willebrand syndrome type 1 and a decrease in factors V, VII, VIII, IX, and X

Diagnosis [2]

Any patient presenting with a depressed mental state or coma along with hypothermia, hyponatremia, and hypercapnia should be evaluated for myxedema coma.

Laboratory investigation [7]

In primary hypothyroidism, serum TSH concentration is very high and serum T4 is very low. Patients with central hypothyroidism have associated hypopituitarism along with secondary adrenal insufficiency.

Expected abnormalities in Routine investigations

- Anemia
- Elevated CPK
- Elevated creatinine
- Elevated transaminases
- Hypercapnia
- Hyperlipidemia
- Hypoglycemia
- Hyponatremia
- Hypoxia
- Leukopenia
- Respiratory acidosis

Diagnostic scoring system

There are 21 parameters which include the degree of hypothermia, lethargy, obtundation, stupor or coma, anorexia, reduced intestinal mobility/ paralytic ileus, presence of precipitating event, bradycardia, ECG changes, pericardial or pleural effusion, cardiomegaly or hypertension, hyponatremia, hypoglycemia, hypoxemia, hypercapnia or reduced GFR.

Treatment [8-12]

- Thyroid hormone – According to the most recent American Thyroid Association (ATA) guidelines- 200-400 mcg T4 intravenously followed by 1.6 mcg/kg/day, reduced to 75% when given IV as a preferred route (50-100 microgram until the patient can take orally).
- T3 intravenously can be given 5-20 mcg followed by 2.5-10 mcg every 8 hours
- Measure T4 and T3 every one to two days
- Once there is an improvement in mental state and cardiac and pulmonary function, it can be converted into oral dosing.
- Glucocorticoids – in view of the possibility of adrenal insufficiency, hydrocortisone can be initiated at 100 mg every eighth hour.

<u>Recent Updates –</u>

In 2017, a case report used a split dose of levothyroxine to 200 mcg LT4 every 8th hour in five consecutive doses (total dose of 1 mg). It was observed that it caused significant restoration of depleted thyroid status and clinical improvement within 48 hours after treatment initiation. [13] In 2019, another case report treated the patient with a combination of levothyroxine of 200 mcg with liothyronine 50 mcg for five days, with a successful improvement of the patient's condition, so some reports recommended starting with 200 to 300 mcg levothyroxine with 10 to 25 mcg liothyronine as an alternative initial treatment. [14]

Differential Diagnosis (15)

- Sepsis
- Shock
- Stroke
- Drug overdose
- Diabetic ketoacidosis
- Seizure
- Hypothermia

Reference

1. Yafit D, Carmel-Neiderman NN, Levy N, et al. Postoperative myxedema coma in patients undergoing major surgery: Case series. Auris Nasus Larynx 2019; 46:605.

2. Kwaku MP, Burman KD. Myxedema coma. J Intensive Care Med 2007; 22:224.

3. Jansen HJ, Doebé SR, Louwerse ES, et al. Status epilepticus caused by a myxoedema coma. Neth J Med 2006; 64:202.

4. Fjølner J, Søndergaard E, Kampmann U, Nielsen S. Complete recovery after severe myxoedema coma complicated by status epilepticus. BMJ Case Rep 2015; 2015.

5. Zwillich CW, Pierson DJ, Hofeldt FD, et al. Ventilatory control in myxedema and hypothyroidism. N Engl J Med 1975; 292:662.

6. Klein I. Thyroid hormone and the cardiovascular system. Am J Med 1990; 88:631.

7. Popoveniuc G, Chandra T, Sud A, et al. A diagnostic scoring system for myxedema coma. Endocr Pract 2014; 20:808.

8. Holvey dn, Goodner cj, Nicoloff jt, Dowling jt. Treatment of myxedema coma with intravenous thyroxine. Arch Intern Med 1964; 113:89.

9. Jonklaas J, Bianco AC, Bauer AJ, et al. Guidelines for the treatment of hypothyroidism: prepared by the american thyroid association task force on thyroid hormone replacement. Thyroid 2014; 24:1670.

10. Ladenson PW, Goldenheim PD, Ridgway EC. Rapid pituitary and peripheral tissue responses to intravenous L-triiodothyronine in hypothyroidism. J Clin Endocrinol Metab 1983; 56:1252.

11. Zaninovich AA, el Tamer E, el Tamer S, et al. Multicompartmental analysis of triiodothyronine kinetics in hypothyroid patients treated orally or intravenously with triiodothyronine. Thyroid 1994; 4:285.

12. Bigos ST, Ridgway EC, Kourides IA, Maloof F. Spectrum of pituitary alterations with mild and severe thyroid impairment. J Clin Endocrinol Metab 1978; 46:317.

13. Charoensri S, Sriphrapradang C, Nimitphong H. Split high-dose oral levothyroxine treatment as a successful therapy option in myxedema coma. Clin Case Rep. 2017 Oct;5(10):1706-1711.

14. Ueda K, Kiyota A, Tsuchida M, Okazaki M, Ozaki N. Successful treatment of myxedema coma with a combination of levothyroxine and liothyronine. Endocr J. 2019 May 28;66(5):469-474.

15. Mazonson PD, Williams ML, Cantley LK, Dalldorf FG, Utiger RD, Foster JR. Myxedema coma during long-term amiodarone therapy. Am J Med. 1984 Oct;77(4):751-4.

Diabetic Ketoacidosis and Hyperosmolar Hyperglycemic State

Diabetic Ketoacidosis (DKA) and Hyperosmolar hyperglycemic state (HHS) are one of the most serious complications of diabetes mellitus

DKA is characterized by severe hyperglycemia and ketoacidosis, whereas HHS has more severe hyperglycemia without ketoacidosis.

Precipitating factors (1-2)

1. Infections (pneumonia, urinary tract infections)
2. Myocardial infarction, cerebrovascular accident, sepsis, pancreatitis
3. Nonadherence to medication
4. Cocaine use (4)
5. Sodium-glucose Cotransporter 2 (SGLT-2) inhibitors associated with DKA. (5)
6. Non-adherence to insulin
7. Psychological problems including eating disorders (3)
8. Malfunctioning continuous insulin infusion pump

Clinical presentation

1. DKA has more rapid progression whereas HHS develops as a more insidious course.
2. The earliest symptoms can be polyurea polydipsia and polyphagia
3. Neurological manifestations can be in the form of lethargy, obtundation, and focal signs. Coma is a severe manifestation. Both mental obtundation and coma are more common in patients with HHS as compared to DKA. (6)
4. Gastrointestinal manifestations like nausea, vomiting, and abdominal pain (7)

Physical examination

Signs of volume depletion are common in both DKA and HHS. They include decreased skin turgor, dry axilla and oral mucosa, low jugular venous pressure, tachycardia, hypertension

Table 2:

	Plasma glucose (mg/dl)	Arterial pH	Serum bicarbonate (mEq/l)	Urine ketone	Serum osmolarity	Anion gap
DKA						
Mild	>250	7.25- 7.30	15-18	Positive	Variable	>10
Moderate	>250	7- 7.24	10-15	Positive	Variable	>12
Severe	>250	<7.0	<10	Positive	Variable	>12
HHS	>600	> 7.30	>18	Small	>320	Variable

Management

1. Give 0.9% saline, 15 to 20 ml/kg/hr for the first few hours. (8)
2. Once the intravascular volume is restored, start 0.45% saline at the rate of 4 to 14 ml/kg/hour
3. Add glucose when blood sugar reaches 200 milligram/dl.
4. If potassium is less than 3.3 mEq/L, start potassium infusion at the rate of 20-40 mEq/hr IV infusion.
5. If potassium is between 3.3 to 5.3 mEq/L, give potassium 20 to 30 mEq/L IV fluid and maintain potassium between 4-5 mEq/L.
6. Do not give potassium when serum potassium is more than 5.3 mEq/L.
7. Omit insulin when serum potassium is less than 3.3 mEq/L.
8. When potassium is more than 3.3 mEq/L, 0.1 units/kg IV bolus to be given followed by 0.1 units/kg/hour. (9)
9. If the serum glucose does not fall by 50-70 mg/dl, double the dose of insulin infusion.
10. When blood sugar reaches 200 mg/dl, decrease the infusion rate to 0.02 to 0.05 units/kg/hr.
11. Insulin infusion should be continued till ketoacidosis is resolved.
12. Sodium bicarbonate is only indicated when arterial pH is lesser than 6.9.

Converting IV insulin to subcutaneous dosing

In patients with newer onset of type 1 diabetes mellitus, the total dose of subcutaneous insulin (0.5 unit/kg) can be divided into 50% basal and 50% pre-meal regular insulin. It should be converted when ketoacidosis resolves and the patient starts taking orally.

Complications of DKA and HHS [11, 12]

- Hypoglycemia and hypokalemia due to an overzealous treatment of insulin and bicarbonate.
- Hyperchloremic acidosis can occur as a consequence of loss of a large amount of ketoanions and also infusion of excess chloride containing fluids.

- 0.7 to 1 % of children with new-onset diabetes mellitus present with cerebral edema.

- Headache is the most common manifestation of cerebral edema. It is characterized by sudden alteration in the level of consciousness, lethargy, and coma.

- Other manifestations include seizures, pupillary changes, urinary incontinence, bradycardia, and respiratory depression or arrest. Mannitol infusion should to be initiated in those patients.

Euglycemic Diabetic Ketoacidosis (EDKA)

It was first described by Munro et al. It is characterized by ketonuria and high anion gap metabolic acidosis with normoglycemia. Patients with type 1 diabetes mellitus, Latent Autoimmune Diabetes in Adults (LADA), type 2 diabetes mellitus on SGLT-2 inhibitors, pregnancy, alcoholism, and severe liver disease are at increased risk of Euglycemic diabetic ketoacidosis. Most of the patients are young.

Landmark trials on the association of SGLT-2 inhibitors use in EDKA in type 1 DM

- 'EASE' TRIAL – SGLT-2 inhibitor used was empagliflozin. [13]
- DEPICIT-1 and 2 – Dapagliflozin was the used agent. The reported event rate per 1000 patient-year was 58.3 and 47.6 events. [14, 15]
- 52 week and 24 week study – Dapagliflozin 5mg and 10 mg were used. The reported event rate per 1000 patient-year was 58.3 and 47.6 percent. [16,17]
- TANDEM-1 and 2 study – Sotagliflozin 200 mg and 400 mg were used. The reported event rate per 1000 patient-year was 30-34 events. [18,19]
- FAERS DATA – Canagliflozin, empagliflozin, and dapagliflozin drugs were compared. [9]

Pathophysiology of EDKA on SGLT-2 inhibitors

The lower insulin to glucagon ratio stimulates lipolysis at the expense of reduced carbohydrate oxidation. Increased lipolysis and decreased insulin levels favour ketogenesis and ketosis. SGLT-2 inhibitors lead to increased glucosuria and decreased serum glucose.

Differential diagnosis of DKA/ HHS/ EDKA [19]

- Lactic acidosis
- Alcoholic ketoacidosis
- Salicylate poisoning
- Paracetamol overdose
- Toxic substance ingestion
- Stroke
- Uremic acidosis

Markers of severity defining HDU/ ICU admission in patients with DKA/ HHS/ EDKA

- Venous pH < 7.1

- Blood ketones > 6 mmol/l in DKA or >1 mmol/l in HHS.

- Sodium bicarbonate <5 mmol/l, anion gap >16 mmol/l.

- Potassium < 3.5 mmol/l or >6mmol/l.

- SBP < 90 mm Hg, Pulse rate >100 or <60 beats per minute.

- Urine output < 0.5 ml/kg/hr, evidence of AKI.

- Mental status- GCS <12; SpO_2 <92%

- Sodium > 160 mmol/l; osmolality >350 mOsm/kg in HHS.

- Comorbidities such as hypothermia, ACS, stroke.

CLINICAL PEARLS

As per NICE-SUGAR trial in 2009, an increased mortality risk was observed in patients with intensive insulin therapy in critically ill patients. (20) Iatrogenic hypoglycemia risk was highlighted by various randomized trials. In 2009, an ADA and American Association of Clinical Endocrinologists (AACE) task force recommended a target glucose of 7.8–10.0 mmol/L (140–180 mg/dL) in patients in critical care settings. Similar guidelines have come up by the Society of Critical Care Medicine with a target blood glucose concentration of 8.3 mmol/L (150 mg/dL) or higher, thus minimizing the risk of hypoglycemia. (22) Subcutaneous sliding scale insulin or correctional insulin, used to treat hyperglycemia after it has already occurred, is widely used in some hospitals despite condemnation in clinical guidelines. The use of sliding scale insulin is associated with clinically significant hyperglycemia in many patients, and its use has been discouraged.

Figure 1: Non critically ill patients with diabetes

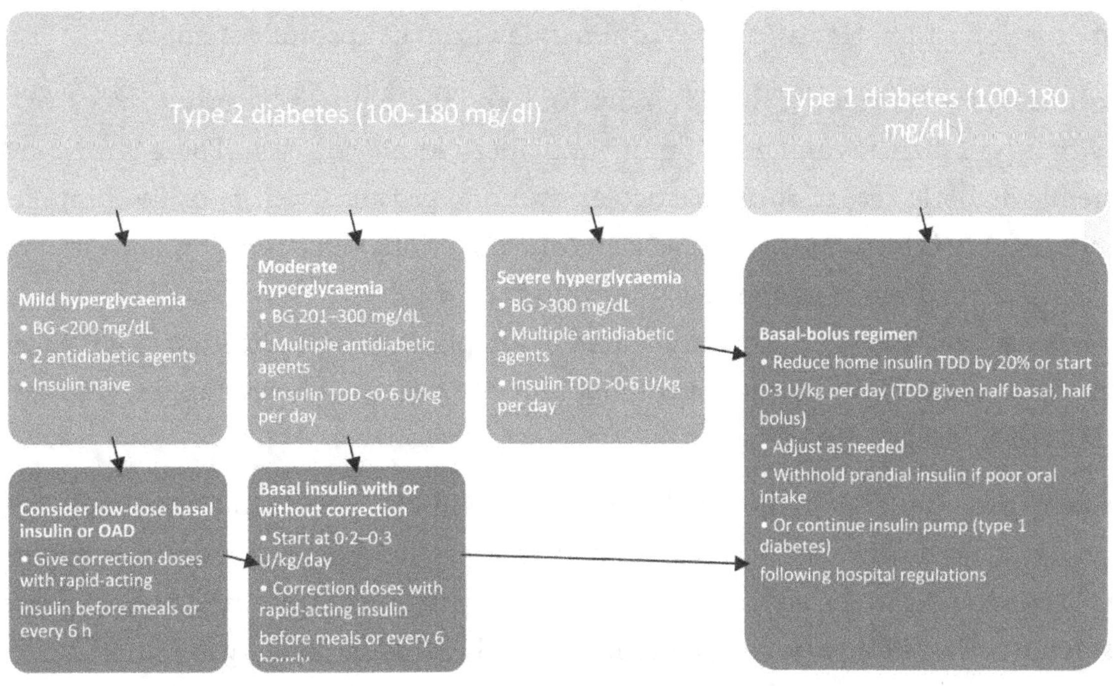

Figure 2: Critically ill patients with diabetes

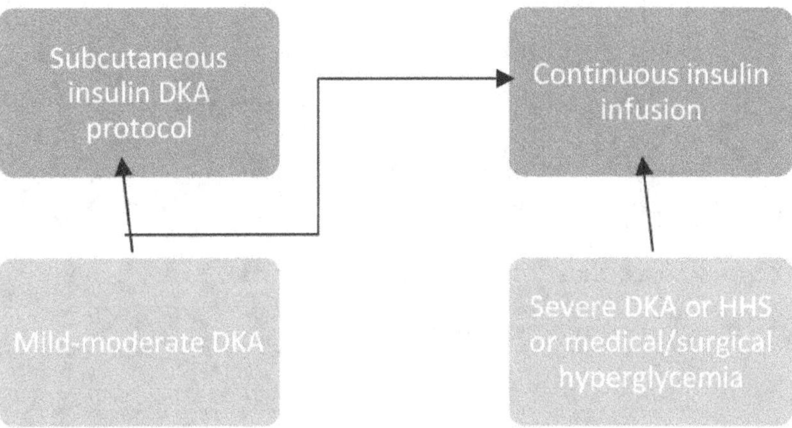

Non-insulin drugs (23-28)

Metformin – Dose modification is required if the estimated glomerular filtration rate (eGFR) is 30–45 mL/min per 1·73 m². However, metformin should be stopped if the eGFR is below 30 mL/min per 1·73 m². Metformin increases the risk for lactic acidosis (i.e., acute kidney injury, hypoxia, shock). It should be discontinued before an iodinated contrast imaging procedure in patients with reduced eGFR.

Sulfonylureas – Hypoglycemia is the most common reported complication of sulfonylureas. It is more commonly associated with older age, concurrent treatment with insulin, and renal impairment. Professional societies recommend against the use of sulfonylureas in the hospital because of the potential risk of sustained hypoglycemia.

Thiazolidinediones – There is a potential risk of fluid retention and risk of heart failure, as well as delayed onset of action. Hence, not a recommended drug in hospital settings.

SGLT2 inhibitors – Currently, SGLT2 inhibitors are the glucose-lowering drugs of choice in patients with type 2 diabetes and heart failure or diabetic kidney disease. There is an increased risk of euglycaemic diabetic ketoacidosis (particularly among patients with poor food intake) and the risk of genitourinary infections (particularly mycotic infections). In a recent pilot randomized trial, empagliflozin did not improve dyspnoea, N-terminal pro-B-type natriuretic peptide concentrations, diuretic response, or length of stay compared with placebo. However, empagliflozin use was associated with a reduction in a combined endpoint of worsening heart failure, rehospitalization for heart failure, or death at 60 days.

DPP-4 inhibitors – DPP-4 inhibitors have been found to be well-tolerated and effective for glycaemic control, with a low risk of hypoglycemia in patients with mild-to-moderate hyperglycemia. They have been reported to be effective alone or in combination with basal insulin in patients with type 2 diabetes with mild hyperglycemia unit change in HbA1c (odds ratio 1·3, 95% CI 1·2–1·5).

Linagliptin results in a substantial reduction in the incidence of hypoglycemia compared with basal-bolus therapy (2 [2%] of 128 vs. 14 [11%] of 122; p=0·001; 86% relative risk reduction). Similar results were reported in a study of saxagliptin versus basal-bolus therapy in patients with type 2 diabetes with very mild hyperglycemia.

GLP-1 receptor agonists- Recent guidelines have recommended the use of GLP-1 receptor agonists as first-line drugs in patients with type 2 diabetes and established atherosclerotic cardiovascular disease.82 Both GLP-1 receptor agonists and native GLP-1 have been tested in the inpatient setting.

Reference

1. Kitabchi AE, Ayyagari V, Guerra SM. The efficacy of low-dose versus conventional therapy of insulin for treatment of diabetic ketoacidosis. Ann Intern Med 1976; 84:633.

2. Wolfsdorf J, Glaser N, Sperling MA, American Diabetes Association. Diabetic ketoacidosis in infants, children, and adolescents: A consensus statement from the American Diabetes Association. Diabetes Care 2006; 29:1150.

3. Rosenstock J, Marquard J, Laffel LM, et al. Empagliflozin as Adjunctive to Insulin Therapy in Type 1 Diabetes: The EASE Trials. Diabetes Care 2018; 41(12): 2560–9.

4. Dandona P, Mathieu C, Phillip M, et al. Efficacy and safety of dapagliflozin in patients with inadequately controlled type 1 diabetes (DEPICT-1): 24 week results from a multicentre, double-blind, phase 3, randomised controlled trial. Lancet Diabetes Endocrinol 2017; 5(11): 864–76.

5. Dandona P, Mathieu C, Phillip M, et al. Efficacy and Safety of Dapagliflozin in Patients With Inadequately Controlled Type 1 Diabetes: The DEPICT-1 52-Week Study. Diabetes Care 2018; 41(12): 2552–9. [PubMed] [Google Scholar]

6. Mathieu C, Dandona P, Gillard P, et al. Efficacy and Safety of Dapagliflozin in Patients With Inadequately Controlled Type 1 Diabetes (the DEPICT-2 Study): 24-Week Results From a Randomized Controlled Trial. Diabetes Care 2018; 41(9): 1938–46.

7. Buse JB, Garg SK, Rosenstock J, et al. Sotagliflozin in Combination With Optimized Insulin Therapy in Adults With Type 1 Diabetes: The North American inTandem1 Study. Diabetes Care 2018; 41(9): 1970–80.

8. Danne T, Cariou B, Banks P, et al. HbA1c and Hypoglycemia Reductions at 24 and 52 Weeks With Sotagliflozin in Combination With Insulin in Adults With Type 1 Diabetes: The European inTandem2 Study. Diabetes Care. 2018;41(9):1981-1990.

9. Blau JE, Tella SH, Taylor SI, Rother KI. Ketoacidosis associated with SGLT2 inhibitor treatment: Analysis of FAERS data. Diabetes Metab Res Rev. 2017;33(8):10.1002/dmrr.2924.

10. Shah P, Isley WL. Ketoacidosis during a low-carbohydrate diet. N Engl J Med 2006; 354:97.

11. Kitabchi AE, Umpierrez GE, Miles JM, Fisher JN. Hyperglycemic crises in adult patients with diabetes. Diabetes Care. 2009 Jul;32(7):1335-43. doi: 10.2337/dc09-9032. PMID: 19564476; PMCID: PMC2699725.

12. Kitabchi AE, Razavi L.Hyperglycemic Crises: Diabetic Ketoacidosis (DKA), And Hyperglycemic Hyperosmolar State (HHS). In: http://www.endotext.org/diabetes/diabetes24/ diabetesframe24.htm (Accessed on January 30, 2013)

13. Randall L, Begovic J, Hudson M, Smiley D, Peng L, Pitre N, Umpierrez D, Umpierrez G. Recurrent diabetic ketoacidosis in inner-city minority patients: behavioral, socioeconomic, and psychosocial factors. Diabetes Care. 2011 Sep;34(9):1891-6. doi: 10.2337/dc11-0701. Epub 2011 Jul 20. PMID: 21775761; PMCID: PMC3161256.

14. Warner EA, Greene GS, Buchsbaum MS, Cooper DS, Robinson BE. Diabetic ketoacidosis associated with cocaine use. Arch Intern Med. 1998 Sep 14;158(16):1799-802. doi: 10.1001/ archinte.158.16.1799. PMID: 9738609.

15. Taylor SI, Blau JE, Rother KI. SGLT2 Inhibitors May Predispose to Ketoacidosis. J Clin Endocrinol Metab. 2015 Aug;100(8):2849-52. doi: 10.1210/jc.2015-1884. Epub 2015 Jun 18. PMID: 26086329; PMCID: PMC4525004.

16. Lorber D. Nonketotic hypertonicity in diabetes mellitus. Med Clin North Am. 1995 Jan;79(1):39-52. doi: 10.1016/s0025-7125(16)30083-9. PMID: 7808094.

17. Umpierrez G, Freire AX. Abdominal pain in patients with hyperglycemic crises. J Crit Care. 2002 Mar;17(1):63-7. doi: 10.1053/jcrc.2002.33030. PMID: 12040551.

18. Kitabchi AE, Umpierrez GE, Miles JM, Fisher JN. Hyperglycemic crises in adult patients with diabetes. Diabetes Care. 2009 Jul;32(7):1335-43. doi: 10.2337/dc09-9032. PMID: 19564476; PMCID: PMC2699725.

19. Beigelman PM. Potassium in severe diabetic ketoacidosis. Am J Med. 1973 Apr;54(4):419-20. doi: 10.1016/0002-9343(73)90037-5. PMID: 4633105.

20. The NICE-SUGAR Study Investigators. Intensive versus conventional glucose control in critically ill patients. N Engl J Med 2009; 360: 1283–97

21. Moghissi ES, Korytkowski MT, DiNardo M, et al. American Association of Clinical Endocrinologists and American Diabetes Association consensus statement on inpatient glycemic control. Diabetes Care 2009; 32: 1119–31.

22. Jacobi J, Bircher N, Krinsley J, et al. Guidelines for the use of an insulin infusion for the management of hyperglycemia in critically ill patients. Crit Care Med 2012; 40: 3251–76.

23. Satpathy SV, Datta S, Upreti B. Utilization study of antidiabetic agents in a teaching hospital of Sikkim and adherence to current standard treatment guidelines. J Pharm Bioallied Sci 2016; 8: 223–28.

24. Montejano L, Vo L, McMorrow D. Transitions of care for people with type 2 diabetes: utilization of antihyperglycemic agents pre- and post-hospitalization. Diabetes Ther 2016; 7: 91–103.

25. Bolen S, Feldman L, Vassy J, et al. Systematic review: comparative effectiveness and safety of oral medications for type 2 diabetes mellitus. Ann Intern Med 2007; 147: 386–99.

26. Damman K, Beusekamp JC, Boorsma EM, et al. Randomized, double-blind, placebo-controlled, multicentre pilot study on the effects of empagliflozin on clinical outcomes in patients with acute decompensated heart failure (EMPA-RESPONSE-AHF). Eur J Heart Fail 2020; 22: 713–22.

27. Pasquel FJ, Gomez-Huelgas R, Anzola I, et al. Predictive value of admission hemoglobin A1c on inpatient glycemic control and response to insulin therapy in medicine and surgery patients with type 2 diabetes. Diabetes Care 2015; 38: e202–03.

28. Nyström T, Gutniak MK, Zhang Q, et al. Effects of glucagon-like peptide-1 on endothelial function in type 2 diabetes patients with stable coronary artery disease. Am J Physiol Endocrinol Metab 2004; 287: E1209–15

Adrenal Insufficiency

Introduction

The clinical presentation of adrenal insufficiency can be variable. The clinical presentation can be acute in the form of adrenal crisis and chronic, when the symptoms are more insidious in onset.

Causes of primary adrenal insufficiency

I. Addison disease

- Autoimmune adrenalitis
- Isolated adrenal insufficiency
- Polyglandular autoimmune syndrome type-I
- Polyglandular autoimmune syndrome type-II

II. Infections adrenalitis

- Tuberculosis, Disseminated fungal infection, HIV and AIDS, syphilis

III. Metastatic or cancer

IV. Adrenal hemorrhage of infection ketoconazole, fluconazole, rifampicin, phenytoin, barbiturates.

V. Others

- Congenital adrenal hypoplasia
- Familial glucocorticoid deficiency
- Familial glucocorticoid resistance

Causes of secondary Adrenal insufficiency

I. Panhypopituitarism

- Mass lesions
- Post- radiation
- Infiltrative - sarcoidosis, Langerhans cell histiocytosis
- Infection - tuberculum meningitis
- others - Traumatic brain injury stroke.
- Apoplexy
- Empty Sella syndrome
- Pituitary, infarction - Sheehan's syndrome

- Pituitary surgery
- Pituitary radiation
- hypophysitis /Hemochromatosis

II. Isolated ACTH deficiency

III. Autoimmune causes

IV. Mutation in POMC gene

V. TPIT gene mentation

VI. Traumatic brain injury

VII. Drugs like High dose progestins and opiates

Causes of Tertiary Adrenal Insufficiency

- Abrupt Cessation of high dose glucocorticoid therapy
- correction (cure) of hypercortisolism (Cushing's syndrome)

Clinical manifestations

- Adrenal crisis
  - Anorexia
  - nausea
  - vomiting
  - abdominal pain
  - weakness, fatigue, lethargy, fever, confusion, coma
- Common features of chronic primary adrenal insufficiency
  - Fatigue
  - weight loss,
  - nausea, vomiting, abdominal pain
  - muscle and joint pain
  - skin hyperpigmentation due to increased production of proopiomelanocortin (POMC)
  - Postural hypotension
  - salt cravings
- Hyperpigmentation is more prominent on the face, back of the hand and neck, and areas exposed to chronic friction such as elbows, knees, spine, waist, shoulders, midriff. Other areas of hyperpigmentation are the outer border of lips, patchy pigmentation on the inner lip, and buccal mucosa along the line of dental occlusion. Existing freckles may become dark, scars may get darkened, and generalized buccal, vaginal or mucosal membrane hyperpigmentation.

Precipitating factors

Serious infection, major stress, insufficient daily doses of glucocorticoid therapy, failure to take more glucocorticoid therapy during infection or major illness, or persistent vomiting or dose shoots leading to decreased absorption.

Laboratory findings

The most common laboratory findings are hyponatremia, hyperkalemia, and hypoglycemia. Psychiatry manifestations in the form of confusion, delirium, and stupor may also occur.

Laboratory Investigations

1. serum cortisol concentration

    Caution should be taken while interpreting the results in patients with abnormalities of cortisol binding proteins, nephrotic syndrome, cirrhosis, and those taking estrogen.

    Serum cortisol is highest at 6:00 am, ranging from 10 to 20 mcg/dl. Demonstration of low serum cortisol (less than 3meg/dl) strongly suggests adrenal insufficiency.

2. Morning salivary cortisol concentration.

3. Afternoon serum cortisol concentration - at 4:00 pm (serum cortisol ranges from 3 to 10 mcg/dl)

4. Subnormal response to ACTH stimulation

    Short ACTH stimulation test - synthetic ACTH (1-24) (cosyntropin) is used as per endocrine society 2016 clinical practice guidelines, 250mcg IV standard high dose test is used.

Figure 4: Short ACTH stimulation test

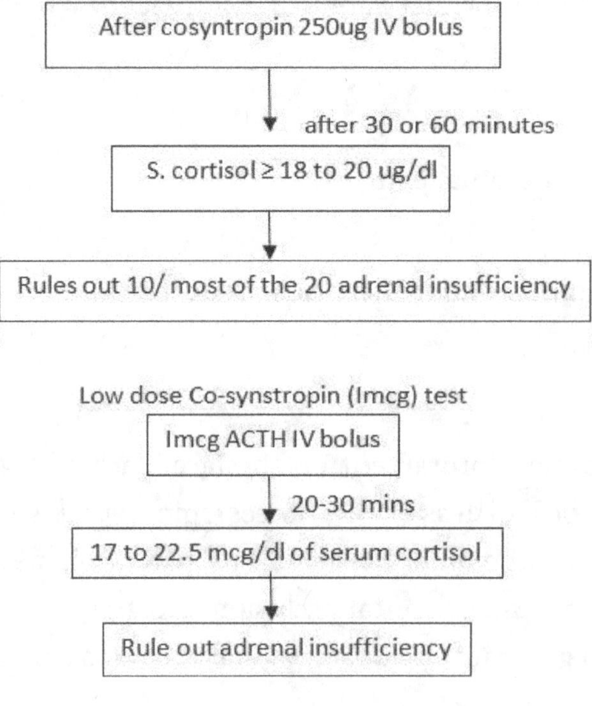

5. Other tests - Basal plasma ACTH, Serum, aldosterone concentration, response to prolonged ACTH stimulation, prolonged ACTH Stimulation, metyrapone tests insulin induced hypoglycemia test, Co-syntrophin releasing hormone test.

Treatment of Acute adrenal insufficiency

1. Establish intravenous access with a large-gauge needle
2. Measure serum electrolyte, glucose, plasma cortisol, ACTH
3. Give isotonic saline 2-3 litres or 5% dextrose in isotonic saline as quickly as possible.
4. Give hydrocortisone (100mg intravenous bolus) following by 50 mg intravenously every 6th hours
5. It hydrocortisone is enviable, alt relatives include prednisolone, prednisolone and dexamethasone
6. search and triggers of adrenal rises in the form of infectious diseases.
7. Determine the type of adrenal insufficiency
8. Tape parenteral glucocorticoid over 1 to 3 days, once the patient stabilizes.
9. Perform a short ACTH stimulation test to confirm the diagnosis of adrenal insufficiency
10. Begin mineralocorticoid replacement with fludrocortisone 0.1 mg orally in patients with primary adrenal insufficiency once. saline infusion is slopped.

Endocrine and Haematology landmark trials

1. SCOPE-DKA: Normal Saline vs Plasmalyte in Severe DKA-In this trial, it was evaluated that if administration of plasmalyte result in faster resolution of critically ill patients with severe DKA and not increase ketone generation compared to the administration of sodium chloride. The Outcomes of the study were

Primary

Change in base excess to $\geq$ -3 mEq/L at 48-hours post ICU admission

Sensitivity analyses for primary outcome were the following:

Change in base excess to $\geq$ -3 mEq/L at 24-hours post ICU admission

DKA resolution at 24-hours post ICU admission per American Diabetes Association criteria:

Plasma glucose < 11.1 mmol/L and two of the following:

Bicarbonate $\geq$ 15 mmol/L

Venous pH > 7.3

Anion gap $\leq$ 12 mEq/L

Secondary

- ICU mortality and length of stay
- Hospital mortality and length of stay
- Organ support (ie. invasive and non-invasive ventilation, CRRT)
- Cumulative urine output and fluid balance at 24-, 48- and 72-hours post-ICU admission
- Biochemical outcomes (ie. serum potassium, chloride, pH, pCO_2, base excess, anion gap, blood glucose and ketone concentrations) at 6-, 12-, 18-, 24-, 36-, 48- and 72-hours post-ICU admission
- The authors concluded that plasmalyte-148, compared to sodium chloride 0.9%, may lead to faster resolution of metabolic acidosis in patients with DKA without an increase in ketosis. These findings need confirmation in a large, Phase 3 trial.

2. **The PLUS Trial – Balanced vs Unbalanced Fluids in the Critically Ill- The trial studied if** balanced multicelctrolyte solutions (BMES) reduce death in critically ill patients in the ICU vs 0.9% saline solution. The **Outcomes of the study were**

   - **Primary:** Death from any cause within 90 days after randomization
   - **Secondary:**
     - Receipt of new renal replacement therapy
     - Maximum increase in creatinine level during ICU stay

       The authors concluded that no evidence exists that the risk of death or acute kidney injury among critically ill adults in the ICU was lower the use of BMES than with saline."

3. Andexanet Alfa Vs. Four-Factor PCC: Is Andexanet Alfa Worth The Hype?- How does andexanet alfa compare to four-factor PCC in the treatment of patients with FXi associated intracranial hemorrhage?

   - This is a retrospective observational study done at a single center
   - Included a consecutive series of adult patients admitted to Yale New Haven Health System from July 2018 to April 2019 presenting with life-threatening ICH in the setting of oral FXi therapy.
   - Patients were treated with one dose of either AA or 4F-PCC
   - Patients had a CT scan at 6 and 24 hours post-administration of AA or 4F-PCC

Outcomes measured were

- **_Primary outcome:_** Stable head CT at 6 hours and 24 hours post-administration of reversal agent

- Defined as
  - No significant increase in volume of bleed (<6mL or 33% from baseline volume) for IPH
  - Stable CT as determined by "an experienced provider" for all other bleeds
- ***Secondary outcomes:***
  - Good functional outcome at discharge (Modified Rankin Score of 0-3)
  - In-hospital thrombotic events after reversal therapy
  - Short-term mortality (in-hospital mortality or discharge to hospice)
  - Length of stay (hospital and ICU)
  - Disposition on discharge

The author concluded that there was no significant difference in the degree of achieved hemostasis based on CT stability, functional outcomes at discharge and thrombotic events during admission when comparing AA and 4F-PCC for the reversal of oral FXi in the setting of ICH.

References

1. Ramanan M, Attokaran A, Murray L, Bhadange N, Stewart D, Rajendran G, Pusapati R, Petty M, Garrett P, Kruger P, Peake S, Billot L, Venkatesh B; SCOPE-DKA Collaborators and Queensland Critical Care Research Network (QCCRN). Sodium chloride or Plasma Lyte-148 evaluation in severe diabetic ketoacidosis (SCOPE-DKA): a cluster, crossover, randomized, controlled trial. Intensive Care Med. 2021 Nov;47(11):1248-1257. doi: 10.1007/s00134-021-06480-5. Epub 2021 Oct 5. PMID: 34609547.

2. Hammond NE, Bellomo R, Gallagher M, Gattas D, Glass P, Mackle D, Micallef S, Myburgh J, Saxena M, Taylor C, Young P, Finfer S. The Plasma-Lyte 148 v Saline (PLUS) study protocol: a multicentre, randomised controlled trial of the effect of intensive care fluid therapy on mortality. Crit Care Resusc. 2017 Sep;19(3):239-246. PMID: 28866974.

3. Stevens VM, Trujillo TC, Kiser TH, MacLaren R, Reynolds PM, Mueller SW. Retrospective Comparison of Andexanet Alfa and 4-Factor Prothrombin Complex for Reversal of Factor Xa-Inhibitor Related Bleeding. Clin Appl Thromb Hemost. 2021 Jan-Dec;27:10760296211039020. doi: 10.1177/10760296211039020. PMID: 34541920; PMCID: PMC864

Nerve Blocks in Emergency

Contributors

1. Dr. Rohan Bhatia,
2. Dr. Ruhi Vaid

Contents

1. US guided nerve blocks
2. Lower extremity Blocks
3. Upper extremity blocks
4. Chest blocks

US Guided Nerve Blocks

INTRODUCTION

Recent advances in various surgical techniques and the development of more minimally invasive procedures lead to an increase in outpatient procedures. With these developments, it requires that analgesic techniques keep pace with these surgical advancements. Studies have shown that nerve blocks are usually well-tolerated and provide regional analgesia superior to other modalities such as oral pain medications or general anesthesia in emergency department.(2,3)

Pain management is an important but often challenging task for emergency people.Patients often receive suboptimal pain management in the Emergency department.Ultrasound-guided nerve blocks offer effective and safe alternatives to systemic analgesics to manage pain. Studies have shown that with good training, emergency providers can perform nerve blocks successfully in both pediatric and adult patients. Ultrasound-guided nerve blocks also can be performed quickly and require only basic equipment that is already available in most emergency departments. Most importantly, the administration of nerve blocks for some injuries (hip fractures) is associated with improved analgesia, decreased intravenous narcotic use, and improved morbidity and mortality when compared to use of intravenous analgesics alone.

PATIENT SELECTION

Ultrasound-guided nerve blocks are safe and effective in most patients, including children. In addition, given that they require minimal supplies, ultrasound-guided nerve blocks can be performed in a variety of settings, including in calamity. An important contraindication to nerve blocks is allergy to local anesthetic and patient refusal.

<u>Nerve blocks should be performed only on</u>:

- Awake and alert patients.
- Patients should understand the risks and benefits of the nerve block, provide consent, and be able to report any pain or paresthesia during the nerve block.
- Patients should be able to report unpredicted changes in sensory function.
- Some blocks are technically challenging and require that the patient remain still and follow instructions.

Taking a detailed medical history is necessary to determine conditions like coagulopathy or respiratory compromise that may impact the decision to perform a block. A thorough physical exam is necessary to determine pre existing sensory or motor deficits in the distribution of the block. Studies show that patients with preexisting sensory or motor deficits are more likely to develop new deficits following a block than patients without pre existing deficits. Following the history and physical, the patient should be made familiar with the risks, benefits, and care needed during the recovery phase of the block.

Also, intravenous access should be obtained due to the risk of potential complications like vasovagal events, local anesthetic toxicity, and the possible use of general anesthetics.

<u>GENERAL TECHNIQUE</u>

Prior to starting any nerve block, adjust the height of the bed and position the patient and ultrasound machine to facilitate the procedure. Identify the nerve on ultrasound at the anticipated site of injection and then follow the nerve both proximally and distally.

Equipment Required to Perform an Ultrasound-guided Nerve Block

- Ultrasound machine with probe (usually a high-frequency linear probe)
- Sterile ultrasound probe cover and gel
- Sterile gloves
- Skin disinfectant and antiseptic (e.g., chlorhexidine or povidone-iodine)
- Local anesthetic
- Syringe (size will depend on type of block being performed)
- 18-gauge needle to draw up anesthetic
- 25- to 30-gauge needle to place skin wheal
- Blunt needle for nerve block

A rapid-onset, short-acting anesthetic, such as lidocaine, is adequate for quick procedures, such as suturing or reductions. Long-acting anesthetics, such as bupivacaine and ropivacaine, are preferred to manage pain associated with fractures, including hip fractures. Remember, mepivacaine and bupivacaine may cross the placenta and are contraindicated in pregnancy.

Common Anesthetics Used to Perform Nerve Blocks

Anesthetic	Onset Time	Duration	Maximum Dose (maximum total)
3% 2-Chloroprocaine	5-10 min	≤ 1 hour	11 mg/kg (800 mg)
1% Lidocaine without epinephrine	1-2 min	≤ 1 hour	4 mg/kg (300 mg)
1% Lidocaine with epinephrine	1-2 min	2 hours	7 mg/kg (500 mg)
1.5% Mepivacaine	3-20 min	2-3 hours	7 mg/kg (400 mg)
0.5% Bupivacaine	2-10 min	2-6 hours	2 mg/kg (175 mg)
1% Ropivacaine	15-30 min	4-8 hour	3 mg/kg (300mg)

- Documentation

All ultrasound-guided nerve blocks require proper documentation in the medical record. This includes the clinical examinations pre and post the nerve blocks, sterile preparation, the type and amount of anesthetic used, the time of injection (to monitor longer blocks), and any complications.

<u>Ultrasound-Guided Nerve Blocks-</u> Nerve blocks are a simple-to-learn, non-opioid analgesic technique that can result in optimal pain management for the acutely injured patient.

Ultrasound-Guided Regional Nerve Blocks	
Nerve Block	**Injury/Affected Tissue**
Lower Extremities	
Tibial	Calcaneal fracture, foreign body/laceration to the sole
Distal Sciatic in the Popliteal Fossa	Ankle dislocation, Achilles tendon rupture
Superficial Peroneal	Dorsal lateral foot
Femoral	Hip/femur/proximal tibia fractures, patellar subluxation, anteromedial thigh abscess/laceration
Head/Neck	
Superficial Cervical	Clavicle fracture, IJ central line placement, submandibular abscess, lateral neck laceration
Greater Auricular	Laceration/abscess to ear lobe
Trunk	
Supraclavicular Brachial Plexus	Elbow or wrist dislocation
Serratus Anterior Plane	Acute anterior and lateral rib fractures, burns, chest wall abscesses, thoracic zoster
Interscalene	Shoulder dislocation
Transverse Abdominal Plane	Pre-procedural abdominal surgery
Dorsal Penile Nerve	Priapism, Paraphimosis

Femoral Nerve Block

Indication

The ultrasound-guided femoral nerve block is an ideal adjunct in the emergency department treatment of femoral neck, intertrochanteric and shaft fractures. This block will also provide analgesia for large thigh lacerations, abscesses, and even in knee injuries. Hip fractures are particularly ideal for performing a block, since most patients with this injury pattern are elderly.

Technique

Once the area is cleaned with chlorhexidine, place a 1-2 mL skin wheal of anesthetic lateral to the probe. Using an in-plane lateral to medial approach, advance the needle tip under the fascia iliaca (lateral to medial), and gently inject 1-2 mL of normal saline. Anechoic fluid should be visible spreading under the fascia iliaca. The anesthetic solution can then be gently injected after aspiration. The anechoic anesthetic should track under the fascia iliaca and toward the femoral nerve bundle. The fluid will separate the superficial adipose tissue from the femoral nerve that is adjacent to iliopsoas muscle.

Figure 1: The femoral nerve sits lateral to the femoral artery (FA) and under the fascia iliaca. Note the fascia iliaca holds the femoral nerve close to the iliopsoas muscle.

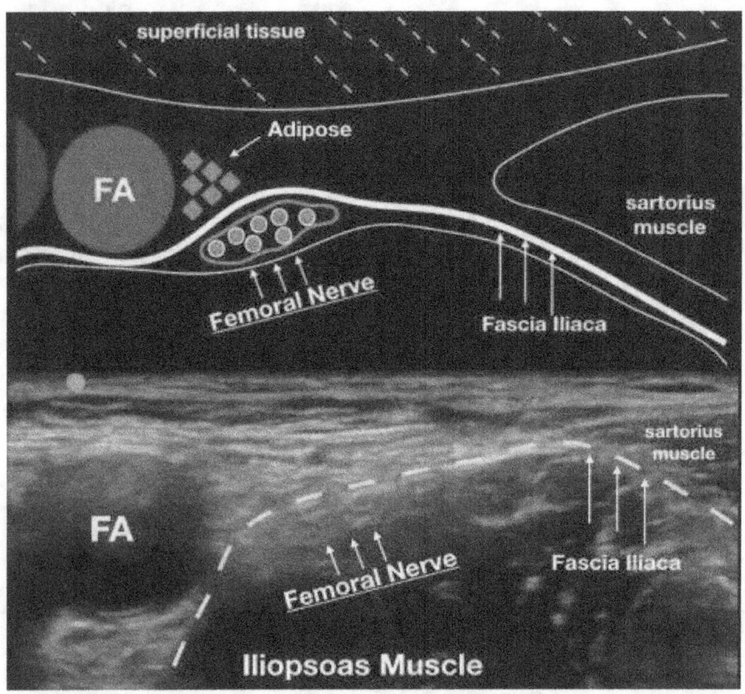

Figure 2: Anatomic landmarks for femoral nerve block. The needle insertion site (X) is located just below the inguinal crease, 1–2 cm lateral to the pulse of the femoral artery.

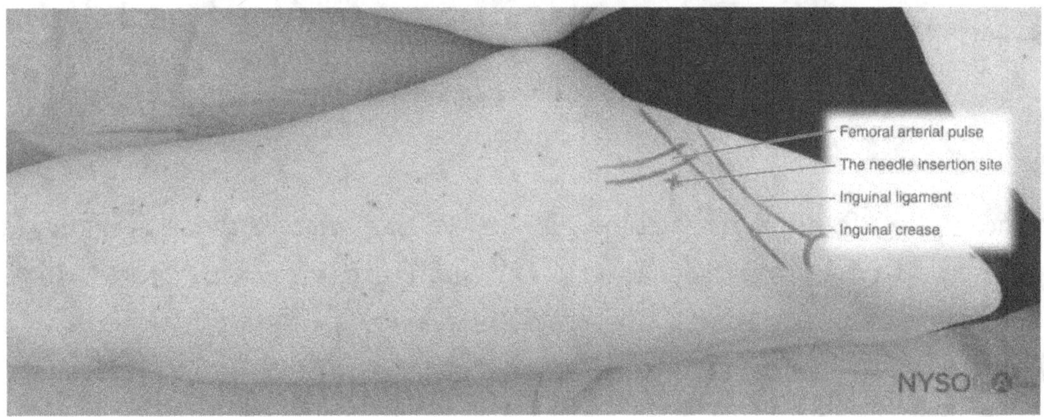

Fascia iliaca block:

The patient is placed in a supine position where using ultrasound, the probe is placed transversely to the leg at the junction of the middle and lateral thirds (between the ASIS and pubic tubercle) to identify the fascia lata, iliacus muscle, and fascia iliaca. The needle is introduced in-plane inferior to the inguinal ligament and guided beneath the fascia iliaca, and 30 cc of local anesthetic is injected in 5 cc increments. (fig3).Before injection, however, aspiration should be performed to ensure there is no blood.(2,5)

Figure 3: Sonoanatomy of infrainguinal approach to fascia iliaca compartment block. FA, femoral artery; FN, femoral nerve; FI, fascia iliaca; IM, iliacus muscle; IPM, iliopsoas muscle.

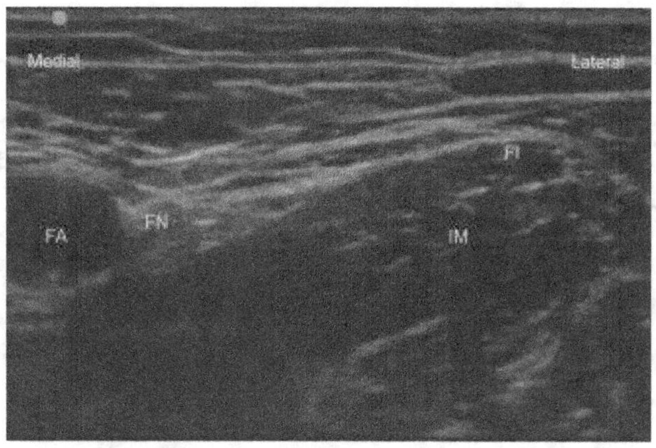

Obturator nerve block:

The patient is placed in the supine position with the leg externally rotated. Using an ultrasound probe, it is placed in the inguinal crease, and the femoral vein is identified. The probe is then moved medially to visualize the pectineus and adductor longus muscles. The needle is inserted in-plane or out of plane and is directed to the fascial plane between the adductor brevis and adductor magnus, and 5 cc to 10 cc of local anesthetic is injected. Before injection, aspiration should be performed to ensure there is no blood.

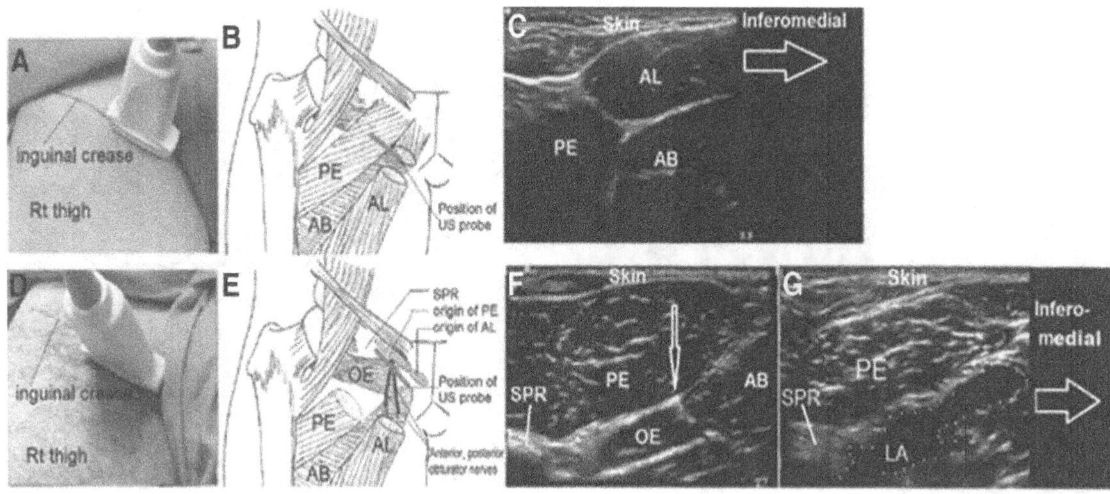

The ultrasound (US)-guided obturator nerve block technique. A and B, The US probe was placed on the medial aspect of the inguinal crease and aimed posteriorly. C, The letter Y and the pectineus (PE) muscle were identified. D and E, The US probe was tilted, while following the pectineus muscle, until the superior pubic ramus (SPR) was visualized (F). In this plane, a needle was advanced toward the most medial part (the arrow) of the fascia separating the pectineus and obturator externus (OE) muscles. G, LA was injected to achieve spread within the intermuscular fascial layer deep to the pectineus muscle. AB = adductor brevis; AL = adductor longus. SourceUltrasound-Guided Obturator Nerve Block: A Proximal Interfascial Technique Anesthesia & Analgesia114(1):236-239, January 2012.

Sciatic nerve block:

The patient is placed in the lateral decubitus position with the hip flexed at 45 degrees and the knee at 90 degrees for the posterior approach. The ultrasound probe is held transverse to the course of the nerve. The nerve is found lateral to the ischial tuberosity and deep to the gluteus maximus muscle. The needle is inserted in-plane from the lateral aspect of the transducer and positioned with the tip of the needle adjacent to the nerve as shown in fig(4,5). About 20 cc of local anesthetic is injected with gentle aspirations between injections, to ensure that there is no blood.

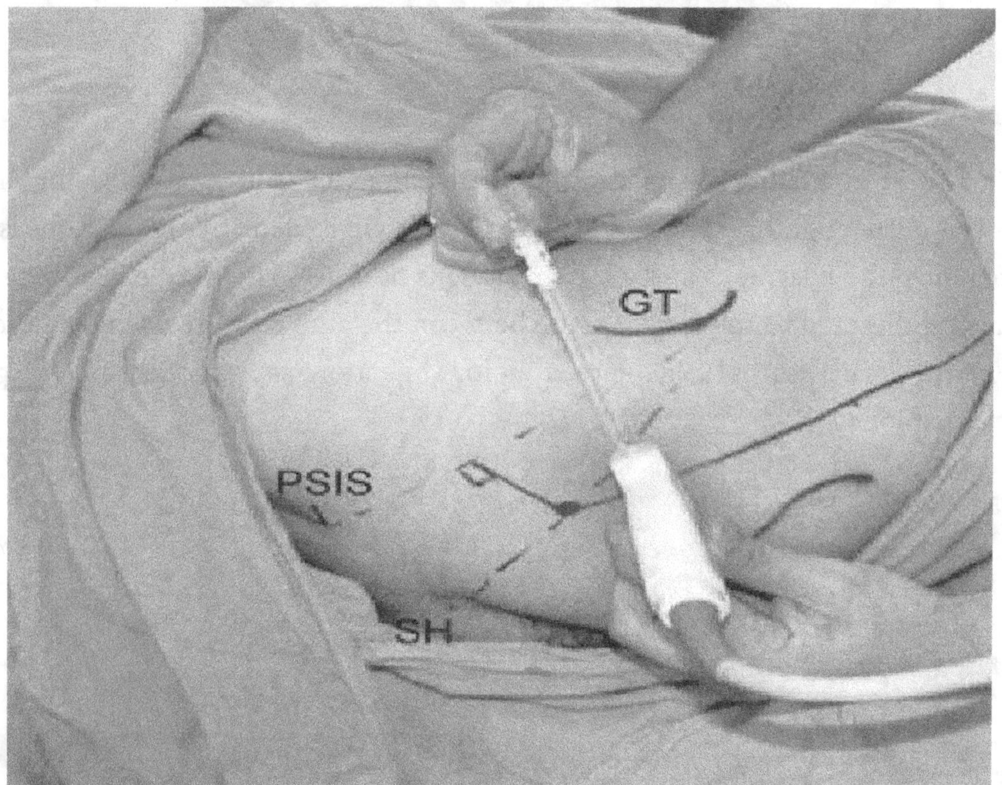

fig(4)

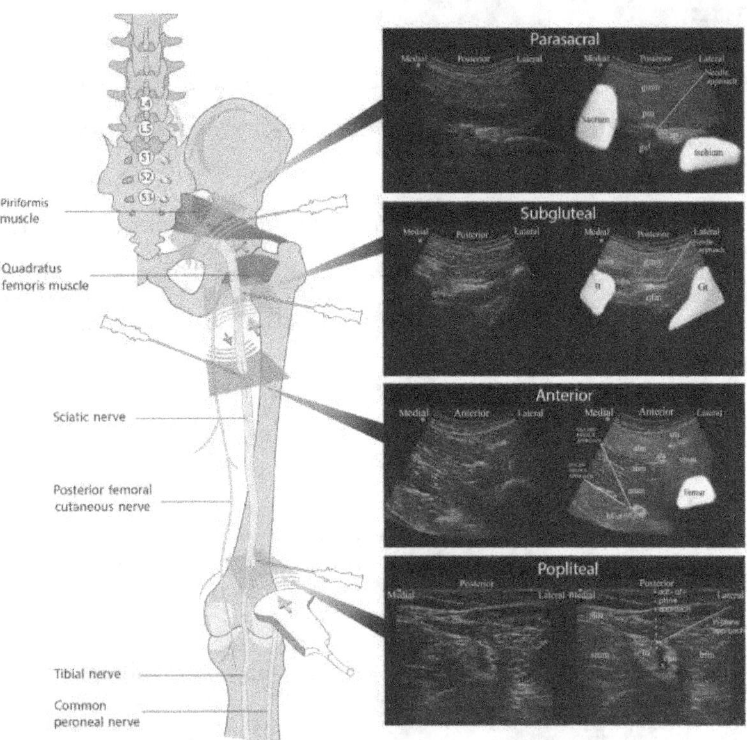

fig(5)

Popliteal nerve block:

The patient can be placed in either prone, lateral decubitus or supine. There are two approaches. For the posterior approach, the biceps femoris and semitendinosus / semimembranosus tendons are palpated. The ultrasound probe is placed transverse to the thigh and in the popliteal crease. The popliteal artery is used as the landmark, and the tibial nerve is found superficial and lateral to the popliteal artery. The nerve is then followed cephalad to the point where the common fibular nerve joins the tibial nerve from the lateral side to form the sciatic nerve. The sciatic nerve is blocked proximal to this to ensure that both the common fibular and tibial nerves are anesthetized

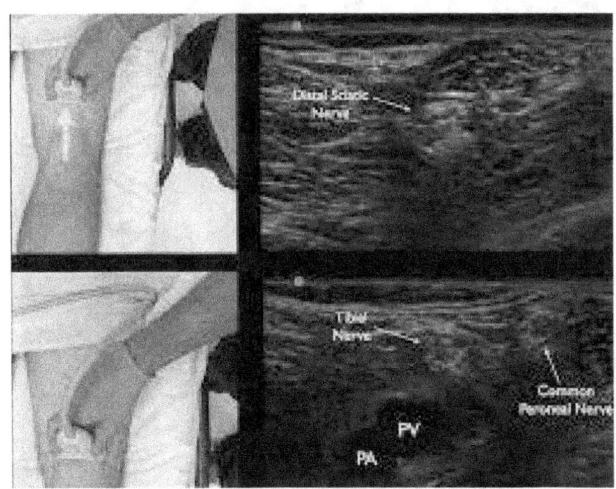

fig(6)

Saphenous nerve block:

The patient is positioned supine with the leg straight. Using the ultrasound probe, it is placed perpendicularly to the thigh at the midpoint between the anterior superior iliac spine and the distal end of the femur (fig7,8) The nerve is identified as it exits from the adductor canal adjacent to the femoral artery. As it is followed distally, it becomes more superficial, traveling with an arterial branch just deep to the sartorius muscle. Using an in-plane approach 10 cc of local anesthetic is injected deep into the sartorius muscle at the lateral border of the artery.

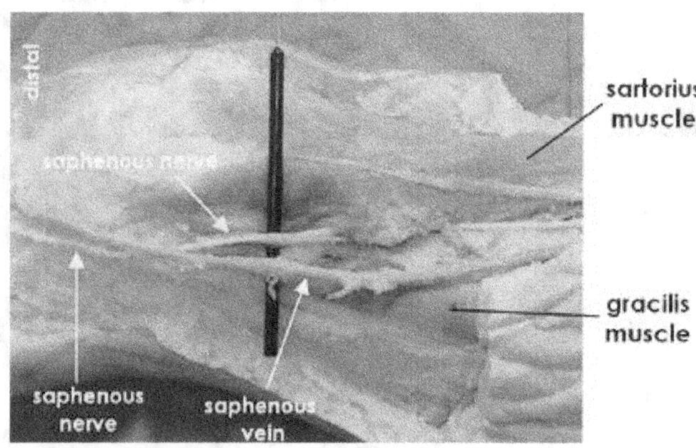

fig(7)

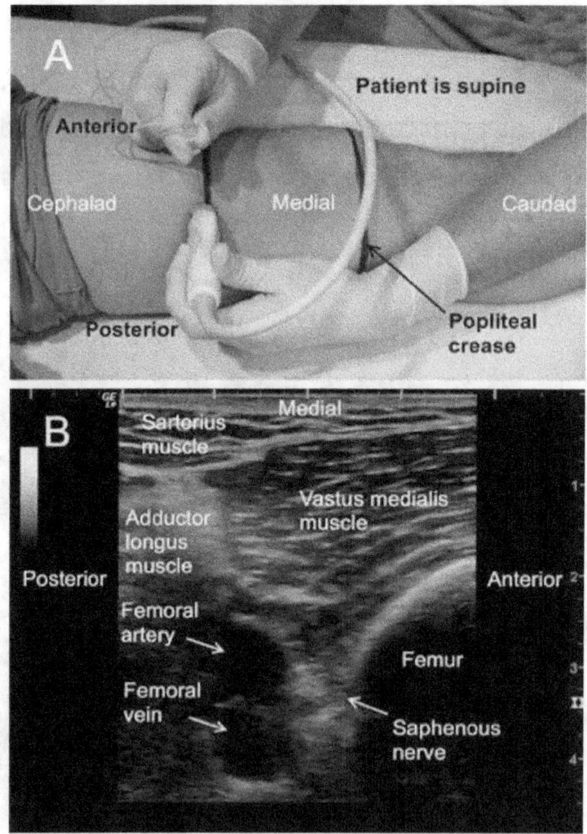

fig(8)

RECENT ADVANCES

- ### PENG block:

  The pericapsular nerve group (PENG) block is an interfascial plane block which block articular branches supplied by femoral, obturator, and accessory obturator nerves. This block is indicated for anterior hip arthroplasties, lateral hip arthroplasties, and for hip fractures. It is performed in supine position by depositing 15-20 ml of local anesthetic in the plane between the psoas tendon and the pubic ramus under direct ultrasound visualization. Femoral nerve block, fascia iliaca compartment block, or lumbar plexus block have been used to manage post-operative analgesia in hip surgeries. These blocks result in weakness of quadriceps muscles and thus predispose to fall.. The main advantage of PENG block is that it provides better analgesia of the hip without causing any muscle weakness. As there is no muscle weakness so the patient can participate in physical therapy early.(3,10)

Figure 9: PENG BLOCK SONOANATOMY ((FA= femoral artery; FV = femoral vein; FN= femoral nerve AIIS = antero inferior iliac spine; IPE = iliopubic emminece. Contributed by Beric Berlioz, MD)

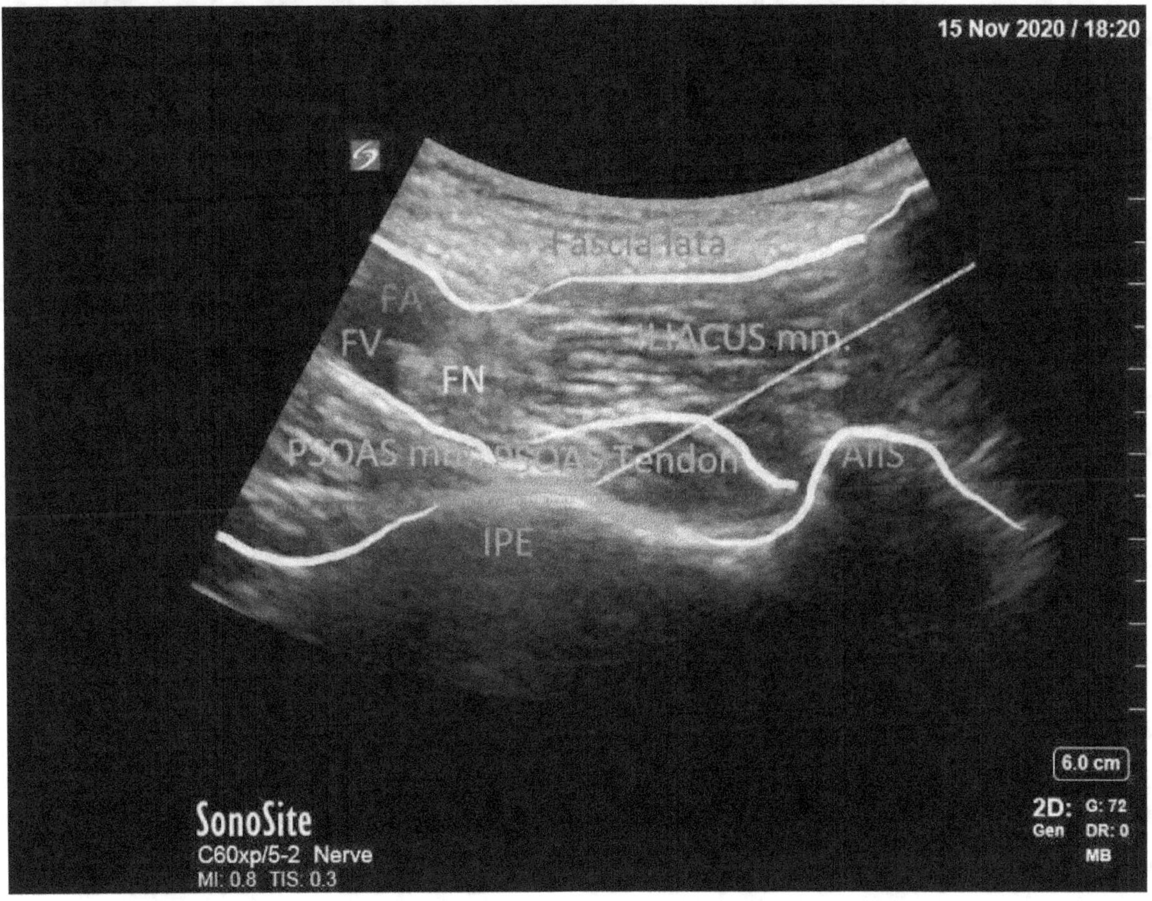

• **IPACK block:**

IPACK block states for infiltration of local anesthetic into the interspace between the popliteal artery and the posterior capsule of the knee. This was first introduced by Dr. Sanjay K Sinha at the American Society of Regional Anesthesia (ASRA) meeting in 2012. iPACK block is used for postoperative analgesia for total knee arthroplasty and cruciate ligament repair. Posterior knee pain is mediated by articular branches arising mainly from the tibial nerve with contributions from the obturator nerve. In iPACK block, 15-20 ml of local anesthetic is deposited under ultrasound guidance in tissue plane femoral artery and posterior aspect of the capsule of the knee joint. The main advantage of iPACK block is that it is a muscle strength sparing block and doesn't result in foot drop or loss of sensorimotor function of leg and foot.(9)

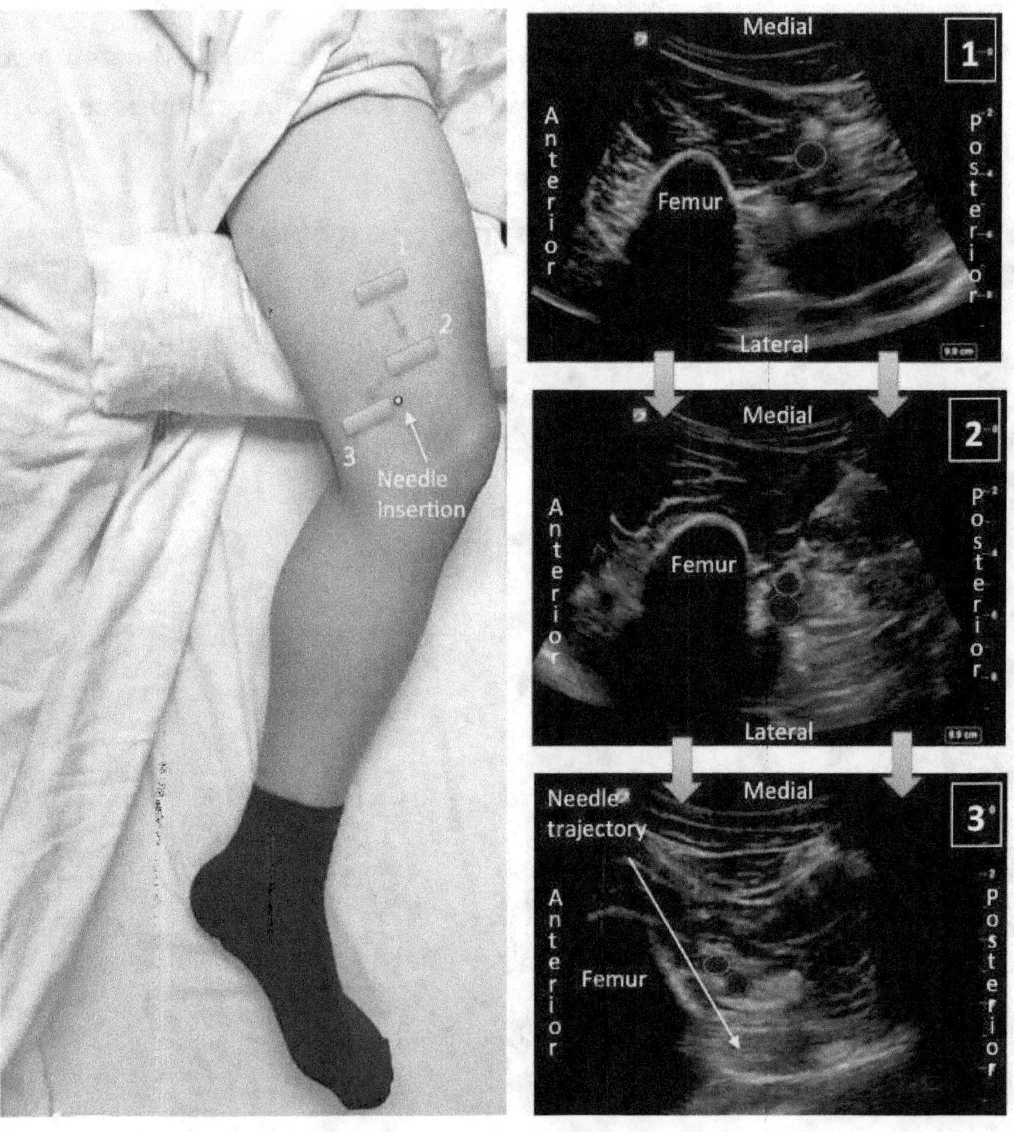

fig(10) IPACK BLOCK

- ### **Supraclavicular block:**

  The patient is placed in the supine position with arms by the sides and the head turned away from the side of the block. The probe is placed in a transverse position just above the clavicle using ultrasound. The carotid artery and internal jugular vein are visualized. The needle is inserted in-plane (parallel to the probe), and a local anesthetic is injected to hydro dissect between the nerves until the tip reaches an area bordered by the first rib, subclavian artery, and brachial plexus. 20 cc to 30 cc of local anesthetic is injected. Before injection, however, aspiration should be performed to ensure there is no blood.(3,8)

- ### **Infraclavicular block:**

  The patient is placed in the supine position with the head turned away from the side of the block. The arm is abducted with the elbow flexed to identify the coracoid process. The axillary artery is identified, and the cords of the brachial plexus are visualized adjacent to the artery using ultrasound. The needle is placed adjacent to the axillary artery in the cranio-posterior quadrant, and 30 to 40 cc of local anesthetic is administered. Before injection, however, aspiration should be performed to ensure there is no blood.

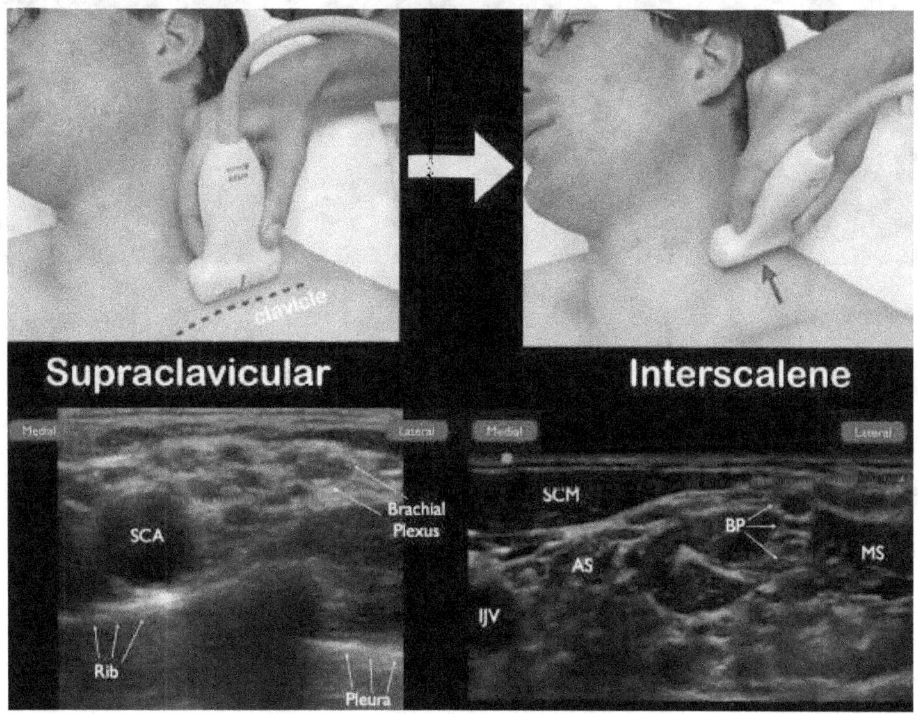

fig(11)

- ### **Axillary block:**

  This block is used to anesthetize nerves of the brachial plexus at the level of the individual nerves and requires multiple injections. The patient is positioned supine with the arm abducted 90 degrees, and the elbow is flexed(fig12). The transducer is placed transversely in the axilla using ultrasound. The needle is introduced perpendicular to the skin and advanced until the tip is next to each nerve.

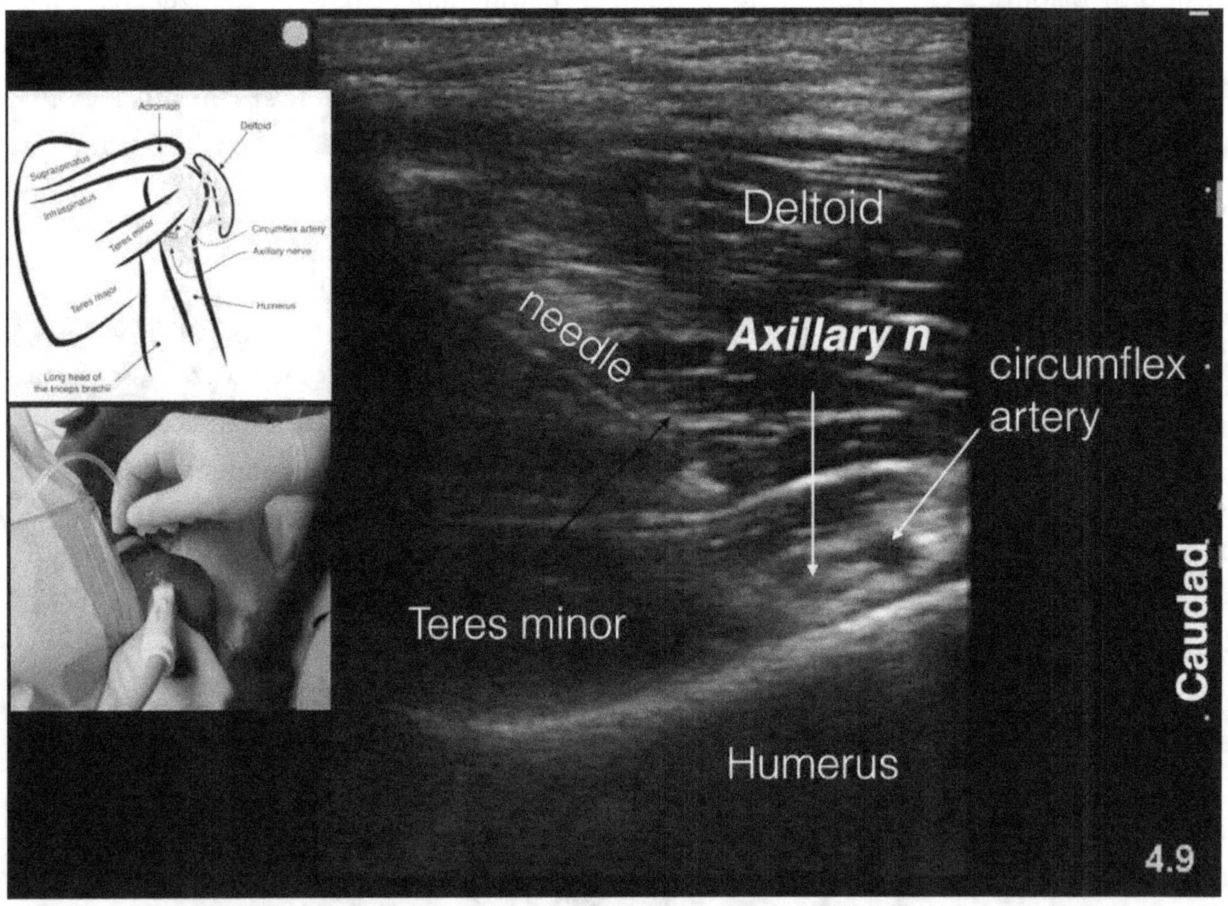

fig(12)

- **<u>Intercostobrachial block:</u>**

The patient is positioned supine with the arm abducted to expose the axillary fossa. The intercostobrachial nerve runs in the subcutaneous tissue of the medial upper arm. The needle is advanced subcutaneously across the medial aspect of the arm while injecting 5 cc to 10 cc of local anesthetic.(3,11)

- **<u>Radial nerve block:</u>**

Radial nerve emerges between the brachioradialis tendon and the radius, just proximal to the styloid process. The needle is inserted subcutaneously, just proximal to the styloid process of the radius, aiming medially, and 3 cc to 5cc of local anesthetic is injected.

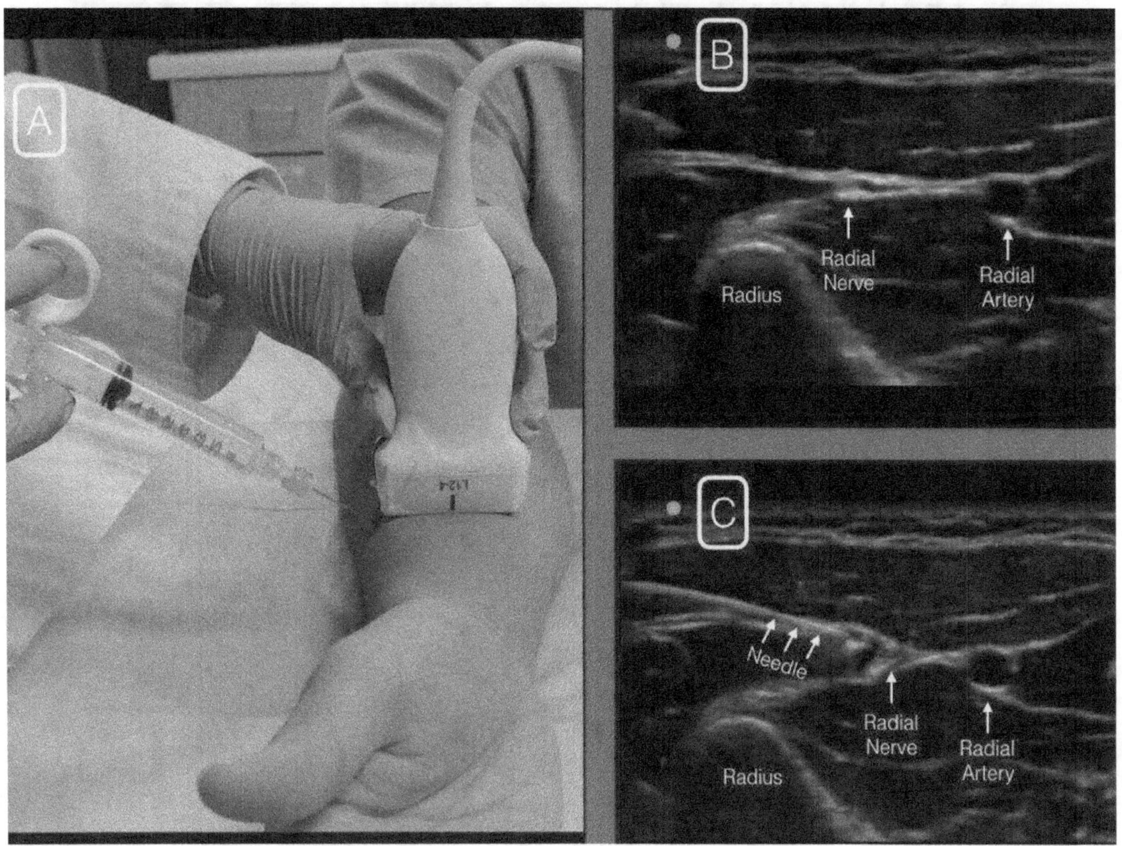

fig(13)

For the radial nerve block, starting at the wrist with the linear ultrasound probe in a transverse position over the radial artery (A), scan proximally until the nerve can be visualized separating from the radial artery (B). Locate the radial nerve between the brachioradialis and brachialis muscles. insert your needle from the radial (lateral) aspect of the probe.

- **<u>The median nerve block</u>**

    Median nerve is located between the tendons of the flexor palmaris longus and the flexor carpi radialis. The needle is inserted between the two tendons until it penetrates the fascia and advanced until contact is made with bone. The needle should be redirected and local anesthetic injected in lateral and medial directions.

    Fig(14) For the median nerve block, place the linear ultrasound probe in a transverse position at the wrist crease on the volar surface of the distal forearm. Scan proximally to the mid-forearm (A) and look for the classic "honeycomb" appearance of a nervous structure at the junction of several fascial planes (B). insert your needle from whichever side is most comfortable.

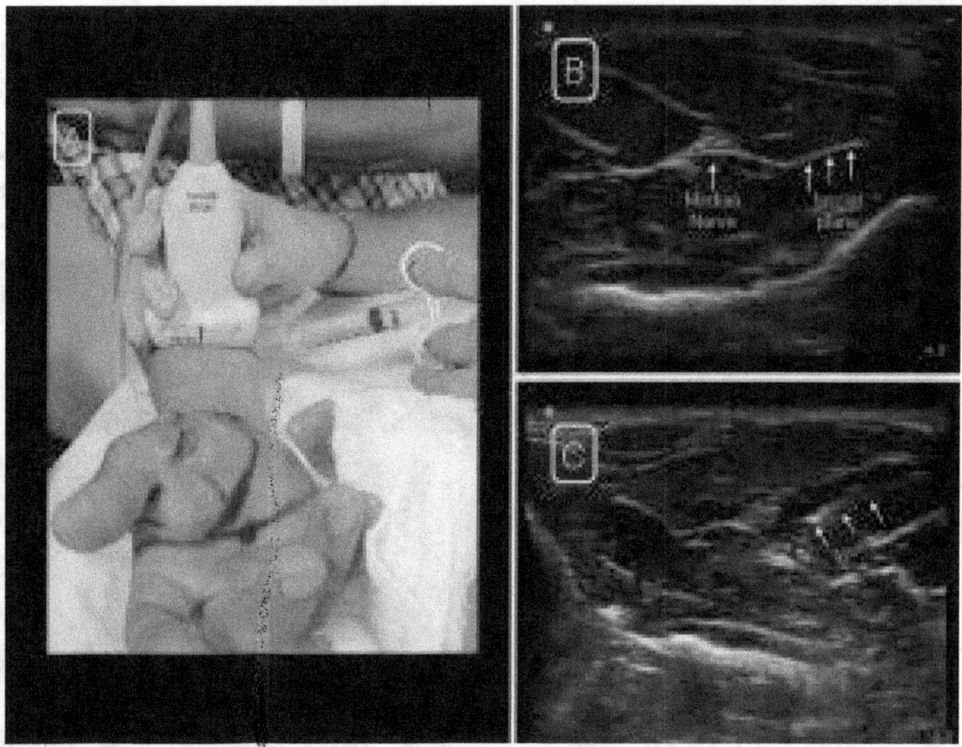

<u>Complications-</u> Potential complications and side effects are dependent upon the type of block performed.

Complications include –

- Peripheral nerve injury (although not common, the rate may be as high as 8% to 10%),
- Hematoma
- Local anesthetic systemic toxicity
- Allergic reaction,
- Infection,
- Secondary injury, which includes reduced sensation after nerve block.

References

1. Chang A, Dua A, Singh K, et al. Peripheral Nerve Blocks. [Updated 2022 Feb 6]. In: StatPearls [Internet]. Treasure Island (FL): StatPearls Publishing; 2022 Jan

2. Sohoni A, Nagdev A, Takhar S, Stone M. Forearm ultrasound-guided nerve blocks vs landmark-based wrist blocks for hand anesthesia in healthy volunteers. The American Journal of Emergency Medicine. 2016 Apr 1;34(4):730-4.

3. Raj N. Regional anesthesia for sternotomy and bypass- Beyond the epidural. Paediatr Anaesth. 2019 May;29(5):519-529.

4. Donado C, Solodiuk J, Rangel SJ, Nelson CP, Heeney MM, Mahan ST, Ullrich C, Tsegaye B, Berde CB. Patient- and Nurse-Controlled Analgesia: 22-Year Experience in a Pediatric Hospital. Hosp Pediatr. 2019 Feb;9(2):129-133.

5. Saranteas T, Koliantzaki I, Savvidou O, Tsoumpa M, Eustathiou G, Kontogeorgakos V, Souvatzoglou R. Acute pain management in trauma: anatomy, ultrasound-guided peripheral nerve blocks and special considerations. Minerva Anestesiol. 2019 Jul;85(7):763-773.

6. Tran DQ, Salinas FV, Benzon HT, Neal JM. Lower extremity regional anesthesia: essentials of our current understanding. Reg Anesth Pain Med. 2019 Jan 11

7. Dickman E, Pushkar I, Likourezos A, et al. Ultrasound-guided nerve blocks for intracapsular and extracapsular hip fractures. *Am J Emerg Med*. 2016;34(3):586-589.

8. Beaudoin FL, Haran JP, Liebmann O. A comparison of ultrasound-guided three-in-one femoral nerve block versus parenteral opioids alone for analgesia in emergency department patients with hip fractures: a randomized controlled trial. *Acad Emerg Med*. 2013;20(6):584-591.

9. Caballero-Lozada AF, Gómez JM, Ramírez JA, Posso M, Zorrilla-Vaca A, Lasso LF. IPACK block: emerging complementary analgesic technique for total knee arthroplasty. Colombian Journal of Anesthesiology. 2020 Jun;48(2):78-84.

10. Berlioz BE, Bojaxhi E. PENG Regional Block.

11. Magazzeni P, Jochum D, Iohom G, Mekler G, Albuisson E, Bouaziz H. Ultrasound-guided selective versus conventional block of the medial brachial cutaneous and the intercostobrachial nerves: a randomized clinical trial. Regional Anesthesia & Pain Medicine. 2018 Nov 1;43(8):832-7.

Toxicology Updates

Contributors

1. Dr. Aravind Ranjan CA
2. Dr. Varsha Shinde
3. Dr. Ashima Sharma
4. Dr. Anitha Sharma

Chapters-

1. Toxidromes and updates
2. Snakebite

Toxidromes and Updates

Introduction

Incidence of acute drug intoxications – continuously rising. Due to the absence of well-designed randomised control trials, it is necessary for the emergency physicians to be aware about the recent advances happening in the field of toxicology

The table covers the toxidromes seen commonly.

Toxidrome	Vital Signs	Mental Status	Pupils	Other Findings	Examples
Anticholinergic	Hyperthermia, Hypertension Tachycardia, tachypnea	Agitated, Hallucinations	Mydriasis	Dry, flushed skin, urinary retention	Antihistamines, TCA, Atropine, Scopolamine, Antispasmodics
Cholinergic	Bradycardia, tachycardia, Hypertension	Confused, Coma	Miosis	SLUDGE- Salivation, Lacrimation, Urination, Diarrhea, Gi upset, Emesis	Organophosphate pesticides, nerve agents
Hallucinogen	Hyperthermia, Tachycardia, hypertension	Hallucination, Synaesthesia, Agitation	Mydriasis	Nystagmus	PCP, LSD, Mescaline
Opioid	Hypothermia bradycardia, hypotension, bradypnea	CNS depression, coma	Miosis	Hyporeflexia, Pulmonary edema	Opioids – heroine, morphine, methadone
Sedative-Hypnotic	Hypothermia bradycardia, hypotension, bradypnea	CNS depression, coma	Miosis	Hyporeflexia	Benzodiazepine, Barbiturates, Alcohol

Serotonin Syndrome	Hyperthermia, Tachycardia, hypertension, tachypnea	Confused, agitated, coma	Mydriasis	Tremor, myoclonus, diaphoresis, hyperreflexia, trismus, rigidity	MAOI, SSRI, Meperidine, Dextromethorphan
Sympathomimetic	Hyperthermia, Tachycardia, hypertension, tachypnea	Agitated, hyperalert	Mydriasis	Diaphoresis, Tremors, Hyperreflexia, Seizures	Cocaine, Amphetamines, Pseudoephedrine

1. **Systematic review on the use of activated charcoal for gastrointestinal decontamination following acute oral overdose.** Clinical toxicology (Philadelphia, Pa.), 59(12), 1196–1227. Hoegberg, L., Shepherd, G., Wood, D. M., Johnson, J., Hoffman

   – Main objective - Does oral activated charcoal given to adults or children prevent toxicity or improve clinical outcome and survival of poisoned patients compared to those who do not receive charcoal?

   – Secondary objectives - evaluate pharmacokinetic outcomes, the role of cathartics, and adverse events to charcoal administration

   – 90 studies were judged to be of Moderate or High GRADE. The higher-GRADE studies reported on the following drugs: acetaminophen, phenobarbital, carbamazepine, cardiac glycosides (digoxin and oleander), ethanol, iron, salicylates, theophylline, tricyclic antidepressants, and valproate. Data on newer pharmaceuticals such as quetiapine, olanzapine, citalopram, and Factor Xa inhibitors were included

   – Study found that there was evidence that the activity of activated charcoal extended beyond the traditional 1 hour in certain clinical scenarios

2. **The NACSTOP Trial**: A Multicenter, Cluster-Controlled Trial of Early Cessation of Acetylcysteine in Acetaminophen Overdose. Hepatology (Baltimore, Md.), 69(2), 774–784 Wong, A., McNulty, R., Taylor, D., Sivilotti, M., Greene (2019)

   – A 12 hour treatment regimen of Acetylcysteine was investigated in a selected low risk patient with acetaminophen overdose.

   – Patients with single or staggered acetaminophen overdose with normal serum alanine transaminase (ALT) and creatinine on presentation and at 12 hours, and acetaminophen <20 mg/L at 12 hours were included in the study.

   – Primary outcome: incidence of "hepatic injury" 20 hours post-initiation of acetylcysteine treatment; defined as ALT doubling and peak ALT > 100 IU/L.

– Secondary outcomes: incidence of hepatotoxicity (ALT > 1000 IU/L), peak INR and adverse drug reactions

– 100 patients included

– There was no difference in ALT (18 IU/L vs 16 IU/L or INR (1.2 vs 1.2) 20 hours after starting acetylcysteine between groups.

– No patients developed hepatic injury or hepatotoxicity in either group (OR 1·0 [95% CI 0.02,50]).

– No patients re-presented with liver injury, none died and were well at 14-day telephone follow-up

– Conclusion: Discontinuing acetylcysteine based on laboratory testing after 12 hours of treatment is feasible and likely safe in selected patients at very low risk of liver injury from acetaminophen overdose.

3. **POP TRIAL**- Principal results of a randomised open label exploratory, safety and tolerability study with calmangafodipir in patients treated with a 12 h regimen of N-acetylcysteine for paracetamol overdose (POP trial). Morrison, E. E., Oatey, K., Gallagher, B., Grahamslaw, J., O'Brien, R., Black, P., Oosthuyzen, W., Lee, R. J., Weir, C. J., Henriksen, D., Dear, J. W., & POP Trial Investigators (2019). EBioMedicine

– Explored the safety and tolerability of calmangafodipir (superoxide dismutase mimetic) co-treatment with n-acetylcysteine (NAC) for paracetamol overdose

– Adults within 24 h of a paracetamol overdose that required NAC were included in the study

– Participants were randomly assigned, with concealed allocation, to NAC and a single intravenous calmangafodipir dose or NAC alone.

– Primary outcome was safety and tolerability.

– Secondary outcomes were ALT, INR, keratin-18, caspase-cleaved keratin-18 (ccK18), microRNA-122, and glutamate dehydrogenase (GLDH) levels

– No adverse effects or serious adverse effects were probably or calmangafodipir-related.

– Secondary safety outcomes demonstrated no differences between groups

– Conclusion - Calmangafodipir was tolerated when combined with NAC and may reduce biomarkers of paracetamol toxicity.

4. **Prediction Rule for Adverse Cardio-Vascular Events from Drug Overdose.** Validation of a Prediction Rule for Adverse Cardiovascular Events from Drug Overdose - Manini AF, Brent J, Campleman S, Judge BS, Kao L, Loo G, Pizon AF, Ruha A, Wiegand T, Wax P, Toxicology Investigators Consortium (ToxIC) Study Group – Annals of Emergency Medicine, October 2020

Adverse Cardio-Vascular Events (ACVE), defined as any of the following:

- Myocardial injury (elevated cardiac troponin I)
- Shock (requiring vasopressors)
- Ventricular dysrhythmia (VT/VF/TdP), or cardiac arrest (pulselessness requiring CPR).

Risk Prediction rule included 3 factors:

1. Any prior cardiac disease (CAD or CHF)
2. Initial QTc ≥ 500ms
3. Initial serum bicarbonate ≤ 20 mmol/L

    - The validation study confirmed the following independent predictors of ACVE: QTc ≥ 500 msec (OR 2.6, p<0.001), bicarbonate ≤20 mmol/L (OR 3.3, p<0.001), and prior cardiac disease (OR 2.3, p<0.001).
    - Prediction rule performance in 5500 patients with documentation of all 3 factors was the following: 61.4% sensitivity, 78.8% specificity, and 95.4% negative predictive value.
    - The presence of 2+ risk factors was 96.4% specific with an LR+ of 4.33 and 5.8-fold increased odds of ACVE (p<0.001).

5. **Prognostic Utility of Initial Lactate Levels in Patients with Acute Drug Overd**ose. Cheung, R., Hoffman, R. S., Vlahov, D., & Manini, A. F. (2018). Prognostic Utility of Initial Lactate in Patients With Acute Drug Overdose: A Validation Cohort. Annals of emergency medicine, 72(1)

- Study was conducted to formally validate the prognostic utility of the initial lactate concentration in patients with acute drug overdose.
- Primary outcome – inpatient fatality
- 1406 patients were analysed
- Difference in mean initial lactate concentration was 5.9 mmol/L (higher in patients who died compared with survivors.
- Area under the curve for prediction of fatality was 0.85 (95% CI 0.73 to 0.95)
- Optimal lactate cut point for fatality was greater than or equal to 5.0 (odds ratio 34.2; 95% CI 13.7 to 84.2; 94.7% specificity).
- Drug classes for which lactate had the highest utility were salicylates, sympathomimetics, acetaminophen, and opioids (all area under the curve ≥0.97); lowest utility was for diuretics and angiotensin-converting enzyme inhibitors.
- Study concluded that initial lactate concentration is a useful biomarker for early clinical decision making in ED patients with acute drug overdose. Studies of lactate-tailored management for these patient populations are warranted.

6. **METHYLENE BLUE**

   – Primarily used in the treatment of patients with methemoglobinemia and refractory shock from a variety of causes

   – Also described as an option for treatment in vasodilatory shock in Calcium Channel Blocker (CCB) Poisoning

   – More effective in Dihydropyridine CCB poisoning due to its mechanism of action

   – Also effective in refractory shock due to metformin, beta blockers, and/or mixed drug overdose

   – CCBs cause an increase in nitric oxide release by increasing nitric oxide synthase activity, which in turn increases the generation of cGMP by activation of guanylate cyclase – Increase in cGMP causes vasodilation

   – Methylene Blue inhibits guanylate cyclase activity, scavenges nitric oxide, and inhibits nitric oxide synthesis

   – Preferred dosing regimen - 1 to 2 mg/kg bolus followed by a low-dose infusion

   – of 0.25 to 1 mg/kg/h.

   – Currently, there is no high-level evidence to support routine use of Methylene Blue prior to conventional treatment. As a result, it should be considered only after traditional treatment modalities such as vasopressor administration, high dose insulin euglycemia therapy, intravenous lipid emulsion therapy, and extracorporeal therapies have been exhausted

7. **Test-mate ChE 400 Kit in Acute Organophosphate Poisoning**

   – Levels of plasma and/or RBC cholinesterase enzyme may be measured in OP poisoning.

   – Most readily available, is the test for plasma (or pseudo) cholinesterase. Because this can be affected by other disorders, it does not confirm the diagnosis.

   – Mild intoxication is diagnosed when RBC cholinesterase inhibition is less than 50% of normal. Depression of this value by 25% or more is confirmatory.

   – Test-mate ChE 400 is a portable field kit used to detect occupational organophosphorus exposure - The test measures RBC AChE and plasma cholinesterase (PChE) within 4 minutes.

   – A study of patients with acute OP poisoning compared Test-mate ChE results to reference laboratory and found good agreement between the two.

8. **The Role of Sodium Bicarbonate in the Management of Some Toxic Ingestions.**

   Mirrakhimov, A et al International journal of nephrology, 2017

Mechanism of Action-Sodium bicarbonate when given, dissociates into sodium and bicarbonate. Bicarbonate in turn binds hydrogen converting into carbonic acid which dissociates into carbon dioxide and water. Carbon dioxide under intact lung perfusion and ventilation is exhaled, and thus maintains the acid-base equilibrium.

INDICATIONS

1. Sodium Channel Blocker Toxicity
2. Salicylate Toxicity
3. Methanol and Ethylene Glycol Poisoning
4. Miscellaneous drugs such as methotrexate, phenobarbital, chlorpropamide and metformin

Sodium Channel Blocker Toxicity

- Sodium channel blockade may lead to serious cardiac dysfunction – cardiac dysrhythmias and hemodynamic instability – e.g. - TCA
- Associated metabolic acidosis – potentiates sodium channel blocking
- Use of sodium bicarbonate especially in TCA overdose – increases pH and increases extracellular sodium levels which in turn attenuates the TCA blocking of sodium channels
- Literature is limited as RCTs are precluded due to ethical reasons
- IV sodium bicarbonate should be considered in the cases of suspected sodium channel blocker toxicity associated with hemodynamic and ECG abnormalities, given the very high risk of adverse outcome without aggressive treatment.

Salicylate Toxicity

- Mechanism of action of aspirin - inhibition of cyclooxygenase enzyme, resulting in decreased production of thromboxane A2 and various prostaglandins
- With higher dosages - uncoupling of oxidative phosphorylation in the electro transport chain - decrease in the blood pH will favor formation of lipid soluble salicylic acid which easily penetrates blood-brain barrier and undergoes renal reabsorption.
- Sodium bicarbonate – causes metabolic alkalosis that decreases the amount of lipid soluble salicylate resulting in decreased penetration into central nervous system and in increased urinary clearance

Methanol and Ethylene Glycol Poisoning

- Acidemia leads to protonation of methanol and ethylene glycol metabolites to uncharged molecules (e.g., formic acid and oxalic acid), making them more likely to penetrate end-organ tissues such as the retina and more likely to be reabsorbed across the renal epithelium from the urine.

- Sodium bicarbonate – prevents acidemia and enhances urinary clearance of toxic metabolites like formate

Miscellaneous Drug Toxicities

- IV sodium bicarbonate may result in enhanced urinary excretion of certain chemicals through urinary alkalinization - methotrexate, phenobarbital, chlorpropamide, and fluoride
- Metformin associated lactic acidosis with pH < 7.1 – Sodium bicarbonate used – but less literature available on the same

Complications of Sodium Bicarbonate

1. Under conditions such as shock states and impaired ventilation, carbon dioxide may accumulate, leading to worsening acidosis. CO_2 penetrates cellular membranes easily, and exacerbate intracellular acidosis

2. By correcting systemic acidosis, sodium bicarbonate reduces respiratory drive leading to accumulation of CO_2 in the central nervous system and associated adverse neurological sequelae

3. Complications secondary to excess sodium content and osmolality – cellular dehydration and systemic hypervolemia

4. Alkaline pH - Ionized calcium may be decreased, which may cause tetany, decrease cardiac contractility, and potentially predispose to cardiac arrhythmias via prolongation of QT interval

5. Lactic acid production may be increased via alkalosis dependent activation of 6-phosphofructokinase enzymes and ketone bodies production may be enhanced.

6. Serious skin injuries can occur due to extravasation of hypertonic bicarbonate solutions, and whenever possible it should be administered through large bore iv lines or central venous lines.

9. **HaVOC Trial**-Intravenous Haloperidol Versus Ondansetron for Cannabis Hyperemesis Syndrome (HaVOC): A Randomized, Controlled Trial. Ruberto, A. J et al Annals of emergency medicine, 77(6) 2021

   - Compared haloperidol with ondansetron for cannabis hyperemesis syndrome.
   - Randomized cannabis users with active emesis to either haloperidol 0.05 or 0.1 mg/kg or ondansetron 8 mg IV
   - Haloperidol at either dose was superior to ondansetron:

     1. Similar improvements in both pain and nausea
     2. Less use of rescue antiemetics
     3. Shorter time to emergency department (ED) departure

10. **Aluminium Phosphide Poisoning**-A. K. Pannu, A. Bhalla, J. Gantala, N. Sharma, S. Kumar & D. P. Dhibar (2020) Glucose-insulin-potassium infusion for the treatment of acute aluminum phosphide poisoning: an open-label pilot study, Clinical Toxicology, 58:10, 1004-1009

    — Aluminium phosphide releases phosphine – inhibits cytochrome c oxidase – cellular hypoxia – GI upset, and cardiopulmonary failure ensues.

    — Phosphine induced production of free radicals and oxidative stress results in insulin resistance and hyperglycemia

    — In this study, Glucose-insulin-potassium (GIK) was administered based on the benefit of GIK in improving cardiac contractility in patients with calcium channel and beta blocker toxicity – Regular insulin used.

    — Primary outcome - in-hospital case fatality – significantly lower in GIK group

    — Secondary outcomes - duration of hospital stay, the requirement of mechanical ventilation, and the change in hemodynamic and metabolic parameters

        1. Duration of hospital stay – significantly higher in GIK group

        2. Mechanical ventilation – significantly less in GIK group

        3. Hemodynamic parameters such as SBP, DBP and MAP – significantly improved in GIK group

    Conclusion – Addition of GIK to standard supportive treatment reduced both CFR and severity of the toxicity. A further large multicentre trial required to confirm and clarify the magnitude of GIK infusion benefit in aluminium phosphide poisoning.

11. Anbalagan, L. C., Arora, N., & Pannu, A. K. (2021). Management of **Acute Aluminum Phosphide Poisoning**: Has Anything Changed?. Drug metabolism letters, 14(2)

    — Easy availability, rapid and severe toxicity and no specific antidote – Makes Aluminium phosphide poisoning lethal

    — Very high fatality rate with no definitive treatment

    — Literature review done in the study

    — Glucose-insulin-potassium infusion and lipid emulsion – given a new hope in the complete recovery in this fatal poisoning

12. Pannu AK, Bhalla A, Sharma A, Sharma N. **"PGI Score"**: A Simplified Three-point Prognostic Score for Acute Aluminum Phosphide Poisoning. Indian J Crit Care Med. 2020

    — A reliable and accurate prognostic scoring tool will help in appropriate triaging, guide clinical decision-making, and to evaluate the efficacy of therapeutic interventions for the patients with Aluminium Phosphide toxicity

- 3 parameters:

  1. pH <7.25
  2. GCS <13
  3. Systolic blood pressure (SBP) <87 mm Hg

  These 3 were found to be most important predictors of case fatality rate

- Based on these parameters - 1 point to each, a prognostic score was developed, ranging from 0 to 3 points.
- Score of 3 - 98.2% specificity and a positive predictive value of 96.4%
- Score ≤1 - 100% sensitivity and 100% negative predictive value.

POCUS IN TOXICOLOGY

1. **Hypotension and Shock associated with Toxin Intake**

   - Visualisation of IVC helps to evaluate the patient hydration and volume status
   - Cardiac status – LV and RV function

2. **Assessment of need for gastric lavage**

   - Gastric Lavage should not be used regularly in the treatment of intoxicated patients – Ultrasound visualisation of ingested pills/drugs

3. **Snake Bite**

   - Subcutaneous tissue edema – Most common finding
   - Able to evaluate the deeper muscle content in case of diffuse leg edema
   - In case of finger involvement – swelling and tendon injury – visualised using water bath procedure

4. **Lead poisoning**

   - Trans cranial sonography can be used to examine congenital lead poisoning in infant with lead encephalopathy
   - Increase in systolic function and decrease in diastolic function observed in lead toxicity

5. **Rhabdomyolysis**

   - Muscle necrosis – observed through sonography - decreased echogenicity and increased thickness and disorganization of muscular structure without local defect over the muscle

ECMO IN TOXICOLOGY

- Leading cause of death in acute toxic ingestions is cardiovascular failure
- Various methods like parenteral calcium, hyper-insulinemic-euglycemic therapy, intravenous lipid emulsion, and vasopressors have been used in cardiac failure associated with acute toxic ingestions. But they are of no use in severe cardiovascular toxicity
- There comes the use of ExtraCorporeal Membrane Oxygenation (ECMO) as the only measure to prevent mortality – ECMO provides adequate time to allow metabolism of drug, its elimination, and cardiac recovery.
- VA-ECMO – provides both cardiac and pulmonary support whereas VV-ECMO provides circulatory support
- Severe lung injury with adequate cardiac function – VV-ECMO and if hemodynamic compromise – VA-ECMO
- ECMO is contraindicated in

    1. Patients with irreversible multiorgan failure
    2. Patients with severe neurological damage
    3. Patients who have had prolonged periods of end-organ hypoperfusion

- ECMO may affect drug metabolism and elimination. Drugs which are lipophilic drugs and protein bound drugs are significantly sequestered in the circuit, whereas hydrophilic drugs are affected by haemodilution and other pathophysiologic changes that occur during ECMO
- ECMO has been used in patients poisoned with flecainide, tricyclic antidepressants, b-adrenergic receptor antagonists, calcium channel antagonists, digoxin, and bupropion etc.
- Potential complications include

    1. Limb ischemia and compartment syndrome
    2. AKI
    3. Bleeding
    4. Emboli and stroke
    5. Infection.

- Fat deposition can occur within the ECMO circuit in patients who were previously treated with intravenous lipid emulsion therapy
- Though only less data available, its best to consider ECMO early, in poisoned patients with refractory cardiac arrest or hemodynamic compromise who have not yet undergone irreversible organ failure

HEMODIALYSIS IN TOXICOLOGY

- Extracorporeal treatments for drug removal include intermittent hemodialysis (IHD), hemoperfusion, and/or hemofiltration.

  Most Common - IHD

- Most important determinant of effective removal by hemodialysis-drug's volume of distribution – Smaller volume of distribution – easily removed
- High-efficiency high-flux IHD - meaning larger membrane pore size, dialyzers with diffusive modalities are capable of clearing poisons in the middle MW range
- New high-cutoff and middle-cutoff membranes may remove poisons up to 50 000 Da.
- Previously, clearance of drugs such as valproic acid, carbamazepine, and theophylline was only possible by charcoal hemoperfusion. High-flux IHD has shown to be just as effect as hemoperfusion and has made hemoperfusion an obsolete choice in clearance of drugs
- Continuous renal replacement therapies such as continuous venovenous hemofiltration, continuous venovenous hemodialysis, and continuous venovenous hemodiafiltration are also utilised for toxin clearance especially in:

  1. Patients who are hemodynamically unstable
  2. HD for toxins that undergo redistribution – this prevents rebound

  But it can't remove toxins rapidly unlike conventional HD.

Snake Bite

<u>Introduction</u> Snakebite is an acute life-threatening, time sensitive medical emergency. It is a preventable public health hazard often faced by the rural populace in tropical and subtropical countries. Fatalities are often due to the inability of the victim to reach the hospital in time where definitive treatment can be administered. [1]

WHO has formally re-listed snakebite as a neglected tropical disease (NTD) in June of 2017 [2]. It has also implemented various measures to improve the awareness of health regulation authorities and policy makers regarding the appropriate approach to the management of snakebites.

<u>Epidemiology</u> It is estimated that there are over 10,00,000 snakebites in India alone causing 58,000 deaths annually and about four times that number survive and but are left with significant and permanent disabilities [3]

The National Health Profile (2019) data on snakebites, however, only reported 1,64,031 snakebite cases and 885 deaths in 2018. [4] Thus, there is a discrepancy between WHO estimates and the reported figures.

According to WHO data, around 1,00,000 people die each year worldwide because of snakebite. There is a huge gap between the number of snakebite deaths reported from direct surveys and official data. Only 7.23% snakebite deaths were officially reported [5]. Annual snakebite deaths were greatest in the states of Uttar Pradesh, Andhra Pradesh, and Bihar. Other Indian states with high incidence of snakebites cases are

Tamil Nadu, West Bengal, Maharashtra and Kerala. Approximately half of global snakebite deaths occur on the Indian subcontinent. Because a large proportion of global totals of snakebites arise from India, global snakebite totals might also be underestimated.

Snakebite deaths and disability remain a major public health challenge also for poor rural communities in many parts of Asia, Africa, Latin America and Oceania [3]. A Snakebite Envenoming Working Group was established that tasked with informing the development of a strategic WHO road map on snakebites. This strategy focuses on a 50% reduction in mortality and disability caused by snakebite envenoming by 2030. [2]

<u>Types-</u> There are about 300 known species of snakes in India, most of which are non-venomous and are not expected to cause significant harm. The four most common deadly venomous snakes in India include Cobra (Naja naja), Russell's viper (Dabiola russelii), Saw-scaled viper (Echis carinatus), Common krait (Bungarus caeruleus). Most of these are widely distributed on the plains and low hills where most of the rural population lives.

Kraits are notorious for being active during the night, often biting a person sleeping on a floor bed, whereas vipers and cobras are known to bite during the day or in early darkness.

<u>Clinical Presentation:</u>

Clinical presentation of snakebite victim depends upon species of snake, amount of venom injected, season of the bite, whether snake is fed or unfed, site of bite, area covered or uncovered, dry or incomplete bite, multiple bites, venom injection in vessel, weight of the victim. Venom

concentration and constitution depends on environmental conditions as well as snake's maturity and darkness of colour of snake.[1]

The four main clinical syndromes seen are progressive weakness (neuroparalytic), bleeding (vasculotoxic / haemotoxic), myotoxic and painful progressive swelling. Patients can present either as one of the four main clinical syndromes or as a mixed clinical picture.

While eliciting a history of snake bite is prudent, clinicians should be aware that the history of snake bite is often missing. Emergency physicians should always consider occult poisonous snake bite as a differential when the clinical situation demands. Many-a-time snake bites are misdiagnosed as abdominal colic or vomiting due to indigestion, appendicitis, stroke, trismus, Guillain Barre syndrome, hysteria.[6].

Unexplained respiratory distress in children in the presence of ptosis or sudden onset of acute flaccid paralysis in a child (locked-in syndrome) are highly suspicious symptoms in endemic areas particularly of Krait bite envenomation. Sometimes patients may present with throat pain or chest pain also.

<u>Neuroparalytic snakebite patients</u> present with typical symptoms within 30 min– 6 hours in case of Cobra bite and 6 – 24 hours for Krait bite.

These symptoms can be remembered as 5 Ds and 2 Ps.

- 5 Ds – dyspnea, dysphonia, dysarthria, diplopia, dysphagia
- 2 Ps – ptosis, paralysis

To identify impending respiratory failure bedside lung function test in adults viz.

- Single breath count – number of digits counted in one exhalation - >30 normal
- Breath holding time – breath held in inspiration – normal > 45 sec
- Ability to complete one sentence in one breath.

It is very important to note that bilaterally dilated, poorly or a non reacting pupil is not the sign of brain death in elapid envenoming.

<u>Vasculotoxic (haemotoxic or Bleeding)</u> bites are due to viper species. They can have local manifestations as well as systemic manifestations.

Local manifestations are in the form of local swelling, bleeding, blistering, and necrosis. Pain at the bite site and severe swelling can lead to compartment syndrome. Pain on passive movement, absence of peripheral pulses and hypoesthesia over the nerve passing through the compartment helps to diagnose compartment syndrome.

Systemic manifestations include visible systemic bleeding like gingival bleeding, epistaxis, ecchymotic patches, vomiting, hematemesis, hemoptysis, bleeding per rectum, subconjunctival hemorrhages, continuous bleeding from the bite site or bleeding from pre-existing conditions e.g. haemorrhoids or from freshly healed wounds.

The skin and mucous membranes may show evidence of petechiae, purpura, ecchymoses, blebs and gangrene. Acute abdominal tenderness may suggest gastro-intestinal or retro peritoneal bleeding. Lateralizing neurological symptoms such as asymmetrical pupils may be indicative of intracranial bleeding. Consumption coagulopathy detectable by 20WBCT, develops as early as within 30 minutes from time of bite but may be delayed

<u>Life threatening complications</u>

Neuroparalytic snake bite can cause **central apnea** due to bulbar palsy and death if not treated.

Acute Kidney Injury – It may present as declining or no urine output, rising serum creatinine, urea or potassium. Patients present with hematuria, hemoglobinuria, myoglobinuria, bilateral renal tenderness followed by oliguria and anuria. Hypotension due to hypovolemia or direct vasodilatation or direct cardiotoxicity aggravates acute kidney injury. It may present as cardiac arrhythmias due to hyperkalemia secondary to kidney injury.

Long term sequelae e.g. pituitary insufficiency with Russell's viper, Sheehan's syndrome or amenorrhea in females.

Painful progressive swelling:

Local necrosis often has a rancid smell. Limb is swollen and the skin is taut and shiny. Blistering with reddish black fluid at and around the bite site. Skip lesions around main lesion are also seen

- Ecchymoses due to venom action destroying the blood vessel wall.
- Significant painful swelling potentially involving the whole limb and extending onto the trunk with regional tender lymphadenopathy

Myotoxic

Patient presents with muscle aches, muscle swelling, involuntary contractions of muscles, passage of dark brown urine.

Occult snake bite:

Krait has nocturnal habitat and has fine slender teeth. Hence bite marks usually cannot be identified even on close examination. Typical presenting history is that the patient was healthy at night, in the morning gets up with severe epigastric/umbilical pain with vomiting persisting for 3-4 hours and followed by typical neuroparalytic symptoms within the next 4-6 hours. There is no history of snakebite.

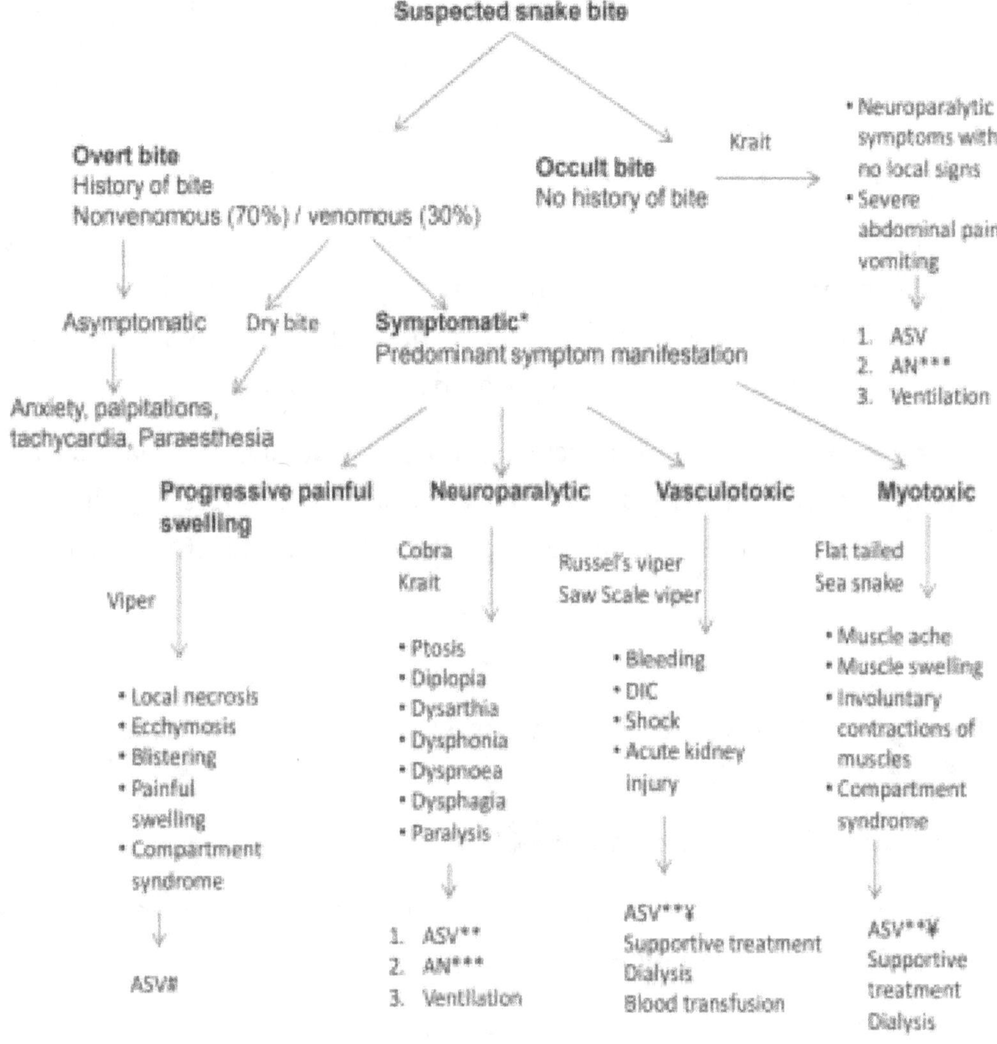

*   Even though present as predominant manifestation but there may be overlap of syndrome as well.

\#   ASV indicated in rapidly developing swelling only. Purely localized swelling with or without bite marks is not an indication of ASV.

**   For reaction to antisnake venom (ASV) Dose of Adrenaline 0.5 mg IM (in children 0.01 mg/kg)

¥   Specific ASV for sea snake and Pit viper bite is not available in India. However, available ASV may have some advantage by cross reaction.

***   Atropine 0.6 mg followed by neostigmine (1.5mg) to be given IV stat (In children Inj. Atropine 0.05 mg/kg followed by Inj. Neostigmine 0.04 mg/kg IV.) Repeat neostigmine dose 0.5 mg (in children 0.01mg/kg) with atropine every 30 minutes for 5 doses. Thereafter taper dose at 1 hour, 2 hour, 6 hours and 12 hour. Positive response is measured as 50% or more recovery of the ptosis in one hour. If no response after 3rd dose. Stop AN injection.

From standard guidelines on snake bite by the Ministry of Health and Family welfare, Jan 2016.

<u>Pathophysiology:</u> Snake venom is a complex enzyme mixture that causes local tissue injury, systemic vascular damage, hemolysis, fibrinolysis, and neuromuscular dysfunction, resulting in a mixture of local and systemic effects. It quickly alters blood vessel permeability; this leads to loss of plasma and blood into the surrounding tissue, which causes hypovolemia. It activates and consumes fibrinogen and platelets, causing coagulopathy.

The lymphatic system may be damaged by the various enzymes contained in the venom leading to edema.

Snake venom may cause myotoxicity via the enzyme phospholipase A2 which disrupts the plasma membrane of muscle cells. This damage to muscle cells causes rhabdomyolysis.

Toxins in snake venom cause nephrotoxicity via inflammatory cytokines. The toxins cause direct damage to the glomeruli in the kidneys as well as causing protein deposits in Bowman's capsule. The kidneys may also be indirectly damaged by envenomation due to shock, clearance of toxic substances such as immune complexes or blood degradation products.

Snake venom is known to cause neuromuscular paralysis, usually as a flaccid paralysis that is **descending**; starting at the facial muscles, causing ptosis or drooping eyelids and dysarthria descending to the respiratory muscles causing respiratory compromise.Cobra causes postsynaptic transmission block whereas Krait causes presynaptic.

<u>Diagnosis:</u>

It is based on the history of snake bite, fang marks with signs of systemic envenomation or local tissue injury. Occult bite need to be kept in mind.

20 minute whole blood clotting test (20 WBCT):

It is a point of care test. Place 2 ml of freshly sampled venous blood in a small glass test tube and leave undisturbed for 20 minutes at ambient temperature.

Gently tilt the test tube to see if the blood is still liquid; the patient has hypofibrinogenemia. If there is any doubt, repeat the test in duplicate, including a "control" (blood from a healthy person).

We need to counsel patients and relatives in the beginning that 20 WBCT may be repeated several times before giving any medication.

If clotted, the test should be carried out every 1 h from admission for three hours and then 6 hourly for 24 hours. In case the test is non-clotting, repeat 6 hour after administration of the loading dose of ASV. In case of neurotoxic envenomation repeat clotting test after 6 hours.

Other lab investigations

Prothrombin time, platelet count, clot retraction time, liver function test (LFT), Renal Function test (RFT), Serum Amylase, Blood sugar, ECG, Abdominal ultrasound, 2D Echo

Management as per National guidelines:

Polyvalent ASV is the only scientifically validated treatment for poisonous snake bite.

Each millilitre of ASV neutralizes 0.6 mg of D. russelii and N. naja venoms and 0.45 mg venom of B. caeruleus and E. carinatus. Each vial contains 10 ml of ASV which in effect should neutralize ten times the above-mentioned amounts of venom. The average ASV required is about 20 vials for a victim.

ASV is scarce, costly and can have anaphylactic reactions. Hence it is administered only when there are signs of **systemic envenomation** like coagulopathy primarily detected by 20 WBCT or visible spontaneous systemic bleeding. Evidence of neurotoxicity like ptosis,

ophthalmoplegia, muscle paralysis, inability to lift neck. Cardiovascular abnormalities like shock, hypotension, cardiac arrhythmias and persistent severe abdominal pain and vomiting. It is indicated only when local swelling is rapidly increasing. There are no absolute contraindications to ASV.

Precautions during ASV Administration – ASV should be given only by the IV route, and should be given slowly, with the physician at the bedside during the initial period to intervene immediately at the first sign of any reaction.

The rate of infusion can be increased gradually in the absence of a reaction until the full starting dose has been administered (over a period of ~1 hour). Epinephrine (adrenaline) should always be drawn up in readiness before ASV is administered.

ASV must NEVER be given by the IM route because of poor bioavailability by this route. Also do NOT inject the ASV locally at the bite site since it is not effective, is extremely painful and may increase intra-compartmental pressure. Take all aseptic precautions before starting ASV to prevent any pyrogenic reactions to ASV.

Dose of ASV

Neuroparalytic snake bite – ASV 10 vials stat as infusion over 30 minutes followed by 2nd dose of 10 vials after 1 hour if no improvement within 1st hour.

Vasculotoxic snake bite - Two regimens

Low dose infusion therapy and high dose intermittent bolus therapy can be used. Low dose infusion therapy is as effective as high dose intermittent bolus therapy and also saves scarce ASV doses.

Low Dose infusion therapy – 10 vials for Russel's viper or 6 vials for Saw scaled viper as stat as infusion over 30 minutes followed by 2 vials every 6 hours as infusion in 100 ml of normal saline till clotting time normalizes or for 3 days whichever is earlier.

High dose intermittent bolus therapy - 10 vials of polyvalent ASV stat over 30 minutes as infusion, followed by 6 vials 6 hourly as bolus therapy till clotting time normalizes and/or local swelling subsides.

No ASV for Sea snakebite or pit viper bite as available ASV does not contain antibodies against them. Existing polyvalent ASV can be used due to cross reactivity.

The range of venom injected is 5 mg-147 mg. The total required dose range between 10 and 30 vials as each vial neutralizes 6 mg of Russell's Viper venom. Depending on the patient's condition, additional vials can be considered.

Repeat dose: Vasculotoxic envenomation

Repeat clotting test every 6 hours until coagulation is restored. Administer ASV every 6 h until coagulation is restored. If 30 vials of ASV have been administered, reconsider whether continued administration of ASV is serving any purpose, particularly in the absence of proven systemic bleeding.

Repeat dose: Neuroparalytic envenomation

Repeat ASV when there is worsening neurotoxic or cardiovascular signs even after 1–2 h. Maximum dose 20 vials of ASV for neurotoxically

envenomed patients. If large doses have been administered and the coagulation abnormality persists, give fresh frozen plasma (FFP) or cryoprecipitate (fibrinogen, factor VIII), fresh whole blood, if FFP not available or platelet concentrate.

Children also are given exactly the same dose of ASV as adults as snakes inject the same amount of venom into children and adults. Infusion: liquid or reconstituted ASV is diluted in 5-10 ml/kg body weight of normal saline. However, reduce the amount of fluid in the running bottle to 200 ml to avoid fluid overload.

ASV reaction – No test dose is needed.

Pyrogenic reactions usually develop 1–2 h after treatment. It is treated with paracetamol. Early anaphylactic reactions occur within 10–180 min of the start of therapy and are characterized by itching, urticaria, dry cough, nausea and vomiting, abdominal colic, diarrhoea, tachycardia. ASV is still administered in such cases.

Desensitizing procedure is undertaken only in cases of severe anaphylactic reaction following ASV.

Late (serum sickness–type) reactions develop 1–12 (mean 7) days after treatment. Clinical features include fever, nausea, vomiting, diarrhoea, itching, recurrent urticaria, arthralgia, myalgia, lymphadenopathy, immune complex nephritis and, rarely, encephalopathy.

Neurotoxic envenomation

Atropine neostigmine (AN) dosage schedule – Atropine 0.6 mg followed by neostigmine (1.5mg) to be given IV stat and repeat dose of neostigmine 0.5 mg with atropine every 30 minutes for 5 doses (In children, Inj. Atropine 0.05 mg/kg followed by Inj. Neostigmine 0.04 mg/kg Intravenous and repeat dose 0.01 mg/kg every 30 minutes for 5 doses). A fixed dose combination of Neostigmine and glycopyrrolate IV can also be used.

Thereafter to be given as tapering dose at 1 hour, 2 hour, 6 hours and 12 hour. Majority of patients improve within the first 5 doses. Observe the patient closely observed for 1 hour to determine if the neostigmine is effective. After 30 minutes, any improvement should be visible by an improvement in ptosis.

Positive response to "AN" trial is measured as 50% or more recovery of the ptosis in one hour. Stop Atropine neostigmine (AN) dosage schedule if patient has complete recovery from neuroparalysis, patient shows side effects in the form of fasciculations or bradycardia. or if there is no improvement after 3 doses.

Compartment syndrome

Compartment syndrome is diagnosed with 5 'P'. They are pain (severe) on passive stretch, pallor, paraesthesia, pulselessness, paralysis or weakness of compartment muscle.

Fasciotomy in a bitten limb with compartment syndrome is undertaken only when haemostatic abnormalities have been corrected otherwise the patient may bleed to death. Intra-compartmental pressure should be >40 mmHg of normal saline (in adults). Timely fasciotomy decreases the need for repeated dialysis.

Summary

It is vital that the emergency physician considers occult snake bite as a differential; in presentations with altered sensorium, paralysis, unexplained bleeding, abdominal pain, vomiting, shock, respiratory distress or acute kidney injury. Polyvalent anti-snake venom administration is the only scientifically validated treatment for symptomatic venomous snake bites. Children should receive the same dose as adults.Dilated and fixed pupils are not a sign of brain death in neurotoxic snake bites. Supportive management in the form of adequate oxygenation, fluid resuscitation is important.

Recent Advances:

Snakebite was re-designated as a neglected tropical disease (NTD), category A, in 2017, which was removed from the list in 2013, re considering the problem of snakebite in developing and tropical countries, which contributes 95 per cent of the total snakebites of the world by WHO. It is known that the available polyvalent ASV acts best in snakebites from the southern and western parts of India and not as well in the northern and eastern parts of the country.

Road map towards mitigation of the problem of venomous snakebite

SVDK (snake venom diagnostic kit) maybe developed by using any of the available methods – ELISA, lateral flow, optical immunoassay, fluorescence immunoassay, reverse latex agglutination, polymerase chain reaction-based assays, Aptamer-based assays *etc*. The major disadvantage of the syndromic approach is that treatment starts only after envenomation is confirmed from the signs and symptoms of systemic toxicity, which happens after the venom has already bound to receptors in tissues. ASV neutralizes only the free fractions of venom in the blood and does not have an effect on venom fractions which have been bound to tissue. With an SVDK, we would be able to confirm the presence of venom from a swab from the bite site even immediately after the bite, which would help identify the biting species.

Availability of an SVDK would also help ascertain as to which species has inflicted the bite, which would pave the way for the availability and manufacturing of monovalent ASV in the future. Treatment with monovalent ASV would help decrease the quantum of ASV being used, thereby decreasing adverse reactions as also making the treatment far more effective and concerted.

Awareness and Media outreach

Appropriate information on snakes, snakebite prevention and first-aid should be shared with all the vulnerable groups through campaigns, social media and public broadcasting.

Basic preventive measures of snakebite including Do's and Dont's such as wearing footwear, using a flashlight and a walking stick at night, not putting ones hand into holes in the ground, keeping the premises and the boundary of the house clear from litter/grass, keeping the hen coop and shed a little distance from the house, not stacking firewood against the side of the house and doing so some distance away and using a mosquito net well tucked in under the mat while sleeping at night are some of the easily implementable measures to prevent snake bite at home.

Setting up a 24×7 snakebite helpline to answer queries with relation to snakes and snakebite.

A concerted effort on the part of all concerned namely policymakers, health authorities, public servants, ASV manufacturers, forest departments and health caregivers including treating doctors, non-governmental organizations, basic scientists, herpetologists and the lay public would lead to a fall in mortality and morbidity related to this eminently preventable cause of death and disability.

Future therapies for poisonous snake bite

Various technological approaches are being pursued by different research groups[4] It included the use of small molecule inhibitors against enzymatic toxins. The most promising of these small molecule inhibitors, varespladib, may have the potential to become a broad spectrum orally administered first line of treatment for snakebite victims, or possibly an anti-PLA2-specific supplement to conventional antivenom therapy. While small molecule inhibitors might be particularly well-suited for targeting enzymatic toxins, such as PLA2s and proteinases, smaller non-enzymatic toxins (such as three-finger toxins) may better be targeted by antibody-based or antibody-like therapeutics. It is therefore likely that increased research efforts on nanobodies and human antibody formats will occur within the next few years. This not only represents an opportunity for innovation within snakebite antivenoms, but it may also facilitate more research efforts on the development of therapies against envenomings by other animals, such as scorpions and spiders.

References

1. Standard Treatment Guidelines on the Management of Snake Bites. Ministry of Health & Family Welfare, Government of India. 2016. [accessed on April 20, 2022]. Available from: https://nhm.gov.in/images/pdf/guidelines/nrhm guidelines/stg/Snakebite_QRG.pdf.

2. Fact sheet: Snake Bite envenomation[Internet]. WHO; 17 May 2021]. Available from: https://www.who.int/news-room/factsheets/detail/snakebite-envenoming

3. Mohapatra B, Warrell DA, Suraweera W, BhatiaP, Dhingra N, Jotkar RM, Rodriguez PS, Mishra K, Whitaker R, Jha P. Snakebite mortality in India: A Nationally Representativ: e Mortality Survey. PLOS Negl Trop Dis, 2011.5 (4): e 1018

4. Central Bureau of Health Intelligence: National Health Profile. 2019accessed on May 22, 2020:151–2 Available from: http://www.cbhidghs.nic.in/showfile.php?lid=1147

5. Majumder D, Sinha A, Bhattacharya SK, Ram R, Dasgupta U, Ram A. Epidemiological profile of snake bite in south 24 Parganas district of West Bengal with focus on underreporting of snake bite deaths. *Indian J Public Health*. 2014;58(1):17-21. doi:10.4103/0019- 557X.128158

6. Bawaskar HS, Bawaskar PH, Punde DP, Inamdar MK, Dongare RB and Bhoite RR. Profile of snakebite envenoming in rural Maharashtra, India. J Assoc Physicians India 2008; 56: 88–95.

7. Mohapatra B, Warrell DA, Suraweera W, BhatiaP, Dhingra N, Jotkar RM, Rodriguez PS, Mishra K, Whitaker R, Jha P. Snakebite mortality in India: A Nationally Representativ: e Mortality Survey. PLOS Negl Trop Dis, 2011.5 (4): e 1018

8. Seifert, Steven A; James O; Sanchez, Elda E. (6 January 2022)."Snake Envenomation".New England Journal of Medicine.386 (1): 68-78

9. Spawls S, Branch B (1997). The Dangerous Snakes of Africa. Johannesburg: Southern Book Publishers. P. 192. ISBN 978-1-86812- 575-3

10. Shibendu Ghosh, Prabuddha Mukhopadhyay, Tanmoy Chatterji.

11. Management of Snake Bite in India. Journal of Association of Physicians of India Vol 64, issue – Editorial. ISSN 0004 – 5772 August 2016.

Psychiatric Emergencies

Contributors

1. Dr. Vikram Singh Rawat
2. Dr. Tanve Garg

Chapters

1. Psychosocial emergencies
2. Behavioral emergencies

Psychosocial Emergencies

<u>**OUTLINE**</u>

- Introduction
- Clinical presentations:
  - Agitated patient
  - Depressive and suicidal patient
  - Substance use and withdrawal
- General guidelines of management
- Management based on clinical presentations
- Updates

<u>**INTRODUCTION**</u>

Emergency care staff are responsible for managing patients with a plethora of presentations having diverse etiologies. Considering that emergency departments are frontline and often the first contact for patients, the staff need to be prepared for handling a variety of emergencies. This situation is often compounded by excess patient load and shortage of staff and / or resources. Patients admitted for medical emergencies may develop an add on behavioural emergency which can strain the team by adding workload (Example – New onset Delirium in a patient admitted for the evaluation and treatment of fever). Alternatively, a patient may present with a medical issue that has an underlying psychiatric issue which needs to be addressed (Example – Paracetamol overdose consequent to an underlying psychiatric or psychosocial cause). The other possibility remains of a psychiatric emergency presenting directly like an agitated patient of bipolar disorder in a manic episode. Hence, emergency staff, including physicians, are responsible for managing patients throughout the day which inevitably also includes patients with behavioural disturbances warranting a need for basic psychiatric training in primary evaluation, assessment and management of such cases.

The American Psychiatric Association characterises a psychiatric emergency as "an acute disturbance in thought, behaviour, mood, or social relationship, which requires immediate intervention as defined by the patient, family, or social unit." Emergency department of a hospital may be the area of first contact of a psychiatric patient with medical care services for behavioural problems in many cases. Major apparent reasons for the same being convenience of 24-hour availability of healthcare team, acutely agitated & unmanageable patients, and other not so apparent reasons like lack of knowledge about appropriate department for consultation, denial about psychological nature of presentation or avoidance of psychiatry outpatient consequent to an apprehension of being considered and labelled as mentally unwell.

An emergency staff must be vigilant enough to assess and manage the behavioural symptoms of a patient, and dispose of the patient within a limited time span given the high patient turnover rate in most emergency settings. This requires a breadth of knowledge encompassing psychiatry, addiction medicine, general medicine, neurology, psychology as well as about social and legal issues. Careful history from the patient as well as relatives / family members available at sight must be taken followed by physical examination and mental status examination (MSE) including a cognitive screen. This chapter attempts to detail the behavioural (psychiatric) emergencies that are encountered in emergency settings and discuss updates in this context.

Psychiatry emergencies can be divided based on common presentations into the following three categories which shall be further discussed in detail within the chapter.

1. Agitation
2. Depression and suicidality
3. Substance use and withdrawal

AGITATION

Agitation can be defined as abnormal and excessive verbal, physically aggressive, or purposeless motor behaviours, heightened arousal, and clinically significant disruption of the patient's functioning. This may be accompanied by verbal or physical violence in certain conditions especially if the patient feels threatened by his surroundings and is trying to resist any interventions. Such patients may present with bizarre, disorganised, and / or paranoid thinking, perceptual disturbances, intense inappropriate emotional expressions and odd exaggerated behaviours putting them and everyone around them at the risk of harm.

An attempt to gather history of the illness from the patient must be made, however, they might not be receptive / attentive enough to converse in most cases. When little information is available, try to reach out to the relatives and attendants available with the patient and gather as much collateral information as possible about the patient and his illness. Agitation can be assessed using the Agitation Behaviour Scale or the Behavioural Activity Ratings Scale. A violence risk assessment must be undertaken before proceeding further with the patient.

There are various conditions that can manifest with agitation in a patient, most common psychiatric diagnoses being acute mania, psychosis (schizophrenia / bipolar disorder), anxiety / panic attacks, dissociative disorders and personality disorders. Important medical conditions like delirium, meningitis, medication induced or neurological conditions might also present with unmanageable agitation and may mimic a psychiatric disorder if not evaluated cautiously. We will discuss each of these conditions briefly.

ACUTE MANIA - These patients require careful assessment for past manic / depressive symptoms, their onset, nature, duration and remission with particular focus on finding a recent stressor if possible. Some of the prominent features expected on MSE in patients of mania are increased goal directed activity, pressured speech, increased talkativeness, elevated mood, grandiose ideas, flight of ideas and sometimes abnormalities of beliefs resulting in grandiose delusions and rarely even perceptual disturbances like hallucinations.

The severity of symptoms can be inferred by the disruption caused to daily rhythms and activities which can disrupt personal life and work. The YMRS (Young Mania Rating Scale) may help in quantifying the severity of the episode by providing an objective score.

Manic disorder can also be a manifestation of an underlying medical condition which should be considered while obtaining a careful history and during initial physical examination. Such conditions include varied etiologies like thyrotoxicosis, SLE, Steroid /drug induced, Wilson's disease, Multiple sclerosis, Huntington disease, cerebrovascular accident, diencephalic and third ventricular tumours, head trauma, complex partial seizures, syphilis and AIDS. These etiologies are often missed or overlooked in the emergency settings and also an ever growing list of causative influences keep accumulating as many newer medications are approved for use. For example - TNF-alpha inhibitors and association with psychiatric conditions like hypomania and mania as has been reported in a systematic review.

These concepts emphasize the need for clinicians to be aware of secondary mania (mania as a manifestation of an underlying medical or surgical condition or induced by medication or substance) and assess every patient with an unbiased perspective. Often newer medications and newer medical illnesses have undocumented effects which result in an oversight and potentially missed diagnoses. The psychiatric manifestation is seen in isolation from the rest of medical conditions leading to a loss of understanding and potentially inappropriate treatment.

PSYCHOSIS - These patients may further have an underlying medical condition resulting in the presentation or a psychiatric disorder such as Schizophrenia / Acute and Transient Psychotic Disorders/ Delusional disorder etc. The aim of emergency psychiatric care is not to reach an immediate psychiatric diagnosis, but to identify any underlying medical cause, risk assessment, the details of current behavioural manifestations and manage it appropriately by seeking consultations from various specialties. These patients might present with common features of agitation, impaired reality testing, paranoia, delusions, hallucinations (mostly auditory), perplexed affect and disorganised thinking.

Some medical causes of psychotic disorders include AIDS/HIV, Dementia due to pick's disease or Alzheimer's disease, endocrine diseases, frontal lobe neoplasms, drug induced psychosis, temporal lobe epilepsy and syphilis. All of these need to be considered and carefully ruled out in order to arrive at a psychiatric diagnosis.

ANXIETY/ PANIC ATTACKS - These patients often end up seeking emergency consultation for an exacerbation of anxiety that results in uncomfortable symptoms. The autonomic manifestations can result in a dramatic presentation. For example - A patient with a panic attack may present to the emergency stating that he is about to have a heart attack. This feeling of impending doom is often accompanied by palpitations, restlessness, chest discomfort, shortness of breath, sweating, goose flesh and choking sensations. These patients may be seen pacing around or gasping for breath and appear to be agitated consequent to the intense anxiety.

Such patients need careful evaluation to rule out underlying medical conditions such as encephalitis, epilepsy, hypertension, hyperthyroidism, hypoglycemia, hypokalemia, internal haemorrhage, cardiac arrhythmias, pheochromocytoma, pulmonary embolism and endocarditis. A careful history and physical examination including a MSE are important along with appropriate investigations.

OTHER CONDITIONS - certain personality disorders especially antisocial PD, Borderline PD, might be repeatedly visiting ED due to their frequent involvement in violent activities. Sometimes dissociative disorder, particularly dissociative convulsions might present as an acutely agitated patient with heightened activity levels.

DEPRESSION AND SUICIDALITY:

Self harm and suicidal attempts are a common presentation to the ED. Most frequently as drug overdose especially with analgesics / benzodiazepines or psychotropics. A physician must never miss asking the patient about circumstances of the act and the prevailing mental state before, during and after the attempt. Particular attention must be given to the extent of planning, intent of the act (harming self or threat or intending to kill self) and the exact mode of self-harm. A majority of the patients indicate or forewarn of their suicidal intent before committing an act. Despite the apprehensions of emergency staff, they are less likely to initiate a suicidal idea in a patient by enquiring about if they want to die. The patient can be asked direct questions in this context and to elicit the intent and the lethality of the suicidal ideation. Infact, it might help to relieve the patient by discussing his problems. Establishing a good therapeutic alliance with the patient might help further.

Specific plans of the patient should be assessed and correlated with actual lethality of the plan.

Assessment of suicide risk is one of the major responsibilities of attending physician to take a decision regarding further management of the patient.

Many Scales can be used for assessment of suicidality in the ED like modified SAD PERSONS scale, Beck scale for suicide Ideation and risk of suicide questionnaire. Depression in a patient can be rated on HAM-S or BDI scale. However, these scales only assess the risk for suicide, the cut off scores should not be used strictly to warrant admission and treatment of the patient.

Clinical judgement of the physician comes into picture while assessing a case for risk of suicide in the ED.

Some risk factors that enhance the proneness to suicidality are-

1. Past history of suicide attempt
2. Family history of suicide
3. Current psychiatric illness of major depressive disorder
4. Expressed suicidal ideations, with well-formed plan
5. Current crisis situation such as serious medical illness / disfiguring surgery
6. Presence of command hallucinations
7. Easily available means of suicide
8. Low perceived / actual social support
9. Suicide note preparation or preparation of a will

The assessment for depression or suicidality is incomplete without ruling out the differentials of medical disorders for depression which include substance withdrawal states, major neurocognitive disorder, hepatitis, hypokalemia, hypothyroidism, infectious mononucleosis, occult malignancy, post viral syndromes and vascular dementia.

Substance use and withdrawal:

Patients with substance intoxication or withdrawal are frequently brought to EDs in either a state of altered mental status or a state of heightened activity, agitation and loss of control. It becomes important for the physician to separate the signs of intoxication from withdrawal and also separate signs of various illicit psychoactive substances that might present with similar manifestations.

The assessment for suspected substance use must include a thorough history from the patient or the family members regarding the last use of illicit substance, amount of use and past history regarding the same. Also a urine drug screen (UDS) is helpful in finding out the suspected drug of abuse.

Behavioural manifestations of a few common substances are given below.

Alcohol: Acute alcohol intoxication can present as violent, disruptive patient, aggressive behaviour, impaired judgement, incoordination, psychomotor agitation, transient hallucinations and unsteady gait who might even have suicidal ideations. Medical complications might include nausea, vomiting, GI bleeding, vitamin deficiencies and malnutrition. Death may occur due to aspiration or respiratory depression. All intoxicated patients must be evaluated for BAC levels and then correlated clinically to guide further management.

BAC LEVEL -

- ▶ 30 mg/dL: Euphoria and inattention
- ▶ 50 mg/dL: Unsteady gait and problems with coordination
- ▶ 100 mg/dL: Memory disturbances and ataxia
- ▶ 200 mg/dL: Confusion and stupor
- ▶ >400 mg/dL: Seizures/ Coma/ Death

Most cases of alcohol intoxication can be managed conservatively, once the BAC has reached within a low range, the patient starts improving.

Alcohol withdrawal on the other hand can be a serious life threatening condition and a psychiatric emergency. The symptoms for withdrawal start appearing within 2-10 days after the last dose of alcohol, peak within 1-2 days and subside after 5-6 days completely. Death may occur in about 4-20% cases following complications like hyperthermia or aspiration. For detection of alcohol withdrawal look for signs of disorientation, violent agitation, decreased attention, along with autonomic instability including tachycardia, hypertension, sweating, tremors, vomiting and occasionally generalised seizures. These patients might present with hallucinations, generally tactile in nature with complaints of insects crawling under the skin. In some cases, olfactory or auditory hallucinations might also be prominent.

Complicated alcohol withdrawal might present to ED with seizures or Delirium Tremens. Alcohol withdrawal delirium is a variety of delirium where benzodiazepines are the treatment of choice unlike in other medical causes of delirium. Therefore, it is important to take alcohol use history in all patients in ED presenting in the status of delirium or seizures.

CIWA-Ar scale or AUDIT scale can be used for assessment of alcohol withdrawal in emergency settings.

Alcohol withdrawal delirium, an extreme form of alcohol withdrawal state, is a variety of delirium where benzodiazepines are the treatment of choice unlike in other medical causes of delirium.

Opioids: Common features of opioid intoxication are drowsiness, pinpoint pupils, respiratory depression, slurring of speech, may result in complications such as seizures, arrhythmias and even coma. Pulmonary or cerebral edema could also be life threatening in certain cases.

Unlike alcohol withdrawal, opioid withdrawal is not life threatening. Onset of withdrawal symptoms occur within 7-8 hours, peak at 36-72 hours and last upto a week with symptoms of withdrawal being Nausea, Vomiting, Diarrhoea, Tremors, Sweating, Piloerection, Generalised weakness, Abdominal cramps, Muscle aches, frequent yawning and increased lacrimation to enlist a few. COWS (Clinical Opiate Withdrawal Scale) can be used to assess severity of opioid withdrawal quickly in the ED.

Sedative hypnotics - Benzodiazepines are common drugs of misuse. Acute intoxication with benzodiazepine may present as excessive drowsiness, impaired control, social disinhibition, slurred speech, incoordination, unsteady gait, areflexia, muscle hypotonicity, hypotension, and hypothermia. These patients require urgent medical attention and should be admitted to ICU until stabilisation of medical condition.

Onset of Withdrawal from BZD occurs after 12-24 hours after last dose, peaks at 24-72 hours and lasts upto 5-8 days with prominent features of tremors, palpitations, anxiety, nausea, vomiting, loss of appetite, and even result in seizures or delirium. The symptoms can be remarkably similar to any other depressant withdrawal state (example – Alcohol withdrawal).

Withdrawal from benzodiazepines can be assessed using CIWA-B scale.

Management of psychiatric emergency

Ensure safety of self, followed by safety of others including patient as well as staff and bystanders

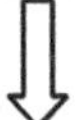

Assess (history, physical exam and investigations) and consider potential medical causes of the behavioural manifestations.

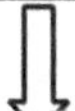

Detailed psychiatric evaluation and assessment and triage the patient according to imminent conditions.

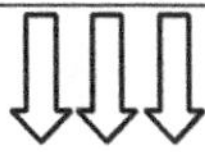

Agitated/ Violent patient	Depressive/ suicidal patient	Substance use or withdrawal
• Verbal de escalation • Oral Sedatives/ antipsychotics • Injectable sedatives/ antipsychotics • Physical restraint	• Assess severity based on history, exam and impairment of functioning • Psychotherapy • No-harm contract • Oral sedatives / antidepressants • Observation in ward	• Antidote for intoxication if available • Oral sedatives (BZD) preferred for withdrawal management

Risk assessment – Assessing risk of any kind of harm (to person or objects or possessions) is an important part of a psychiatric emergency and must be carried out in all cases. This must be documented clearly in terms of the imminent nature of the risk and further evaluation initiated at once.

General management strategies for a psychiatric emergency

1. Precautions – Ensure safety of the evaluation area for self, other emergency staff and the patient as well as the bystanders so that there is no harm. Ensure easy access to a safe exit in case the situation becomes unmanageable due to worsening of violence, keep a distance of more than arm's length during evaluation (at least two arm length). Communicate in a clear and firm manner with eye contact while ensuring that it does not appear intimidating or threatening. Availability of security personnel and ancillary staff for further assistance is an important aspect while also ensuring that there is no crowding or cornering of the patient. CCTV cameras and training the staff may be necessary with environmental modifications that prevent worsening of aggression or any untowards injury. Agitated patients may be interviewed away from non-agitated patients in the emergency if possible.

2. Assessment – Obtain a focussed history including a thorough general physical examination followed by relevant systemic examination and investigations. The assessment is an ongoing process as more information becomes available from history and / or exam and / or investigations. It is critical to ensure that medical causes of patient's behavioural symptoms are excluded and any other illness that needs immediate care is identified as soon as possible. It is also important to determine the patient's cognitive functioning during the mental status examination. Cognitive functions of a patient can be tested in the shortest time using tools like HMSE (Hindi mental status examination), CAM (Confusion Assessment Method) and clock drawing test etc.

Initially CBC, Random blood sugar, Serum electrolytes, ECG, Urine Drug Screen, Breath Alcohol Concentration and for females Urine Pregnancy Test may be indicated.

Physical examination and history must aid in deciding about the need for imaging, especially the brain and any other organ system.

- Consider possible medical causes in extremes of age, patients with history of fever, seizures, loss of consciousness, head injury, underlying endocrine dysfunction, acute onset symptoms, impaired cognition, first episode without any past or family history of psychiatric conditions, presence of substance use.

Whenever the diagnosis is unclear even after initial assessment and investigations, advanced diagnostic tests may be required such as NCCT head, MRI brain which might help to explain the current behavioural symptoms especially in cases of head trauma/ CVA/ other infectious causes.

3. <u>Detailed psychiatric assessment and triaging</u> - It is challenging to obtain history from an agitated or mute patient or patient with cognitive impairment. In such situations, a physician should try to obtain as much collateral information as possible from family members / police personnel / staff and past medical records when available. Out of all the patients with psychiatric manifestations coming to the ED almost 20% patients have risk of harm to self and about 10% patients pose risk of harm to others and 40% patients out of the total require admission into a psychiatric ward <u>(synopsis)</u>. But to decide whether a patient is in need of hospitalisation or not and to guide further management plans, it is important to triage the psychiatric patients coming to ED, much like other routine cases in the ED.

Foremost step before triaging is to make an assessment of risk of the patients. Doing a suicidal risk assessment, assessment for homicidal ideations and violence risk assessment including risk factors, protective factors, support system and overall risk stratification should be considered as and when deemed appropriate.

Patients who are agitated or suicidal may need immediate attention (within minutes) whereas patients who are psychotic or depressed and have a potential to become agitated may be attended urgently (within 30 minutes). Patients with Delirium also may need immediate attention for prompt evaluation and avoiding inappropriate medication or treatment errors by other staff.

Patients with an established psychiatric disorder presenting with relapse and not showing any likely agitation or self-harm risk and medically stable can be attended in a relaxed manner (in an hour) after sorting more urgent issues in the ED.

Patients with accompanying escorts must be assessed as early initially while getting as much information from the escort (as often escorts may leave or take turns in ED).

The triage can be carried out by the emergency physician while simultaneously seeking appropriate inputs from other specialties as well as psychiatry. It may be necessary to involve a counsellor or social worker or a clinical psychologist or more than one member in cases of psychosocial issues that are presenting to the emergency.

Management of the case based on triaging -

AGITATED AND VIOLENT PATIENTS -

1. Psychotherapeutic management - It is important for an examiner to build a working relationship with the patient in order to ensure any psychotherapeutic approach in a short span of time, which is very difficult in an emergency setting. Therefore, it becomes necessary to ask direct questions to the patient about psychopathology. Whenever a patient describes a perceptual abnormality, it is important to get a full description, without challenging their experiences as it might provoke them further leading to increased violent behaviours. One should always have an empathetic approach towards these patients without getting over involved with them. A paranoid patient needs to be handled very tactfully since they might feel unsafe in the new environment of the ED. a safe distance must be kept, usually about 2 steps or a leg's distance from the patient.

    While interviewing the patient, keep in mind to give them repeated reassurance from time to time to keep them calm and try verbal de-escalation techniques that might be helpful to reduce the agitation and decrease the danger of violence without requiring pharmacotherapy.

    If there is no improvement with psychotherapeutic intervention, try to ascertain authority over the patient with a show of force by 2-3 security guards which might make the patient cooperate for the interview and treatment.

2. Psychopharmacological management - The National Institute for health and Care Excellence (NICE), stated that "the aim of drug treatment in agitated patients is to calm the person and reduce the risk of violence and harm" and that "an optimal response would be a reduction in agitation or aggression without sedation, allowing the service user to participate in further assessment and treatment."

    The most frequently used strategies are use of BZDs, SGAs and Haloperidol amongst the FGAs alone or along with a BZD, commonly being Lorazepam. Generally, a patient should be given the option of route of preferred administration and the use of oral dissolving tablets and liquid formulations is encouraged over parenteral routes as these are the least invasive options available, however it might not be possible in many cases considering the heightened psychomotor activity of the patient.

    Options that can be considered are -

    -   Oral first line for agitation - oral mouth dissolving risperidone (2mg) with or without Lorazepam (2mg) or oral mouth dissolving olanzapine alone (5-10mg)

- Parenteral first line for agitation without psychosis - IM Lorazepam (2 mg) for cases without psychosis
- Parenteral first line for agitation with psychosis - IM Ziprasidone (20 mg) + IM Lorazepam (2mg)
- Parenteral second line for agitation with psychosis - IM Haloperidol (5mg) + IM Lorazepam (2mg) or IM Olanzapine alone (5-10mg). *Lorazepam should be avoided to use with olanzapine due to risk of cardiorespiratory depression.
- Some clinicians prefer to use IV route for rapid effects for which IV Diazepam (5-10 mg) or IV Lorazepam (2-4mg) can be given slowly over 2 mins, however it is best avoided as it might cause overmedication and sedation.

Medication doses can be repeated once every 1 hour, maximum upto 3-4 times per day until the patient is calm enough to participate in the assessment, however most patients don't need heavy dosing.

Most common medication in psychiatric emergency has been use of combination of IM Haloperidol (5mg) + IM Lorazepam (2mg) as it is well tolerated as compared to Haloperidol alone, achieves adequate sedation and also reduces the adverse effects of Haloperidol.

The most common side effects with parenteral antipsychotics could be acute dystonia, akathisia and other EPS which can be controlled by IM Benztropine (2mg). Acute dystonia can range from oculogyric crisis, torticollis to even laryngospasm, therefore the team must be prepared to manage the side effects swiftly and intube if necessary.

For patients with insomnia, agitation, panic attacks, or psychic anxiety, benzodiazepines can be used on a short-term basis; however, when used, long-acting benzodiazepines (like T Diazepam 5-10 mg or Tab Clonazepam 0.25-0.5 mg) are preferable and should be tapered. If benzodiazepines are not desired, other calming medications, such as trazadone, low doses of second-generation antipsychotics, and anticonvulsants can be used.

The expert consensus guidelines for treatment of behavioural emergencies (2005) recommend the following options for specified causes of agitation: -

SUSPECTED DISORDER	ORAL	PARENTERAL
Delirium	Haloperidol/Risperidone	IM - Haloperidol/ olanzapine/ ziprasidone
Acute mania	Antipsychotic + BZD First line - Olanzapine/Risperidone Second line - Haloperidol/ Quetiapine/ Ziprasidone Mood stabiliser - Divalproex	Antipsychotic + BZD IM first line - olanzapine alone or haloperidol + BZD IM second line - ziprasidone + BZD

Primary psychotic disorder	First line - Risperidone/ Olanzapine alone or Haloperidol/Risperidone + BZD Second line - Quetiapine/ Ziprasidone	IM first line - olanzapine or haloperidol + BZD or ziprasidone + BZD

Dose & freq - oral lorazepam (1–3 mg), I.M. lorazepam (0.5–3 mg), oral or I.M. haloperidol (2.5–10 mg), oral risperidone (1–3 mg), oral olanzapine (5–20 mg), I.M. olanzapine (5–10 mg), and I.M. ziprasidone (10–20 mg). Oral Divalproex (30 mg/kg/day starting dose, followed by 20 mg/kg/day)

Medical comorbidities	Medication	Avoid to use
Chronic Obstructive Pulmonary Disease	Typical antipsychotic > Atypical antipsychotic	Benzodiazepines (Respiratory depression)
Cardiac arrhythmias	Benzodiazepine > Typical/Atypical antipsychotics	
Delirium	Typical antipsychotic > Atypical antipsychotic	Benzodiazepines and Anticholinergics.
Delirium Tremens/ History of substance use.	Benzodiazepines	
Elderly	Atypical antipsychotic > Typical antipsychotic	Benzodiazepines
History of seizures	Benzodiazepines > Atypical antipsychotics	

3. Use of restraint - One must bear in mind that use of restraint is a compromise to a person's autonomy and can be devastating for therapeutic alliance, therefore its use must be restricted for the utmost difficult patients, that too for the least possible time. While using a physical restraint, always maintain privacy and dignity of the patient and the medical staff should be adequately trained regarding its safe use and monitoring. It should only be commenced after a proper written consent from the attendants of the patient, explaining to them the need for it.

A checklist for guidelines to be followed during use of restraint for a patient should be made in every ED and followed thoroughly.

It is contraindicated in certain medical comorbidities such as cardiac disorders, metabolic illnesses, respiratory disorders, orthopaedic problems. Also rigorous attention is required to a restrained patient with observation every 15 mins to ensure circulation, respiration and regular recording of vitals and screening for thromboembolism, reduced respiratory function, pressure sores or urinary and bowel incontinence.

FOR DEPRESSIVE OR SUICIDAL PATIENT:

Establishing a rapport as described above is a pre requisite for psychotherapy in suicidal patients. In case a physician does not know what to say, it is best to listen to the patient empathetically. Let the patient talk uninterrupted and indulge them to discuss their crisis situations in depth. Try to identify the intent, plan and lethality of the attempt and the remorse after the attempt. Most importantly assess any current suicidality that indicates an urgent admission to psychiatric ward. Discuss the treatment options with the patient oral as well as injectables and need for medication to keep them calm.

A common tool used in the outpatient setting is the no-harm contract in which the person makes a contract with the physician to contact them as soon as he has a self-harm thought. However, it should not defer the required evaluation and management of agitated/impulsive patients who require immediate intervention and admission. If identified, treat the underlying cause of the suicidality.

FOR SUBSTANCE USE AND WITHDRAWAL PATIENTS:

Different substances might require slightly different approaches.

Alcohol withdrawal is best managed with Benzodiazepines preferably Chlordiazepoxide (25-100 mg) or Diazepam (5-10 mg) or Lorazepam (1-2 mg) particularly in patients with hepatic impairment, which can be repeated every 4-6 hours as required, until the patient is sedated. Apart from this, also add Thiamine upto 300 mg via oral or parenteral route for replenishment of vitamin B1 in case of chronic alcohol users.

For the treatment of Benzodiazepine withdrawal, start treatment with giving the equivalent dose of benzodiazepine as was being used by the patient previously in either the same form and taper gradually over next few weeks, or use a longer acting benzodiazepine substitute such as Diazepam or Clonazepam and taper over the next few weeks. Patients with complicated withdrawal with seizures may need to be admitted to an addiction treatment facility.

For patients with opioid withdrawal, methadone substitution or buprenorphine substitution therapy can be initiated in coordination with addiction treatment facilities and also, clonidine can be given for symptomatic treatment.

References:

1. Sadock BJ, Sadock VA, Ruiz P, Kaplan HI. Kaplan and Sadock's comprehensive textbook of psychiatry. 2017.

2. Gelder M, Gath D, Mayou R. Oxford textbook of psychiatry, 2nd ed. New York, NY, US: Oxford University Press; 1989. xiv, 1079 p. (Oxford textbook of psychiatry, 2nd ed).

3. Kaplan & Sadock's Synopsis of Psychiatry [Internet]. [cited 2022 May 2]. Available from: https://www.wolterskluwer.com/en/solutions/ovid/kaplan--sadocks-synopsis-of-psychiatry-2253

4. Slade M, Taber D, Clarke MM, Johnson C, Kapoor D, Leikin JB, et al. Best Practices for the Treatment of Patients with Mental and Substance Use Illnesses in the Emergency Department. Disease-a-Month. 2007 Nov 1;53(11):536–80.

5. Zun LS. Pitfalls in the Care of the Psychiatric Patient in the Emergency Department. The Journal of Emergency Medicine. 2012 Nov 1;43(5):829–35.

6. Brown JF. Psychiatric Emergency Services: A Review of the Literature and a Proposed Research Agenda. Psychiatr Q. 2005 Apr 1;76(2):139–65.

7. Allen MH, Currier GW, Carpenter D, Ross RW, Docherty JP, Expert Consensus Panel for Behavioral Emergencies 2005. The expert consensus guideline series. Treatment of behavioral emergencies 2005. J Psychiatr Pract. 2005 Nov;11 Suppl 1:5–108; quiz 110–2.

CPR Updates

Contributors

1. Dr. K Shailaja
2. Dr. Nithya Shreya Meghana
3. Dr. Ashima Sharma

Chapters

1. PALS
2. Peri arrest updates

Pediatric Cardiopulmonary Resuscitation

Introduction

The American Heart Association started developing a course in pediatric advanced life support (PALS) in 1983, owing to the need for separate resuscitation guidelines and training for children. These differed from adult and newborn guidelines due to differences in the etiology of cardiopulmonary arrest (CPA), anatomy, and physiology among them. PALS courses were started in 1988, and in 1989 the European Resuscitation Council was formed.

In 1992 International Liaison Committee On Resuscitation (ILCOR) formed, which managed to bring about liaison between principal resuscitation organizations to a common forum over the years. Experts from various countries contribute to the worldwide Consensus On Science and Treatment Recommendations (CoSTR).

Indian Resuscitation Council Federation is in the process of joining ILCOR and is actively advocating adult as well as pediatric resuscitation guidelines that suit the needs of the Indian subcontinent.

Epidemiology

The prehospital and hospital setting pediatric cardiopulmonary arrests have differing prognoses, with prehospital CPA having lower survival rates. Higher survival rates have been associated with increasing age, early recognition and life support, shockable rhythms, emergency medical care, automatic external defibrillator (AED) usage, telephone dispatcher-assisted cardiopulmonary resuscitation (CPR), and witnessed CPA. Survival was also better when the CPR duration was shorter, when the arrest occurred on weekdays and during the daytime, and in patients undergoing monitoring. Pediatric CPR has a poor prognosis, but with increasing knowledge and efforts, improved survival has been observed over the years, especially in the in-hospital setting.

Implementation of dispatch-assisted CPR appears acceptable and feasible. However, its cost-effectiveness and impact on health equity need to be further evaluated and may present barriers to implementation in under-resourced regions.

Pediatric CPR has progressed considerably, particularly in developed countries. Recognition of the epidemiological factors that influence resuscitation helps direct the efforts towards better and effective management of pediatric CPR in different countries.

Definition

Pediatric Advanced Life Support (PALS) - It is a course conducted by the American Heart Association for healthcare personnel who care for children and infants in the in-hospital as well as out-of-hospital settings.

Pediatric life support courses and guidelines – Courses and guidelines for resuscitation of pediatric patients by health care personnel and lay persons are available for different countries and institutions that are tailored to the particular region's needs.

Pathophysiology

There are several causes of CPA, categorized into respiratory, cardiac, infectious, and traumatic origin.

Respiratory issues are a much more common etiology of CPA in infants and children than primary cardiac events, making effective management of airway take high precedence. However, airway management should not cause undue delay or interruption of chest compressions in any resuscitation efforts.

Table 1: REVERSIBLE CAUSES OF CPA

Hypovolemia	Tamponade Cardiac
Hypoxia	Toxins
H+ Acidosis	Tension Pneumothorax
Hypothermia	Thrombosis Pulmonary
Hypo/Hyperkalemia	Thrombosis Coronary
Hypoglycemia	Trauma

Recent advances in Paediatric Resuscitation

CPA in children, particularly out-of-hospital cardiac arrest (OHCA), has a poor prognosis. High-quality CPR improves outcomes, as seen over the years, but what is deemed the best possible CPR for a particular patient is still based on limited evidence and differs between patients and etiologies. Developing better parameters to guide CPR and adjusting it to the needs of each patient for reviving them is the ultimate goal of resuscitation research. The latest research-based guidelines on pediatric resuscitation, which are advocated by the major resuscitation councils in the world, are discussed here.

ILCOR emphasizes three essential components for good resuscitation outcomes: guidelines based on sound resuscitation science, effective education of the lay public and resuscitation providers, and implementation of a well-functioning chain of survival. These guidelines contain pediatric basic and advanced life support recommendations, excluding the newborn period, and are based on the best available resuscitation science. The chain of survival is now expanded to include recovery from CPA.

Figure 1: PALS CHAIN OF SURVIVAL PEWS-Pediatric Early Warning Scores; PRRT-Pediatric Rapid Response Team; MET-Medical Emergency Team; AED-Automated External Defibrillator

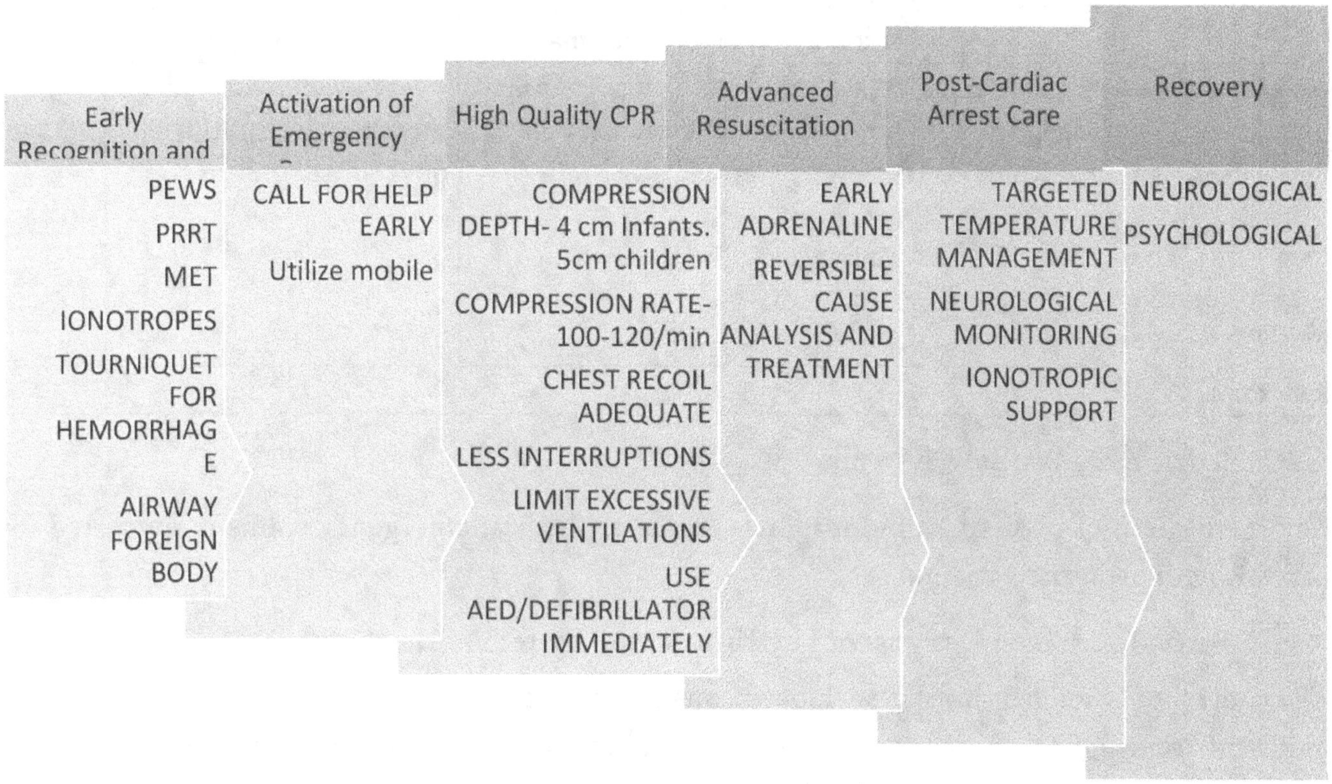

<u>*Pre-Cardiac Arrest Recommendations*</u>

1. Inotropes for Pediatric Septic Shock:

Patient response-based fluid resuscitation with balanced crystalloid, unbalanced crystalloid and colloid fluids with frequent reassessment is needed for resuscitation in cases of sepsis. Epinephrine or norepinephrine infusions can be used for fluid-refractory septic shock. There has not been any recommendation of a specific inotrope or vasopressor for use in pediatric septic shock, and the latest review also suggests no changes to this at present.

2. Pediatric Early Warning Scores (PEWS):

The use of PEWS is suggested to recognize any deterioration in hospitalized pediatric patients, but its ability to predict CPA cannot be recommended with the available data.

Table 2: PEWS CHART

	0	1	2	3	Score
Behavior/Neuro	Playing/ Appropriate	Sleepy	Irritable	Lethargic/ Confused/ Reduced response to pain	
Cardiovascular	Pink/Capillary refill 1-2 seconds	Pale/ Capillary refill 3 seconds	Grey/ Capillary refill 4 seconds/ Heart Rate > 20 above normal	Grey/ Mottled/ Capillary refill ≥5 seconds/ Heart Rate > 30 above normal/Bradycardia	
Respiratory	Within normal range, No retractions	> 10 above normal, using accessory muscles/ 30% FiO_2/≥ 3l/min	>20 above normal/ Retractions/ 40% FiO_2 ≥ 6l/min	< 5 below normal with retractions/ Grunting/ 50% FiO_2 or ≥ 8l/min	
Total score					

3. Pediatric Early Warning Systems:

The organization of pediatric rapid response teams or medical emergency teams is suggested for hospitals with pediatric patients.

4. Pediatric Tourniquet Designs for Life-threatening Extremity Hemorrhage:

Early control of blood loss must be achieved considering the lower blood volumes in children. The designs of tourniquets at present are not optimal, especially those needed for younger children below two years. Direct pressure should be used when feasible to control the bleeding. Further betterment of tourniquet design and usage is necessary. A manufactured windlass tourniquet can be utilized for managing large volume extremity bleeds.

5. Removal of foreign body airway obstruction (FBAO):

Back Slaps can be utilized, followed by abdominal thrusts if needed, in cases of FBAO in a child with ineffective cough.

The rescuer can manually remove visible FBAO, but blindly searching for the foreign body is prohibited. The use of Magill forceps is suggested for rescuers capable of handling it. Bystanders can try maneuvers to support the airway foreign body removal as soon as it is recognized.

Cardiac Arrest Recommendations

1. High-quality CPR:

High-quality CPR forms the basis for successful resuscitation. New data reaffirm the essential components of high-quality CPR, i.e., providing adequate chest compression rate and depth (100-

120/minute; 4cm in infants, 5cm in children), decreasing interruptions in CPR, full chest recoil between compressions, and avoiding excessive ventilation.

2. Starting CPR (ABC vs. CAB):

No further human or manikin studies have been published since the 2015 ILCOR systematic review. Starting CPR with compressions rather than ventilations is recommended at present.

3. Pediatric Chest Compression Depth:

Recent literature shows that it is difficult to achieve the chest compression depth requirements set presently i.e., 4cm for infants and 5cm for children. But with the use of CPR feedback devices and proper training, the target depth can be achieved. Further studies using better feedback devices are needed for a review of the present guidelines.

4. CPR: Chest Compression to Ventilation Ratio - for bystander:

Previous studies indicated that the outcome was better when ventilation was given along with compressions (30:2 for single-rescuer and 15:2 for two-rescuer compressions and ventilations ratio), but the latest studies do not suggest so. According to recent studies, compression-only CPR seems to be as good as compressions with ventilation. Still, ILCOR guidelines suggest there is insufficient evidence to change the current practice. The primary CPA etiology in the pediatric population being respiratory; this stand seems valid.

5. Public Access Defibrillation programs including infants, children, and adolescents:

Suggestion has been made for the use of an AED by the lay rescuer for children above one year. For children below one year having non-traumatic cardiac arrests, there are no recommendations for or against AED use.

6. Emergency medical dispatch centers:

Regarding dispatch-assisted CPR, the guidelines suggest instructions to be given for presumed pediatric CPA and where bystander CPR has not started but make no recommendation for or against when bystander CPR is already in progress.

7. Airway:

A respiratory rate of 20-30 breaths per minute is advocated for infants and children receiving CPR with an advanced airway or receiving rescue breathing and having a pulse.

Advanced airways do not seem to be associated with better outcomes. In out-of-hospital situations, it is suggested to use bag-mask ventilation (BMV) over the advanced airway. Owing to the paucity of evidence, recommendations could not be made about the use of advanced airways in the in-hospital situations. Time should not be wasted in trying advanced airway placement for prolonged periods.

The use of cricoid pressure does not reduce the risk of regurgitation during bag-mask ventilation and may reduce intubation success. When intubation is done, cuffed endotracheal tube usage decreases the need for endotracheal tube changes. Endotracheal tube size, position, and cuff pressures (<20-25 cm of H2O) should be managed appropriately.

8. Drugs

Two doses of amiodarone or lignocaine can be used for shock refractory ventricular fibrillation and pulseless ventricular tachycardia. No specific preference is suggested for one over the other.

The earlier epinephrine is given after CPR initiation, the more likely the patient benefits and survives in cases with non-shockable rhythms.

Opioid overdose can be treated with naloxone, but there is a lack of evidence that it benefits patients in cardiac arrest as much as it does in patients with palpable pulse.

Table 3: CPR DRUGS

CPR DRUG	DOSE	REMARKS
Adrenaline	10 mcg/kg	0.1 ml/kg of 1 in 10,000 solution every 3-5 min
Amiodarone	5 mg/kg	After second shock
Lignocaine	1 mg/kg	After second shock

9. Oxygen titration during pediatric CPA:

The titration of oxygen during or immediately post-CPA was reviewed, but there is insufficient data on this. Maintaining 100% oxygen during resuscitation and immediately after, followed by titrating according to saturation in the post circulation restoration phase, is suggested.

10. Point-of-Care Cardiac Ultrasound (POCUS) during Pediatric CPA:

Cost of the ultrasound machine and the learning curve associated with its use are the main deterrents in hospitals with low resources. Also, care must be taken not to interrupt compressions while trying to analyze the cause of arrest with the help of POCUS. Caution is suggested when using POCUS for ultrasound based on adult observations as there are anatomical variations and different usage modalities. Based on all these, no new recommendation could be made regarding its use in pediatric CPR presently.

11. Prone CPR:

CPA can rarely happen in pediatric patients undergoing surgeries in the prone position or undergoing prone ventilation in pediatric ICUs. Prone CPR can be done in such cases with the available monitors like arterial blood pressure or the $ETCO_2$ monitoring guiding the effectiveness of the CPR. Immediate supination can be done where an advanced airway is not in place to give ventilations along with compressions. Supination can be done after a period of prone CPR when an advanced airway is in place, with proper care of the lines and surgical site. Defibrillation (2 J/kg initial shock; 4J/kg increasing up to 10J/kg or maximum of 200J) is also feasible in the prone position. Compressions can be done according to the existing guidelines except the position of compressions will be in between the scapulae.

Figure 2: PRONE CPR - COMPRESSIONS IN AN INFANT (A) IF THERE IS A MIDLINE SURGICAL INCISION (B) WITHOUT SURGICAL INCISION

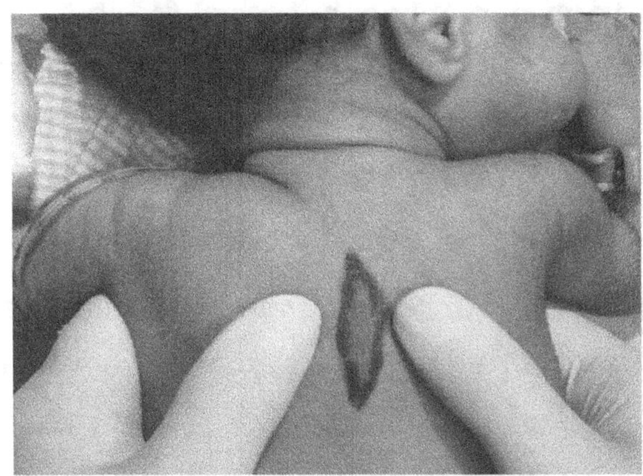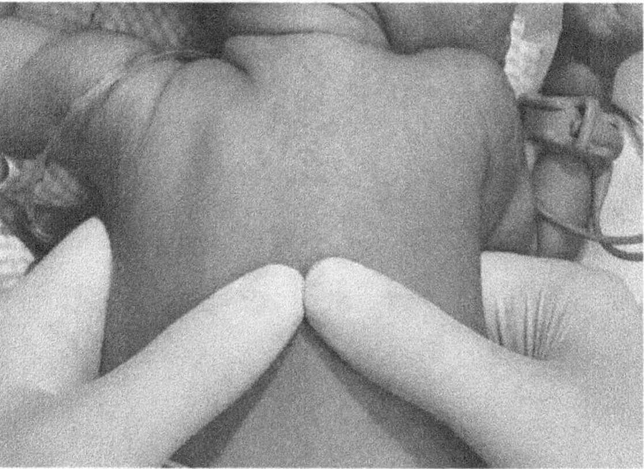

12. Value of Blood Pressure (BP) monitoring during pediatric cardiac arrest:

The value of a specific BP goal based on which a particular child's CPR can be adjusted is yet to be determined.

13. Value of End-tidal CO_2 measurement during pediatric cardiac arrest:

$EtCO_2$ may be of value in pediatric arrest assessment when the patient is already intubated, as in the pediatric ICU or during surgery. Compressions take precedence over advanced airway placement during CPR. Not much research has happened in this area in recent times to prompt any change in the existing guidelines.

14. Value of near-infrared spectroscopy during pediatric in- and out-of-hospital cardiac arrest:

The use of near-infrared spectroscopy during pediatric CPR in both in-hospital and out-of-hospital situations needs to be considered for individualized care of children in CPA.

15. Extracorporeal cardiopulmonary resuscitation (ECPR) for cardiac arrest:

ECPR can be considered for specific in-hospital pediatric cardiac arrests where there is a facility for its quick implementation. There is a lack of evidence for out-of-hospital settings to suggest its use.

16. Drowning:

No previous treatment recommendations exist on prehospital oxygen use, advanced airway placement and mechanical ventilation, AED or ECMO usage after drowning. The present general BLS

ALS Task Force recommendations for these interventions can be utilized until specific guidelines are available for drowning.

The use of prehospital oxygen in drowning has the potential to reverse hypoxemia and may improve outcomes. Direct evidence to guide the prehospital use of oxygen therapy in drowning is unavailable. However, as the primary cause of death from drowning is insufficient oxygen delivery to the heart and brain, prompt restoration of oxygen delivery is essential. Pulse oximetry can be unreliable in this situation, particularly after cold-water immersion, but when feasible can enable continuous titration of FIO_2 after ROSC. Tracheal intubation can be done after a water submersion incident. There is an association between tracheal intubation and poor outcomes in the studies, which may be because tracheal intubation is limited to more severe drowning.

Better outcomes were observed for patients who required ECMO for respiratory support rather than conventional ECPR. Extracorporeal oxygenation to treat CPA or severe respiratory failure caused by drowning is feasible, but further research is required to refine the indications and optimal timing for initiating ECMO.

17. COVID-19 Infection Risk from patients in Cardiorespiratory Arrest:

No change to Treatment Recommendation has been made since 5th August 2020.

A significant consideration in developing treatment recommendations is the importance of rescuer safety. During chest compressions, aerosol generation may happen minimally. Whether defibrillation does or does not generate aerosols is still unknown. Also, the person performing chest compressions being in physical contact with the patient and close to their airway is prone to infection. Health care professionals may use PPE for aerosol-generating procedures during resuscitation. Health care providers may consider defibrillation before donning PPE in situations where the provider assesses that the benefits may exceed the risks. Lay rescuers can consider chest compressions and public-access defibrillation. It is suggested that lay rescuers may consider providing breaths to the patient along with chest compressions if they are willing, trained, and able to do so.

COVID-19 working group of ILCOR has carefully tried to balance the benefit of early treatment with chest compressions and defibrillation (before donning PPE) with the possible harm to the rescuers, the people around, and the wider community.

The impact of COVID-19 varies across regions and countries. When applying these treatment recommendations to their local context, regional and national resuscitation councils should consider the preferences of their local communities, prevalence of disease, vaccination status, availability of PPE, training needs of their workforce, and infrastructure and resources to provide ongoing care for patients resuscitated after CPA.

The use of adhesive pads is encouraged for defibrillation to be delivered without direct contact between the defibrillator operator and the patient.

Prevention of aerosol generation with supraglottic airway and bag-mask ventilation is not reliable. A supraglottic airway may provide a better airway seal than a facemask. For ventilation with a bag-mask or supraglottic airway, pause chest compressions for ventilation.

Minimize the duration of bag-mask ventilation. Both hands can be used to hold the mask and ensure a good mask seal for bag-mask ventilation.

Mechanical chest compression devices can be used where available.

Post Cardiac Arrest Recommendations

1. Pediatric Targeted Temperature Management (TTM) Post Cardiac Arrest:

Successful resuscitation does not end with the return of spontaneous circulation (ROSC). Excellent post-cardiac arrest care is vital to achieving the best patient outcomes. Post ROSC comatose children may be given TTM of 32-34°C or 36-37.5°C.

2. Oxygen and carbon dioxide levels in patients with ROSC:

These need to be tailored to the specific patient condition in case it is known, or else targeting normoxia either by PaO2 or SpO2 (94-99%) is suggested. Normocapnia is also suggested unless the child has any condition precluding it, such as chronic lung disease, congenital heart disease with a single ventricle, and increased intracranial pressure. Preventing and treating hypotension, hyperoxia or hypoxia, and hypercapnia or hypocapnia is essential to decrease secondary damage.

Appropriate management of pre-arrest conditions (treatable causes), high-quality CPR when cardiac arrest happens, and good post ROSC care based on current recommendations are necessary to improve outcomes. Even after discharge from the hospital, cardiac arrest survivors can have physical, cognitive, and emotional challenges and may need ongoing therapies and interventions. Knowledge gaps still exist and most of the current guidelines are based on weak recommendations, which can be strengthened by good-quality research from across the world.

PALS FLOW CHART

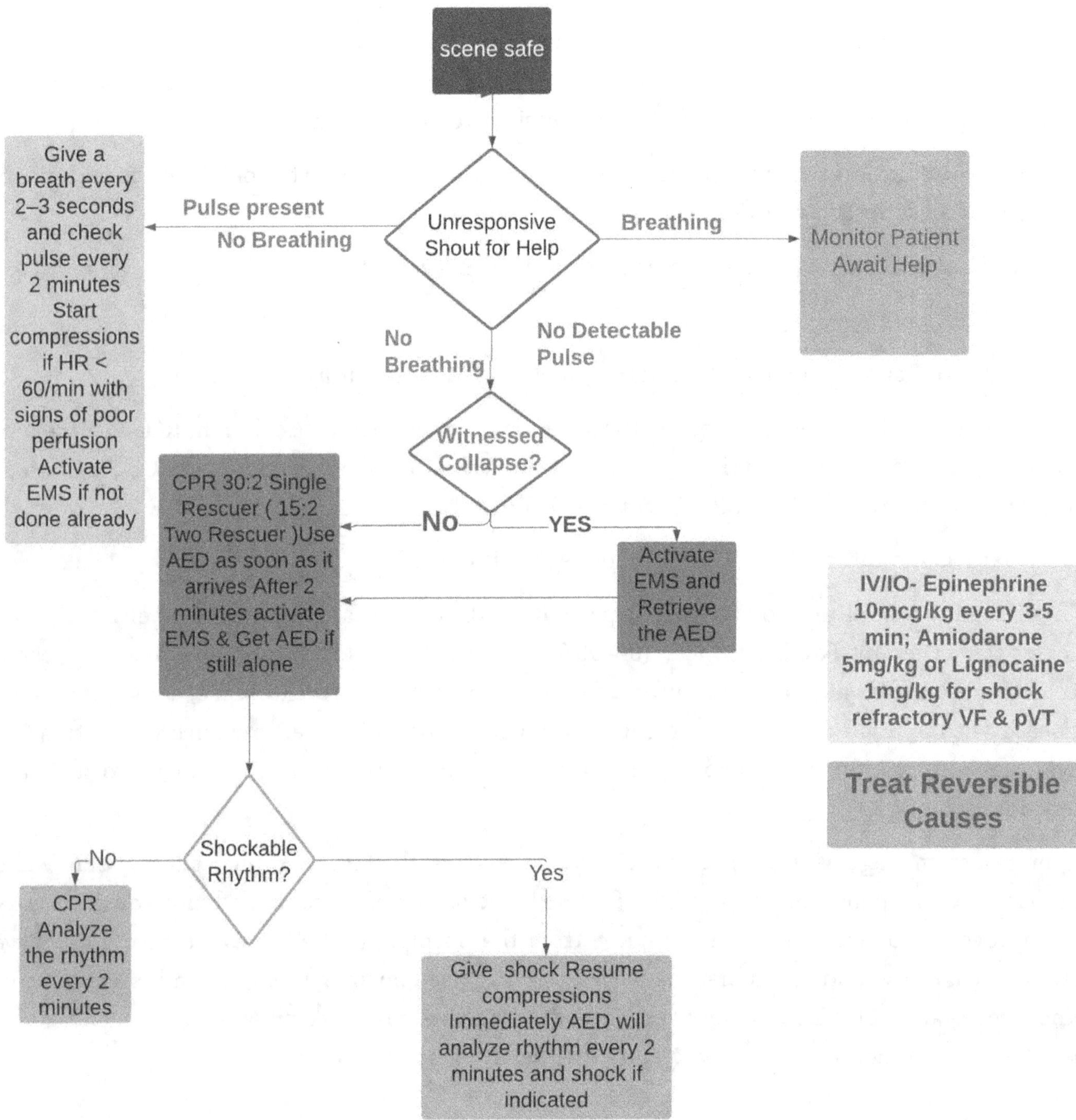

VF- Ventricular Fibrillation; pVT- pulseless Ventricular Tachycardia; HR- Heart Rate; EMS- Emergency Medical System

References

1. Tania Miyuki Shimoda-Sakano, Cláudio Schvartsman, Amélia Gorete Reis. Epidemiology of pediatric cardiopulmonary resuscitation. J Pediatr (Rio J) Jul-Aug 2020;96(4):409-421. doi: 10.1016/j.jped.2019.08.004. Epub 2019 Sep 30.

2. Part 4: Pediatric Basic and Advanced Life Support. 2020 American Heart Association Guidelines for Cardiopulmonary Resuscitation and Emergency Cardiovascular Care

3. Michael A. Gropper MD, PhD, in Miller's Anesthesia, 2020 Pediatric Advanced Life Support. Cardiopulmonary Resuscitation and Advanced Cardiac Life Support

4. https://costr.ilcor.org

5. ANZCOR Guideline 12.2 – Paediatric Advanced Life Support (PALS)

6. Myra H. Wyckoff, Eunice M. Singletary, Jasmeet Soar, Theresa M. Olasveengen, Robert Greif, Helen G. Liley, David Zideman, Farhan Bhanji, Lars W. Andersen, Suzanne R. Avis, and Collaborators. 2021 International Consensus on Cardiopulmonary Resuscitation and Emergency Cardiovascular Care Science With Treatment Recommendations: Summary From the Basic Life Support; Advanced Life Support; Neonatal Life Support; Education, Implementation, and Teams; First Aid Task Forces; and the COVID-19 Working Group

Resuscitation in Peri-Arrest Situations

There have been many technical modifications to the care of peri arrest patients for a neurologically intact recovery. The concepts have been revised in the recent guidelines by the American Heart Association and the European Society of Cardiology. The application of newer ideas, which have improved the quality of life of cardiac arrest victims in various studies are being discussed below -

1. **Cardiac arrest and Mortality related to intubation procedure in critically ill adult patients: a multicenter cohort study**

   A retrospective analysis was done with objectives of finding the prevalence of cardiac during intubation, mortality of patients with cardiac arrest and risk factors of cardiac arrest.

   The authors De Jong A, et al. concluded that ICU intubation-related cardiac arrest occurs in one of 40 procedures with high immediate and 28-day mortality. Five independent risk factors for cardiac arrest, which are hypoxemia prior to intubation, absence of preoxygenation, obesity, age >75 and low arterial blood pressure prior to intubation, were identified - three of which are modifiable, to decrease intubation-related cardiac arrest prevalence and 28-day ICU mortality

2. **Risk factors for Peri-intubation Cardiac Arrest in a Pediatric Emergency Department**

   This was a retrospective, nested case control done at a tertiary children's hospital to identify risk factors that predict peri-intubation cardiac arrest in a pediatric ED.

   The authors, Pokrajac, et al. in their study concluded that hypoxia (or an unobtainable pulse oximetry value) was the strongest predictor for PICA among children after emergent ETI. A simple risk model combining pre-ETI hypoxia and younger than 1 year showed excellent discrimination in this sample.

3. **Peri-intubation in the Emergency Department: A National emergency Airway registry (NEAR) study**

   This was a secondary analysis of NEAR done in 2021, to estimate the prevalence of peri-intubation CA among patients undergoing emergency airway management.

   The authors of the study April MD, et al. concluded that 157 (1%) out of 15776 experienced cardiac arrest, and therefore for patients undergoing ETI in the ED is rare. There is a higher likelihood of arrest in patients with pre-intubation shock or hypoxemia.

4. **Intubation Practices and Adverse Peri-intubation Events in Critically Ill Patients From 29 Countries**

This study was an international prospective cohort study done at 197 centres in 29 countries, to evaluate the incidence and nature of adverse peri-intubation events and to assess current practice of intubation in critically ill patients.

This authors Russotto V, et al. concluded that out of 2964 patients, 45.2% experience at least 1 major adverse event - cardiac arrest (3.1%), cardiovascular instability (42.5%), severe hypoxemia (spo$_2$ <80%) – 9.3%

5. **The PrePARE trial** talks about the effect of a fluid bolus on cardiovascular collapse among critically ill adults undergoing intubation. Administration of IVF bolus during RSI of critically ill patients may not affect incidence of CV collapse. The authors concluded that administration of an intravenous fluid bolus did not decrease the overall incidence of cardiovascular collapse during tracheal intubation of critically ill adults, compared with no fluid bolus in this trial.

6. **Safety of peripheral administration of vasopressor medications: A systematic review**

Reports of the administration of vasopressors via PiVCs, when given for a limited duration, under close observation, suggest that extravasation is uncommon and is unlikely to lead to major complications.

The authors of the study Tian, et al. concluded that administration of vasopressors via peripheral intravenous catheters for a limited duration and under close observation is unlikely to cause major complications, and that extravasation occurred in 3.4% of 1382 patients with no reported incidents of tissue necrosis or limb ischaemia.

7. **The association of rocuronium dosing and first-attempt intubation success in adult emergency department patients**

The recommended dose of rocuronium for rapid sequence intubation is 1.0 mg/kg but evidence from emergency airway management is limited. In In this observational study, the relationship between rocuronium dose and first-attempt success among emergency department (ED) patients undergoing rapid sequence intubation was assessed.

From the 19,071 encounters in this study, the authors, Levin, et al. concluded that Rocuronium dosed ≥1.4 mg/kg was associated with higher first attempt success when using direct laryngoscopy and among patients with pre-intubation hypotension with no increase in adverse events.

8. **Ketamine Versus Etomidate and Peri-intubation Hypotension: A National Emergency Airway Registry Study**

The hemodynamic impact of induction agents is a critically important consideration in emergency intubations. We assessed the relationship between peri-intubation hypotension and the use of ketamine versus etomidate as an induction agent for emergency department (ED) intubation.

The goal of this study is to compare patient outcomes between intubations performed with ketamine versus etomidate using a large prospective observational multicenter ED cohort. Our primary objective is to compare peri-intubation hypotension (systolic blood pressure <100 mm Hg) among normotensive patients undergoing intubation in the ED with ketamine versus etomidate. Our secondary objectives include comparing the incidence of adverse events such as peri-intubation hypotension requiring intervention and mortality.

The authors, April MD et al. suggest that clinicians should not necessarily prioritize ketamine over etomidate based on concern for hemodynamic compromise among ED patients undergoing intubation. Ketamine has myocardial depressant effects that can be unmasked during RSI and result in hypotension.

9. **Association of Timing of Electrocardiogram Acquisition After Return of Spontaneous Circulation With Coronary Angiography Findings in Patients With Out-of-Hospital Cardiac Arrest**

The primary end point of this study was a false-positive ECG findings, defined as the percentage of patients with post-ROSC ECG findings that met STEMI criteria but who did not show obstructive coronary artery disease on angiography that was worthy of percutaneous coronary angioplasty.

These authors suggest that early ECG acquisition after ROSC in patients with OHCA is associated with a higher percentage of false-positive ECG findings for STEMI. Further they suggest that it may be reasonable to delay post-ROSC ECG by at least 8 minutes after ROSC or repeat the acquisition if the first ECG is diagnostic of STEMI and is acquired early after ROSC. In this cohort study of 370 patients who were resuscitated from out-of-hospital cardiac arrest, the percentage of false-positive ECG findings among those performed 7 minutes or less after ROSC (18.5%) was significantly higher than those performed between 8 and 33 minutes (7.2%) and over 33 minutes (5.8%) after ROSC.

10. **COACT TRIAL- Coronary Angiography after Out-of-Hospital Cardiac Arrest without ST-Segment Elevation**

This was a randomised open label trial, done to weigh the benefits of early coronary angiography and revascularization in resuscitated patients without electrocardiographic evidence of ST-segment elevation. Patients-Included adults >30 years of age, OHCA of possible cardiac origin, shockable or non-shockable rhythm and no STEMI on ECG

In this trial, the researchers evaluated if in adult patients who have sustained an out of hospital arrhythmia-associated cardiac arrest without an ST-elevation myocardial infarction, is immediate angiography superior to delayed angiography in improving 90-day survival.

This is the first randomized controlled trial (RCT) assessing early angiography in patients who have an out of hospital cardiac arrest without STEMI. Two further RCTs are currently recruiting patients in an attempt to answer this question ACCESS trial; DISCO trial.

Patients were randomised in a 1:1 ratio with the use of a web-based randomisation system. Study powered at 85% power to detect a 40% relative difference in 90-day survival between the immediate angiography and delayed angiography groups. Adaptive design was used that allowed for an increase in sample size if survival benefit was substantial but smaller than the 40% relative difference.

Following are the inclusion and exclusion criteria of the patients-

Inclusion: Patients who had an out of hospital arrest with an initial shockable rhythm and who were unconscious after return of spontaneous circulation (ROSC).

Exclusion:

- Signs of STEMI on the ECG at the emergency department (including new LBBB or isolated ST depression in V1-V3 due to an true posterior infarct)
- Hemodynamic instability unresponsive to medical therapy
  - Defined as a prolonged (>30 min) systolic blood pressure <90 mmHg at the time of screening
- An obvious or suspected non-coronary cause of the arrest
- A known severe renal dysfunction (GFR<30 ml/min)
- Obvious or suspected pregnancy
- Suspected or confirmed acute intracranial bleeding
- Suspected or confirmed acute stroke
- Known limitations in therapy or DO Not Resuscitate-order
- Known pre-arrest Cerebral Performance Category 3 or 4
- >4 hours (from return of spontaneous circulation to screening)
- Refractory ventricular arrhythmia
- Known inability to complete 90-day follow-up

- Intervention planned was coronary angiography as soon as possible and initiated within 2 hours after randomization. No statistical difference in survival at 90 days was observed. No difference was observed in survival with good cerebral performance- Immediate angiography (62.9%) vs delayed angiography (64.4%).
- No difference in the following:
  - Survival to ICU discharge
  - Major bleeding
  - Recurrence of arrhythmia
  - Time of inotrope support
  - Duration of mechanical ventilation
  - Need for renal replacement therapy
- The immediate angiography group took longer to achieve targeted temperature than the delayed angiography group

The authors of this study, Desch, et al. concluded that among patients with resuscitated out-of-hospital cardiac arrest without ST-segment elevation, a strategy of performing immediate angiography provided no benefit over a delayed or selective strategy with respect to the 30-day risk of death from any cause.

11. **Hypothermia versus Normothermia after Out-of-Hospital Cardiac Arrest-TTM2**

    This was an open-label, randomised, superiority trial done in 14 countries to assess benefits of hypothermia vs normothermia and early fever treatment in OHCA patients. Patients included adults >18 years of age, OHCA of presumed cardiac or unknown causes, any initial rhythm, >20min of ROSC or unconscious, unable to obey verbal commands. Patients were randomized to TH of 33°C versus targeted normothermia (goal temperature: <37.5°C). Overall, there was no difference in survival at 6 months (50% vs. 48%, P = 0.37) and no difference in survival with severe disability on the modified Rankin scale (55% vs. 55%; RR 1.00; 95% CI, 0.92-1.09). There was also no difference in health-related quality of life between the groups, but a higher incidence of arrhythmias with the use of hypothermia. These findings are in direct contrast to the original RCTs published in 2002 and the HYPERION trial, but do align with the findings reported in the TTM trial.

    This study that included 1861 patients concluded that in patients with coma after out-of-hospital cardiac arrest, targeted hypothermia did not lead to a lower incidence of death by 6 months than targeted normothermia.

12. **Adult Basic and Advanced Life Support: 2020 American Heart Association Guidelines for Cardiopulmonary Resuscitation and Emergency Cardiovascular Care**

Post-Arrest goals should be to optimise neurological resuscitation and to prevent secondary injury due to cardiac arrest. Post-Arrest Care is defined as management Of O_2 and CO_2 levels, optimising CPP/MAP, detection of seizures, emergent PCI and TTM.

Goals for

1. <u>oxygenation:</u>

   - Avoid Hypoxia
   - Avoid Hyperoxia
   - Titrate FiO_2 to maintain SpO_2 92-98%

2. <u>Ventilation</u>

   - Maintain $PaCO_2$ 35-45mmHg

3. <u>Blood Pressure Management</u>

   - Avoid hypotension
   - Optimal MAP not clear
   - Maintain SBP of 90 mmHg or MAP of 65 mmHg
   - Trends towards benefit when targeting MAP of 80 mmHg

4. <u>Seizures:</u>

   - Promptly perform an ECG in all comatose patients after ROSC
   - ILCOR systemic review did not address timing and method
   - Non-Convulsive seizures are common
   - Seizure prophylaxis in adults post arrest patients NOT recommended

5. <u>PCI</u>

6. The recommendation is to perform PCI on all post arrest patients with suspected cardiac etiology and a STEMI on ECG.

7. <u>Targeted Temperature Management:</u>

   - Initiate TTM for adults who do not follow commands after ROSC from OHCA
   - Select and maintain temp 32-36 C
   - Reasonable to maintain for at least 24hrs
   - For others- treat fever

To summarize,

1. Risk factors for peri intubation CA can be peri intubation hypoxemia, peri intubation hypotension and altered shock index.

2. Administration of IVF bolus during RSI of critically ill patients may not affect incidence of CV collapse.

3. Use of peripheral vasopressors showed low rate of extravasation and injury when used via 18 or 20 G iv in antecubital fossa or proximal

4. Ketamine has myocardial depressant effects that can be unmasked during RSI and result in hypotension.

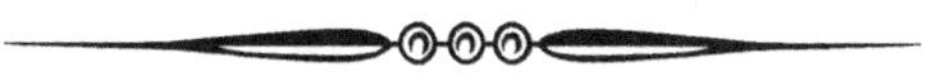

Covidology and Newer Drugs

Contributors

1. Dr. Manisha Bisht
2. Dr. Nidhi Kaeley
3. Dr. Ashima Sharma
4. Dr. Sarat Chandra Uppaluri
5. Dr. G Dharani Reddy

Chapters

1. Covid 19 infection
2. Covid cardiology
3. Covid neurology
4. Covid pulmonology
5. Pharmacology

Update on Covid-19 Infection - Clinical Features, Pathogenesis and Management

Introduction

The COVID-19 virus or severe acute respiratory syndrome coronavirus 2 (SARS-CoV-2) was first reported in Hubei Province of China in December 2019. Since then it has been rapidly spreading in the rest of the world. The outbreak was declared a public health emergency of international concern on 30th January 2020. In India, on August 1, 2020 till 8am, there were 19,97,054 cases and 36,551 deaths due to SARS-COV2 infection. Out of which, 57,486 new cases and 764 new deaths were added in one day.

The corona viruses are major causative pathogens of respiratory illness outbreaks. They are positive sense single stranded RNA viruses. These viruses cause a wide spectrum of respiratory diseases ranging from common cold to severe pneumonia such as MERS (Middle East Respiratory Syndrome) and SARS (Severe Acute Respiratory Syndrome) outbreaks in the past [1]. Currently, there is a speculation that SARS-CoV-2 has an animal origin. World scientists are working tirelessly to understand clinical spectrum, pathogenesis, transmission, diagnostic criteria, treatment modalities as well as preventive strategies aiming at reducing further transmission in the community. The increasing spread of the virus is mounting pressure on the medical resources of the country in the form of ventilators, personal protective equipment (PPE) and health care professionals. This continued pressure had overburdened clinics, hospitals especially the emergency departments leading to increased use of web based systems such as telemedicine services for stable patients. Almost all the nations of the world has declared country wide lockdowns affecting the global trade and small scale businesses. In this review, we discuss the etiology, pathogenesis, clinical features and treatment modalities available for SARS-CoV-2 pneumonia.

Etiology

SARS-CoV-2 is a positive sense RNA virus. It belongs to the genus betacorona virus. Phylogenetic analysis reveals that SARS-CoV-2 closely resembles the two bat derived corona viruses namely bat-SL-CoV ZC 45 (Gen bank accession No MG772933.1) and bat-SL-CoVZXC21 (Gen bank accession no MG772934.1). It has been found to have around 79% similarity with SARS-CoV and around 50% similarity with middle east respiratory coronavirus (MERS-CoV) [2,3].

The other genera of coronaviruses are alpha coronavirus, delta corona virus and gamma coronavirus. Coronaviruses constitute a large family of viruses causing multiorgan manifestations. It is estimated that these viruses cause approximately 5-10% of acute respiratory infections. Common human coronaviruses, HCoV-OC43 and HCoV- HKu1 belonging to beta coronaviruses of A lineage, cause self-limiting upper respiratory tract infections. The other human corona viruses such as SARS-CoV, SARS-CoV-2 and MERS-CoV belonging to the B and C lineage of betacoronavirus have been found to cause severe pneumonia and multi organ dysfunction [4].

SARS-CoV-2 virus has a diameter of around 60-140 nm with round or elliptical shape and pleomorphic form. The coronaviruses have open reading frames (ORFs). Open reading frames-ORF1a and ORF1b undergo translation to form polyprotein 1a(PP1a) and PP1b. These polyproteins undergo further processing by viral proteases to form 16 new structural proteins. These proteins contain RNA dependent RNA polymerase enzyme (RdRp) which aids in transcription of viral RNA to minus strand templates. On further replication,6-9 sub genomic mRNAs are released which undergo translation to form accessory and structural proteins. The virus has been found to be inactivated by 75% ether, ethanol, chlorine containing disinfectants, peroxyacetic acid and chloroform.

Transmission

In December 2019, people at Wuhan city of China had started reporting to hospitals with features suggestive of severe pneumonia, cause being of unknown origin. On 31st December, China notified the outbreak to WHO and consequently, on 1st January 2020 WHO closed the local seafood market of Wuhan. On 7th January the causative organism was identified as coronavirus [6]. Similar to other respiratory viruses, SARS-CoV-2 spreads via respiratory droplets including aerosol transmission in closed spaces and contact transmission. It is believed that spread is maximum from symptomatic patients. However, now there are reports that the virus also spreads from asymptomatic patients. The incubation period is generally between 3 to 7 days extended up to 2 weeks [7]. The data revealed that the novel epidemic is doubling every seven days. However, the basic reproduction rate (R0-R naught) of the epidemic has been found to be 2.2. The basic reproduction rate of SARS-CoV in the year 2002-2003 was 3 [8].

Furthermore, it must be emphasized that the pandemic is still spreading. Thus more studies are needed to understand the incubation period, clinical course, pathogenesis, transmission rate and treatment of the disease.

Epidemiology

As per covid19india.org in India, on August 1, 2020 till 8am, there were 19,97,054 cases and 36,551 deaths due to SARS-COV2 infection. Out of which, 57,486 new cases and 764 new deaths were added in one day.

Pathophysiology

As discussed, the primary pathogen responsible for COVID-19 is SARS-CoV-2. It is a highly contagious virus and belongs to the coronaviridae family. It is a positive sense RNA virus with size 50-200nm. Among the known corona viruses, SARS-CoV-2 and MERS (Middle east respiratory syndrome coronavirus) have been found to cause severe respiratory diseases and fatalities. SARS-CoV-2 affects alveolar epithelial cells of the lung using angiotensin converting enzyme 2 receptor (ACE 2 R) mediated endocytosis. Patients with subclinical COVID-19 infection who underwent lobectomy were found to have exudate deposition, scattered large protein globules, alveolar wall expansion, proliferating fibroblasts in the interstitium, macrophages infiltrating the airspaces and hyperplasia of type II pneumocytes. [9,10,11]. It has been observed that the affinity of SARS-CoV-2 to bind ACE 2 receptors is 10 to 20 times more than SARS-CoV. This explains the contagious nature of SARS-CoV-2 over SARS-CoV [12]. Another contributory factor which adds to the mortality and morbidity of cases of COVID-19 patients is coinfection with bacterial pathogens. Du et al observed in a retrospective analysis of fatal 85 cases of SARS-CoV-2 pneumonia, coinfection with other pathogens is a contributory factor of mortality in these patients [13]. SARS-CoV-2 virus in severe cases leads to rapid development of pneumonia and acute respiratory distress syndrome (ARDS). It not only affects lungs but multiple organs such as liver, heart and kidneys [14,15]. ACE-2-the primary binding protein of COVID-19 which is present in lung tissue is also present in other tissues such as digestive, cardiovascular and urogenital systems [16]. Another contributory factor which causes multi organ dysfunction is production of large quantities of cytokines also called cytokine storm [17]. The cytokine storm leads to the release of various proinflammatory cytokines such as IL-2, IL-7, IL-10. G-CSF, MCP-1, MCP1A AND NF-Alpha. These cytokines result in inflammation induced lung injury leading to complications such as pneumonitis, acute respiratory distress syndrome, organ failure and even death [20]. Similar cytokine response was observed in patients with SARS-CoV and MERS. In a retrospective analysis conducted at Wuhan, it was observed that patients with COVID-19 admitted in ICU had higher levels of neutrophils, low lymphocyte levels, higher levels of cytokines such as IP-10, MCP-1, MIP1A and TNF as compared to patients not admitted in ICU [17]. The most likely intermediate host was found to be pangolins as the genetic sequences of viruses from these animals and humans during the outbreaks in February, 2020 showed around 99% match. Based on previous studies conducted around 80% of patients of COVID-19 are asymptomatic while remaining present as severe pneumonia. It has been observed that approximate spread of COVID-19 infection in pre-symptomatic stage is 48%to 62% [18,19].

Innate immune response to SARS-CoV-2

Effective innate immune response against viral infection depends upon type 1 interferon response and its downstream cascade. Innate immune cells recognize invasion of viruses by pathogen associated molecular patterns (PAMPs). In case of RNA viruses, PAMPs are either viral genomic RNA or intermediates during viral replication such as dsRNA. These are further recognized by endosomal RNA receptors such as TLR 3 and TLR 7 on cytosolic RNA sensors such as RIG-1/MDA-5. Consequently, the downstream signaling pathway NF-KB and IRF-3 is activated which leads to nuclear translocation. In the nucleus, there is induction of expression of type 1 IFN which in turn activates JAK-STAT pathway [21]. It was observed that response to viral infection is suppressed by interfering with action of type 1 IFN [22].

The genomic sequence of SARS-CoV-2 has been found to have 68% similarity with that of SARS-CoV virus. Thus, it was found to use the same strategies to modulate the innate immune system by down regulating type 1 IFN response.

Adaptive immune response

The Th1 type immune system, part of adaptive immunity, plays a crucial role against viral infections. The cytokines released by antigen presenting cells direct the helper T Cells. The cytotoxic T cells kill the virus infected cells. Humoral immune response plays an important role by producing neutralizing antibodies which aid in limiting the infection in the later phase. Thus, it has been suggested that Th1 type immune response is not only responsible for control of SARS-CoV and MERS but also SARS-CoV-2.

Clinical features

The patients of COVID-19 present with wide spectrum of symptoms. They range from asymptomatic to mildly symptomatic to severe pneumonia and acute respiratory distress syndrome (ARDS). Huang el al reported a case series of 41 SARS-CoV-2 patients who had fever, dry cough, dyspnea and malaise. It was observed that all the patients had abnormal chest computerized tomography findings [23]. The median incubation period of SARs-COV-2 is 4.5 days before the symptom's onset. It has been observed that 97.5% patients develop symptoms within 11.5 days. [41,42,43,44]. The viral load reaches maximum within 5-6 days of symptoms onset. [45]. In a study conducted by Jang et al, a retrospective analysis was done of 52 critically ill patients of SARS-CoV-2. It was observed that fever (n=51,98%) was the most common symptom followed by dry cough (n=40, 77%), dyspnea (n=33. 63.5%) and malaise (n=18,35%). The other uncommon symptoms were myalgia, rhinorrhea, arthralgia, chest pain, headache, loss of smell, diarrhea and fatigability. It was observed that complications such as ARDS, kidney injury, cardiac injury, liver dysfunction, hyperglycemia, gastrointestinal hemorrhage and pneumothorax were more common in the non survivors group [24].

According to previous studies symptoms of COVID-19 can be sub- divided as [25,26]

1. Mild or uncomplicated illness – These patients have dry cough, nasal congestion, mild fever, malaise, headache, muscle pain. Dyspnea is absent.

2. Moderate pneumonia- These patient have cough and shortness of breath (tachypnea in children, SpO_2 - 90% to less than equal to 93% in moderate disease.

3. Severe pneumonia- These patients have fever, severe dyspnea, tachypnea (73 breaths/min) and hypoxia (spo_2 <90% on room air). Cyanosis may be present in children.

4. These category patients can develop ARDS categorized as mild, moderate and severe ARDS [25,26].

Evaluation

The national center for disease control, India has given the following definitions of patients with severe acute respiratory illness (SARI) suspected of novel coronavirus in the emergency department.

SARI is defined as an acute respiratory illness with a history of fever or measured temperature >38C and cough, onset within the last 10 days and requiring hospitalization. However, the absence of fever does not exclude viral infection.

Suspected Case

A suspected case is defined as a patient with acute respiratory illness that is with fever and at least one sign/symptom of respiratory disease(cough, shortness of breath) and history of travel to or residence in a location reporting community transmission.

Or

A patient with any respiratory illness and have been in contact with a confirmed or probable covid-19 case in the last 14 days prior to symptom onset.

Or

A patient with severe acute respiratory illness (fever and at least one sign/ symptom of respiratory disease like cough, shortness of breath) and requiring hospitalization and in the absence of an alternative diagnosis that fully explains the clinical presentation.

Probable case

Probable case is defined as

A: A suspected case for whom testing for the covid-19 virus is inconclusive or

B: A suspected case for whom testing could not be performed due to any reason. A confirmed case is defined as a person with laboratory confirmation of covid-19 infection, irrespective of clinical signs and symptoms [27].

Laboratory diagnosis

According to NCDC, India, specimens from both upper respiratory tract (nasopharyngeal and oropharyngeal) and lower respiratory tract (expectorated sputum, endotracheal aspirate or bronchoalveolar lavage) should be collected for novel coronavirus testing by RT PCR technique. During sample collection use of personal protective equipment (PPE) is mandatory. SARS-CoV-2 can also be tested using serum. However, only 151 cases have been detected using serum RNA [23]. The initial handling as specimens collected should be performed at biosafety level -3 (BSL-3) until the specimen is declared safe and non-infectious by lysis technique [28]. SARS-CoV-2 can be grown in primary monkey cells and cell lines such as Vero and LLC-MK2. However, it should not be routinely performed due to biosafety reasons [29]. Rapid antigen tests, although providing faster results, have poor sensitivity [30]. Serological tests are not routinely used for diagnostic purposes. But these tests are used for the purpose of clinical trials and regulatory review processes. These tests are also useful in confirming the burden of the disease by detecting asymptomatic patients [31]. The real time reverse transcriptase polymerase chain reaction (RT-PCR) is highly specific for diagnosing SARS-CoV-2 infection, although false positive tests can also occur. The sensitivity of RT-PCR is varying. It can be as low as 60% [33]. As per the recommendations two negative tests at 24 hours interval rules out COVID-19 infection [34]. All the sample stored for long term purpose should be appropriately labelled and should be kept at -80° Celsius deep freezer. The ICMR advises that the sample testing positive should be retained for at least 30 days from the date of testing before being destroyed. As per the recommendation of ICMR, all the covid-19 testing labs have been mapped to QC (Quality Control) labs.

All the labs are supposed to send five random positive and five negative samples to QC labs.

As per the ICMR guidelines, the US-FDA approved COVID-19 diagnostic kits do not require validation whereas for CE- IVD approved non US-FDA approved kits, first batch will require validation, there after two batches should be tested in four months' time.

The various tests available are RT-PCR kits, RNA extraction and VTM kits and rapid antibody tests, ELISA and CUA kits.

The gold standard diagnostic frontline test for covid-19 is real-time RT-PCR.

Currently, miscellaneous open and closed RT-PCR systems are available.

The open system RT-PCR machines are True Nat and CBNAAT.

The minimum time taken for each test is 2 to 5 hours. The only available point of care rapid antigen test is standard Q COVID-19 Ag detection kit. It is a rapid chromatographic immunoassay for qualitative detection of specific antigens to SARS-COV-2.

The sample collected for the same is nasopharyngeal swab. Maximum duration for interpreting a positive or negative test is 30 minutes. The test is independently evaluated by two agencies, ICMR and AIIMS, New Delhi. The specificity of the test is 99.3 to 100% whereas the sensitivity of the tests is 50.6% to 84%. In view of higher specificity and lower sensitivity of the test the ICMR recommends the test as a point of care marker along with a combination of RT-PCR gold test.

Treatment

The patients with SARS-CoV2 infection have higher levels of cytokines such as IL-1B, IL-1A, IL-2, IL-10, fibroblast growth factor (FGF), granulocyte colony stimulating factor (G-CSF), tumor necrosis factor (TNF), platelet derived growth factor (PDGF) and vascular endothelial growth factor (VEGF). Thus, multiple anti-rheumatoid drugs are under trial for the treatment of the same. Various preliminary trials have highlighted their anti-viral properties (Table 1). At present the patients with severe acute respiratory illness should be considered as SARS-CoV-2 carriers and investigated and treated accordingly [32].

Table 1: Agents for COVID-19 Management

AGENTS	PROPERTIES
Hydroxychloroquine / Chloroquine	Anti-inflammatory and immunomodulator. [35-40, 47-50]
Remdesivir	The dose under investigation is 200mg intravenous on day 1 followed by 100 mg IV for 10 days, infused over 30-60 minutes.[46-47]
Lopinavir/Ritonavir (LPV/r)	Lopinavir is a protease inhibitor and ritonavir, CYP3A4 inhibitor, boosts lopinavir concentration. The fixed dose combination inhibits viral replication. The dose used for trial for lopinavir/ritonavir is 400mg/100mg twice orally for not more than 10 days.[51-55]
Nitazoxanide	It has demonstrated potent in vitro activity against SARs-COV-2 with an EC50 at 48 hours of 2.12uM in vero E6 cells (56). It interferes with viral replication by affecting the host regulated pathways. The dose used in clinical trial is 600mg twice daily.[56-57]
Tocilizumab	It is a humanized monoclonal antibody that inhibits IL-6 receptors. As it is known that severe SARS-COV-2 infection is associated with cytokine storm including elevated levels of IL-6, this drug is currently under trial [58]. The recommended dose used in one of trial in China is 4-8mg/kg or 400mg IV once, re-started after 12 hrs.[58-60]
Oseltamivir and Baloxavir	Oseltamivir is a neuraminidase inhibitor. Since corona viruses do not inhibit neuraminidase enzyme, none of the neuraminidase inhibiting agents have been found to be effective against SARs. COV-2 infection.[61]
Anakinra –	IL-1 receptor antagonist. No clinical trial in China, USA has enrolled the drug.
Arbidol	Antiviral drug used in China, Russia, no clinical data available about the use of the drug for SARs-COV-2.
Baricitinib	A Janus Kinase family enzyme inhibitor, no clinical data exists[62].
Convalescent Plasma	It has been used with success for viral infections SARs-COV-1, MERS, H1N1 and Ebola infection. However, it is under trial for SARs-COV-2 infection. [63-64]

Corticosteroids	The data on the use of corticosteroids is confusing. A recent study on SARS-CoV2 patients has demonstrated a decrease in mortality in patients with ARDS (59). As per Indian guidelines use of dexamethasone has been approved in severe infection[59].
Ribavirin with and without interferon	Wang et al evaluated the efficacy of ribavarin. It has been found to be 100 times more potent than remdesivir. Interferon (alpha and beta), although has substantial innate antiviral properties but is associated with substantial toxicities such as cytopenias and hepatotoxicity[56].

Management

The management of mild cases includes isolation of the patient at covid care centres, first referral units (FRus), community health centre (CHCs), sub District or district hospitals or home isolation. Proper vital monitoring and spo_2 recording should be done in all the patients. The management of moderate cases involves delivering oxygen therapy, maintaining SpO_2 (92-96%), daily ECG recording and follow up with CRP, D -dimer and ferritin every 48 to 72 hourly. Complete blood count, kidney and liver function tests should be done daily. Tablet hydroxychloroquine (400 mg twice daily on the first day followed by 200 mg twice daily for 3 days) and for severe infection methylprednisolone (0.5 to 1 mg/ kg for 3 days) can also be given. Management of severe cases involves symptomatic treatment of ARDS, septic shock, methylprednisolone and prophylactic dose of LMWH or unfractionated heparin can be given. Investigational therapies in the form of remdesivir, convalescent plasma and tocilizumab can be given.

Biomarkers of COVID-19 infection

Severe COVID-19 infection can lead to complications such as respiratory failure, liver failure and kidney injury as well as cardiac complications. A recent study published at Wuhan showed that older age, co-morbidities such as diabetes, hypertension, higher SOFA scores, and D-dimer more than 1microgram per ml were associated with higher mortality. The other biochemical parameters associated with poorer prognosis were thrombocytopenia and raised LDH and serum creatinine levels (65).Guo et al published MuLBSTA score to assess prognosis in patients with COVID-19 infection. It incorporates multilobar infilterates, lymphocytes less than $0.8x10^9$ per litre, bacterial infection, smoking status, hypertension and age more than 60 years of age (66).Ducca et al published Brescia COVID Respiratory Severity Scale (BRSS) which incorporates a)patients wheezing or unable to speak at rest or with minimal effort, b) Respiratory Rate more than 22 per minutes, c) PaO_2 less than 65 mmof hg or SpO_2 less than 90%, d) Repeat chest x ray showing significant worsening (67). The other prognostic biomarkers are serum ferritin, LDH, D-dimer, ESR, high sensitivity troponinI, IL-6 and procalcitonin levels (68). A study using artificial intelligence has reported raised ALT, myalgias and elevated hemoglobin levels as strong predictors of ARDS, having 70 to 80%

accuracy (69).Hypokalemia is also noted in patients with COVID-19 as a consequence of continuous degradation of ACE-2 (70).

Stepwise management of COVID-19 patients in the Emergency Department

1. As soon as the patients with hypoxia with COVID-19 infection, arrives in ED, supplemental oxygen should be initiated via nasal cannula or face mask. Inorder to diagnose occult or silent hypoxia, patients with normal oxygen saturation should be given ambulatory pulse oximeter at least for 60 seconds (71).

2. Patients with hypoxemic respiratory failure who fail to maintain normal oxygenation with a face mask or nasal cannula should be considered for high flow nasal cannula. Some physicians consider giving non-invasive positive pressure ventilation instead.However, closed loop set up or negative pressure is required for the same.

3. If the patient develops deteriorating ARDS even on advanced setting mechanical ventilation, prone positioning should be considered which aids in improved lung recruitment (72).

4. When the decision of intubation is considered, most experienced emergency physicians should do it by taking proper precautions. Also, video laryngoscopy should be considered.

    Gattinoni et al has described two subtypes of COVID-19 respiratory failures. The first type is L type, one with lower elastance, lung weight and lung recruitability. The second type is one with higher elastance, lung weight and lung recruitability. Patients with L type respiratory failure respond well to nasal cannula and face mask oxygenation, HFNC and NIPPV whereas H type should be managed traditionally like severe ARDS (73).

5. In patients with advanced respiratory failure, not responding to mechanical ventilation and prone positioning, ECMO (extracorporeal membrane oxygenation) should be considered.

Special circumstances

COVID-19 and pregnancy

Pregnancy is a state of lower immunity and thus, there are increased chances of infection. The symptoms described remain the same. Pregnancy is associated with physiological dyspnea and thus it is difficult to differentiate it from pathological dyspnea due to COVID-19 infection. Till date the data supporting vertical transmission is lacking(74,75). The reported complications COVID-19 infection in pregnant females are intra-uterine growth retardation, pre-term delivery and miscarriages (76). In view of limited resources in developing counteries, it is difficult to test all pregnant females.However, testing of symptomatic pregnant females should be considered.

COVID-19 and Diabetes Mellitus

Patients with type 1 and type2 diabetes mellitus are susceptible to infections. The underlying pathogenesis is dysfunction, decreasing T cell response and altered humoral immunity. Thus, hyperglycemia in any patient with pneumonia on admission is a poor predictor of mortality (77). Diabetes Mellitus has been labelled as a strong predictor of mortality in both SARS-CoV and MERS epidemic (78,79). As per the available evidence, diabetes mellitus, hypertension, coronary artery disease and cerebrovascular disease were present in 16.2%,23.7%, 5.8% and 2.3% respectively in patients with severe COVID-19 infection (80). The other risk factors described are immunocompromised state, obesity and smoking (81,82). The receptor binding domain of SARS-CoV-2 fuses with viral and host cell membranes using ACE2 receptor of the host under normal conditions. ACE-2 has lower expression in the lung tissue.However, infection and lung injury upregulates the ACE-2 expression in the lung (83). It was observed that SARS-CoV binds to ACE-2 in the pancreatic islet cells leading to damaging them and causing hyperglycemia. A similar mechanism has been postulated in SARS-CoV-2 infection (84). ACE-2 is not inhibited by ACE-I.On the contrary, it has been observed that ACEI and angiotensin receptor blockers (ARBs) upregulate ACE2 expression (85). Thus, ACEI and ARB might stimulate SARS-CoV-2 infection (86).Patient with SARS-CoV-2 infection suffering from diabetes mellitus present with similar symptoms and signs.However, they frequently present in the emergency with hyperglycemic emergencies such as diabetic ketoacidosis (DKA) (87).Management of diabetes mellitus involves lifestyle modification including diet protocol and regular exercise, timely intake of medications and frequent doctor visits for blood sugar monitoring. But in lockdown, patients with Diabetes Mellitus especially the geriatric population are frequently facing problems in carrying out the above activities. Patients should be encouraged to use continuous glucose monitoring devices(CGM). The foremost step in management of patients with COVID-19 infection is good glycemic control. Following points should be kept in mind while managing hyperglycemia in patients with COVID-19 infection (88-92).

a. Metformin increases the risk of lactic acidosis.Hence, it should be avoided in critically ill patients with hypoxia.

b. Insulin is the drug of choice in treating critically ill patients of COVID-19 infection with Diabetes Mellitus.

c. SGL-2 inhibitors increase the risk of dehydration and euglycemic ketoacidosis and should be deferred in critically ill patients.

d. DPP4 inhibitors have lower risk of hyperglycemia and thus it can be continued in patients with mild infection.

e. Sulfonylureas increase the risk of hypoglycemia and should be avoided.

f. It is known that pioglitazone causes fluid retention and consequently increases the risk in hemodynamically unstable patients.

RECENT UPDATES ON TREATMENT OF COVID -19

Pharmacological Therapy Tried in Management of COVID

Pharmacological agents tried for the management of COVID-19 infection can be classified into three major classes according to the stage of infection.

Stage I is the early infection phase characterised by upper respiratory tract symptoms. The treatment goal during this phase is to provide symptomatic management according to patient's clinical presentation. Symptomatic management involves the use of analgesics, antipyretics and antihistaminic and cough suppressant. Apart from medications adequate hydration, rest, self-proning, ambulation and education on breathing exercise is also recommended.

Stage II is the pulmonary phase where patient develops pneumonia and associated symptoms like a worsened cough, fever, dyspnea and decreased oxygen levels. Most patients require hospitalization during this stage. Management during this phase is aimed at inhibiting viral entry or replication by antiviral therapy or any other agent. [1] Table 1 summarises the list of agents tried in this phase.

Stage III is the most severe phase known as the hyperinflammation phase. During this phase, inflammation extends beyond lungs and systemic hyperinflammatory syndrome (cytokine storm) sets in. This phase is characterised by development of acute respiratory distress syndrome (ADRS), sepsis and multi-organ failure. Since this phase is characterized by elevation in inflammatory mediators like IL-2, IL-6, IL-7, TNF- alpha, C reactive protein, pharmacological management is targeted to suppress the immune response. Table 2 summarises agents tried Stage 3 for managing the cytokine release syndrome.

Since the beginning of COVID-19 pandemic many pharmacological agents have been tested for COVID infection. There is a great deal of both research and misinformation regarding the effective treatments for COVID-19. Hence the guidelines for management of COVID -19 is also changing frequently in relation to emerging evidence from RCTs on existing and new drug treatments for COVID-19.

Current Treatment Guidelines for COVID-19 Management

Recently WHO has released a recent guidelines based on accumulating evidence for COVID -19 management. [2] Several treatment alternatives are available for all categories of COVID-19 patients (non-severe to severe or critical COVID-19). Some of the agents can be used in combination (i.e. as for severe or critical COVID-19) or as an alternative. Preferred agent of choice depends on availability of the drugs, routes of administration (only intravenous for remdesivir and the monoclonal antibodies), duration of treatment, and time from onset of symptoms. Table 3 summarise the recent guidelines recommended by WHO. The guidelines recommend the use of

Nirmatrelvir and ritonavir for mild cases and Corticosteroids and IL-6 blockers or Baricitinib for severe to critical cases.

Prevention of SARS-COV-2 Infection

Apart from general preventive measures, vaccination is the most effective way to prevent SARS-CoV-2 infection and should be considered as first line of prevention. At present, 10 Vaccines are approved for use in India, out of which, Covishield (AstraZeneca's vaccine manufactured by Serum Institute of India), Covaxin (manufactured by Bharat Biotech Limited) and CorbeVax (manufactured by Biological E. Limited) are used in National COVID Vaccination Program in India. Table 1 compares various vaccines available for use in India.

Drugs with Strong Recommendation for Use in COVID-19 Infection

Nirmatrelvir-ritonavir [3]

It is a combination of two orally bioavailable protease inhibitors where ritonavir is used as pharmacokinetic enhancer.

Mechanism – Nirmatrelvir blocks the activity of the SARS-CoV-2-3CL protease enzyme which is required for viral replication, and coadministration with low dose ritonavir inhibits the metabolism of nirmatrelvir thereby enhancing its duration and concentrations to the target therapeutic range.

ADME – Nirmatrelvir-ritonavir is an inhibitor of CYP3A enzyme (predominantly because of the ritonavir component) as well as a substrate of CYP3A. Dose modification is required in case of reduced kidney function. It is not recommended for patients with severe hepatic impairment (i.e., Child-Pugh Class C.)

Dose – The dose is 300 mg nirmatrelvir (two 150 mg tablets) with one 100 mg ritonavir tablet taken together orally twice daily for 5 days. It should be initiated as soon as possible following COVID-19 diagnosis and within five days of symptom onset.

Monitoring and Adverse Effects

Most frequently observed adverse effects with ritonavir-boosted nirmatrelvir were diarrhea, dysgeusia, hypertension and myalgia.

Drug-Drug Interactions

Presence of Ritonavir component of the combination leads to chance of significant drug-drug interactions. It may increase the concentrations of certain concomitant medications, thereby increasing the potential for serious and sometimes life-threatening drug toxicities. Hence medications with narrow therapeutic index that are mainly metabolised by CYP3A should not be coadministration with nirmatrelvir-ritonavir [4]

IL-6 inhibitors [3]

There are two classes of Food and Drug Administration (FDA)-approved IL-6 inhibitors: anti-IL-6 receptor monoclonal antibodies (mAbs) (e.g., sarilumab, tocilizumab) and anti-IL-6 mAbs (i.e., siltuximab).

Tocilizumab

Tocilizumab is a recombinant humanized anti-IL-6 receptor mAb primarily used in patients with rheumatologic disorders and cytokine release syndrome induced by chimeric antigen receptor T cell (CAR T-cell) therapy. It is also recommended for use in severe to critical COVID-19 patients.

Dose – Tocilizumab can be dosed as 8 mg/kg as a single intravenous dose. It is used in patients who are also taking dexamethasone (or another glucocorticoid).

Adverse Effects

Tocilizumab is associated with elevated liver enzyme levels that appear to be dose dependent. Additional adverse effects like serious infections (e.g., tuberculosis [TB], bacterial or fungal infections) and bowel perforation have also been reported with use of Tocilizumab.

Corticosteroids [3]

The COVID-19 Treatment Guidelines Panel's recommends the use of corticosteroids esp. dexamethasone in hospitalized patients with COVID-19. Corticosteroids presumably act by mitigating the COVID-19-induced systemic inflammatory response that can lead to lung injury and multisystem organ dysfunction.

Dose – Dexamethasone is used at a dose of 6 mg daily for 10 days or until discharge, whichever is shorter. In case of unavailability of dexamethasone, other glucocorticoids at equivalent doses (eg, total daily doses of hydrocortisone 150 mg, methylprednisolone 32 mg, or prednisone 40 mg) can also be used.

Adverse effects – Patients receiving glucocorticoids should be monitored for adverse effects. In severely ill patients, these include hyperglycemia, psychiatric effects, avascular necrosis and an increased risk of infections (including bacterial, fungal, and Strongyloides infections)

Table 1: Comparison of vaccines approved for use in India

Vaccine	Manufacturer	Type of vaccine	Route and doses	Efficacy	Adverse drug reaction
Covaxin	Bharat biotech I.M	Inactivated	I.M. 2 doses 4 weeks apart	77.8%	Injection site pain, Swelling, Redness, Itching, Headache, Fever, Malaise, body ache, Nausea, Vomiting, Rashes
Covishield	Serum Institute of India Pvt.Ltd	Non replicating viral vector	I.M. 2 doses 12-16 weeks apart	70.42%	Headache, nausea, myalgia, arthralgia, fatigue, malaise, feverishness, chills, fever, and local injection site reactions
Corbevax	Biological E limited	Protein subunit	I.M. 2 doses 4 weeks apart	90%	Injection site pain, Swelling, Redness, Itching, Headache, Fever, Malaise, body ache, Nausea
Covovax	Serum Institute of India Pvt.Ltd	Protein subunit	I.M. 2 doses 3 weeks apart	90%	Injection site Tenderness, Pain, Fatigue, Malaise, headache, Nausea or vomiting, arthralgia
Ad26. COV2.S	Janssen pharmaceutical	Non replicating viral vector	I.M 1	66.9%	Headache, Nausea, Myalgia, Fatigue; injection site pain, Arthralgia, Cough, Pyrexia; injection site erythema; injection site swelling; chills, anaphylaxis.
Vaxzevria	Oxford/ AstraZeneca	Non replicating viral vector	I.M. 2 doses 12-16 weeks apart	62.6%	Headache, nausea, myalgia, arthralgia, fatigue, malaise, feverishness, chills, fever, and local injection site reactions
Sputnik V	Gamaleya	Non replicating viral vector	I.M. 2 doses 3 weeks apart	91.6%	Flu-like syndrome (chills, fever, arthralgia, myalgia, asthenia, general discomfort, headache) or local (injection site tenderness, hyperemia, swelling
Sputnik Light	Gamaleya	Non replicating viral vector	I.M. Single dose	79.4%	Flu-like syndrome (chills, fever, arthralgia, myalgia, asthenia, general discomfort, headache) or local (injection site tenderness, hyperemia, swelling

| Spikevax | Moderna | RNA | I.M. 2 doses, 4 weeks apart. | 94.1% | pain at the injection site, fatigue, headache, myalgia, chills |
| ZyCoV-D | Zydus Cadila | DNA | Intradermal 3 dose 28 days apart | 66.6% | injection site pain, pruritus, pyrexia, arthralgia and diarrhea |

Table 2: Pharmacological agents tried for the management of COVID-19 infection

Stage	Disease severity	Postulated mechanism	Treatment options tried
Stage I Early infection phase	Mild	Symptom relief	• Adequate hydration • Acetaminophen • Nonsteroidal anti-inflammatory drug (NSAID) • Self-proning • Breathing exercises education • Cough medications
Stage II Pulmonary phase	Moderate	Inhibition of viral fusion and replication	• Ivermectin • Hydroxychloroquine • Antiviral • Monoclonal antibodies, • Nanobodies • Famotidine • Baricitinib • camostat mesylate • Boceprevir • Remdesivir • Zotatifin • Plitidepsin
Stage III hyperinflammation phase	Severe	Anti-inflammatory effect by reducing important proinflammatory cytokines immunomodulatory agents	• Dexamethasone • Monoclonal antibody tocilizumab, • Selective serotonin reuptake inhibitors (SSRI), • Melatonin

Table 3: Current treatment guidelines for COVID-19 management

Disease severity	Clinical profile	Strong recommendation in favour	Weak or conditional recommendation in favour	Weak or conditional recommendation against	Strong recommendation against
Mild	Absence of signs of severe disease	Nirmatrelvir-ritonavir	Molnupiravir Sotrovimab Remdesivir Casirivimab and imdevimab	Corticosteroids Ivermectin	Convalescent Plasma Hydroxychloroquine Lopinavir ritonavir
Severe	Oxygen saturation <90% on room air Signs of pneumonia Sign of respiratory distress	Corticosteroids IL-6 blockers Or Baricitinib	Casirivimab and imdevimab	Ivermectin Ruxolitinib and tofacitinib Convalescent Plasma	Hydroxychloroquine Lopinavir ritonavir
Critical	Require life sustaining treatment Acute respiratory distress syndrome Sepsis Septic shock	Corticosteroids IL-6 blockers Or Baricitinib	Casirivimab and imdevimab	Ivermectin Ruxolitinib and tofacitinib Convalescent Plasma	Hydroxychloroquine Lopinavir ritonavir

Table 4: Recommended dose of anticoagulant in hospitalised COVID-19 patients

Low molecular weight heparin/ Unfractionated heparin	Dose
Enoxaparin	creatinine clearance (CrCl) >30 mL/min, 4000 units once daily; CrCl 15 to 30 mL/min, 3000 Units once daily.
Dalteparin	5000 units once daily.
Nadroparin	≤70 kg, 3800 anti-factor Xa units once daily; >70 kg, 5700 units once daily.
Tinzaparin	4500 anti-factor Xa units once daily.
Sub cutaneous unfractionated heparin	5,000 units every 8 hours

COVID - Cardiology

COVID 19 was declared as pandemic on March 11th, 2020. The lung is the most commonly affected organ but the heart and other organs are also affected.

The spike protein of coronavirus interacts with Angiotensin converting enzyme 2 (ACE 2) receptors on the host cells thereby gaining entry into the cells. ACE 2 receptors are expressed more in lungs and heart which explains the disease predilection.

Hyper-inflammation and cytokine storm causing cardiac injury, respiratory failure and hypoxemia damaging the myocytes and hypercoagulability leading to thrombosis are other proposed mechanisms that ultimately lead to cardiac dysfunction in COVID 19 disease.

SARS- CoV2 can cause various cardiovascular manifestations like myocardial injury or myocarditis, arrhythmias, acute coronary syndromes and thromboembolism.

Myocardial injury during the course of COVID 19 is independently associated with higher mortality. Pre-existing cardiovascular disease increases the severity of COVID 19 by aggravating and decompensation of underlying cardiac pathology.

Acute cardiac injury may be manifested by increased blood levels of cardiac biomarkers like troponins.

Studies:

1. The INSPIRATION trial: Sadeghipour P, Talasaz AH, et al. JAMA, March 2021.

Effect of Intermediate-Dose vs. Standard-Dose Prophylactic Anticoagulation on Thrombotic Events, Extracorporeal Membrane Oxygenation Treatment, or Mortality Among Patients With COVID-19 Admitted to the Intensive Care Unit.

- Open-label, multi center, randomized trial.
- Patients were enrolled from 10 academic centers in Iran
- Participants were randomized in a 1:1 ratio to receive an intermediate dose of enoxaparin (1 mg/kg daily) or the standard prophylactic dose of enoxaparin (40 mg daily) for 30 days. Patients with severe kidney disease were given unfractionated heparin.
- Primary Outcome (Composite outcome at the end of 30 days):
  - Venous thromboembolism
  - Arterial thrombosis
  - Treatment with extracorporeal membrane oxygenation (ECMO)
  - All-cause mortality

- Secondary Outcomes:
  - All-cause mortality
  - Venous thromboembolism
  - Ventilator free days
- Principal Safety Outcomes:
  - Major bleeding according to the Bleeding Academic Research Consortium criteria.
  - Thrombocytopenia

Results:1692 patients were screened for eligibility and 562 patients were finally included in the analysis.

Following were the results

	Intermediate Dose	Standard Prophylactic Dose	Absolute Risk Diff [CI 95%]	Odds Ratio [CI 95%]	P-Value
Composite Primary Outcome	126/276 (45.7%)	126/286 (44.1%)	1.5 [-6.6 to 9.8]	1.06 [0.76 to 1.48]	0.70
All Cause Mortality	119/276 (43.1%)	117/286 (40.9%)	2.2 [-5.9 to 10.3]	1.09 [0.78 to 1.53]	0.50
VTE Events	3.3%	3.5%	-0.2 [-3.2 to 2.7]	0.93 [0.37 to 2.32]	0.87
Ventilatory Free Days (median)	30	30	0	N/A	0.50
Safety Outcomes					
Severe Thrombocytopenia	6/276 (2.2%)	0/286 (0%)	2.2%		0.01

Author's conclusion: Among patients with COVID-19 admitted to the ICU, intermediate-dose prophylactic anticoagulation, compared with standard-dose prophylactic anticoagulation, did not result in a significant difference in the primary outcome of a composite of venous or arterial thrombosis, treatment with ECMO, or mortality within 30 days. These results do not support the routine empirical use of intermediate-dose prophylactic anticoagulation in unselected patients with COVID-19 admitted to the ICU."

2. The ACTION trial:

Lopes RD, de Barros E Silva PGM, Furtado RHM, et al. The Lancet, June, 2021.

Therapeutic versus prophylactic anticoagulation for patients admitted to hospital with COVID-19 and elevated D-dimer concentration (ACTION): an open-label, multicentre, randomised, controlled trial.

- Pragmatic, open-label, multicenter, randomized controlled trial in patients hospitalized with COVID-19 with elevated D-dimer.
- Patients were randomly assigned to receive
    - Therapeutic anticoagulation for 30 days
    - Stable patients received rivaroxaban
    - Unstable received enoxaparin or heparin
- (OR) prophylactic anticoagulation with enoxaparin or heparin

Primary Outcome:

- Hierarchical Composite through 30 days:
    - Time to death
    - Duration of hospitalization
    - Duration of supplemental oxygen

Results: Out of the 3331 patients screened, 615 patients were enrolled and were randomised into treatment and control group.

- NO DIFFERENCE in time to death
- NO DIFFERENCE in the duration of hospitalization
- NO DIFFERENCE in supplemental oxygen

To conclude, In this trial, therapeutic dose rivaroxaban did not improve clinical outcomes and increased bleeding compared to a prophylactic dose anticoagulation strategy with enoxaparin or heparin.

3. Therapeutic anticoagulant ion with heparin in critically ill patients with COVID 19.

By the investigators of REMAP CAP, ACTIV 4a and the ATTACC trial. NEJM, August 2021.

It is an open-label, adaptive, multi-platform, randomized clinical trial. Intervention: Critically ill patients with severe Covid-19 were randomly assigned to a pragmatically defined regimen of either therapeutic-dose anticoagulation with heparin or pharmacologic thromboprophylaxis in accordance with local usual care.

	Therapeutic AC Group	Prophylactic AC Group	Effect (95% CI)	P value
Efficacy Outcome				
Heirarchical Composite Outcome	28,899 (35%)	34,288 (41%)	Win Ratio 0.86 (0.59-1.22)	0.40
Composite Thrombotic Outcome	23 (7%)	30 (10%)	RR 0.75 (0.45-1.26)	0.32
Composite Thrombotic Outcome and Death	46 (15%)	44 (14%)	RR 1.03 (0.70-1.50)	0.91
Death	35 (11%)	23 (8%)	RR 1.49 (0.90-2.46)	0.13
Rehospitalization	2 (1%)	5 (2%)	RR 0.39 (0.08-2.01)	0.28
WHO 8-point scale			OR 1.35 (0.85-2.16)	0.21
Safety Outcomes				
Major or clinically relevant non-major bleeding	26 (8%)	7 (2%)	RR 3.64 (1.61-8.27)	0.0010
Combined Efficacy and Safety Outcome				
Net Benefit	56 (18%)	47 (15%)	RR 1.17 (0.82-1.66)	0.45

Primary Outcome: Organ support–free days, evaluated on an ordinal scale that combined in-hospital death and the number of days free of cardiovascular or respiratory organ support up to day 21 among patients who survived to hospital discharge.

Results: 1098 patients were randomized into two arms of the study. 534 assigned to therapeutic-dose anticoagulation and 564 assigned to usual-care thromboprophylaxis.

The trial was stopped when the pre-specified criterion for futility was met for therapeutic-dose anticoagulation.

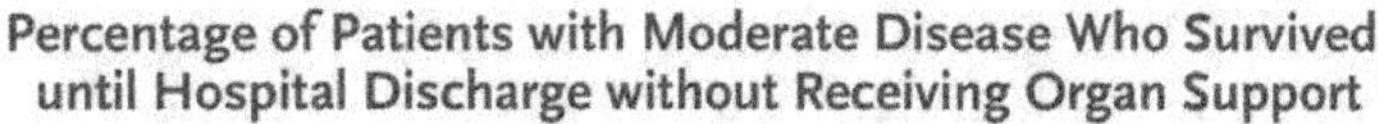

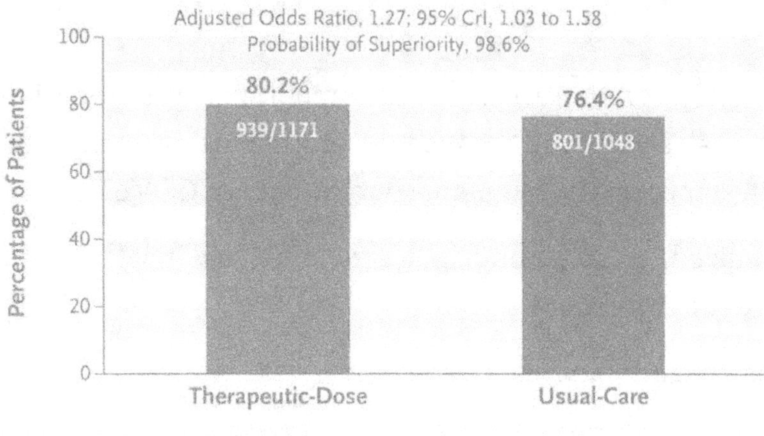

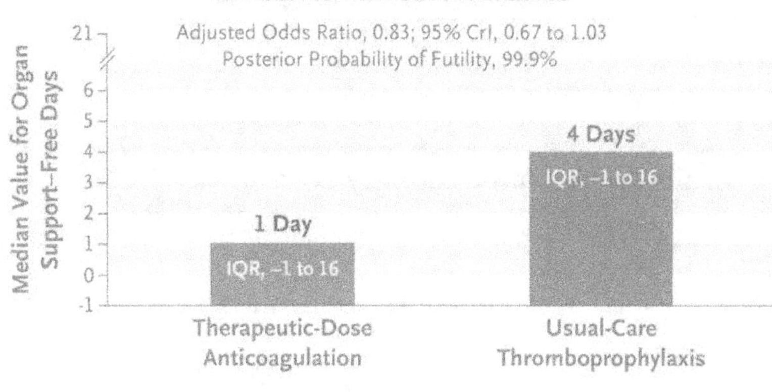

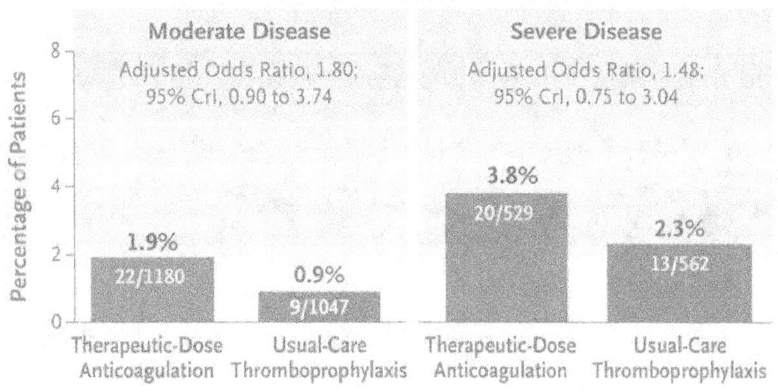

Conclusion: In critically ill patients with Covid-19, an initial strategy of therapeutic-dose anticoagulation with heparin did not result in a greater probability of survival to hospital discharge or a greater number of days free of cardiovascular or respiratory organ support than did usual-care pharmacologic thromboprophylaxis.

4. The ACTIV- 4b Trial. Connors, J. M. et al. JAMA, August 2021.

Effect of antithrombotic therapy on clinical outcomes in outpatients with clinically stable symptomatic COVID-19.

Multiple studies have investigated the use of antithrombotic agents in patients with COVID-19 admitted to various hospital settings. The authors of this study looked into the benefits of antithrombotic therapy in symptomatic but stable outpatients of COVID 19.

It is an adaptive, randomized, double-blind, placebo-controlled trial.52 centers were included throughout the US for patient enrollment.

Primary Outcome: Composite endpoint of-

- Symptomatic DVT
- Pulmonary embolism
- Arterial thromboembolism
- Myocardial infarction
- Ischemic stroke
- Hospitalization for a cardiovascular or pulmonary event
- All-cause mortality within 45 days

Results:Patients randomized 1:1:1:1. Treatment with aspirin (81 mg daily) with matching placebo (placebo to create twice daily dosing)

- Prophylactic dose of apixaban (2.5 mg twice daily)
- Therapeutic dose of apixaban (5 mg twice daily)
- Placebo (twice daily)

657 patients were included in the study. It was terminated early due to low event rates.

	ASA 81mg	Prophylactic Apixaban (2.5mg BID)	Therapeutic Apixaban (5mg BID)	Placebo
Composite Primary Endpoint	0	0.7%	1.4%	0%
Risk Difference vs Placebo	0.0%	0.7% (95% CI -2.1 to 4.1)	1.4% (95% CI -1.5 to 5.0)	---

To conclude, the preliminary evidence in this study demonstrates no benefit from aspirin or apixaban for thromboprophylaxis in symptomatic patients who are clinically stable for outpatient management.

5. The HEP- COVID Trial. Spyropoulos AC et al. JAMA, October 2021.

Efficacy and Safety of Therapeutic-Dose Heparin vs Standard Prophylactic or Intermediate-Dose Heparins for Thromboprophylaxis in High-risk Hospitalized Patients With COVID-19

It is a multicenter, pseudo-open labeled, active control randomized clinical trial.

Patients in the therapeutic-dose group received enoxaparin at a dose of 1 mg/kg subcutaneously twice daily if CrCl was ≥30 mL/min/1.73 m2 or 0.5 mg/kg twice daily if CrCl was 15-29 mL/min/1.73 m2. If CrCl fell below 15 mL/min/ 1.73 m2, enoxaparin was converted to treatment-dose intravenous UFH until kidney function improved to CrCl greater than 15 mL/min/1.73 m2, when blinded-dose subcutaneous enoxaparin was resumed

Patients in the standard-dose group received prophylactic or intermediate-dose heparin regimens per local institutional standard and could include:

- UFH, up to 22,500 IU subcutaneously (divided twice or three times daily)
- Enoxaparin 30 mg or 40 mg subcutaneously once or twice daily (weight-based enoxaparin 0.5 mg/kg subcutaneously twice daily was permitted but strongly discouraged)
- Dalteparin, 2500 IU or 5000 IU subcutaneously daily

Primary Outcome: composite of

1. All types of VTEs including DVTs, PTE, CSVT and splanchnic venous thrombosis
2. All arterial thromboembolisms like MI, Ischemic stroke, peripheral and systemic arterial thrombosis.
3. All cause mortality in 30 days.

Results: Out of the 11,649 patients screened for eligibility, 253 patients were finally included in the analysis.

The authors concluded that the therapeutic-dose LMWH reduced the composite of thromboembolism and death compared with standard heparin thromboprophylaxis without increased major bleeding among hospitalized patients with COVID-19 with very elevated D-dimer levels. The treatment effect was not seen in ICU patients.

This small trial showed promising evidence that therapeutic-dose LMWH reduced the composite outcome of death and thromboembolism when compared to the standard-dose in patients with markedly elevated D-dimer levels who were on oxygen therapy and not treated in an ICU. The outcome was driven by the reduction in thromboembolism with no statistically significant difference in mortality.

Clinical Outcomes During the 30-Day Postrandomization Phase

Outcome	No./total No. (%)		RR (95% CI)	P value[a]
	Therapeutic dose (n = 129)	Standard dose (n = 124)		
Primary efficacy outcome				
VTE, ATE, or death	37/129 (28.7)	52/124 (41.9)	0.68 (0.49-0.96)	.03
Non-ICU stratum	14/84 (16.7)	31/86 (36.1)	0.46 (0.27-0.81)	.004
ICU stratum	23/45 (51.1)	21/38 (55.3)	0.92 (0.62-1.39)	.71
VTE + ATE	14/129 (10.9)	36/124 (29.0)	0.37 (0.21-0.66)	<.001
Death	25/129 (19.4)	31/124 (25.0)	0.78 (0.49-1.23)	.28
Secondary efficacy outcomes				
Primary efficacy outcome at day 14	30/129 (23.3)	45/124 (36.3)	0.64 (0.43-0.95)	.02
Principal safety outcome				
Major bleeding	6/129 (4.7)	2/124 (1.6)	2.88 (0.59-14.02)	.28
Non-ICU stratum	2/84 (2.4)	2/86 (2.3)	1.02 (0.15-7.10)	>.99
ICU stratum	4/45 (8.9)	0	7.62 (0.42-137.03)	.12

6. The MICHELLE Trial. Ramacciotti E, Barile Agati L, Calderaro D, et al. The Lancet, January 2022. Rivaroxaban versus no anticoagulation for post-discharge thromboprophylaxis after hospitalization for COVID-19 (MICHELLE).

Methodology: Pragmatic, open-label, multi-center, randomized control trial. Patients enrolled from 14 hospitals in Brazil. Participants were randomized in a 1:1 ratio to receive either 10 mg rivaroxaban per day or no anticoagulation (without placebo) for 35 days.

Primary Outcomes:Composite endpoint at day 35 of:

- Symptomatic venous thromboembolism (VTE)
- VTE related death
- Asymptomatic VTE detected via venous duplex of bilateral lower extremities or CT pulmonary angiogram.
- Symptomatic arterial thromboembolism (ATE) including myocardial infarction, non-hemorrhagic stroke, or major adverse limb event
- Cardiovascular death

Results: Out of 997 patients initially screened, 320 were finally randomised into the two arms of the study. Two of them withdrew consent and hence 318 were finally analysed.

The authors of MICHELLE concluded that in patients at high risk discharged after hospitalization due to COVID-19, evidence suggests that thromboprophylaxis with rivaroxaban 10 mg/day through 35 days improved clinical outcomes, reducing thrombotic events, compared with no post-discharge anticoagulation.

Although the study gave a statistically significant benefit in the composite outcomes, there was no significant difference in the individual endpoints. Also, the study was an open labelled trial without placebo which can introduce a potential bias.

	Rivaroxaban (n=159)	Control (n=159)	Relative risk (95% CI)	p values (two-sided)
Primary efficacy outcome	5/159 (3·14%)	15/159 (9·43%)	0·33 (0·13–0·90)	0·0293
Secondary efficacy outcomes				
Symptomatic and fatal VTE	1/159 (0·63%)	8/159 (5·03%)	0·13 (0·02–0·99)	0·0487
Symptomatic VTE and all-cause mortality	4/159 (2·52%)	9/159 (5·66%)	0·44 (0·14–1·41)	0·1696
Composite of symptomatic VTE, myocardial infarction, stroke, and cardiovascular death	1/159 (0·63%)	9/159 (5·66%)	0·11 (0·01–0·87)	0·0360
Components of the primary outcome				
Symptomatic DVT	0	3 (1·89%)	0·14 (0·01–2·74)	0·1968
Symptomatic pulmonary embolism	1 (0·63%)	2 (1·26%)	0·50 (0·05–5·46)	0·5698
Fatal pulmonary embolism	0	3 (1·89%)	0·14 (0·01–2·74)	0·1968
Asymptomatic DVT on duplex scan	3 (1·89%)	1 (0·63%)	3·00 (0·32–28·53)	0·3391
Asymptomatic pulmonary embolism on CT pulmonary angiogram	1 (0·63%)	4 (2·52%)	0·25 (0·03–2·21)	0·2127
Symptomatic arterial thrombosis	0	1 (0·63%)	0·33 (0·01–8·12)	0·5001
Myocardial infarction	0	0	NA	NA
Non-haemorrhagic stroke	0	0	NA	NA
Major adverse limb event	0	0	NA	NA
Cardiovascular death	0	1 (0·63%)	0·33 (0·01–8·12)	0·5001

Data are n/N (%), or n (%), unless otherwise specified. CRNM=clinically relevant non-major. DVT=deep vein thrombosis. NA=not applicable. VTE=venous thromboembolism.

Table 2: **Efficacy and safety outcomes (intention-to-treat analysis)**

7. Cardiac Manifestations in patients with COVID 19: A Scoping Review. Peiris S et al. Global heart, 2022.

The overall aim of this review was to provide an in-depth description of the available literature related to the cardiac system and COVID-19 infection.

Out of the 1312 records identified through database search, 63 were finally included in qualitative synthesis. The overall frequency of acute cardiac injury ranged from 15% to 33% in the reporting studies. The main cardiac complications were

- Arrhythmias (3.1% to 6.9% in non-severe patients, 33.0% to 48.0% in severe disease),
- Acute coronary syndromes (6% to 33% in severe disease), and -Myocarditis.

Most studies found no association with the use of Renin- angiotensin-aldosterone system inhibitors (RAASI) with COVID-19 outcomes such as susceptibility to infection, hospitalization, severity, and mortality.

These trials will be influencing our treatment protocols for management of cardiac complications in covid 19 infection.

Neurological Manifestations in COVID 19 Illness

A meta-analysis of various studies done and published in July 2021 in the American Chemical Society (ACS) included prospective and retrospective observational cohort studies, cross-sectional and case-control studies.

The exact pathophysiologic basis of neuronal insults remains unclear; however, they are hypothesized to be caused by multiple factors such as damage to specific receptors, secondary hypoxia, cytokine-related injury, and retrograde travel along the olfactory nerve and bulb. Additionally, global inflammatory markers (IL-6, 12, 15, TNF alpha) can activate glial cells and produce an inflammatory response. These systemic consequences, coupled with alveolar lung damage, cause severe hypoxia leading to cerebrovascular vasodilatation, cerebral edema, and ischemia.

The neurologic manifestations in COVID 19 illness can be classified into non-specific, central nervous system, and peripheral nervous system, depending upon symptoms. The most common symptoms reported in COVID 19 illness were the non-specific symptoms such as headache, dizziness, nausea, and vomiting, which were significant with a pooled proportion of around 15%.

Central nervous system manifestations were also highly reported in COVID-19 patients. Significantly reported manifestations included altered mental status, agitation, confusion, seizures of new-onset, cerebrovascular diseases, encephalitis, encephalopathy, and movement disorder in the decreasing order of their incidence. Among peripheral nervous system manifestations, smell and taste disturbances have been widely reported; A pooled proportion of 27.2% and 26.4% for gustatory dysfunction and olfactory dysfunction, respectively. Other significant manifestations include Guillain Barre Syndrome (GBS), arthralgia, and neuralgia.

GBS reported in COVID 19 illness has satisfied Brighton level 1 or level 2 of diagnostic certainty. Cases of GBS were also noted within four weeks of COVID 19 vaccination, especially after receiving the BNT162b2 vaccine (commonly Pfizer, BioNTech).

A well-known Johnson and Johnson product, AstraZeneca adenoviral vaccine, used in COVID 19 illness prevention, was also found to be associated with post vaccine GBS.

Management of hypoxemic covid 19 patient

Covid 19 infection involves the lung primarily either as endotheliitis, pneumonia and severe ARDS. The requirement of oxygen is present for almost all patients as the disease progresses.

Pathophysiology- The major morbidity and mortality from coronavirus disease 2019 (COVID-19) is largely due to acute viral pneumonia that evolves to acute respiratory distress syndrome.

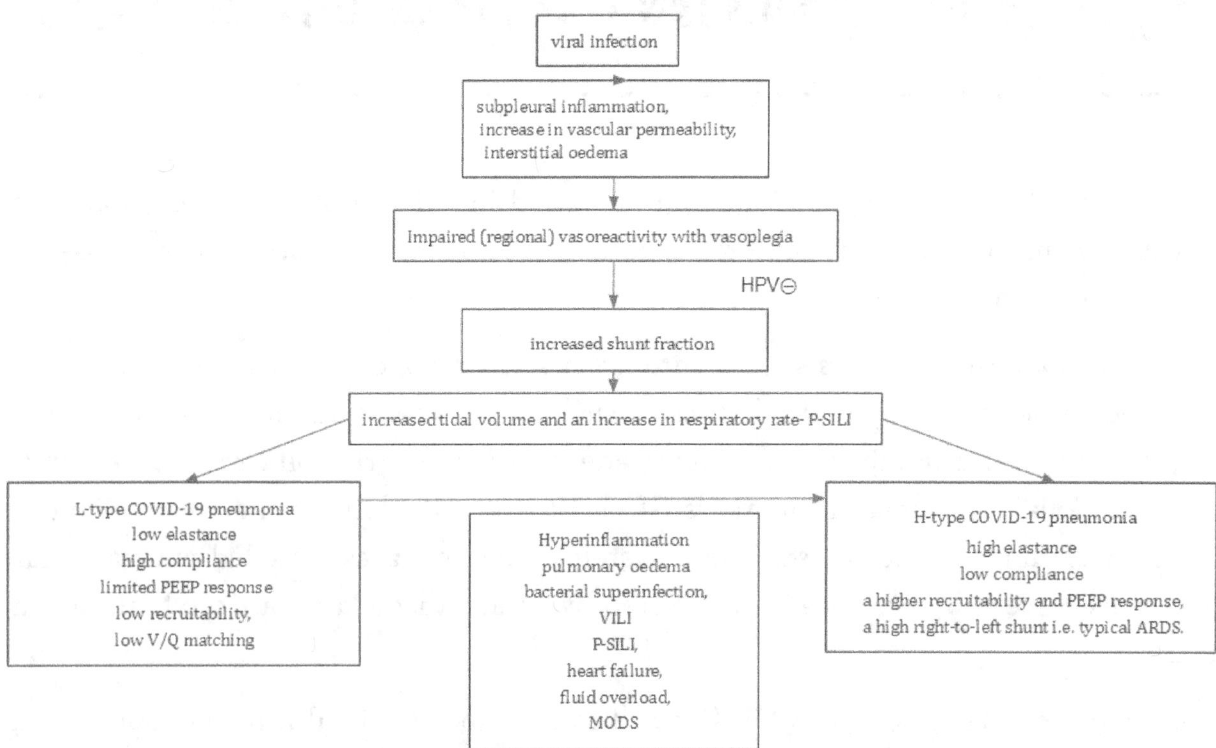

Recommendations for a covid 19 patients who are receiving oxygen or noninvasive modalities of support (including low-flow oxygen, HFNC or NIV

Awake Pronation	Spend as much time as is feasible and safe in the prone position. Typically 6 to 8 hours everyday. No benefit if hypoxemia is due to pulmonary edema, pulmonary embolism
Target SPO_2	Target peripheral oxygen saturation (SpO_2) of ≥94% during initial resuscitation and ≥90% for maintenance oxygenation. Prefer the lowest possible FiO_2 necessary to meet oxygenation goals Hyperoxia should be avoided. Individualization of the goal is important, eg, patients with a concomitant acute Type II respiratory failure from COPD require lower SPO_2 whereas Pregnant females require a higher target.
Monitoring	Respiratory- First ABG after 2 h, thereafter on a daily basis and SOS. Low threshold for intubation should be practiced. Fluid and nutrition – Monitor for dehydration and malnutrition. Nasogastric feeding is advised No need for extra protein, vitamin C or D or trace element supplementation over and above the usual recommended daily doses.
Duration of treatment	No set duration for a trial period of either modality. Few patients tolerate therapy for 7-10 days. No factors that reliably predict which course a patient will take.

The dilemma of choosing between HFNC and NIV- In retrospective cohorts, rates for HFNC use ranged from 14 to 63 percent, while 11 to 56 percent were treated with NIV. It is advocated that these modalities will prevent intubations but it is not entirely true. There may be some patients who will respond with better SPO_2s and ABG. The intubation threshold is kept high with some improvement and this is clinically judged a prevention of IMV with appropriate application of NIV or HFNC. Others who could be benefitted were Patients with acute exacerbation of COPD, acute cardiogenic pulmonary edema, underlying sleep-disordered breathing [eg, obstructive sleep apnea or obesity hypoventilation], or respiratory muscle weakness. In the absence of such comorbidities, either modality is acceptable. The tolerability of the device and patient comfort are often the determining factors. HFNC is arguably associated with fewer adverse events and is a more comfortable and practical mode of support, during which patients can continue to converse and eat when compared with NIV. In some cases, we may transition between HFNC and NIV for short periods (eg, during sleep, acute episodes of acute pulmonary edema) and occasionally cycle between both modalities until the patient improves or deteriorates. The data to support NIV is direct evidence as it has been used in Covid patients whereas data for HFNC is majorly from its beneficial effects in non covid patients.

Studies-

1. Ehrmann S, Li J, Ibarra-Estrada M, Perez Y, Pavlov I, McNicholas B, Roca O, Mirza S, Vines D, Garcia-Salcido R, Aguirre-Avalos G, Trump MW, Nay MA, Dellamonica J, Nseir S, Mogri I, Cosgrave D, Jayaraman D, Masclans JR, Laffey JG, Tavernier E, Awake Prone Positioning Meta-Trial Group. **Awake prone positioning for COVID-19 acute hypoxaemic respiratory failure**: a randomised, controlled, multinational, open-label meta-trial.Lancet Respir Med. 2021;9(12):1387. Epub 2021 Aug 20.

The authors aimed to evaluate the efficacy of awake prone positioning to prevent intubation or death in patients with severe COVID-19 in a large-scale randomized trial.1126 adults who required respiratory support with high-flow nasal cannula for acute hypoxaemic respiratory failure due to COVID-19 were randomly assigned to awake prone positioning or standard care. The primary composite outcome was treatment failure, defined as the proportion of patients intubated or dying within 28 days of enrolment. Treatment failure occurred in 223 (40%) of 564 patients assigned to awake prone positioning and in 257 (46%) of 557 patients assigned to standard care (RR 0·86 [95% CI 0·75-0·98]). The hazard ratio (HR) for intubation was 0·75 (0·62-0·91), and the HR for mortality was 0·87 (0·68-1·11) with awake prone positioning compared with standard care within 28 days of enrolment. The incidence of prespecified adverse events was low and similar in both groups. These results support routine awake prone positioning of patients with COVID-19 who require support with high-flow nasal cannula.

2. Ospina-Tascón GA, Calderón-Tapia LE, García AF, Zarama V, Gómez-Álvarez F, Álvarez-Saa T, Pardo-Otálvaro S, Bautista-Rincón DF, Vargas MP, Aldana-Díaz JL, MarulandaÁ, Gutiérrez A, Varón J, Gómez M, Ochoa ME, Escobar E, Umaña M, Díez J, Tobón GJ, Albornoz LL, Celemín Flórez CA, Ruiz GO, Cáceres EL, Reyes LF, Damiani LP, Cavalcanti AB, HiFLo-Covid Investigators. **Effect of High-Flow Oxygen Therapy vs Conventional Oxygen Therapy** on Invasive Mechanical Ventilation and Clinical Recovery in Patients With Severe COVID-19: A Randomized Clinical Trial. JAMA. 2021;326(21):2161.

The authors planned to determine the effect of high-flow oxygen therapy through a nasal cannula compared with conventional oxygen therapy on need for endotracheal intubation and clinical recovery in severe COVID-19. A total of 220 adults with respiratory distress and a PaO_2/FiO_2 ratio < 200 were randomly assigned to receive high-flow oxygen through a nasal cannula (n = 109) or conventional oxygen therapy (n = 111). The co-primary outcomes were need for intubation and time to clinical recovery until day 28 as assessed by a 7-category ordinal scale (range, 1-7, with higher scores indicating a worse condition). Intubation occurred in 34 (34.3%) randomized to high-flow oxygen therapy and in 51 (51.0%) randomized to conventional oxygen therapy. The median time to clinical recovery within 28 days was 11 (IQR, 9-14) days in patients randomized to high-flow oxygen therapy vs 14 (IQR, 11-19) days in those randomized to conventional oxygen therapy. Suspected bacterial pneumonia occurred in 13 patients (13.1%) randomized to high-flow oxygen and in 17 (17.0%) of those randomized to conventional oxygen therapy, while bacteremia was detected in 7 (7.1%) vs 11 (11.0%), respectively. They concluded that among patients with severe COVID-19, use of high-flow oxygen through a nasal cannula significantly decreased need for mechanical ventilation support and time to clinical recovery compared with conventional low-flow oxygen therapy.

3. Perkins GD, Ji C, Connolly BA, Couper K, Lall R, Baillie JK, Bradley JM, Dark P, Dave C, De Soyza A, Dennis AV, Devrell A, Fairbairn S, Ghani H, Gorman EA, Green CA, Hart N, Hee SW, Kimbley Z, Madathil S, McGowan N, Messer B, Naisbitt J, Norman C, Parekh D, Parkin EM, Patel J, Regan SE, Ross C, Rostron AJ, Saim M, Simonds AK, Skilton E, Stallard N, Steiner M, Vancheeswaran R, Yeung J, McAuley DF, RECOVERY-RS Collaborators. Effect of **Noninvasive Respiratory Strategies on Intubation or Mortality** Among Patients With Acute Hypoxemic Respiratory Failure and COVID-19: The RECOVERY-RS Randomized Clinical Trial.JAMA. 2022;327(6):546.

CPAP and HFNO have been recommended for acute hypoxemic respiratory failure in patients with COVID-19. The authors aimed to determine whether either CPAP or HFNO, compared with conventional oxygen therapy, improves clinical outcomes in hospitalized patients with COVID-19-related acute hypoxemic respiratory failure. Adult patients were randomized to receive CPAP (n = 380), HFNO (n = 418), or conventional oxygen therapy (n = 475). The primary outcome was a composite of tracheal intubation or mortality within 30 days. Of the 1273 randomized patients (mean age, 57.4 [95% CI, 56.7 to 58.1]years; 66% male; 65% White race), primary outcome data were available for 1260. Crossover between interventions occurred in 17.1% of participants (15.3% in the CPAP group, 11.5% in the HFNO group, and 23.6% in the conventional oxygen therapy group). The requirement for tracheal intubation or mortality within 30 days was significantly lower with CPAP (36.3%) vs conventional oxygen therapy (44.4%) but was not significantly different with HFNO (44.3%) vs conventional oxygen therapy (45.1%). Adverse events occurred in 34.2% (130/380) of participants in the CPAP group, 20.6% (86/418) in the HFNO group, and 13.9% (66/475) in the conventional oxygen therapy group. The group concluded that among patients with acute hypoxemic respiratory failure due to COVID-19, an initial strategy of CPAP significantly reduced the risk of tracheal intubation or mortality compared with conventional oxygen therapy, but there was no significant difference between an initial strategy of HFNO compared with conventional oxygen therapy.

Key points- In patients with COVID-19 and acute hypoxemic respiratory failure despite conventional oxygen therapy, the best approach to escalation of noninvasive respiratory support is unknown. For patients with COVID-19 who have increasing oxygen needs and do not have conditions best treated with noninvasive ventilation (NIV; hypercapnic respiratory failure due to an exacerbation of chronic obstructive pulmonary disease or acute cardiogenic pulmonary edema), we trial NIV (CPAP or bilevel positive airway pressure), HFNC, or cycle between both until patients demonstrate improvement or deterioration. The tolerability of the device and patient comfort often determine the best modality.

Invasive Ventilation in COVID 19 Pneumonia

Upto 15% of patients with covid 19 infection progress to develop serious respiratory issues such as ARDS. These patients should be early recognized and offered intubation and invasive mechanical ventilation. It is noticed that there are no 100% full proof criteria to recognize a deteriorating patient, however application of standard ARDS criteria identifies the majority of them. Many scores like COVID-SOFA, COVID GRAM and 4C scores have been utilized for estimating the progression and morbidity and mortality from the disease.

Indications for institution of IMV

1	Patients with rapid progression over hours
2	Patients with a persistent need for high flows/FiO_2 (eg, >60 L/minute and an FiO_2 >0.6) with High flow machine or NIV
3	Patients with increasing PCO_2, increasing work of breathing, decreasing spontaneous tidal volume, worsening mental status, increasing duration and degree of fall in SPO_2
4	Patients with unstable vitals and MODS

The algorithm of intubation and mechanical ventilation with evidence based interventions is detailed below-

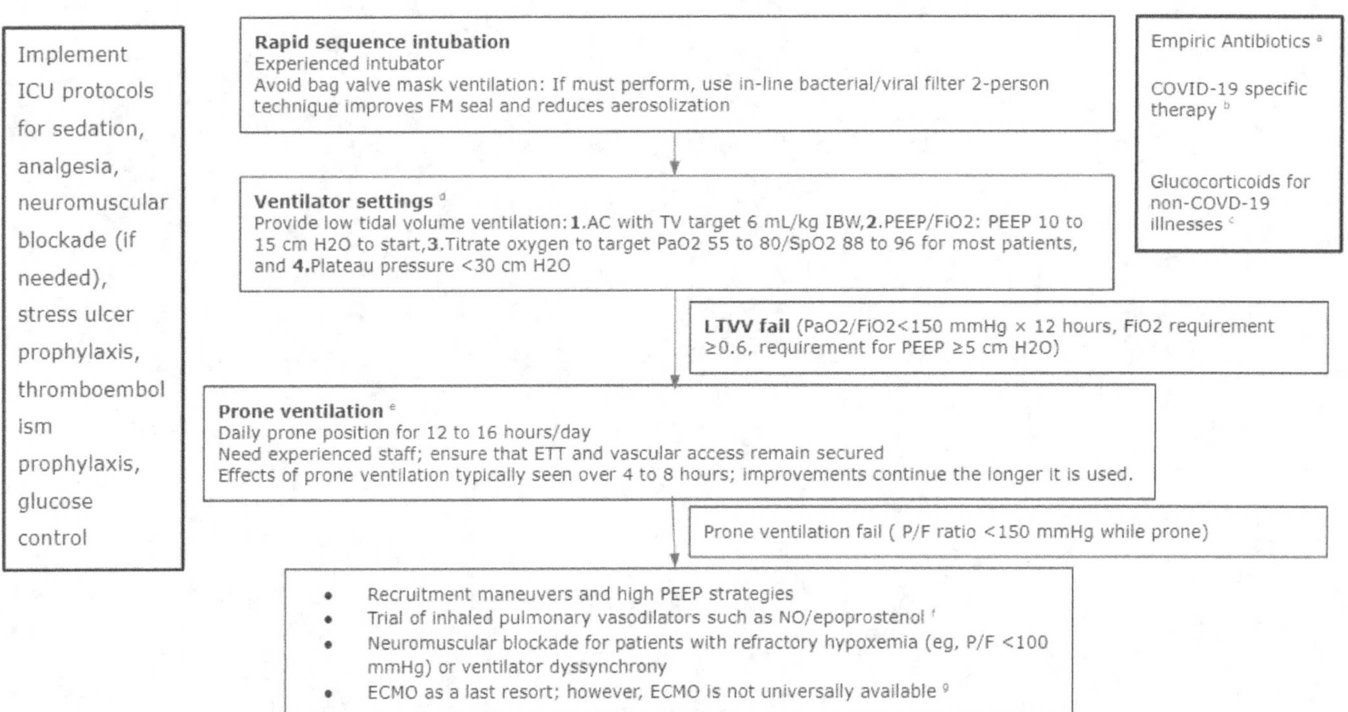

a. For suspected bacterial co-infection (eg, elevated WBC, positive sputum culture, positive urinary antigen, atypical chest imaging), administer empiric coverage for community-acquired or healthcare-associated pneumonia.

b. Dexamethasone, Remdesivir, and interleukin-6 inhibitors should be considered.

c. Give glucocorticoids for other indications (eg, asthma, COPD)

d. The response to LTVV should be assessed within the first four hours of ventilation. The clinicians have a low threshold to start with a higher level of PEEP (eg, 10 to 15 cm H2O) and use PEEP levels at the higher end of the range for the fraction of inspired oxygen (FiO2).

e. Pronation is more likely to be beneficial in the earlier phases of ARDS (eg, first 4 to 12 hours). Should deterioration in oxygenation occur in the later phases of ARDS, the benefits are less clear.

f. Pulmonary vasodilators should **not** be administered unless a specific protocol and staff experienced in their administration are in place as epoprostenol can clog the filters. Inhaled vasodilators may increase aerosolization.Numerical improvement due to pulmonary vasodilators should not prevent prone positioning when otherwise indicated. The dose of iNO is 30PPM for one hour.

g. ECMO can reduce the lymphocyte count and raise the interleukin-6 level, thereby interfering with the interpretation of these laboratory results.

Guidelines for additional COVID-19-specific ventilator equipment precautions —

1	Maintain tight seals for all ventilator circuitry and equipment. ETT cuff pressure between 20 and 30 cm H2O
2	Avoid unnecessary disconnection with the ETT or tracheostomy. In-line suction devices and in-line adapters for bronchoscopy are preferred If disconnection is necessary (eg, during transfer or manual bagging), the ETT or tracheostomy should be temporarily clamped during disconnection and unclamped after reconnection, provided the patient is not spontaneously breathing
3	Use a dual limb ventilator circuit with filters placed at the exhalation outlets. HME should be placed between the exhalation port and the ETT Use appropriate filters and filter change schedule
4	An airborne isolation room is Preferred when aerosol generating procedures take place (eg, extubation, bronchoscopy).
5	Obtain endotracheal aspirates rather than bronchoalveolar lavage via bronchoscopy. Nonbronchoscopic alveolar lavage ("mini-BAL") may also be performed as an alternative to bronchoscopy. Use of smaller aliquots of lavage fluid is safer (eg, three 10 mL aliquots to obtain 2 to 3 mL of fluid).

Extubation pearls-

1	Use of closed systems and not spontaneous breathing trial on T Piece
2	SBT for 2-4 hours rather than 2 h
3	Cuff leak test in an airborne isolation room
4	administer glucocorticoids (eg, methylprednisolone 20 mg intravenously every four hours for a total of four doses if not already receiving dexamethasone) to patients with COVID-19 before extubation

Studies-

1. Botta M, Tsonas AM, Pillay J, Boers LS, Algera AG, Bos LDJ, Dongelmans DA, Hollmann MW, Horn J, Vlaar APJ, Schultz MJ, Neto AS, Paulus F, **PRoVENT-COVID** Collaborative Group. Ventilation management and clinical outcomes in invasively ventilated patients with COVID-19 (PRoVENT-COVID): a national, multicentre, observational cohort study. Lancet Respir Med. 2021;9(2):139. Epub 2020 Oct 23.

The study was done during the first month of covid outbreak taking into consideration that at that time little was known about the practice of ventilation management in patients with COVID-19. PRoVENT-COVID was a national, multicentre, retrospective observational study done at 18 intensive care units (ICUs) in the Netherlands. Consecutive patients aged at least 18 years were eligible for participation if they had received invasive ventilation for COVID-19 at a participating ICU.. The primary outcome was a combination of ventilator variables and parameters over the first 4 calendar days of ventilation: tidal volume, positive end-expiratory pressure (PEEP), respiratory system compliance, and driving pressure. Secondary outcomes included the use of adjunctive treatments for refractory hypoxaemia and ICU complications. Patient-centred outcomes were ventilator-free days at day 28, duration of ventilation, duration of ICU and hospital stay, and mortality. The total number of patients included in the study were 530. Median tidal volume was 6·3 mL/kg PBW (IQR 5·7-7·1), PEEP was 14·0 cm H2O (IQR 11·0-15·0), and driving pressure was 14·0 cm H2O (11·2-16·0). Median respiratory system compliance was 31·9 mL/cm H2O (26·0-39·9). Of the adjunctive treatments for refractory hypoxaemia, prone positioning was most often used in the first 4 days of ventilation ([53%). The median number of ventilator-free days at day 28 was 0 (IQR 0-15); 186 (35%) of 530 patients had died by day 28. Predictors of 28-day mortality were gender, age, tidal volume, respiratory system compliance, arterial pH, and heart rate on the first day of invasive ventilation.

2. Shelhamer MC, Wesson PD, Solari IL, Jensen DL, Steele WA, Dimitrov VG, Kelly JD, Aziz S, Gutierrez VP, Vittinghoff E, Chung KK, Menon VP, Ambris HA, Baxi SM.**Prone Positioning in Moderate to Severe Acute Respiratory Distress Syndrome Due to COVID-19:** A Cohort Study and Analysis of Physiology...J Intensive Care Med. 2021;36(2):241.

The authors studied whether prone positioning improves outcomes in mechanically ventilated patients with moderate to severe ARDS due to COVID-19. The primary outcome was in-hospital death. Secondary outcomes included changes in physiologic parameters. Out of 335 participants who were intubated and mechanically ventilated, 62 underwent prone positioning, Prone positioning was significantly associated with reduced mortality (SHR 0.61, 95% CI 0.46-0.80, P<0.005). The oxygenation-saturation index was significantly improved during days 1-3 (P<0.01) whereas oxygenation-saturation index (OSI), oxygenation-index (OI) and arterial oxygen partial pressure to fractional inspired oxygen (PaO_2: FiO_2) were significantly improved during days 4-7 (P<0.05 for all).. The authors concluded that prone positioning in patients with moderate to severe ARDS due to COVID-19 is associated with reduced mortality and improved physiologic parameters. One in-hospital death could be averted for every 8 patients treated.

3. Weiss TT, Cerda F, Scott JB, Kaur R, Sungurlu S, Mirza SH, Alolaiwat AA, Kaur R, Augustynovich AE, Li J. **Prone positioning for patients intubated for severe acute respiratory distress syndrome (ARDS) secondary to COVID-19**: a retrospective observational cohort study.Br J Anaesth. 2021;126(1):48. Epub 2020 Oct 10.

The authors studied the role of repeated prone positioning in intubated subjects with ARDS caused by COVID-19. The primary outcome was considered as positive if there was an increase in PaO_2/FiO_2 ratio≥20%. Treatment failure of prone positioning was defined as death or requirement for ECMO. Forty-two subjects (29 males; age: 59 [52-69]yr) were eligible for analysis. Nine subjects were placed in the prone position only once, with 25 requiring prone positioning on three or more occasions. A total of 31/42 (74%) subjects survived to discharge, with five requiring ECMO.. After the first prone positioning session, PaO_2/FiO_2 ratio increased from 17.9 kPa (7.2) to 28.2 kPa (12.2) (P<0.01). After the initial prone positioning session, subjects who were discharged from hospital were more likely to have an improvement in PaO_2/FiO_2 ratio≥20%, compared with those requiring ECMO or who died. They concluded that patients with COVID-19 acute respiratory distress syndrome frequently responded to initial prone positioning with improved oxygenation. Subsequent prone positioning in subjects discharged from hospital was associated with greater improvements in oxygenation.

4. Johansson PI, Søe-Jensen P, Bestle MH, Clausen NE, Kristiansen KT, Lange T, Stensballe J, Perner A. **Prostacyclin in Intubated Patients with COVID-19 and Severe Endotheliopathy:** A Multicenter, Randomized Clinical Trial. Am J Respir Crit Care Med. 2022;205(3):324.

The mortality in patients infected with severe ARDS-SARS-CoV-2 who require mechanical ventilation remains high, and endotheliopathy has been implicated. The authors aimed to determine the effect of prostacyclin infusion in mechanically ventilated patients infected with SARS-CoV-2 with severe endotheliopathy. Adults infected with coronavirus disease (COVID-19) who required mechanical ventilation and had a plasma level of thrombomodulin>4 ng/ml were randomized to 72-hour infusion of prostacyclin 1 ng/kg/min or placebo. The main outcome was the number of days alive and without mechanical ventilation within 28 days. Key secondary outcomes were 28-day mortality and serious adverse events within 7 days. Eighty patients were randomized (41 prostacyclin and 39 placebo). The median number of days alive without mechanical ventilation at 28 days was 16.0 days (SD, 12) versus 5.0 days (SD, 10) in the prostacyclin and the placebo groups, respectively. The 28-day mortality was 21.9% versus 43.6% in the prostacyclin and the placebo groups, respectively (risk ratio, 0.50; 95% CI, 0.24 to 0.96; P = 0.06). The incidence of serious adverse events within 7 days was 2.4%versus 12.8% (risk ratio, 0.19; 95% CI, 0.001 to 1.11; P = 0.10) in the prostacyclin and the placebo groups, respectively. This showed that Prostacyclin was not associated with a significant reduction in the number of days alive and without mechanical ventilation within 28 days. The point estimates, however, favored the prostacyclin group in all analyses, including 28-day mortality,.

5. Bagate F, Tuffet S, Masi P, Perier F, Razazi K, de Prost N, Carteaux G, Payen D, Mekontso Dessap A. **Rescue therapy with inhaled nitric oxide and almitrine in COVID-19 patients with severe acute respiratory distress syndrome**. Ann Intensive Care. 2020;10(1):151. Epub 2020 Nov 4.

In COVID-19 patients with severe ARDS, the relatively preserved respiratory system compliance despite severe hypoxemia, with specific pulmonary vascular dysfunction, suggests a possible hemodynamic mechanism for VA/Q mismatch, as hypoxic vasoconstriction alteration. This study aimed to evaluate the capacity of inhaled nitric oxide (iNO)-almitrine combination to restore oxygenation in severe COVID-19 ARDS (C-ARDS) patients. Respiratory mechanics was assessed after a prone session. Then, patients received iNO (10 ppm) alone and in association with almitrine (10 μg/kg/min) during 30 min in each step. Echocardiographic and blood gases measurements were performed at baseline, during iNO alone, and in an iNO-almitrine combination. Ten severe C-ARDS patients were assessed (7 males and 3 females), with a median age of 60 [52-72]years. Combination of iNO and almitrine outperformed iNO alone for oxygenation improvement. The median of PaO_2/FiO_2 ratio varied from 102 [89-134]mmHg at baseline, to 124 [108-146]mmHg after iNO (p = 0.13) and 180 [132-206]mmHg after iNO and almitrine (p < 0.01). We found no correlation between the increase in oxygenation caused by iNO-almitrine combination and that caused by proning. In this pilot study of severe C-ARDS patients, iNO-almitrine combination was associated with rapid and significant improvement of oxygenation. These findings highlight the role of pulmonary vascular function in COVID-19 pathophysiology.

6. Avari H, Hiebert RJ, Ryzynski AA, Levy A, Nardi J, Kanji-Jaffer H, Kiiza P, Pinto R, Plenderleith SW, Fowler RA, Mbareche H, Mubareka S. **Quantitative Assessment of Viral Dispersion Associated with Respiratory Support Devices in a Simulated Critical Care Environment.** Am J Respir Crit Care Med. 2021;203(9):1112.

It is unclear whether some respiratory support devices may increase the dispersion of infectious bioaerosols and thereby place healthcare workers at increased risk of infection with severe acute respiratory syndrome coronavirus 2 (SARS-CoV-2). This study used a simulated ICU room with a breathing-patient simulator exhaling nebulized bacteriophages from the lower respiratory tract with various respiratory support modalities: invasive ventilation (through an endotracheal tube with an inflated cuff connected to a mechanical ventilator), helmet ventilation with a positive end-expiratory pressure (PEEP) valve, noninvasive bilevel positive-pressure ventilation, nonrebreather face masks, high-flow nasal oxygen (HFNO), and nasal prongs. Invasive ventilation and helmet ventilation with a PEEP valve were associated with the lowest bacteriophage concentrations in the air, and HFNO and nasal prongs were associated with the highest concentrations. At the intubating position, bacteriophage concentrations associated with HFNO (2.66×104 plaque-forming units [PFU]/L of air sampled), nasal prongs (1.60×104 PFU/L of air sampled), nonrebreather face masks (7.87×102 PFU/L of air sampled), and bilevel positive airway pressure (1.91×102 PFU/L of air sampled) were significantly higher than those associated with invasive ventilation ($P < 0.05$ for each). The difference between bacteriophage concentrations associated with helmet ventilation with a PEEP valve ($4.29 \times 10\text{-}1$ PFU/L of air sampled) and bacteriophage concentrations associated with invasive ventilation was not statistically significant.Conclusions: These findings highlight the potential differential risk of dispersing virus among respiratory support devices and the importance of appropriate infection prevention and control practices and personal protective equipment for healthcare workers when caring for patients with transmissible respiratory viral infections such as SARS-CoV-2.

7. Ionescu F, Zimmer MS, Petrescu I, Castillo E, Bozyk P, Abbas A, Abplanalp L, Dogra S, Nair GB
Extubation Failure in Critically Ill COVID-19 Patients: Risk Factors and Impact on In-Hospital Mortality.J Intensive Care Med. 2021;36(9):1018. Epub 2021 Jun 2.

The authors conducted a retrospective analysis of 281 patients who were extubated after mechanical ventilation to identify clinical factors that predict extubation failure (reintubation) and its prognostic implications in critically ill COVID-19 patients. The mean age was, 61.0 years [±13.9] with 54.8% males. Reintubation occurred in 93 (33.1%). In multivariate analysis accounting for death, reintubation risk increased with age (hazard ratio.04 per 1-year increase, 95% CI 1.02 -1.06), vasopressors (HR 1.84, 95% CI 1.04-3.60), renal replacement (HR 2.01, 95% CI 1.22-3.29), maximum PEEP (HR 1.07 per 1-unit increase, 95% CI 1.02 -1.12), paralytics (HR 1.48, 95% CI 1.08-2.25) and requiring more than nasal cannula immediately post-extubation (HR 2.19, 95% CI 1.37-3.50). Reintubation was associated with higher mortality (36.6% vs 2.1%; P<0.0001) and risk of inpatient death after adjusting for multiple factors (HR 23.2, 95% CI 6.45-83.33). Prone ventilation, corticosteroids, anticoagulation, remdesivir and tocilizumab did not impact the risk of reintubation or death.Up to 1 in 3 critically ill COVID-19 patients required reintubation. Older age, paralytics, high PEEP, need for greater respiratory support following extubation and non-pulmonary organ failure predicted reintubation. Extubation failure strongly predicted adverse outcomes.

Summary- Though the new variants of SARS-CoV2 are not causing severe ARDS still it is better to evolve your protocols in discussion with intensivists. Newer modes like APRV is shown to be performing well in terms of oxygenation indices in covid 19 paints. Many of the interventions are aerosol generating and safety is mandated to prevent infection transmission.

Newer antibiotics

Plazomicin

It is a broad-spectrum aminoglycoside antibiotic.

Mechanism of action: It has bactericidal action by binding to bacterial 30S ribosomal subunit. Aminoglycosides bind to the ribosomal aminoacyl-tRNA site (A-site) and induce a conformational change to facilitate further the binding of the rRNA and the antibiotic. This will lead to codon misreading and mistranslation of mRNA during bacterial protein synthesis. Plazomicin spectrum includes Enterobacteriaceae, multidrug-resistant phenotypes such as carbapenemase-producing bacteria, and isolates with other aminoglycosides. Its antibacterial activity of it is not inhibited by aminoglycoside modifying enzymes (AMEs) such as acetyltransferases (AACs), phosphotransferases (APHs), and nucleotidyltransferases (ANTs) produced by bacteria.

They are parenterally administered and typically used for moderate-to-severe urinary tract infections or pyelonephritis. Plazomicin has had limited clinical use but has not been linked to serum enzyme elevations during therapy or to instances of clinically apparent liver injury. (1)

Eravacycline

It is a parenterally administered tetracycline - antibiotic. It is used to treat moderate-to-severe intraabdominal infections due to susceptible organisms.

Spectrum- Gram-negative, gram-positive aerobic, and facultative bacteria. This includes most bacteria resistant to cephalosporins, fluoroquinolones, β-lactam/β-lactamase inhibitors, multidrug-resistant strains, carbapenem-resistant Enterobacteriaceae, and the majority of anaerobic pathogens.

Mechanism of action: Eravacycline disturbs bacterial protein synthesis by binding to the 30S ribosomal subunit and preventing the incorporation of amino acid residues into elongating peptide chains. It is bacteriostatic against gram-positive bacteria (e.g., *Staphylococcus aureus* and *Enterococcus faecalis*), but in vitro bactericidal activity was shown against some *Escherichia coli* strains and *Klebsiella pneumoniae*.

The most common adverse reactions include infusion site reactions, nausea, vomiting, palpitations, chest pain, acute pancreatitis, pancreatic necrosis, hypocalcemia, dizziness, dysgeusia, anxiety, insomnia, depression, pleural effusion, dyspnea, rash, and hyperhidrosis. (2)

Sarecycline

Sarecycline is a tetracycline-class Drug. The mechanism of action of sarecycline is as a P-Glycoprotein Inhibitor.

Mechanism of action: Sarecycline targets and inhibits protein synthesis in microbial agents like Cutibacterium acnes pre. Its action mechanism is by inhibiting macromolecular biosynthesis of microbial DNA, RNA, proteins, lipids, and cell walls. It also causes inhibition of microbial macromolecular DNA and protein synthesis. In addition, because Cutibacterium acnes also generates proteins and enzymes capable of causing inflammation, it also has an anti-inflammatory effect via inhibiting such microbial protein synthesis. It is an oral, once-daily, narrow-spectrum tetracycline used to treat moderate-to-severe acne.

Side effects are fetal harm, permanent discoloration of teeth, reversible inhibition of bone growth when administered during pregnancy, and liver impairment. (3)

Omadacycline

It is an oral, tetracycline - antibiotic.

Mechanism of action: It binds to the primary tetracycline binding site on the bacterial 30s ribosomal subunit with high specificity and blocks protein synthesis, disrupting many facets of cellular function and resulting in either cell death or stasis.

Omadacycline is studied in treating Bacterial Pneumonia, Bacterial Infections, Community-Acquired Infections, Skin Structures, and Soft Tissue Infections. Its spectrum includes gram-positive bacteria, such as methicillin-resistant Staphylococcus aureus (MRSA), and gram-negative, atypical, and anaerobic bacteria, including those resistant to currently available classes of antibiotics and known to cause diseases such as pneumonia, skin diseases, urinary tract infections, and blood-borne infections in both the hospital and community settings.

Side effects include thyroid hyperpigmentation, goitrogenicity, thyroid hyperplasia, and adrenal have been noted in multiple animal studies using other tetracycline drugs. (4)

Rifamycin

Rifamycin is a natural antibiotic produced from Streptomyces mediterranei.

Mechanism of action: It inhibits prokaryotic DNA-dependent RNA synthesis and protein synthesis and blocks RNA-polymerase transcription initiation. Rifamycin has a spectrum against Gram-positive and Gram-negative bacteria but is used mainly against Mycobacterium sp. (especially M. tuberculosis) and other agents to overcome resistance. It is a nonabsorbable rifampicin-like antibacterial agent used to treat travelers' diarrhea. Rifamycin has minimal oral absorption and has not been implicated in causing liver test abnormalities or clinically apparent liver injury. (5)

Imipenem/Cilastatin/Relebactam

It is a newly approved anti-infective combination of a well-established β-lactam and a new β-lactamase inhibitor for complicated urinary tract infections (cUTIs), including pyelonephritis and complicated intra-abdominal infections (cIAIs) in patients 18 years of age or older with limited or no alternative treatment options. The antibiotic is also indicated for treating hospital-acquired bacterial pneumonia (HABP) and ventilator-associated bacterial pneumonia (VABP). The antibiotic is active in vitro against many pathogens, including multidrug-resistant (MDR) Pseudomonas aeruginosa and carbapenem-resistant Enterobacterales (CRE) such as Klebsiella pneumoniae carbapenemase. The addition of relebactam does not restore the activity of imipenem against Metallo-β-lactamase (MBL)-producing Enterobacterales and carbapenem-resistant Acinetobacter baumannii. (6)

In clinical trials, commonly reported adverse events included anemia, elevated liver enzymes, electrolyte imbalances, nausea, vomiting, diarrhea, headache, fever, phlebitis, infusion-site reactions, and hypertension.

Lefamulin

It is a new and relatively unique antibiotic used to treat community-acquired pneumonia. Lefamulin has not been linked to an increased rate of transient serum liver test abnormalities during treatment or instances of clinically apparent liver injury.

Side effect-Hepatotoxicity. (7)

Cefiderocol

It is a cephalosporin antibacterial drug and exerts a mechanism of action similar to other β-lactam antibiotics like binding to and inhibiting penicillin-binding proteins (PBPs), preventing cell wall synthesis and ultimately causing the death of the bacterial cell. Unlike other drugs in β-lactam antibiotics, cefiderocol is a siderophore that can actively be transported into the bacterial cell through iron channels. It is also effective against multidrug-resistant strains, including extended-spectrum β-lactamase producers and carbapenemase-producing bacteria

Indications for use include complicated urinary tract infections in patients with limited or no alternative treatments. (8)

Oritavancin

It is a semisynthetic glycopeptide used (as its bisphosphate salt) to treat acute bacterial skin and skin structure infections caused by susceptible isolates of designated Gram-positive microorganisms, including MRSA. It is an antibacterial drug and an antimicrobial agent. It is a disaccharide derivative, a glycopeptide, and a semisynthetic derivative. It derives from a vancomycin aglycone.

Adverse effects- headache, nausea, vomiting, and diarrhea. This drug is not dialyzable, and supportive measures should be undertaken in the case of an overdose. (9)

Dalbavancin

It is a second-generation, semi-synthetic lipoglycopeptide antibiotic with bactericidal activity against various gram-positive bacteriae. Upon administration, it binds to a site different from penicillins and cephalosporins, tightly to the D-alanyl-D-alanine portion of peptidoglycan chains. Hence, preventing peptidoglycan elongation and interfering with bacterial cell wall synthesis leads to activating bacterial autolysins and induces cell wall lysis.

It is used for the treatment of acute bacterial skin, and skin structure infections caused or suspected to be caused by susceptible isolates of Gram-positive microorganisms, including MRSA. (10)

Tedizolid

It is an oxazolidinone antibiotic, similar to linezolid, which has a broad spectrum of activity against gram-positive bacteria, including methicillin-resistant Staphylococcal aureus (MRSA). Tedizolid has been associated with a low rate of transient serum aminotransferase elevations during therapy but has not been linked to instances of clinically apparent acute liver injury.

This product is currently available as an oral tablet and a powder for intravenous injection.

Oxazolidinones are a relatively new class of antibacterials that inhibit protein synthesis and can overcome resistance against other bacterial protein synthesis inhibitors. Earlier studies suggested that they inhibit a step in the initiation of protein synthesis. However, this mechanism was inconsistent with mapped resistance mutations. Later studies involving cross-linking and direct structural determination of the binding site revealed that oxazolidinones, including both linezolid and tedizolid, bind in the A site of the PTC by interacting with the 23S rRNA component. The structural studies also revealed that oxazolidinone binding alters the conformation of a conserved nucleotide in the 23S rRNA (U2585 in Escherichia coli), which renders the PTC non-productive for peptide bond formation. Hence, tedizolid exerts its effect by inhibiting bacterial protein synthesis.

Adverse effects- nausea, headache, dizziness, diarrhea, and vomiting. Symptomatic and supportive measures are recommended. (11)

Newer antitubercular drugs

Pretomanid

It is a nitroimidazooxazine antimycobacterial agent used with other antituberculosis drugs to treat multidrug-resistant tuberculosis. The addition of pretomanid to antituberculosis drug regimens has been linked to an increased rate of transient serum liver test abnormalities during treatment and several instances of mild, clinically apparent liver injury.

Side effects: prolonged Q.T. interval in the case of an overdose. (12)

Newer antifungals

Isavuconazole

It is a water-soluble triazole prodrug with broad-spectrum antifungal activity. Isavuconazole is absorbed quickly, either orally or intravenously, and is hydrolyzed to its active moiety BAL4815 by plasma esterases. BAL4815 inhibits fungal cytochrome P450 lanosterol 14-alpha-demethylase (CYP51) that catalyzes the conversion of lanosterol to ergosterol, an essential component of the fungal cell membrane. Enzyme inhibition by this agent leads to a decrease in the ergosterol pool and therefore disturbs the synthesis of the fungal cell membrane, thereby increasing cell membrane permeability and promoting the loss of essential intracellular elements. This ultimately causes fungal cell lysis and death.

The prodrug formulation of isavuconazole is FDA- and EMA-approved and is marketed under the trade name Cresemba to treat invasive aspergillosis and mucormycosis through oral or intravenous administration. The intravenous formulation is cyclodextrin-free, giving isavuconazole an advantage over other azole antifungals requiring cyclodextrin to facilitate the drug's potential for nephrotoxicity. It is proposed that intravenous and oral dosing be used interchangeably, without a repeat loading dose when transitioning from an IV to an oral formulation.

Adverse reactions included headache, dizziness, paresthesia, somnolence, disturbance in attention, dysgeusia, dry mouth, diarrhea, oral hypoesthesia, vomiting, hot flush, anxiety, restlessness, palpitations, tachycardia, photophobia, and arthralgia. (13)

Brexafemme

- It is a broad-spectrum triterpenoid antifungal.
- Mechanism action: The exact mechanism of echinocandins like inhibiting glucan synthase. It demonstrated *in vitro* activity against all *Candida* species that cause VVC, including azole-resistant strains. When administering BREXAFEMME with potent CYP3A inhibitors, the dose of BREXAFEMME should be reduced to 150 mg twice a day for one day. Avoid administration of BREXAFEMME with strong CYP3A inducers.

The most common adverse reactions observed are diarrhea, nausea, abdominal pain, dizziness, and vomiting. (14)

Ibrexafungerp

It is an intravenous and orally bioavailable semisynthetic derivative of enfumafungin with potential antifungal activity. Upon administration, ibrexafungerp inhibits beta-1,3-D-glucan synthase, an enzyme essential for fungal cell wall synthesis. This weakens the fungal cell wall, leading to osmotic lysis and eventually fungal cell death.

Ibrexafungerp, also known as SCY-078 or MK-3118, is a novel enfumafungin derivative oral triterpene antifungal approved to treat vulvovaginal candidiasis (VVC), also known as a vaginal yeast infection. It was developed to treat fungal infections that may have become resistant to echinocandins or azole antifungals. Ibrexafungerp is orally bioavailable compared to echinocandins. Similar to echinocandins, ibrexafungerp targets the fungal β-1,3-glucan synthase, which is not present in humans, limiting the chance of renal or hepatic toxicity. Ibrexafungerp was granted FDA approval on Jun 1, 2021. (15)

References

1. PubChem. Plazomicin [Internet]. [cited 2022 Feb 25]. Available from: https://pubchem.ncbi. nlm.nih.gov/compound/42613186

2. PubChem. Eravacycline [Internet]. [cited 2022 Feb 25]. Available from: https://pubchem.ncbi. nlm.nih.gov/compound/54726192

3. PubChem. Sarecycline [Internet]. [cited 2022 Feb 25]. Available from: https://pubchem.ncbi. nlm.nih.gov/compound/54681908

4. PubChem. Omadacycline [Internet]. [cited 2022 Feb 25]. Available from: https://pubchem. ncbi.nlm.nih.gov/compound/54697325

5. PubChem. Rifamycin [Internet]. [cited 2022 Feb 25]. Available from: https://pubchem.ncbi. nlm.nih.gov/compound/6324616

6. Mansour H, Ouweini AEL, Chahine EB, Karaoui LR. Imipenem/cilastatin/relebactam: A new carbapenem β-lactamase inhibitor combination. Am J Health-Syst Pharm AJHP Off J Am Soc Health-Syst Pharm. 2021 Mar 31;78(8):674–83.

7. PubChem. Pretomanid [Internet]. [cited 2022 Feb 25]. Available from: https://pubchem.ncbi. nlm.nih.gov/compound/456199

8. PubChem. Lefamulin [Internet]. [cited 2022 Feb 25]. Available from: https://pubchem.ncbi. nlm.nih.gov/compound/25185057

9. PubChem. Cefiderocol [Internet]. [cited 2022 Feb 25]. Available from: https://pubchem.ncbi. nlm.nih.gov/compound/77843966

10. PubChem. Oritavancin [Internet]. [cited 2022 Feb 25]. Available from: https://pubchem.ncbi. nlm.nih.gov/compound/16136912

11. PubChem. Dalbavancin [Internet]. [cited 2022 Feb 25]. Available from: https://pubchem.ncbi.nlm.nih.gov/compound/16134627

12. PubChem. Tedizolid [Internet]. [cited 2022 Feb 25]. Available from: https://pubchem.ncbi.nlm.nih.gov/compound/11234049

13. PubChem. Isavuconazole [Internet]. [cited 2022 Feb 25]. Available from: https://pubchem.ncbi.nlm.nih.gov/compound/6918485

14. PubChem. Brexane [Internet]. [cited 2022 Feb 25]. Available from: https://pubchem.ncbi.nlm.nih.gov/compound/12301639

15. PubChem. Ibrexafungerp [Internet]. [cited 2022 Feb 25]. Available from: https://pubchem.ncbi.nlm.nih.gov/compound/46871657

Trauma Updates

Contributors

1. Dr. Mabel Vasnaik
2. Dr. Ajay Kumar
3. Dr. Madhur Uniyal
4. Dr. Bhaskar Sarkar
5. Dr. Aman Verma
6. Dr. Sarat Chandra Uppaluri
7. Dr. Chidrupi Sharma

Chapters

1. Pediatric Trauma
2. Musculoskeletal trauma
3. Geriatric fracture
4. General management of Fractures
5. Open fractures and Compartment syndrome
6. Pelvic fracture
7. Pregnant trauma victim

Salient Features of Trauma in Infants and Children

Trauma is a common occurrence in children as they are a vulnerable population due to their size as well as diminished reflexes and immaturity. The world over, trauma is one of the leading causes of morbidity and mortality in children. Road traffic accidents are the commonest cause of trauma, however children are

Children appear to be miniature adults. However this statement is not literally true. There are anatomical and physiological differences between children and adults. Trauma is children has to be treated keeping in mind these differences.

In this chapter the features in trauma that are peculiar to children will be emphasized upon. The rest of the trauma assessment and management will be the same as for adults.

Initial Assessment has to be done in all infants and children who come with trauma just as it is done in adult keeping in mind the important anatomical and physiological differences. A systematic approach to the initial assessment helps to rapidly assess injuries without missing out on a life threatening injury, determines management priorities and helps perform the required critical interventions.

The steps of initial assessment of trauma are the same that has to be followed in infants and children as in adults.

1. Preparation:
2. Triage
3. Primary Survey (ABCDE's) with immediate resuscitation and treatment of all life threatening injuries.
4. Adjuncts to Primary Survey with Resuscitation
5. Secondary survey
6. Adjuncts to Secondary Survey
7. Reevaluation
8. Definitive Care

Preparation:

Preparation involves getting the receiving area in the emergency department ready to receive a trauma patient. This is done whenever prior information is received that a trauma patient will be arriving to the department. In such a case one would also be informed about the condition of the patient and the vital parameters. It is then important to keep the necessary personnel and equipment ready to receive the patient.

Since most trauma cases in our set up arrived unannounced, it is essential to have an area identified as a resuscitation or trauma bay with all the facilities to resuscitate a critically ill patient in every emergency department. Patients can then be received in the trauma bay where adequate facilities will be available to treat them.

Triage:

Triage means to sort out. In trauma triage needs to be done both in the field as well as in the emergency department.

In the field depending on the mechanism of injury and the vital parameters of the patient the trauma patient should be transferred to a trauma centre. It is preferable to transfer all paediatric trauma patients to a trauma centre with paediatric facilities and personnel trained to manage paediatric trauma.

Primary Survey:

The primary survey is done in a structured manner in order to identify life threatening injuries and simultaneously manage them. Both assessment and management occur simultaneously during the primary survey. Life threats that are identified should be treated rapidly before moving on to the next step.

The ABCDE of the primary survey is as follows.

A – Airway maintenance with cervical spine protection

B – Breathing and ventilation

C – Circulation with haemorrhage control

D – Disability (neurological evaluation)

E – Exposure

Children tend to suffer emotional trauma when in the presence of unknown adults. Hence it is very important as far as possible to make sure that a child is both examined as well as treated in the presence of either parents of other familiar adults. In the absence of the above it is imperative to make the child comfortable before examining or doing an intervention.

Airway maintenance with cervical spine protection:

Because the child's head is proportionately larger than an adult, airway compromise commonly occurs necessitating aggressive stabilization of the airway and care of breathing.

Maintaining a patent airway always remains the greatest priority in an injured child as in an adult.

In patients with an injury above the clavicle a cervical spine injury should be suspected and an adequate sized cervical collar should be applied until a c spine injury is ruled out. In all unconscious patients a cervical spine injury should be suspected, motion of the C spine should be restricted and the C spine should be immobilized using an appropriately sized C collar.

It is important to provide supplemental oxygen to a patient with a compromised airway. Oxygen can be given vial nasal prongs or mask depending on the saturation, the consciousness of the child and tolerance of the device.

In a child who is obstructing the patency of the airway should be maintain using the jaw thrust maneuver along with the bimanual inline spinal motion restriction. The head tilt, chin lift maneuver should be avoided.

An oral airway should be inserted in a child who is unconscious without a gag reflex. The oral airway should be inserted directly into the oropharynx without causing any trauma. A tongue depressor is useful to facilitate the insertion of the oral airway.

Indications for endotracheal intubation:

- A child with a low GCS due to a head injury or shock and not able to protect the airway.
- A child with ventilatory failure who requires mechanical ventilation.
- Not able to maintain a patient airway due to altered sensorium, obstruction or any other cause.

Because of the anatomical differences in a child, securing an airway can be challenging and the following points should be kept in mind.

Infants have a large tongue which can obscure vision of the oral cavity. The epiglottis is long and overhanging the glottis opening and hence visualization of the vocal cords is impaired. This can be overcome by using a laryngoscope with a straight blade wherein the entire epiglottis is included in the blade so that the vocal cords become visible facilitating intubation.

Children have a funnel shaped larynx which causes accumulation of secretions in the retropharyngeal area. The larynx and vocal cords in a child are anterior, again making visualization of the glottis opening difficult. This also is overcome by using a straight blade which facilitates better visualization.

The narrowest part of the airway in a child is below the cords at the cricoid cartilage. This area therefore forms a seal around the endotracheal tube thus avoiding the need of a cuffed endotracheal tube. However it has been found that cuffed endotracheal tubes even if used in very small children are beneficial in improving ventilation, decreasing the carbon dioxide levels and hence improves cerebral blood flow.

Before intubation is attempted it is mandatory to adequately pre oxygenate the child. Infants have a pronounced vagal response to endotracheal intubation which is worsened with hypoxia. Hence preoxygenation and premedication with atropine helps to minimize this response.

Children have large occiputs and this causes a passive flexion of the cervical spine and difficulty in visualizing the vocal cords. A one inch padding should be placed under the child's entire body in order to maintain neutral alignment of the spinal column. Care must be taken to immobilize the cervical spine during laryngoscopy and intubation.

Most trauma patients have to be considered as having a full stomach, both due to the fact that since trauma occurs at any time the patient might indeed have had something to eat soon before the accident. Also the stress of the trauma would delay gastric emptying also contributing to a full stomach.

Hence it is beneficial to do a rapid sequence intubation using the appropriate drugs in order to secure the airway.

It is mandatory to confirm that the tube is in the trachea and the position of the tube has to be checked after intubation. The trachea of an infant is short and this can cause intubation of the right main bronchus which should be kept in mind. The endotracheal tube should be properly fixed to the sides of the mouth in order to prevent displacement which can occur more often during transfer. Hence it is important to check the position of the tube periodically.

When it is not possible to intubate the child using an endotracheal tube a laryngeal mask airway (LMA) or an intubating LMA can be used. Alternatively in bad facial trauma a needle cricothyroidotomy can be performed. However adequate ventilation is not possible with a needle cricothyroidotomy and it is only a temporizing measure.

Breathing and ventilation:

Infants and children have a delicate and relatively immature trachea bronchial alveolar tree. Hence it is important not to give an excessive volume or pressure while ventilating a child in order to prevent barotrauma. A pediatric bag mask should be used for children less than 30 kgs.

Injuries such as a hemothorax and pneumothorax require insertion of a chest tube in order to decompress the pleura.

In the case of a tension pneumothorax a needle decompression is done in the midclavicular line just above the superior surface of the third rib. The size of the needle should be adequate for the size of the child. A large needle may cause a pneumothorax where there isn't one.

Chest tube insertion should be done using the tunneling technique as children have a thin chest wall. Site of insertion is the fifth intercostal space anterior to the midaxillary line and the tube should be tunneled over the rib above the skin insertion and then directed superiorly and posteriorly along the inside of the chest wall.

Circulation with hemorrhage control:

In children tachycardia and poor skin perfusion help in early recognition of hypovolemia and very often are the only early signs of hypovolemia. The other signs that can occur are given in the table below.

An injured child usually suffers significant blood loss. However children have an increased physiological reserve which is why the blood pressure does not drop initially even in the presence of shock.

Table 1: Systemic responses to blood loss in pediatric patients

System	Mild blood volume loss (< 30%)	Moderate blood volume loss (30%-45%)	Severe blood volume loss (>45%)
CVS	Increased heart rate Weak, thready, peripheral pulses, Normal systolic BP (80-90 + 2 x age in yrs) Normal pulse pressure	Markedly increased heart rate Weak, thready, central pulses, Normal systolic BP (70-80 + 2 x age in yrs) Narrowed pulse pressure	Tachycardia followed by bradycardia. Very weak/absent central pulses Absent peripheral pulses Hypotension (< 70 + 2 x age in yrs) Narrowed pulse pressure/ undetectable diastolic blood pressure
CNS	Anxious, irritable, confused	Lethargic, Dulled response to pain	Comatose
Skin	Cool, mottled Prolonged capillary refill	Cyanotic, markedly prolonged capillary refill	Pale and cold
Urine Output	Low	Minimal	None

Early and adequate fluid resuscitation is essential to stabilize the hemodynamic parameters of a child.

It is important to estimate the weight of the child which can be done using a Broselow tape. A formula that can be used to measure the weight in kgs is {(2 x age in years) + 10}.

Broselow Pediatric emergency tape:

It is important to assess the weight of a child in order to administer the right doses of drugs or to use the right sized equipment. An injured child might not be able to stand on a scale and hence a Broselow tape is a must in every pediatric emergency cart as it helps the clinician to accurately estimate the weight of a child based on the length which can be easily measured. This also gives an approximate respiratory rate, volume of fluid resuscitation and drug dosages.

It is often difficult to obtain peripheral venous access in a child in hemorrhagic shock due to collapse of the peripheral veins. In such a situation intraosseous access can be obtained using an intraosseous needle and fluids can be infused. The preferred site is the proximal tibia below the level of the tibial tuberosity. This route is used till an intravenous access is then obtained. If a peripheral intravenous access is still not possible then a central venous approach using either the femoral, internal jugular or subclavian vein should be done by a clinician with expertise in these procedures.

Weight based fluid resuscitation should be carried out in infants and children.

20ml/kg warmed isotonic crystalloid intravenous fluids have been recommended. This can be followed by one or two additional boluses depending on the child's response. In case the child still has an ongoing bleed after the second or third fluid bolus then 10 ml/kg of packed red blood cells can be given.

The latest practice however has moved away from crystalloid resuscitation in favor of damage control resuscitation. Use of crystalloid is restricted and a balanced ratio of packed red blood cells, fresh frozen plasma and platelets is given early. Studies have found that this approach helps prevent the lethal triad of hypothermia, acidosis and trauma induced coagulopathy and improved outcomes have been noticed.

Initial 20 ml/kg bolus of isotonic crystalloid is administered followed by 10-20 ml/kg of packed red blood cells, fresh frozen plasma and platelets. This is part of the pediatric mass blood transfusion protocol.

Children should be monitored for their response to fluid resuscitation and for the normalization of hemodynamic parameters.

The tachycardia decreases along with the presence of palpable peripheral pulses, the blood pressure improves and pulse pressure improves to more than 20 mm Hg. The color of the skin and temperature improves along with an improved sensorium. The hourly urine output also is found to improve.

One of three responses is noticed:

1. Responders: Children whose hemodynamic parameters improve with the initial fluid or fluid and blood resuscitation.
2. Transient responders: The hemodynamic parameters improve initially with fluid and blood resuscitation but deteriorate after some time.
3. Non responders: These children do not respond to the initial fluid and blood resuscitation indication an ongoing blood loss which needs to be identified and addressed.

Massive blood transfusion protocol should be activated for the transient and non-responders as soon as possible.

Some important values:

Normal systolic Blood Pressure in children is 90 mm Hg + 2 x age in years.

Blood volume:

Infant: 80 ml/kg

Child 1-3 yrs: 75 ml/kg

Children over 3 yrs: 70 ml/kg

Low normal urine output:

Infant: 2 ml/kg/hour

Younger child: 1.5 ml/kg/hour

Older child: 1 ml/kg/hour

Adolescent: 0.5 ml/kg/hour

Table 2: Pediatric Trauma Score

Assessment	+2	+1	-1
Weight	>20 kgs	10-20 kgs	<10 kgs
Airway	Normal	Oral or nasal airway, oxygen	Intubated/cricothyroidotomy/ tracheostomy
Systolic BP	>90mm Hg, Good peripheral pulses, Good perfusion	50-90 mm Hg, carotid/femoral pulses palpable	< 50 mm Hg, weak or not pulses
Level of consciousness	Awake	Obtunded or loss of consciousness	Coma or unresponsive
Fracture	None seen or suspected	Single or closed	Open or multiple
Cutaneous	None visible	Contusion, abrasion, laceration < 7 cm, not through fascia	Tissue loss, any gunshot wound or stab wound through fascia
Total:			

The pediatric trauma score enables assessment of the severity of trauma and thus appropriately formulate a treatment plan.

CPR in children:

It is important to note that children who have had a cardiorespiratory arrest in the field after trauma have a poor prognosis. If they have received CPR for more than 15 minutes before arrival to the Emergency department or if their pupils are fixed on arrival they would not survive. Hence prolonged resuscitative measures have not been found to be of any benefit.

Disability: (neurological evaluation)

A rapid neurological level is now done to find out the level of consciousness, pupillary size and reaction, lateralizing signs and level of spinal cord injury if present.

The Glasgow Coma scale is a quick and accurate method to determine the level of consciousness. The motor score correlates quite accurately with outcome.

Exposure and Environmental Control

It is important to expose the child in order to avoid missing any injury. This should be done in the presence of the parent or caregiver without violating the child's modesty or emotionally traumatizing the child. Cover the child soon after the examination.

Thermoregulation in a child:

Children have a decreased ability to regulate core temperature. This is primarily because of their body surface area to body mass ratio. Children have a thin skin and lack of adequate subcutaneous tissue and an increased metabolic rate all of which contribute to the increased caloric expenditure and heat loss due to evaporation. Due to hypothermia a child can have a delayed response to treatment and increase in the coagulation parameters. Hence it is very important to take all measures to prevent heat loss in a child by covering the child, warming IV fluids and gases and heating the room the child is in.

Adjuncts to Primary Survey with Resuscitation

The following adjuncts should be used during the primary survey in order to help determine the adequacy of resuscitation and guide towards stabilization of a patient.

1. **Monitors:** Continuous electrocardiography, pulse oximetry, capnography and ventilatory rate.

2. **Tubes:**

    Urinary catheters: Hourly monitoring of the urinary output is essential towards gauging the adequacy of volume resuscitation. Transurethral catheter insertion should not be done when a urethral injury is suspected.

    Gastric tube: This helps to decompress the stomach and decrease the risk of aspiration. It also indicates the presence of gastrointestinal hemorrhage. The gastric tube should be inserted through the mouth in the presence of a head injury.

3. **X-rays:** AP chest and AP pelvis
4. **Blood tests:** Arterial blood gas

Secondary Survey:

The secondary survey involves a head to foot examination of the patient to find out all injuries that might be present, however minor.

Secondary survey should only be done once the primary survey has been completed, after the patient has been resuscitated and once the vital parameters of the patient are back to normal.

The patient should be log rolled if not done earlier in order to examine the back and look for any deformities of the spine.

A complete history of the patient should be taken at this stage. This includes the mechanism of injury, other history related to the trauma and past medical history of the patient.

Adjuncts to Secondary Survey:

Additional x-rays are done at this point once the patient has been stabilized. CT scans if required are also done at this time. Any other blood test or special diagnostic tests can also be done.

Reevaluation:

The patient should be constantly monitored and reassessed. The vital signs should be constantly monitored and any deterioration can be picked up. Even though the patient has been resuscitated and stabilized he can deteriorate at any point of time and hence has to be regularly monitored.

Effective analgesia has to be administered for pain management.

Definitive Care:

The patient has to be transferred from the Emergency Department to the intensive care unit, operation theatre or the ward as the case may be.

In case the hospital does not have the capabilities to treat the patient then the patient has to be transferred to another hospital which has the treatment capabilities. The doctor from the receiving hospital has to be spoken to before transfer to make sure that the bed and other facilities are available. The patient should always be transferred accompanied by medical personnel.

Transfer

In children especially following blunt trauma, multi organ injuries are very common because of their anatomy. Because of their smaller body mass the energy that is applied due to a blunt injury has a very great impact. Also because the child has less fat and connective tissue, the organs are more accessible to blunt trauma.

It is very important to shift children to a hospital which had doctors trained in pediatric management. Following trauma most children have stable hemodynamics and do not deteriorate while being treated. However children with multi system injuries do tend to deteriorate rapidly and also develop complications and hence the importance of immediate and appropriate and transfer. Because of the large body surface area to body mass ratio hypothermia develops rapidly hence it is important to both give warm fluids as well as adequately cover the child during transfer.

Trauma specific to certain systems:

Only the differences in children as opposed to adults will be discussed and emphasized upon.

Head injury

Because of the large surface area of the head in children, the brain is involved in a lot of pediatric trauma. Hence airway compromise involving hypoxia, hypoventilation and even apnea occur very commonly. Hemodynamic compromise is less commonly seen. Hence early endotracheal intubation with adequate oxygenation and ventilation is important to avoid further CNS damage.

The brain achieves 80% of adult brain size by 2 years of age. However the subarachnoid space is relatively smaller and hence there is less buoyancy and less protection to the brain. Therefore momentum to the head can cause structural damage to the parenchyma. Cerebral blood flow progressively increases to almost twice that of adult levels by 5 years of age and then decreases. This is why children are more susceptible to cerebral hypoxia and hypercarbia. They are also susceptible to the effects of secondary brain injury due to hypovolemia which causes a decrease in cerebral perfusion, hypoxia and seizures. Therefore it is very important to treat the hypoxia and give the patients adequate fluid resuscitation to maintain the cerebral perfusion pressure.

Because infants have open fontanelles and mobile cranial sutures, swelling of the brain or an expanding intracranial mass lesion remains asymptomatic for a longer time than in an adult. Hence a child with bulging fontanelles or suture diastases need to be seen urgently by a neurosurgeon because their injury is more severe than it appears. Monitoring of the intracranial pressure is important to optimize the cerebral perfusion pressure. This should be done in the following cases

1. Children with a GCS of less than 8 or a motor score of 1 or 2.
2. When the brain injury is also associated with multiple systemic injuries and hypotension.
3. CT scan of the brain shows intracranial hemorrhage, cerebral edema, or transtentorial or cerebellar herniation.

Hypertonic saline and mannitol decrease the edema and intracranial pressure due to their hyperosmolality and increased sodium levels.

Continuous monitoring and reassessment is very essential.

Indications for CT brain:

1. GCS of 14 or less, other signs of altered mental status, or palpable skill fracture or signs of basilar skull fracture.

2. Occipital, parietal or temporal scalp hematoma, or history of LOC more than 5 seconds or a severe mechanism of injury or not acting normally as per the parent. These symptoms are found to be progressively worsening.

3. Persistent vomiting, severe headache, seizures.

Chest trauma

Blunt trauma is the commonest cause of chest injuries in children. Because of the pliable chest wall in a child rib fractures and mediastinal injuries are not common and occur in case the impact is very severe. Pulmonary contusions are commonly seen. The commonest immediate life threatening injury in children is a tension pneumothorax and due to the mobility of the mediastinal structures. This is easily diagnosed by a chest radiograph and easily treated by a tube thoracostomy.

Abdominal trauma:

Examination of the abdomen of a conscious child requires tact because an injured child will be in pain and distress and will not cooperate for examination. It is preferable to keep a parent or caregiver near the child during examination. Explain to the child what is being done and be gentle during the examination. Inspection of the abdomen will reveal the presence or nature of the injury. Ask the child for the presence of pain and assess the tone of the abdominal musculature. It might be beneficial to decompress the stomach by inserting an orogastric tube. Emptying the urinary bladder will facilitate abdominal examination.

Diagnostic tools will aid in making an accurate diagnosis of the abdominal injury.

Focused Assessment Sonography in trauma (FAST) can be easily done at the bedside, is noninvasive and can be repeated multiple times. However it does not identify isolated intraparenchymal injuries which make up nearly one third of solid organ injuries in children. The FAST picks up even a small amount of intra-abdominal blood and this does not correlate with the severity of injury.

Hence computerized tomography (CT) is beneficial if performed preferably with intravenous contrast in order to accurately identify intra-abdominal injuries in children. It would help plan whether the injury could be managed conservatively or whether surgical intervention would be required.

Conservative non operative management is usually the mode of treatment for children with solid organ injuries who are hemodynamically stable. If the child cannot be hemodynamically stabilized and if the diagnostic investigation reveals blood in the abdominal cavity then an exploratory laparotomy is performed to visualize and control the bleeding. Frequent reassessments of the child should be done so that a deterioration can be picked up early.

Small bowel perforations, mesenteric and small bowel avulsion injuries are common in children. The depth of a child's pelvis is shallow making a child more prone to a bladder rupture. Early operative management is required for rupture of a hollow viscus.

Spine trauma:

The anatomical differences in the spine in children should be kept in mind when treating injuries of the spinal cord.

Because of the relatively large heads in children compared to their necks, the angular momentum is greater and the fulcrum is higher in the cervical spine. Therefore children have more injuries at the level of the occiput to C3. The impact of the force on the upper neck is greater than that in an adult.

The growth centers are not completely formed and the growth plates are not closed. These very often appear as fractures on the x-rays.

The joint capsules and interspinous ligaments are more flexible. Hence ligamentous injuries are more common in children.

The vertebral bodies are wedged anteriorly and have a tendency to slide forwards with flexion. They have flat facet joints.

Cervical spine injuries can normally be identified by neurological findings. Careful palpation of the spine will reveal a soft tissue swelling, step deformity or muscle spasm.

Children most often have spinal cord injuries without radiological abnormalities. (SCIWORA). Hence if a spinal cord injury is suspected on clinical examination and neurological findings, it should be assumed that an injury exists irrespective of radiological findings. It is important to restrict spinal motion in these cases.

CT and MRI are not the investigations of choice in suspected spinal injuries in children and x-rays should be done.

Musculoskeletal Trauma

Introduction

Musculoskeletal trauma is one of the most dramatic injuries but rarely causes life-threatening or limb-threatening injuries until associated with major vascular injuries or having crush syndrome. It is a major cause of hemorrhagic shock, death or disability in poly trauma victims. It can affect any part of the human body including; bones, joints, cartilage, ligaments, tendons, muscles, and other soft tissues.

Major musculoskeletal injuries have the potential to distract from more severe internal torso injury. First, surgeons need to recognize and understand their association with severe thoracic and abdominal injuries. Thus surgeons always order the ATLS protocol of ABCDE as taken care of priorities of resuscitation. Major causes of disability and death are:

- Associated major thoracic, abdominal and pelvic injuries with musculoskeletal trauma.
- Renal failure associated with myoglobin deposits in kidneys secondary to rhabdomyolysis from crush injuries.
- Compartment syndrome due to muscle and tissue edema and hypoxia secondary to compromised blood flow, is a major cause of limb threatening situations, needing urgent surgical intervention.
- Pulmonary failure and impaired brain function can occur due to fat embolism.
- Hemorrhage due to major arterial bleed, bilateral femur fractures, pelvic disruption.

Potentially life threatening extremity injuries include major arterial haemorrhage, bilateral femur fractures, and crush syndrome. Thus patients first undergo primary survey and resuscitation of potentially life threatening extremity injuries and then only proceed to secondary survey. So the surgeon must know about the average of blood loss from an isolated bone fracture.

Amount of blood loss from specific fracture given as below:

Bone fractured	Internal blood loss (ml) per fracture
Pelvis	1000-massive
Femur	1000-2000
Tibia- fibula	500-1000
Humerus	500-750
Radius- ulna	250-500
Ribs	125

Surgeons always focused on associated injury as if any injuries missed or extremities injury can lead to distract surgeon from life threatening injury. Always focused on associated injury:

Injury	Associated injury
Clavicle fracture Scapula fracture Facture and/or dislocation of shoulder	Major thoracic injury, especially pulmonary contusion and rib fractures.
Displace thoracic spine fracture	Thoracic aortic rupture
Spine fracture	Intra-abdominal injury
Fracture/dislocation of elbow	Brachial artery injury Median, ulnar and radial nerve injury
Major pelvic disruption	Abdominal, thoracic or head injury Pelvic vascular haemorrhage
Femur fracture and posterior knee dislocation	Acetabular fracture Posterior hip dislocation
Knee dislocation	Popliteal artery and nerve injuries
Calcaneal fracture	Spine injury or fracture Fracture dislocation of hindfoot Tibia plateau fracture

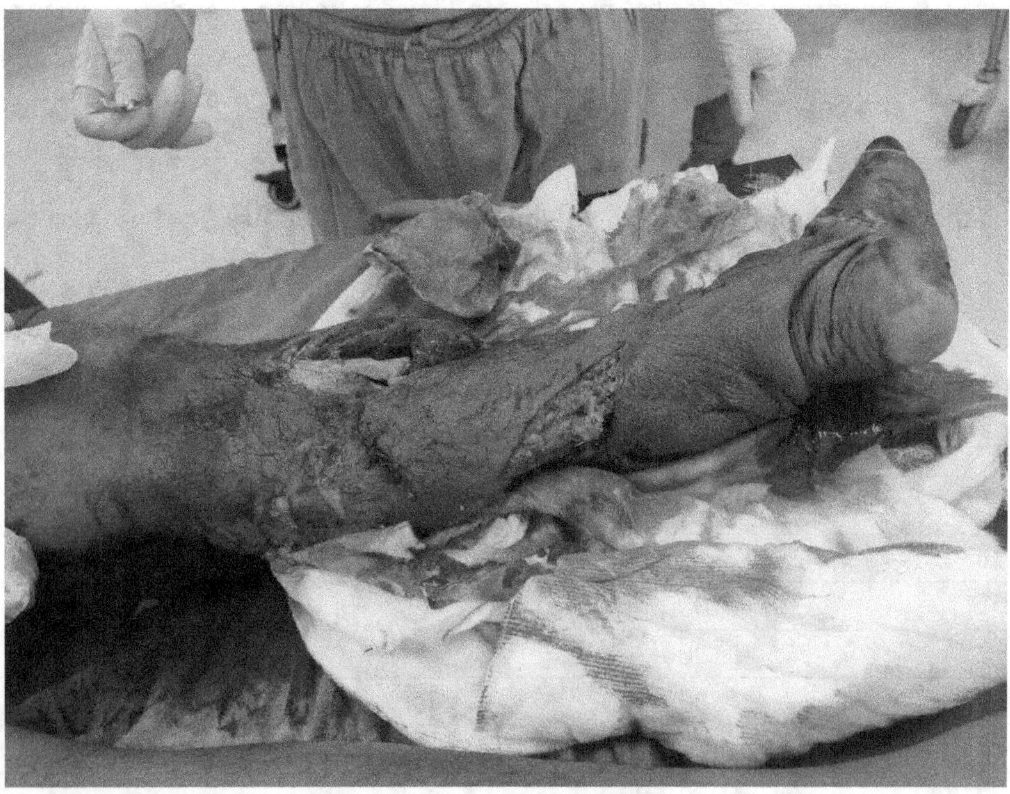

Figure: left lower extremity injury indicates patient sustained significant force with fracture of tibia and fibula with severe soft tissue injury with intact DNVS.

Clinical presentation:

A quick rapid visualisation of the limb will identify the major extremity and vascular injury. The examination includes a complete assessment of the whole limb and comparing the features with the opposite limb. In case of closed fractures, especially femur fractures, large volumes, up to 2 litres, of blood can pool up contributing to shock. History and mechanism of action of trauma help us understand the extent of injuries and possible complications. ABCDE approach is best to prevent death and disability. Assess and examine limbs systematically for distal pulses, symmetry, bony crepitus, deformity, dislocations of joints, open fractures, Degloving injury, range of motion with restriction of motion etc. Logroll can be done as part of assessment. Prolonged entrapped extremities, prolonged tourniquet application, tight splint, can lead to increased pressures, ischemia and necrosis of tissue in a limb compartment. 6Ps of compartment syndrome have to be assessed, which are;

- ○ Pain disproportionate to the injury
- ○ Paresthesias
- ○ Pallor
- ○ Pulselessness
- ○ Paralysis

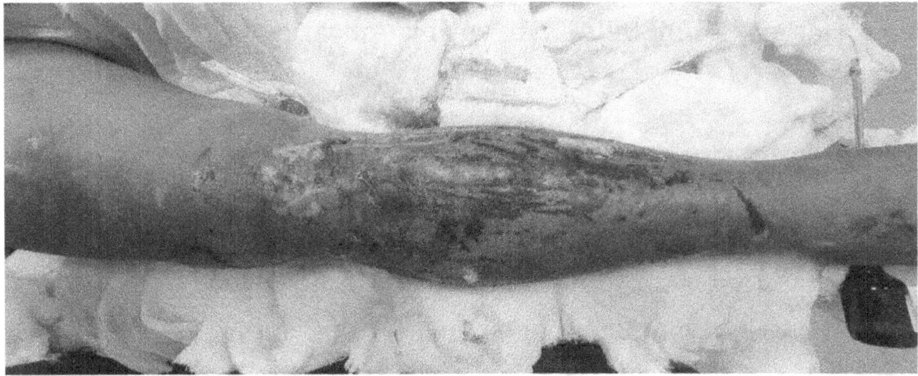

Figure: shows signs of compartment syndrome with blister and discoloration from midthigh

Examine the wounded limbs for external bleeding, the loss of a previously palpable pulse, and changes in pulse quality, Doppler tone, and the ankle/brachial index.

Palpate the extremities to assess skin sensation (i.e., neurologic function) and identify area of tenderness. The loss of pain and touch sensations indicates a spinal or peripheral nerve injury. A muscular contusion or fracture is indicated by tenderness over the muscles. A fracture should be considered if pain, soreness, and swelling are accompanied by deformity or abnormal motion across the bone. A tendon or ligament rupture is indicated by abnormal motion through a joint segment.

A cold, pale, pulseless extremity indicates an interruption in arterial blood supply. A rapidly expanding hematoma suggests a significant vascular injury. Traumatic amputation limb should be directly taken to the operation room if it presents within 6 hours of injury.

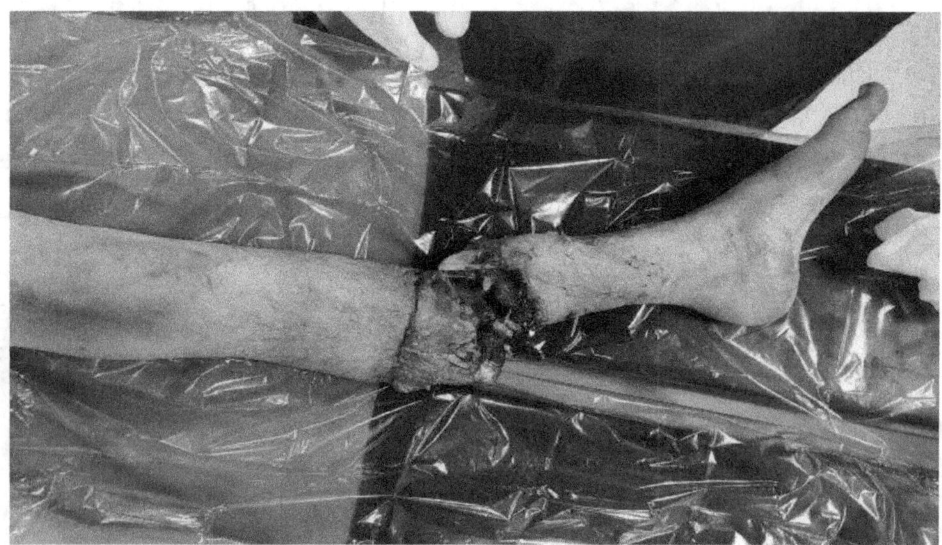

Neurovascular examination should be done in both limbs in every case of musculoskeletal trauma.

Management

The management for musculoskeletal trauma follows the similar principal of ABCDE approach just like any other trauma. Immobilisation with application of splint is the cornerstone of management.

Management of the extremity wound

Wound lavage

Wound lavage with fluid is important for decreasing the bacterial load and removing loose material, and should be a part of routine wound management.

Pain management

Pain management includes both pharmacological and non-pharmacological modalities. Pharmacology includes Intravenous Opioids and NSAIDs. Splints and tractions are included in non-pharmacological methods of pain management. Ultrasound guided peripheral nerve blocks can be a useful modality in management of acute pain in near future. If the amount of pain is not relieved, the splint should be removed and the limb further investigated.

Antibiotic

Dosage and guidelines for open fractures given in table below.

Grade of fracture (Gustilo-Anderson classification)	Open fracture	FIRST-GENERATION CEPHALOSPORINS (GRAM-POSITIVE COVERAGE) CEFAZOLIN	IF ANAPHYLACTIC PENICILLIN ALLERGY (INSTEAD OF FIRST-GENERATION CEPHALOSPORIN) CLINDAMYCIN	AMINOGLYCOCIDE (GRAM-NEGATIVE COVERAGE) GENTAMICIN	Duration
Grade I	Puncture Wound <1 cm; Minimal contamination; Minimal soft tissue damage	<50 kg: 1 gm Q 8 hr 50–100 kg: 2 gm Q 8 hr >100 kg: 3 gm Q 8 hr	<80 kg: 600 mg Q 8 hr >80 kg: 900 mg Q 8 hr		24hrs
Grade II	Laceration 1–10 cm; Moderate soft tissue damage; Adequate bone coverage Minimal comminution	<50 kg: 1 gm Q 8 hr 50–100 kg: 2 gm Q 8 hr >100 kg: 3 gm Q 8 hr	<80 kg: 600 mg Q 8 hr >80 kg: 900 mg Q 8 hr		24hrs
Grade III A	Laceration > 10cm Extensive soft tissue damage; Adequate bone coverage Segmental/ severely comminuted fracture or heavily contaminated wounds	<50 kg: 1 gm Q 8 hr 50–100 kg: 2 gm Q 8 hr >100 kg: 3 gm Q 8 hr	<80 kg: 600 mg Q 8 hr >80 kg: 900 mg Q 8 hr	Loading dose in ER: 2.5 mg/kg for child (or <50 kg) 5 mg/kg for adult)	3 days
Grade III B	As a Gustilo type IIIA injury, but with periosteal stripping and bone exposure	<50 kg: 1 gm Q 8 hr 50–100 kg: 2 gm Q 8 hr >100 kg: 3 gm Q 8 hr	<80 kg: 600 mg Q 8 hr >80 kg: 900 mg Q 8 hr	Loading dose in ER: 2.5 mg/kg for child (or <50 kg) 5 mg/kg for adult)	3 days

Grade III C	Any open fracture with vascular injury requiring repair	<50 kg: 1 gm Q 8 hr 50–100 kg: 2 gm Q 8 hr >100 kg: 3 gm Q 8 hr	<80 kg: 600 mg Q 8 hr >80 kg: 900 mg Q 8 hr	Loading dose in ER: 2.5 mg/kg for child (or <50 kg) 5 mg/kg for adult)	3 days
	Farmyard, soil or standing water, irrespective of wound size or severity	**PIPERACILLIN/ TAZOBACTAM** 3.375 gm Q 6 hr (<100 kg) 4.5 gm Q 6 hr (>100 kg)			3 days

Stabilization of the fracture

1. Traction
2. Hand stabilization
3. Splints
4. Neurovascular Examination- before and after stabilization.

Traction

Traction is applied to restore the anatomical position of the limb. Inline position balances the effect of opposing muscles and prevents further neurovascular bundle injury. Traction also helps in reducing pain and blood loss. The amount of force required for alignment of fractures depends on the site of injury. Usually the fracture distal to elbow and knee joints require gentle traction while the proximal fractures due to large surrounding muscle mass requires significant traction for proper alignment. This is achieved by applying In-line traction to realign the limit and keeping up with traction with an immobilization gadget

Hand Stabilization

Once the extremity has been repositioned, it has to hold gently with help of two hands before the definite stabilization with splint is done. Generally, two persons are required for a good stabilization.

Splint stabilization

The inline splinting of the bones should be done with inline position of the limb and ideally it should immobilize the injured extremity along with the joint proximal and distal to it. For example in case of Tibia fractures the ankle and the knee should be immobilised.

In case of injuries involving the joints the injured joint should be splinted in mid-range position including bones above and below the injury. For example, to splint the elbow joint, the forearm and arm should be splinted.

Characteristics of Good Splint

- It should be well padded, strong and snug
- It should allow to monitor distal Neurovascular bundle
- There should be no movement of the injured bones
- It should not be very large or complex
- It should not inhibit the further examination

Neurovascular examination

Splintage of the limb could not be completed without the assessment of distal neurovascular bundle before and after the procedure. Complete neurological examination as well as the distal pulses should be well documented and assessed at regular intervals. At any time if there are signs of ischemia or the patient develops paraesthesia or excruciating pain, the splint should be opened immediately and again complete examination should be done. If the patient has a low volume pulse then the clinical examination should be aided by POCUS Doppler study of limbs.

Management of vascular injury associated with fracture

Pressure bandaging for a vascular injury without removal of pressure is the key to haemorrhage control. If the bleeding does not control with pressure the tourniquet is to be applied proximal to the fracture site. Recommended pressure of 250 mm Hg in the upper extremity and 400 mm Hg in the lower extremity for 1 hour. There is no role for vascular clamps to be applied in an emergency.

The use of CT angiography and other diagnostic tools are needed for suspected vascular injuries but should not be done in hemodynamically unstable patients; other patients with clear vascular injuries require urgent operation. Incase of diagnosed arterial injury immediately consult a surgeon skilled in vascular repair.

Radiology

X-ray examination should be done in all musculoskeletal injuries. Usually, two views AP and lateral are taken involving one joint above and the other below the fracture site. In case of pediatric injuries, X-ray of the opposite limb should also be taken due to non-closure of epiphysis.CT angiography should be done in all the patients with suspected vascular injuries.

For hemodynamically unstable patients Damage Control Orthopedics is the first line of management.

For patients who are stable, they can be managed with definite fixation with either nailing or plating.

Recent updates:

- Horizontal resuscitation with a new emphasis has been placed on a team approach towards resuscitation.

- Tourniquet application as part of hemorrhage control in severe extremity is recommended. The use of a tourniquet to control severe extremity bleeding is now recommended.
- Prostate examination is not mandatory in the 10th Edition ATLS guidelines.
- Pelvic trauma management has a new flow chart and intraperitoneal packing is recommended.

Chest wall injury society non flail study

Back ground:

we hypothesized that SSRF (surgical stabilisation of rib fracture) improves outcome among patients with displaced rib fractures in absence of flail chest.

Method:

Multicenter, prospective, controlled clinical trial comparing SSRF with in 72hourst to medical management.

Inclusion criteria:

3 or more severely displaced ribfracture without flail chest. The trial involved both randomised and observational arms at patient discretion.

The primary outcome was the NUMERIC PAIN SCORE at 2 week follow up. Narcotic consumption, spirometry, PFT, Respiratory disability related quality of life were also compared.

Results:

110 subjects were enrolled. There were no significant differences between subjects who selected randomisation(n=23) versus observation (n=87). Off the 110 subjects 51 underwent SSRF.

Conclusions:

SSRF performed within 72 hours improved the primary outcome of NPS(numeric pain score) at 2 week follow up. Narcotic consumption also trended toward being lower in operative, RD-QoL was also significantly improved in operative group.

Level of evidence:

Therapeutic, level 2.

Brain Tissue Oxygen Monitoring and Management in Severe Traumatic Brain Injury (BOOST-II): a Phase II Randomized Trial.

Objective

A relationship between reduced brain tissue oxygenation (PbtO2<20mmhg) and poor outcome following severe traumatic brain injury (TBI)(GCS<8).

Method

Randomized prospective clinical trial on 119 severe tbi patients.

Outcomes

The average normal $PbtO_2$ is 23 ± 7 mm Hg. Several observational studies have noted that reduced $PbtO_2$ is common after TBI; $PbtO_2$ values <20mmHg may occur in >70% of monitored patients within the first few days after injury.6-month GOS-E scores were obtained in 106 patients (ICP-only group =53; ICP+$PbtO_2$ group =53) and trended towards lower mortality and better outcomes in the ICP+ PbtO2 management group.

Conclusions

Management of severe TBI informed by multimodal ICP and $PbtO_2$ monitoring reduced brain tissue hypoxia with a trend towards lower mortality and more favorable outcomes than ICP-only treatment.

React 2 trial:- Immediate total body CT scanning versus conventional imaging and selective CT scanning in patients with severe trauma: a randomised controlled trial

A multicentre, randomised controlled trial study done at Level 1 trauma centers in June, 2016. In this the patients aged >/= 18 years with trauma with abnormal vital signs, clinical suspicion of life threatening injuries, or severe injury were randomly assigned to immediate total body CT scan (Interventional group) or to a standard work up with conventional imaging supplemented with selective CT imaging (Control group). The primary objective for the study was in hospital mortality and secondary objectives were radiation exposure, time spent in trauma room, time to complete imaging in ED, time to get the diagnosis, direct medical costs, number of missed injuries found during tertiary survey, life threating event during scanning. The trail showed there was no significant difference seen in in hospital mortality in among both groups. In secondary survey there was significant increase in radiation exposure and reduction of time to get complete imaging and getting a complete diagnosis in interventional group compared to control group.

Resuscitation in shock patients in trauma and emergency

Fluid therapy is a never-ending debate in resuscitative medical science. Several clinical trials and reviews have been published over time in the medical literature. CRISTAL trial was aimed to compare the difference in mortality in ICU patients receiving colloids vs crystalloids. In the multicenter, randomized clinical trial, they found that there was no significant difference in 28-day mortality among both patients. However, 90-day mortality was statistically lower in patients receiving colloids. (1)

Finfer S et al conducted a double-blind, randomized, controlled trial (PLUS trial) and found that there was a lower risk of death and acute kidney injury among critically ill patients receiving BMES than those receiving saline. (2) This can be considered one of the best trials to compare the efficacy of balanced vs unbalanced fluids in critically ill patients.

Another pillar in volume resuscitation is the blood products. Few important studies have been conducted on pre-hospital resuscitation in trauma patients. RePHILL trial studied if packed red blood cells (PRBC) and lyophilised plasma (LyoPlas) transfusion was superior to the use of 0·9% sodium chloride for improving tissue perfusion and reducing mortality in trauma-related haemorrhagic shock. However, they did not find any significant difference in mortality or lactate clearance among patients receiving normal saline vs those receiving Lyso-plas or PRBC in the pre-hospital setting. (3)

Similar results were found in COMBAT trial with pre-hospital plasma transfusion. They studied the 28-day mortality in patients with severe trauma, comparing the effect of prehospital resuscitation with plasma vs normal saline. No significant difference was found between the two. (4)

Contrarily, PAMPer trial, found that prehospital administration of plasma was associated with lower 30-day mortality in trauma patients. However, transportation time was significantly more in the later. Thus, it can be concluded that blood products in prehospital settings can be beneficial if a longer transport time to the definitive care center is expected. (4)

PROPPR trial enrolled 680 and compared two standard interventions of volume resuscitation of severe traumatic hemorrhagic shock patients with Plasma: Platelet: PRBC in the ratio of 1:1:1 vs 1:1:2. They found that there was no significant difference between the two strategies in terms of 24-hour and 30-day mortality. (5)

A non-trauma-related cause of hypovolemic shock is postpartum hemorrhage. Antifibrinolytics have been found to be beneficial in patients with traumatic hemorrhage. Hence, the utility of tranexamic acid is currently being studied in the WOMAN-2 trial for postpartum hemorrhage. The intend to see if giving tranexamic acid can prevent PPH and other severe outcomes in women with moderate and severe anaemia. (6)

References

1. Annane D, Siami S, Jaber S, Martin C, Elatrous S, Declère AD, et al. Effects of fluid resuscitation with colloids vs crystalloids on mortality in critically ill patients presenting with hypovolemic shock: the CRISTAL randomized trial. JAMA. 2013 Nov 6;310(17):1809–17.

2. Finfer S, Micallef S, Hammond N, Navarra L, Bellomo R, Billot L, et al. Balanced Multielectrolyte Solution versus Saline in Critically Ill Adults. N Engl J Med. 2022 Mar 3;386(9):815–26.

3. Crombie N, Doughty HA, Bishop JRB, Desai A, Dixon EF, Hancox JM, et al. Resuscitation with blood products in patients with trauma-related haemorrhagic shock receiving prehospital care (RePHILL): a multicentre, open-label, randomised, controlled, phase 3 trial. Lancet Haematol. 2022 Apr;9(4):e250–61.

4. Pusateri AE, Moore EE, Moore HB, Le TD, Guyette FX, Chapman MP, et al. Association of Prehospital Plasma Transfusion With Survival in Trauma Patients With Hemorrhagic Shock When Transport Times Are Longer Than 20 Minutes: A Post Hoc Analysis of the PAMPer and COMBAT Clinical Trials. JAMA Surg. 2020 Feb 1;155(2):e195085.

5. Baraniuk S, Tilley BC, del Junco DJ, Fox EE, van Belle G, Wade CE, et al. Pragmatic Randomized Optimal Platelet and Plasma Ratios (PROPPR) Trial: design, rationale and implementation. Injury. 2014 Sep;45(9):1287–95.

6. London School of Hygiene and Tropical Medicine. Tranexamic Acid for the Prevention of Postpartum Bleeding in Women With Anaemia: an International, Randomised, Double-blind, Placebo Controlled Trial. [Internet]. clinicaltrials.gov; 2022 Apr [cited 2022 Jun 8]. Report No.: NCT03475342. Available from: https://clinicaltrials.gov/ct2/show/NCT03475342

Geriatric Trauma

Geriatric trauma patients pose a unique challenge to emergency physicians. Trauma is the fifth leading cause of mortality in the elderly population. Although the mechanisms of trauma in elderly may only slightly vary in comparison to their younger counterparts, the anatomic and physiological senescence of existing organ systems and pre existing conditions demand modifications in the usual resuscitative attempts.

The following table summarizes the components and effects of frailty.

	CHANGES	**EFFECTS**
Nutrition	Various degrees of malnutrition	Decreased healing and immune suppression
Skin and Musculoskeletal	Decreased lean mass Increased total body fat Loss of tissue elastance and thinning of skin Osteopenia and osteoporosis	Impaired thermoregulation and more susceptible to hypothermia Less resistance to shearing forces Increased risk of fractures
Neurologic	Neurocognitive decline Peripheral neuropathy (Diabetic) Cerebral atrophy Atherosclerotic vessels Various medications	Decreased ability to auto-regulate More prone to occult injuries Delayed signs of raised ICP More prone to strokes and bleeds.
Cardiovascular	Myocardium is less compliant Fibrosis of conduction system of the heart Drugs (B – blockers, CCBs, Cardiac glycosides)	Reduced cardiac output and less compensation to Hypovolemia. Less responsive to neuro-humoral effects. (Catecholamines) These drugs lead to negative inotropic, dromotropic and chronotropic effects.
Respiratory system	Reduced FRC, TV and TLC Decreased chest wall compliance Decreased mucociliary clearance	Reduced respiratory reserve Limited ability to compensate for hypoxia, hypercarbia, acidosis Atelectasis is common and early in the course More prone to infections and aspiration

Gastrointestinal	Edentulous and loose dentition	Difficulty with BMV or laryngoscopy
	Impaired aerodigestive reflexes	Increased risk of aspiration
	Gastric and intestinal wall integrity is affected as we age	Higher risk of infections and constipation
	Reduced liver function	Hypoalbuminemia and worsening of third spacing. Reduced thrombopoietin production and reduced vitamin K dependent clotting factors.
Genitourinary	Higher rate of urinary incontinence and post voidal residue. Increased rates of prostatism.	Increased risk of infections
		Disturbances in fluid and electrolyte homeostasis.
	Parenchymal loss in kidneys	Creatinine clearance should be borne in mind for certain drugs
	RAAS is downregulated	Less responsive to Hypovolemia and salt retention.
Hematological	Marrow is replaced by fat	Hematopoietic reserves decline.
	Malnutrition causing Iron, B12 or Folate deficiency	Anemia
	Qualitative defects may develop in the blood cells	Functionality of red cells, platelets and leukocytes is affected even though the quantitative values are normal
Immune System	Generalized malnutrition and decrease in immune functions	More prone to infections
Endocrine	May be on steroids or thyroid replacements	There won't be adequate stress response.
		Adrenal suppression

MECHANISMS OF INJURIES

1. **Falls:**

   - These are most common cause of traumatic brain injury in the elderly.

   - Risk factors include advanced age, dementia, unsteady gait, visual impairment, cardiovascular diseases like MI or arrhythmias causing syncope, strokes and other neurologic disorders

   - Environmental factors like loose rugs, slippery surfaces and inadequate lighting increase the risk of falls.

2. **Motor vehicle crashes:**

- Slower reaction times, restricted cervical mobility, larger blind spot and hearing and visual impairment contribute to the risk of accidents.
- Medical conditions like stroke, MI or dysrhythmias may precipitate a collision.

3. **Burns:**

- Mortality rates with burn injuries remain high in elderly.
- Elderly are at increased risk because of decreased reaction times, inability to escape from a burning structure and decreased vision and hearing are certain risk factors
- Spilled hot liquids may result in full thickness burns
- Compensatory mechanisms are also blunted in elderly

4. **Penetrating injuries:**

- Although quite rare, penetrating injuries may occur due to gun shots, assaults or impaled objects in an accidental trauma.

CONSIDERATIONS IN PRIMARY SURVEY

1. **Airway**

- Arthritic changes in mouth and spine and issues with dentition.
- Decreased protective reflexes
- Gauze can be placed between gums and cheek to achieve proper mask seal
- Adjust dosing of RSI drugs

2. **Breathing**

- Kyphoscoliosis, reduced chest wall compliance
- Decreased lung capacities and decreased mucociliary clearance.
- Identify respiratory failure early as there is very limited reserve.
- Manage rib fractures expeditiously and
- Appropriate application of mechanical ventilation.

3. **Circulation**

- Pre existing disorders and use of cardiac medications
- Lack of typical response to Hypovolemia
- Identify and look for hypoperfusion early
- Balanced resuscitation with fluids and early administration of blood products.

4. **Disability**

   - Cerebral atrophy and spinal degeneration
   - Pre existing neurological disorders
   - Liberally use CT scans
   - Early reversal of anticoagulation/ anti platelet therapy

5. **Exposure**

   - Changes in Integumentary system as mentioned above
   - Prevent hypothermia
   - Pad bony prominences as and when appropriate.
   - Early evaluation and liberate patients from spine boards and cervical collars.

SPECIFIC INJURIES

Rib Fractures

- Increased risk for rib fractures even following a ground level fall.
- Pneumonia is a common complication.
- Mortality risk increases with each rib fractured
- Main objectives are pain management and pulmonary hygiene.
- Avoid unwanted narcotic administration which may cause respiratory depression.

Traumatic Brain Injury

- Elderly patients are at highest risk for TBI associated mortality and they have delayed mortality.
- Consider early anticoagulation reversal
- Use CT scan liberally

Pelvic Fractures

- Can result from ground level falls
- Increased risk of osteoporosis and requirement of blood transfusion even for seemingly stable fractures.
- Mortality is quite higher compared to same fractures in young
- They are less likely to return to independent lifestyle.

FRAIL Scale

Easily applied screening tool

Includes *Fatigue*, *Resistance*, *Ambulation*, *Illness* and *Loss of weight*.

Each parameter is cored either 0 or 1. Scores of 3 to 5 are considered frail.

Other Scores for prognostication for in-hospital mortality -

- Geriatric trauma outcome score (GTOS)
- Quick Elderly Mortality After Trauma (qEMAT) – Done after admission
- Full Elderly Mortality After Trauma (fEMAT) – Done after radiological evaluation

ABUSE

There can be Physical maltreatment, Sexual maltreatment, Neglect, Psychological maltreatment, Financial and material exploitation and violation of rights.

Findings suggestive of maltreatment

- Contusions affecting inner arms, inner thighs, palms, soles, scalp, ear, mastoid area, buttocks
- Abrasions to the axillary area or wrists and ankles.
- Oral injury, unusual alopecia pattern
- Untreated fractures, untreated pressure ulcers and injuries in various stages of healing
- Contact burns and scalds.

General Principles of Fracture Management

Orthopedic fractures are a common daily acute health issue. Improper initial management of fractures can lead to significant long-term morbidity and, potentially, mortality. In addition to those fractures sustained from daily crashes and falls, fractures are a common issue in natural disasters.

The most important factors in fracture healing are blood supply and soft-tissue health, and initial management of an injured limb should have the goal of maintaining or improving these. Early fracture management is generally aimed at controlling hemorrhage, providing pain relief, preventing ischemia-reperfusion injury, and removing potential sources of contamination (foreign body and nonviable tissues).

Pathophysiology

- Fractures can heal by two different mechanisms, depending on their position and stability.
- Primary or direct healing is possible when an anatomic reduction with compression is achieved.
- With primary healing, the modeling occurs internally, and no callus is formed.
- Secondary or indirect healing occurs with relative stability when an anatomic reduction is not achieved or compression is not possible. This type of healing involves the formation of a bony callus and then subsequent external remodeling to bridge the gap.

The four phases of indirect fracture healing are as follows

- Fracture and inflammatory phase
- Granulation tissue/soft callus formation
- Hard callus formation, including woven bone creation
- Remodeling, including lamellar bone creation
- Actual fracture injuries to the bone include insult to the bone marrow, periosteum, and local soft tissues. The most important stage in fracture healing is the inflammatory phase and subsequent hematoma formation. It is during this stage that the cellular signaling mechanisms work through chemotaxis and an inflammatory mechanism to attract the cells necessary to initiate the healing response.
- Within 7 days, the body forms granulation tissue between the fracture fragments. Various biochemical signaling substances are involved in the formation of the soft callus, which lasts approximately 2 weeks.
- During hard callus formation, cell proliferation and differentiation begin to produce osteoblasts and chondroblasts in the granulation tissue. The osteoblasts and chondroblasts, respectively,

synthesize the extracellular organic matrices of woven bone and cartilage, and then the newly formed bone is mineralized. This stage requires 4-16 weeks.

- During the fourth stage, the mesh like callus of woven bone is replaced by hard lamellar bone, which is organized parallel to the axis of the bone. This final stage involves remodeling of the bone at the site of the healing fracture by various cellular types such as osteoclasts. Remodeling can take months to years, depending on patient and fracture factors.

- Patient factors that influence fracture healing include age, comorbidities, medication use, social factors, and nutrition. Other factors that affect fracture healing include fracture type, degree of trauma, systemic and local disease, and infection.

History and Physical Examination

Single-limb injury

- A thorough history should be elicited for the mechanism of injury and for any accompanying or associated events surrounding the injury; obtaining a history of any previous injury or fracture is mandatory.

- If the injury involved a fall, the circumstances surrounding the fall should be explored. If a syncopal or presyncopal prodrome occurred, further medical workup is required.

- It is necessary to classify the soft tissues overlying the fracture and to grade any open wounds according to the well-known Gustilo-Anderson system. Compartment syndromes in areas of the body prone to this malady (erg, the forearm and lower leg) must be ruled out by careful examination and documentation and serial assessment.

Multiple traumatic injuries

- Initial assessment of a patient with polytrauma follows the Advanced Trauma Life Support (ATLS) protocols and includes the identification and treatment of life-threatening injuries. The first step is evaluation of the individual's airway, breathing, and circulation (the ABCs). Immediate endotracheal intubation and rapid administration of intravenous fluids may be necessary. Full spinal precautions must be maintained until injury to the complete spine can be excluded clinically and through diagnostic imaging (with radiography or computed tomography [CT]).

Splinting of limb injuries in emergency department

- Reduction and splinting of traumatic injuries (open and closed) in the emergency department (ED) is imperative. Periarticular injuries and dislocations that are not reduced in a timely fashion may cause cartilage necrosis to the affected joints. Splinting reduces pain and deformity and lowers the risk of continued neurovascular injury. Splinting and elevation also enhance nursing care and minimize swelling.

- Open wounds and soft-tissue injuries must be covered with sterile moist dressings after being viewed by a clinician. The injured limb is then splinted by going above and below adjacent joints with adequate soft padding, appropriate cast material (whether plaster of Paris or fiberglass), and tensor bandages.

- The upper extremity is splinted in a standard position, with the shoulder and humerus beside the chest, the elbow at 90° of flexion, and the forearm and wrist in neutral rotation and neutral flexion and extension. The hand is splinted in the "safe position," with the wrist extended, the metacarpal joints flexed to 90°, and the interphalangeal (IP) joints fully extended. To prevent compartment syndrome, splintage should be half-circumferential and should not fully surround the limb.

- The lower extremity also has specific positions for splinting, in that the proximal parts do not lend themselves to casting. To splint an unstable pelvic or femur fracture/dislocation, a distal femoral skeletal traction pin must be placed with 25 lb (~11 kg) of weight off the end of the bed in a pulley system. Knee dislocations and tibial fractures should undergo above-the-knee splinting with half-circumferential dressings and splintage material. Ankle and foot fractures require splintage that includes the whole lower leg up to the knee but does not cross the knee joint.

- Postreduction radiographs should be obtained and neurovascular checks performed in the ED to confirm that the reductions are satisfactory and that it is safe to allow the patient to wait for more definitive care in the operating room. Splinting remains part of good care for all limb injuries and is important for preparing an injured patient for the next step in care, whether that involves nonoperative management or operative fixation.

Classification

The Muller AO (*Arbeitsgemeinschaft für Osteosynthesefragen* [Association for Osteosynthesis])/ OTA (Orthopaedic Trauma Association) comprehensive classification of fractures provides a standardized description of fracture patterns, making communication regarding such injuries more precise and understandable. The various patterns are described as follows:

- Simple fractures are spiral, oblique, or transverse

- A multifragmentary fracture is one that has several breaks in the bone, creating more than two fragments

- Wedge fractures are either spiral (low-energy) or bending (high-energy) and allow the proximal and distal fracture fragments to remain in contact each other

- The complex multifragmentary fracture is a segmental fracture or one in which there is no contact between the proximal and distal fragments without the bone shortening

Soft-tissue involvement

Is the fracture open (formerly referred to as "compound") or closed? Is associated neurologic and/or vascular injury present? Is there muscle damage or is compartment syndrome evident? Gustilo et al described a classification of open fractures comprising the following three types:

- Type I - The wound is smaller than 1 cm, clean, and generally caused by a fracture fragment that pierces the skin (ie, inside-out injury); this is a low-energy injury

- Type II - The wound is longer than 1 cm, minimally contaminated, and without major soft-tissue damage or defect; this is also considered a low-energy injury

- Type III - The wound is longer than 1 cm, with significant soft-tissue disruption; the mechanism often involves high-energy trauma, resulting in a severely unstable fracture with varying degrees of fragmentation

Type III fractures are further divided into the following subtypes:

- IIIA - The wound has sufficient healthy soft tissue to cover the bone without the need for local or distant flap coverage

- IIIB - Disruption of the soft tissue is sufficiently extensive that local or distant flap coverage is necessary to cover the bone (see the first image below); the wound may be contaminated, and serial irrigation and debridement procedures are necessary to ensure a clean surgical wound

- IIIC - Any open fracture associated with an arterial or neurologic injury that requires repair is considered type IIIC (see the second image below); involvement of vascular or plastic surgeons is generally required

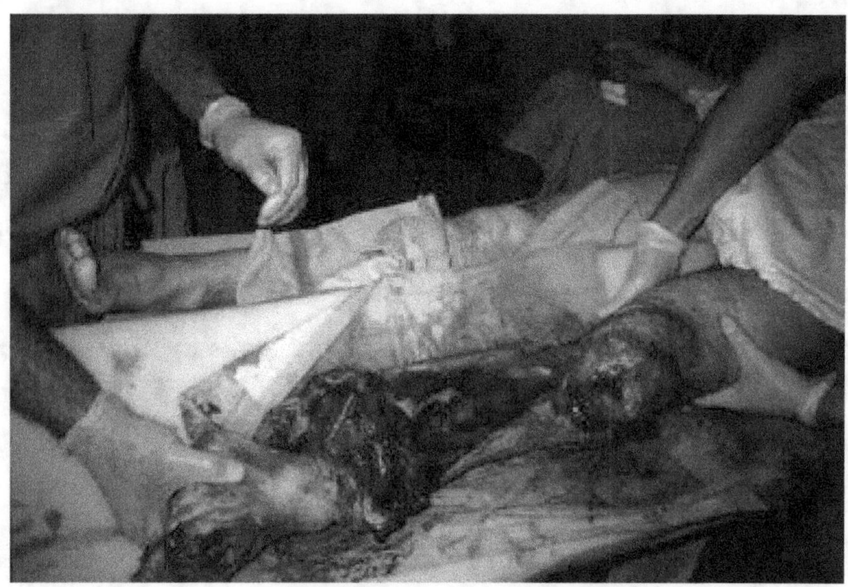

Gustilo type IIIB open fracture.

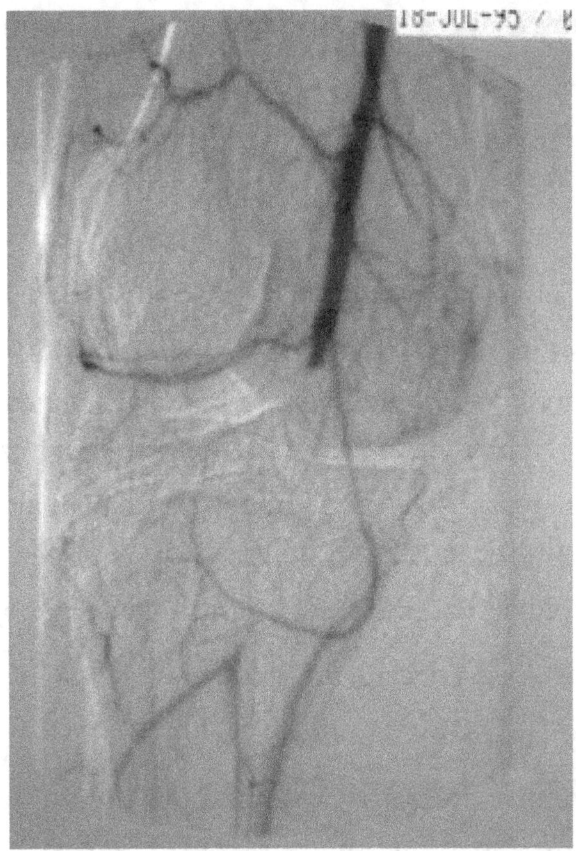

Angiographic evidence of vascular injury after traumatic injury (Gustilo type IIIC open fracture).

- The Gustilo classification has been shown to have only moderate intraobserver and interobserver reliability in terms of fracture classification.

- The Tscherne and Hanover fracture scales are classification systems that allow better evaluation of the soft-tissue injury relative to wound size, area of skin loss, and underlying soft-tissue damage. However, the Gustilo classification remains the system most commonly used.

Management

- Fracture management can be divided into nonoperative and operative techniques.

- The nonoperative approach consists of a closed reduction if required, followed by a period of immobilization with casting or splinting. Closed reduction is needed if the fracture is significantly displaced or angulated. Pediatric fractures are generally much more tolerant of nonoperative management, owing to their significant remodeling potential.

- If closed reduction is inadequate, surgical intervention may be required. Indications for surgical intervention include the following:

  - Failed nonoperative (closed) management

  - Unstable fractures that cannot be adequately maintained in a reduced position

  - Displaced intra-articular fractures (>2 mm)

- Patients with fractures that are known to heal poorly following nonoperative management (eg, <u>femoral neck fractures</u>)
- Large avulsion fractures that disrupt the muscle-tendon or ligamentous function of an affected joint (eg, patella fracture)
- Impending pathologic fractures
- Multiple traumatic injuries with fractures involving the <u>pelvis</u>, <u>femur</u>, or <u>vertebrae</u>
- Unstable open fractures, any type II or type III open fracture
- Fractures in individuals who would poorly tolerate prolonged immobilization required for nonoperative management (eg, elderly patients with <u>proximal femur</u> fractures)
- Fractures in growth areas in skeletally immature individuals that have increased risk for growth arrest (eg, <u>Salter-Harris types III-V</u>)
- Nonunions or malunions that have failed to respond to nonoperative treatment

Contraindications for surgical reconstruction are as follows:

- Active infection (local or systemic) or osteomyelitis
- Soft tissues that compromise the overlying fracture or the surgical approach because of poor soft-tissue quality due to soft-tissue injury or burns, excessive swelling, previous surgical scars, or active infection
- Medical conditions that contraindicate surgery or anesthesia (eg, recent myocardial infarction)
- Cases in which amputation, rather than attempted fracture fixation, would better serve the limb and the patient

Complications

Neurologic and vascular injury

- Neurologic and vascular injuries can occur in any fracture and are more likely in cases with increasing fracture deformity. <u>Peripheral nerve injury</u> is suspected if a patient experiences motor or sensory deficiencies. Management of neurologic injury involves immediate reduction of the fracture and possible nerve exploration, with subsequent follow-up to assess whether or not neurologic function returns.
- Arterial injury is suspected if the patient's pulses are diminished or absent in the affected limb or if the <u>ankle-brachial index</u> (ABI) is less than 0.9 or grossly different from the contralateral limb. If there is evidence of arterial injury, immediate realignment of the limb is performed, and the pulses and perfusion are checked again. If the pulses do not return, angiography is indicated, with concomitant involvement of vascular surgeons. Arterial injuries are especially prevalent in cases of <u>knee dislocations</u>, <u>proximal tibial fractures</u>, and <u>supracondylar humerus fractures</u>.

Compartment syndrome

- <u>Compartment syndrome</u>, initially reported by von Volkmann in 1872, is a potentially limb- and life-threatening condition.

- Compartment syndrome occurs when tissue pressure exceeds perfusion pressure in a closed anatomic space. This condition can occur in any compartment, such as the hand, forearm, upper arm, abdomen, buttock, thigh, and leg, but it most commonly occurs in the anterior compartment of the leg.

Avascular necrosis

- <u>Avascular necrosis</u> (AVN) is caused by disruption of the blood supply to a region of bone. Revascularization of the avascular bone can lead to nonunion, bone collapse, or degenerative changes. AVN is most commonly associated with <u>fractures of the femoral head</u> and neck, scaphoid, talar neck and body, and proximal humerus.

Posttraumatic arthritis

- Posttraumatic arthritis is common in intra-articular fractures, particularly in those that are not adequately reduced. Management of posttraumatic arthritis depends on the joint involved and can include arthroscopic debridement, osteotomy, arthroplasty, or arthrodesis.

Open Fractures and Compartment syndrome

A fracture hematoma is in communication through the skin with the environment called an open fracture.

Classification of open fracture:

Gustilo and Anderson classification of open fracture: Based on

- Size of wound
- Amount of soft tissue injury
- Presence/absence of NV injury
- Degree of contamination

Gustilo Fracture Type	Characteristics	Rates of Infection[32,169,191–193]
Type I	Puncture wound <1 cm Minimal contamination Minimal soft tissue damage	0–2%
Type II	Laceration >1 cm but <10 cm Moderate soft tissue damage Adequate bone coverage Minimal comminution	2–5%
Type IIIA	Laceration >10 cm Extensive soft tissue damage Adequate bone coverage, segmental/ severely comminuted fractures, or heavily contaminated wounds	5–10%
Type IIIB	As a Gustilo Type IIIA injury, but with periosteal stripping and bone exposure	10–50%
Type IIIC	Any open fracture with vascular injury requiring repair	25–50%

* Tibial fractures are associated with twice the infection rate of other bone.

To summarize:

	I	II	III-A	III-B	III-C
Energy of mechanism	Low	Moderate	High	High	High
Wound size	<1 cm	>1 cm	Usually >10 cm	Usually >10 cm	Usually >10 cm
Soft tissue injury	Low	Moderate	Extensive	Extensive	Extensive
Contamination	NO	Low	Severe	Variable	Variable
Conminution/ Fracture pattern	No/ Simple	Some/ Simple	Severe/ Complex	Severe/ Complex	Severe/ Complex
Soft tissue coverage	Yes	Yes	Yes	No, requires reconstructive procedure	Variable
Vacular injury injury	No	No	No	No	Yes, require reparation

Management aim of open fractures:

- Prevent infection
- Ensure # healing
- Restore function

Acute treatment:

- Initial assessment and treatment ATLS
- Remove gross contaminants
- Photograph for records
- Seal from environment
- Splint the extremity
- Antibiotics as soon as possible
- Tetanus prophylaxis
- Analgesia
- Fluid/blood replacement

Surgical treatment: "The solution to pollution is dilution"

- Wash the wound
- Irrigate

- Debride
- Early accurate debridement most important

Which antibiotics?

- BOA/BAPRAS guidelines (2009):

  IV co-amoxiclav 1.2g TDS until 1st debridement (if penicillin-allergic IV clindamycin 600 mg BD)
- At induction of anesthesia:
  - Gentamicin 1.5mg/kg
  - Plus teicoplanin 800mg or vancomycin 1g
- Post-opop continue IV augmentin 1.2g TDS until wound closure or max. of 72 hours

Timing of debridement

- Initial debridement:
  - < 5 hours - 7% infection rate
  - > 5 hours - 38% infection rate
  - Overt manifestations of infection - 4.8 months
- BOA/BAPRAS guidelines lower limb open # (2009)
- Within 24 hours if solitary open fracture.
- However immediately if:
  - Gross contamination
  - Compartment syndrome
  - Devascularized limb
  - Multi-injured patient

Complications

- Wound infection
- Osteomyelitis
- Non-union
- Tetanus infection
- Neurovascular injury
- Compartment syndrome

Summary

- Gustilo-Anderson classification
- Grade I, II, III (A/B/C) dependent on wound size, amount of soft tissue injury, degree of contamination & NV injury
- Take photo & cover wound
- Antibiotics & early debridement

Compartment Syndrome

Compartment Syndrome is an elevation of Interstitial Pressure in a closed Osteofascial Compartment that results in Microvascular Compromise.

It is a true orthopedic emergency.

<u>Etiology:</u>

- Reduced compartment size:
    - Tight dressing:- bandage or cast localized external pressure, lying on limb closure of facial defects.
- Increased compartment size:-
    - Bleeding:- fracture, vascular injury, bleeding disorders.
    - Increased capillary permeability:- ischemia/trauma/burns/exercise/snake bite/drug injection.
- FRACTURE is the first and most common cause
- The incidence is directly proportional to the degree of injury to soft tissue and bone.
- Most common in low energy injury(lack of compartment disruption)

Most common fracture leading to ACS:-

1. Tibial diaphyseal #
2. Distal radius #
3. Forearm #

Second most common cause:- Blunt trauma

<u>Pathophysiology:</u>

Insult to normal local tissue homeostasis

↓

Increased Tissue Pressure

↓

Decreased Capillary Blood Flow

↓

Oxygen Deprivation

↓

Local tissue Necrosis

↓

Tissue Necrosis occurs in normal blood flow if Intra compartmental pressure exceeds 30 mm Hg for longer than 8hrs.

Tissue survival:-

Muscle:

- 3 to 4hours- reversible changes
- 6 hours variable damage
- 8 hours irreversible changes

Nerve:

- 2 hours –looses nerve conduction
- 4 hours – neuropraxia
- 8 hours – irreversible changes

Delayed diagnosis:

- Permanent sensory and motor deficit.
- Contractures Infections
- Amputations

Clinical features:-

- Swelling and tightness(TENSE) compartment involved.
- Severe pain on passive stretching
- 5 p's:
  - Pain out of proportion to the injury
  - Pallor/Cyanosis
  - Hyperaesthesia/Paraesthesia
  - Paralysis
  - Pulselessness

Devices used for measurement of compartment pressure:-

1. Synthes hand-held monitor(most commonly used)
2. Whitesides three-way stopcock apparatus

3. Wick Catheter

4. Stryker STIC catheter (solid-state transducer intercompartmental catheter) for continuous pressure monitoring.

   Newer Non Invasive methods:

   1. Ultrasonography (sensitivity-77%, specificity-93%)

   2. Infrared Imaging

Management-

Fasciotomy:

- A surgical incision or splitting of the fascia to relieve a compartment syndrome
- Principles: Timely and Adequate incisions (skin and fascia)
- Good prognosis:
  - Fasciotomy done in 25 to 30hrs
- Bad prognosis:
  - delayed diagnosis,
  - 3rd or 4th day.
- Indications of Fasciotomy:.
  - Compartment pressure >30mmhg.
  - Arterial disruption for more than 4hrs.
  - Compartment syndrome associated with fracture should be treated at the time of reduction.

Pelvic Fractures

Incidence

- 5% of all skeletal injuries
- 2/3 of all pelvic fractures -RTA
- 10% - visceral injuries
- 10%- mortality rate

Tile Classification

Table 1 - Tile Classification of pelvic ring fractures.

Type A: Pelvic ring stable
  A1: fractures not involving the ring (i.e. avulsions, iliac wing or crest fractures)
  A2: stable minimally displaced fractures of the pelvic ring
Type B: Pelvic ring rotationally unstable, vertically stable
  B1: open book
  B2: lateral compression, ipsilateral
  B3: lateral compression, contralateral or bucket handle-type injury
Type C: Pelvic ring rotationally and vertically unstable
  C1: unilateral
  C2: bilateral
  C3: associated with acetabular fracture

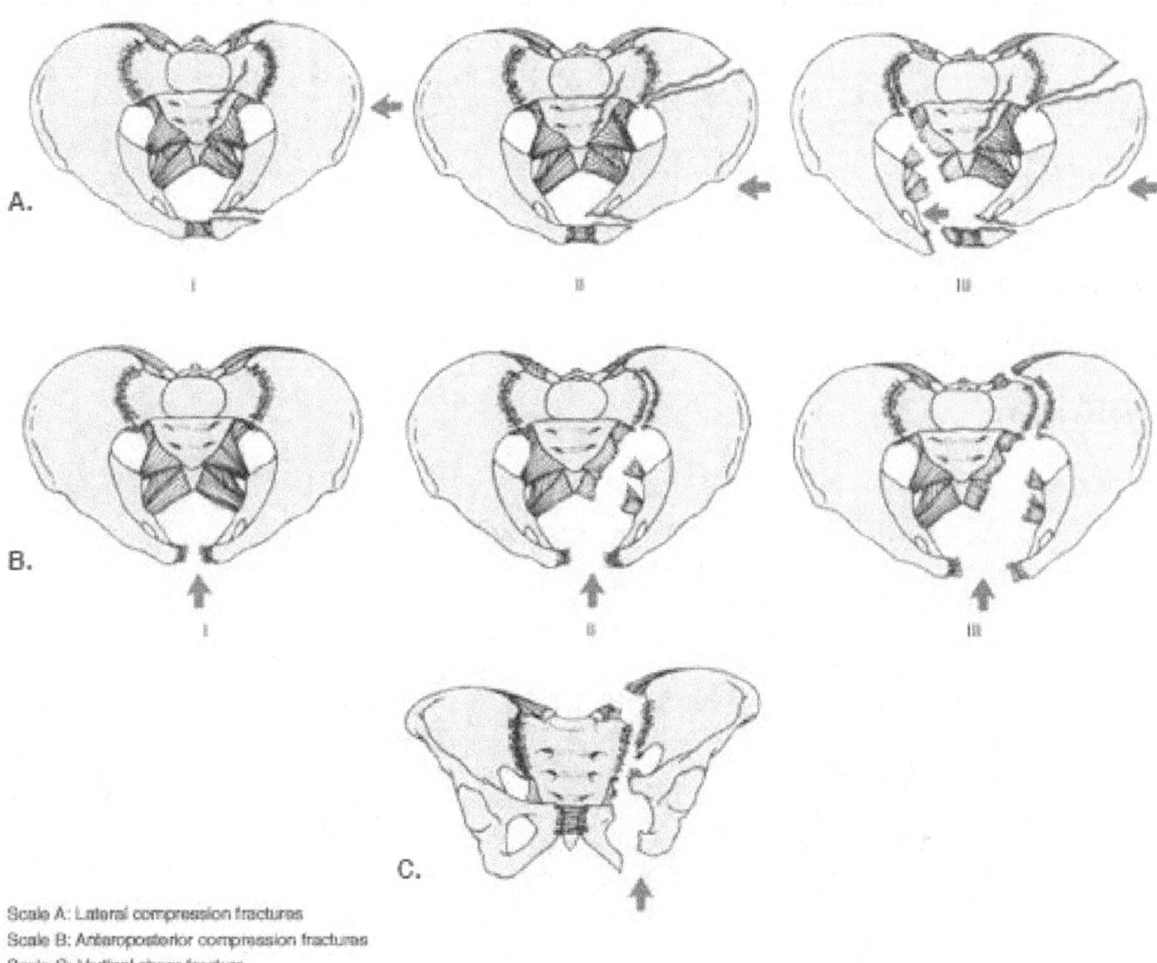

Burgess AR, Eastridge BJ, Young JW, et al. Pelvic ring disruptions: effective classification system and treatment protocols. *Journal of Trauma.* 1990;30:848. Used with permission, Wolters-Kluwer, Lippincott, Williams & Wilkins.

Isolated Fractures

- Avulsion Fractures – A piece of bone is pulled off by violent muscle contraction.
- Commonly in sportsmen and Athletes.
- Sartorius pull off – ASIS
- Rec. Femoris pull off- AIIS
- Add. Longus – A piece of the pubis bone.
- Hams. – part of the ischium
- Direct fractures – a direct blow to the pelvis, usually after fall from the height
- Ex. Ischium, Iliacblade
- Stress fractures – Fracture of the pubic rami

- Ex. Osteoporotic and Osteomalacia patients
- Stress fractures around SI joint – Diagnosis difficult

Acetabular fracture

- Mechanism of injury – when the head of the femur is driven into the pelvis.

Blow on the side.

Blow on the front of the knee –

Dashboard injury

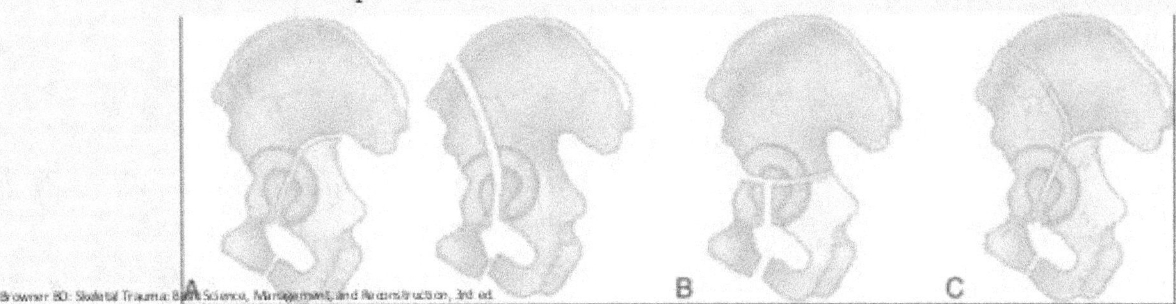

Types of Acetabulum Fractures

- Ant. Column
- Post. Column
- Transverse Fracture
- Complex Fracture

<u>Diagnosis of Pelvic Fractures</u>

History of Significant Trauma:

- RTA
- Fall from height
- Crush Injury

Clinical examination:

- Pelvic fractures suspected in all
- Abdominal or lower limb injuries.
- Swelling or bruising over the lower abdomen, the thigh and the perineum
- severe pain on movement

Bleeding from the urethra or not

- Urine pass or not
- Compression test positive
- Distraction test positive
- Direct pressure test positive
- In abdomen –signs of irritation

Radiological

- AP
- An Inlet view
- An outlet view
- Right oblique view
- Left oblique view

CT Scan

- Posterior pelvic ring disruption
- Complex acetabular fracture

Other Investigations

- USG of abdomen and pelvic region
- Retrograde urethrography and IVU if needed
- Hemogram
- Urine examination

Management

- It includes a combination of assessment and treatment.
- First priority – always assess the general condition of the patient and signs of blood loss > Resuscitation before the examination is completed
- Maintain airways, breathing and circulation = Binder First
- Make patient stable – BP, Pulse, Respiration
- Stop bleeding – IV fluid, blood, compression bandage, splintage
- Treatment of shock
- Treat urethral and abdominal injuries

Type –A

- Bed rest, Traction >4-6 week then crutch walking
- Physiotherapy

Type –B

- < 2.5cm. Gap: bed rest, post sling, Elastic girdle
- > 2.5cm.gap –Ext.fixation, Int.fixation, Plating and screw

Type -C

- More dangerous and difficult to treat-traction +fixator for 10 weeks. If no reduction then open reduction and internal fixation with plating

Treatment of Acetabulum fractures

- Conservative: Traction, Analgesic, Treatment of shock, Physiotherapy
- Surgery: ORIF with plating and screw, ORIF with lag screw, bone graft

Complications of pelvic fractures

- Urethral injury
- Bladder injury
- Injury to rectum and vagina
- Injury to major vessels
- Nerves injury
- Rupture of the diaphragm

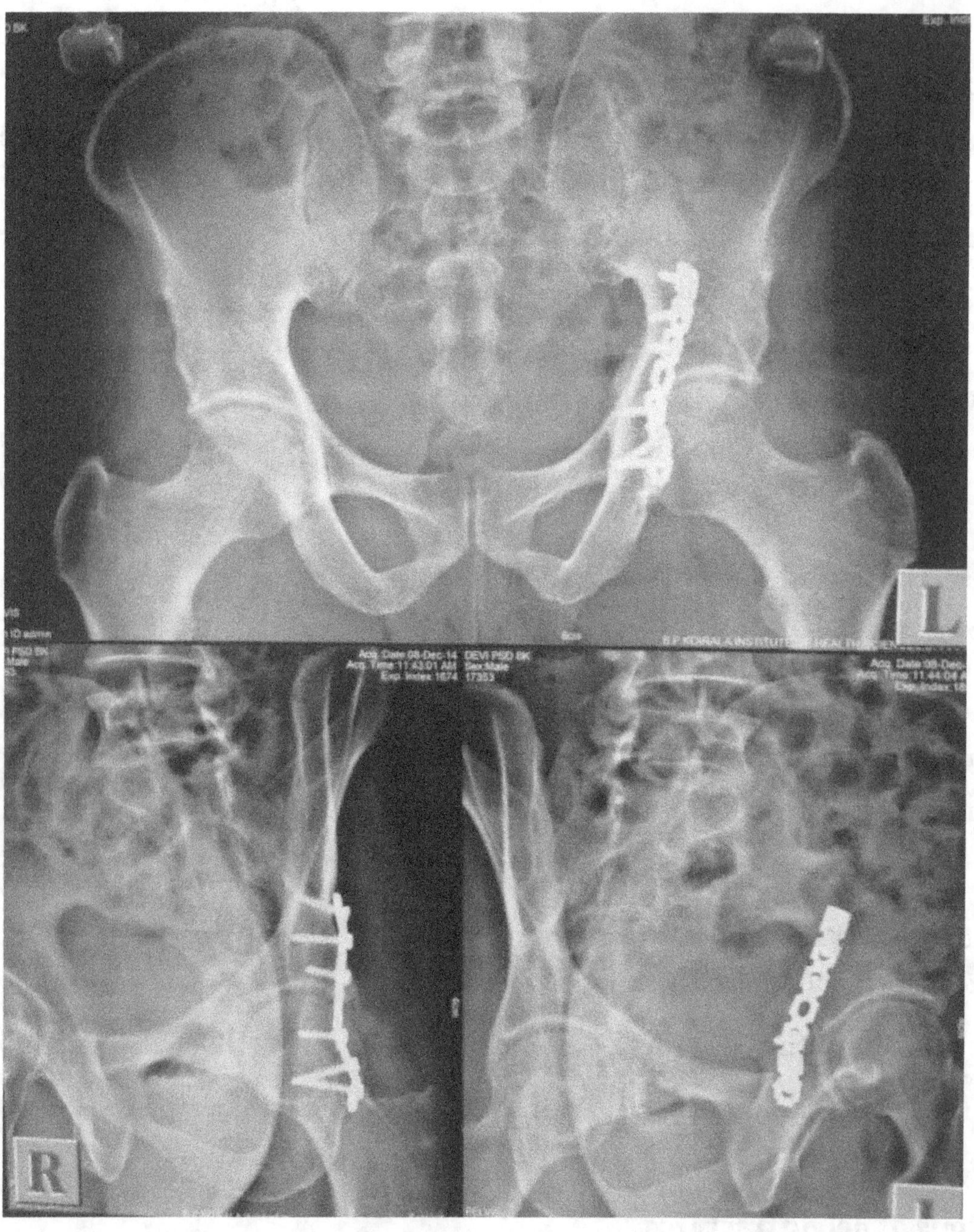

Pregnant Trauma Victim

We all know that a mother's body undergoes various anatomic and physiologic changes during pregnancy and all these should be borne in mind while evaluating a pregnant woman with trauma because these changes have direct impact on the presenting signs, diagnostic tests and the response to resuscitation.

Trauma in pregnancy can occur because of mild injuries like fall from standing height or stumbling over a small piece of furniture or because of major injuries like penetrating injuries or major vehicular accidents. Even a minor trauma in the first or second trimester increases the risk of delivering a child with prematurity or low birth weight.

We must remember that we are dealing with two patients when catering to a pregnant mother: Mother herself and the fetus. It is well iterated and emphasized in all the available literature that the *best maternal resuscitation will also be the best fetal resuscitation.*

The ATLS guidelines state that every female of reproductive age presenting with trauma should be considered pregnant until otherwise proven by a pregnancy test or a pelvic ultrasound. They also advise that a qualified surgeon and an obstetrician should be consulted early in the evaluation of pregnant trauma patient and if not available, early transfer to a trauma centre should be considered.

CHANGES IN PREGNANCY

Pregnancy brings about various changes which are briefly and relevantly summarized in the table below

SYSTEM	CHANGES
Respiratory	• Constant rate but increased TV and therefore increased Minute ventilation leading to chronic respiratory alkalosis [Normal pCO_2 is around 30 mmHg] • Reduced FRC and diaphragm is elevated by 2 to 4 cms [Care during ICD placement
Cardiovascular	• PR increased by 15 to 2o in 3rd T, BP returns to normal in 3rd T. • Increased plasma volume by 50% [Delayed recognition of shock]. Increased cardiac output. • ECG axis may shift left by 15 degrees. Flattened T wave in III and aVF is normal.
Hematological	• Increased plasma volume and red cell mass. Dilutional anemia • Increased coagulation factors and a pro-coagulant state is created. Hence, a normal Fibrinogen level should raise a suspicion of DIC • Increased WBC counts

Airway	• Pregnancy is a difficult airway. Increased chances of Mallampati III to IV. • Increased risk of aspiration due to increased risk of gastric reflux.
Uterus	• Intra pelvic upto 12th week. Peritoneum stretches maximally and is less sensitive to irritation. • Uterine walls become thin and more susceptible to injury.
Gastrointestinal	• Decreased lower esophageal sphincter and reduced gastric motility. Delayed gastric emptying. • Changes in bile composition • Increased production of pro-inflammatory cytokines by liver.
Endocrine	• Increased steroid synthesis • Increased thyroid hormones • Increased beta hCG and estrogen and progesterone.
Neurological	• Seizures can be because of eclampsia. Behavioral changes are common
Skin	• Linea nigra, striae gravidarum, melasma, palmar erythema, spider nevi.
Urinary tract	• Increased GFR, Increased Na and water retention. • Uretero-pelvic dilatation and physiological HDUN. • Flaccid bladder
Musculoskeletal	• Widened pelvis and increased sacro-iliac joint spaces [Important to know while interpreting radiographs]. • Engorged pelvic vessels.

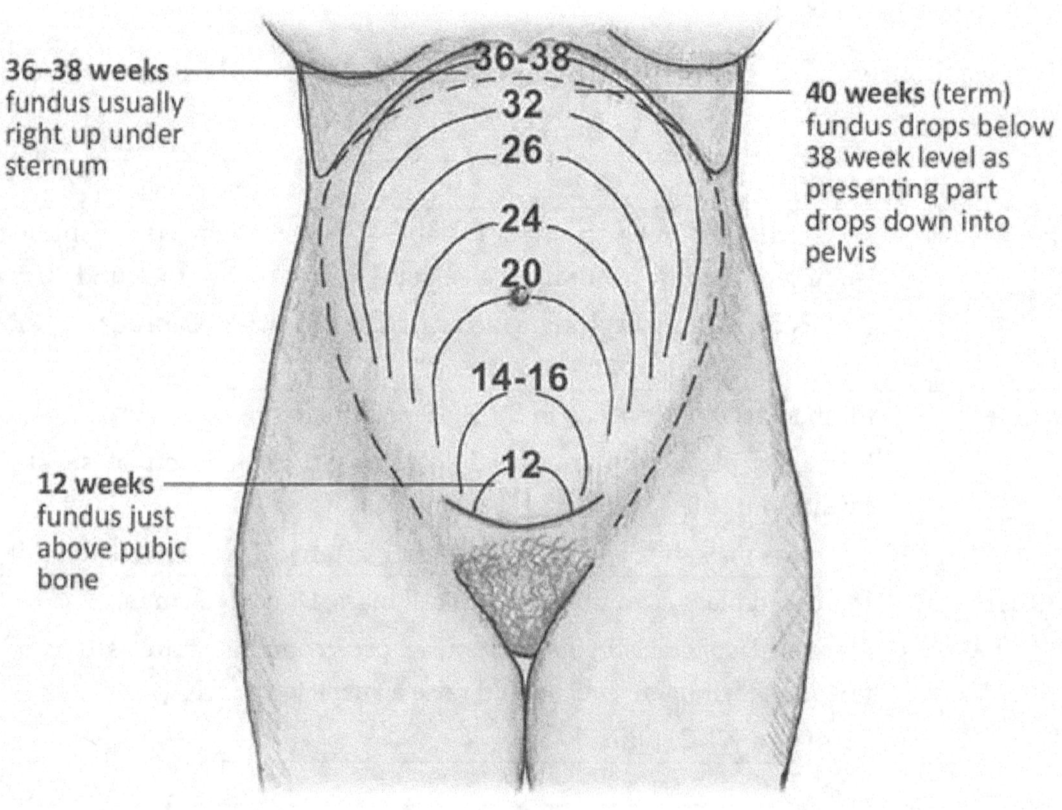

Hematological Findings

TABLE 12-1 NORMAL LABORATORY VALUES: PREGNANT VS. NONPREGNANT		
VALUE	PREGNANT	NONPREGNANT
Hematocrit	32%–42%	36%–47%
WBC count	5,000–12,000 µL	4,000–10,000 µL
Arterial pH	7.40–7.45*	7.35–7.45
Bicarbonate	17–22 mEq/L	22–28 mEq/L
$PaCO_2$	25–30 mm Hg (3.3–4.0 kPa)	30–40 mm Hg (4.0–5.33 kPa)
Fibrinogen	400–450 mg/dL (3rd trimester)	150–400 mg/dL
PaO_2	100–108 mm Hg	95–100 mm Hg
* Compensated respiratory alkalosis and diminished pulmonary reserve		

Source: ATLS 10th edition 1

MECHANISMS OF INJURY

TABLE 12-2 DISTRIBUTION OF MECHANISMS OF INJURY IN PREGNANCY	
MECHANISM	PERCENTAGE
Motor vehicle collision	49
Fall	25
Assault	18
Gunshot wound	4
Burn	1

Source: Chames MC, Pearlman MD. Trauma during pregnancy: outcomes and clinical management. *Clin Obstet Gynecol*, 2008;51:398

TABLE 12-3 DISTRIBUTION OF BLUNT AND PENETRATING ABDOMINAL INJURY IN PREGNANCY

MECHANISM	PERCENTAGE
Blunt	91
Penetrating	9
Gunshot wound	73
Stab wound	23
Shotgun wound	4

Source: Data from Petrone P, Talving P, Browder T, et al. Abdominal injuries in pregnancy: a 155-month study at two level I trauma centers. *Injury.* 2011;42(1):47–49.

Blunt injury

- Fetus is generally protected by abdominal wall, uterus and amniotic fluid which act as buffers to prevent direct fetal injury
- Indirect fetal injuries may occur due to rapid compression, deceleration, contrecoup or shearing injuries

Penetrating injuries

- Uterus acts as a shield to other viscera.
- The dense uterine wall, amniotic fluid and fetus prevent injuries to other viscera. Hence the maternal outcome is excellent but it comes at the cost of poor fetal outcome.

ASSESSMENT AND TREATMENT

Catastrophic outcomes specific to pregnancy related injuries

1. Premature labor
2. Placental Abruption
3. Amniotic fluid embolism
4. Uterine rupture

CONCERNS WITH PRIMARY SURVEY

1. MOTHER

   a. Low threshold for intubation. Increased risk of difficult airway and aspiration.

   b. Maintain PCO_2 at 30 mmHg at late pregnancy. If pCO_2 is more than this value consider respiratory issues.

c. Manually displace the gravid uterus to the left side to relieve the pressure on the inferior vena cava. If a patient requires spinal immobilization and maintenance of supine position, logrolling her to the left by 15 to 30 degrees can help. This can be achieved by elevating the right side with a bolstering device.

d. Pregnant patients can lose a significant amount of blood before tachycardia and hypotension develop. Therefore administer crystalloids and blood products early. *Vasopressors should be an absolute last resort as these can compromise uterine perfusion.*

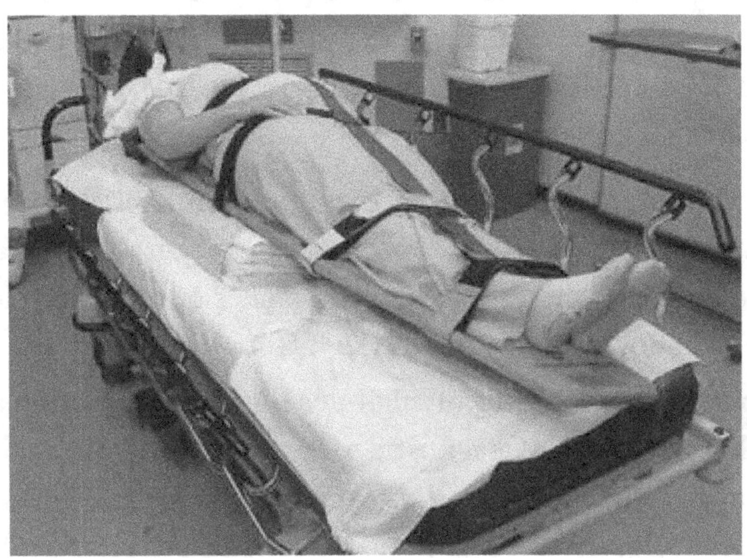

2. FETUS

a. Most common cause of fetal death is maternal shock and maternal death. This is followed by placental abruption

b. Placental abruption is suggested by vaginal bleeding (only in 70%), frequent uterine contractions and uterine tetany

c. Uterine rupture is rare yet catastrophic entity characterized by abdominal tenderness, guarding, and rigidity. Other feature may include an abdominal fetal lie, easy palpation of fetal parts. It may require surgical exploration to diagnose rupture.

d. We should perform continuous fetal monitoring with a tocodynamometer beyond 20 to 24 weeks of gestation.

e. The risk factors for fetal loss are maternal heart rate > 110, fetal heart rate > 160 or <120, injury severity scale of >9, evidence of placental abruption, dangerous mechanisms of injuries like pedestrian collisions, ejection during a motor vehicle crash, etc.

ADJUNCTS TO PRIMARY SURVEY

- All patients should be monitored for fluid status. Blood gases may reveal low bicarbonate as a part of chronic compensating respiratory alkalosis.

- Fetal heart tones should be monitored and arranged for early obstetric consultation. If not available, consider early transfer.

DURING SECONDARY SURVEY

- Adjunct imaging modalities include ultrasonography (US) and magnetic resonance imaging (MRI). US in form of eFAST should still be incorporated during trauma secondary survey.

- Radiographic imaging is often indicated in pregnant patients.

- The fear of radiation exposure should not take precedent over quickly. The risk of a missed injury or delay in diagnosis is much greater to the fetus than the risk of radiation. The American College of Obstetricians and Gynecologists (ACOG) has submit the below guidelines for diagnostic imaging during pregnancy:

  - Women should be counseled that X-ray exposure from a single diagnostic procedure does not result in harmful fetal effects. Specifically, exposure to < 5 rads (50 mGy) has not been associated with an increase in fetal anomalies or pregnancy loss. An abdominal CT approaches a radiation dose of 2.5 rads (25 mGy).

  - Concern about possible effects of high-dose ionizing radiation exposure should not prevent medically indicated diagnostic x-ray procedures from being performed on a pregnant woman. During pregnancy, other imaging procedures not associated with ionizing radiation (eg, ultrasonography, MRI) should be considered when appropriate.

  - Ultrasonography and MRI are not associated with known adverse fetal effects.

  - Consultation with an expert in dosimetry calculation may be helpful in calculating estimated fetal dose when multiple diagnostic x-rays are performed on a pregnant patient.

  - The use of radioactive isotopes of iodine is contraindicated for therapeutic use during pregnancy.

  - Radio-opaque and paramagnetic contrast agents are unlikely to cause harm and may be of diagnostic benefit, but these agents should be used during pregnancy only if the potential benefit justifies the potential risk to the fetus

- A Vaginal examination is mandated as bleeding may indicate disruption of placenta. Repeated examinations should be avoided.

- All pregnant RH negative trauma patients should receive RH immunoglobulin therapy (RhoGam) unless the injury is remote from uterus (E.g., isolated distal extremity injury). It should be instituted within 72 hours of injury.

- As little as 0.01 ml of Rh positive fetal blood will sensitize 70% of Rh negative patients. A Kleihauer betke (KB test) test may detect fetal blood in maternal blood. But a negative test doesn't exclude minor feto-maternal hemorrhage.

PERI MORTEM CESAREAN SECTION

- Limited data exists to support peri-mortem C section.
- At the time of maternal hypovolemic cardiac arrest, the fetus would have already sustained prolonged hypoxia.
- Therefore, for other causes of maternal cardiac arrest, perimortem C section may be occasionally successful if performed within 4 to 5 minutes of the arrest.
- An extensive abdominal incision is given – from xiphi-sternum to pubic symphysis.

MEDICATIONS COMMONLY USED

TREATMENTS (MEDICATIONS LISTED ARE COMMONLY RECOMMENDED)		
Rh-negative	RhIG 1 ampule (300 g) IM	
Tetanus	Td safe	
BP >160 s, >110 d Hypertension	labetalol 10–20 mg IV bolus	
Seizures	Eclamptic	magnesium sulfate 4–6 Gm IV load over 15–20 minutes
	Non-eclamptic	lorazepam 1–2 mg/min IV
CPR ACLS >20 wks	Patient should be in left lateral decubitus position. If no return of spontaneously circulation after 4 minutes of CPR, consider cesarean delivery of viable fetus.	

Source: ATLS 10th edition 2

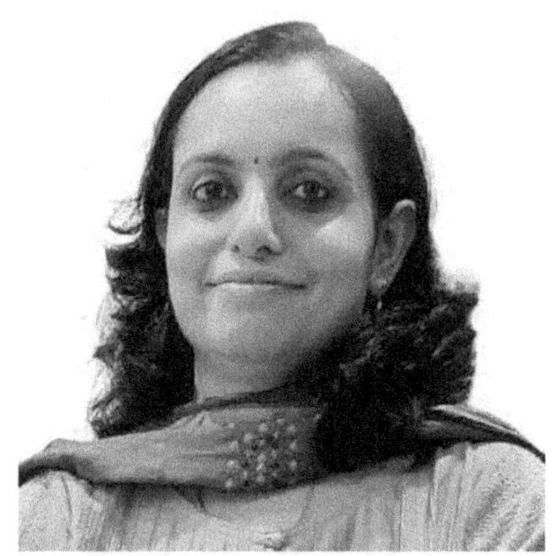
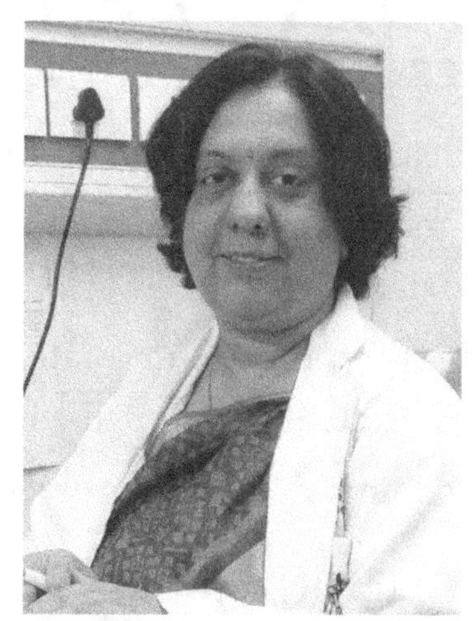
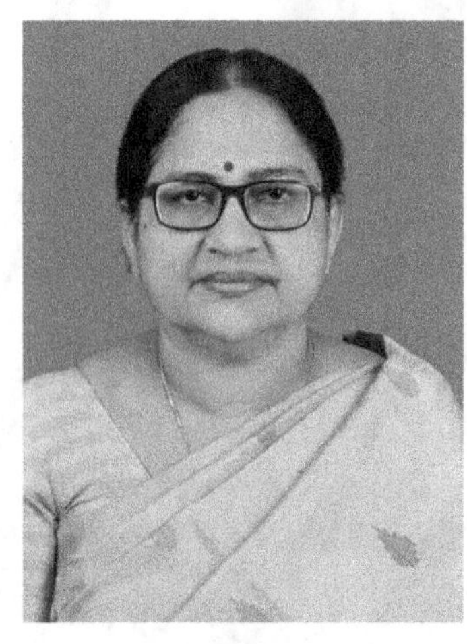
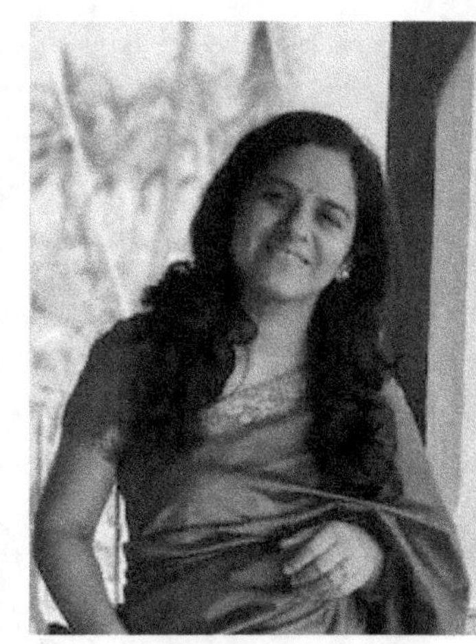
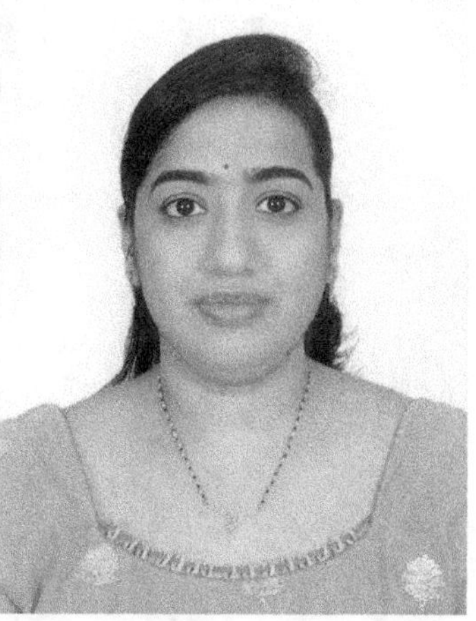
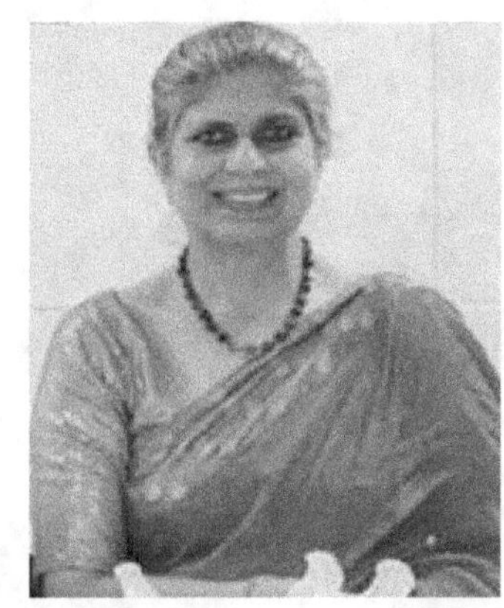
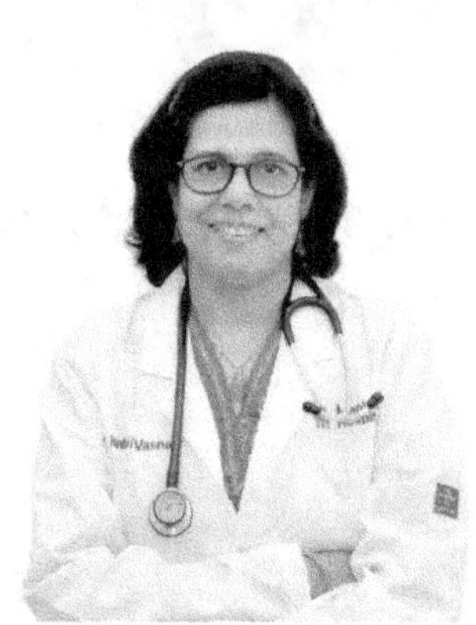
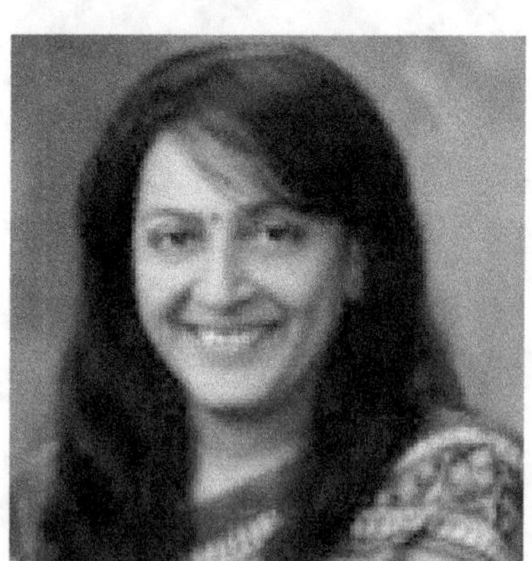
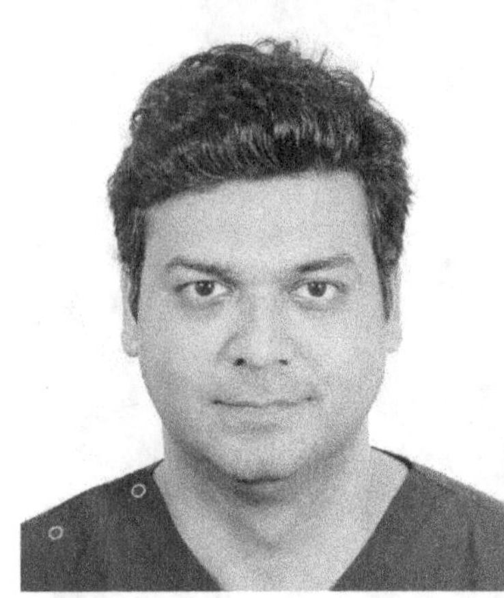
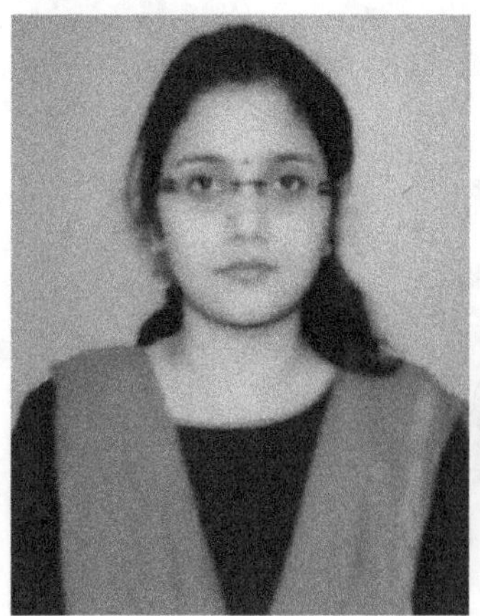
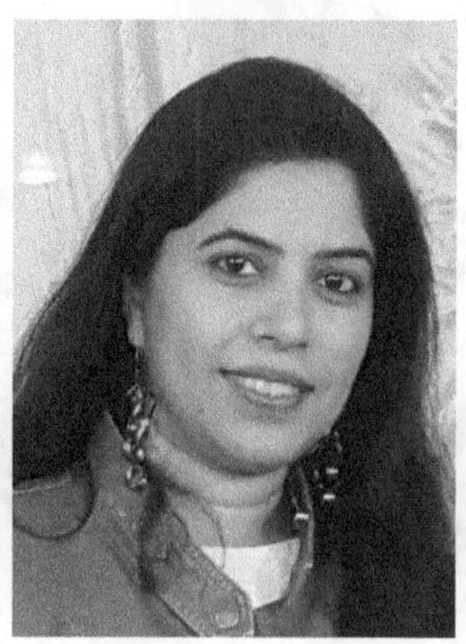
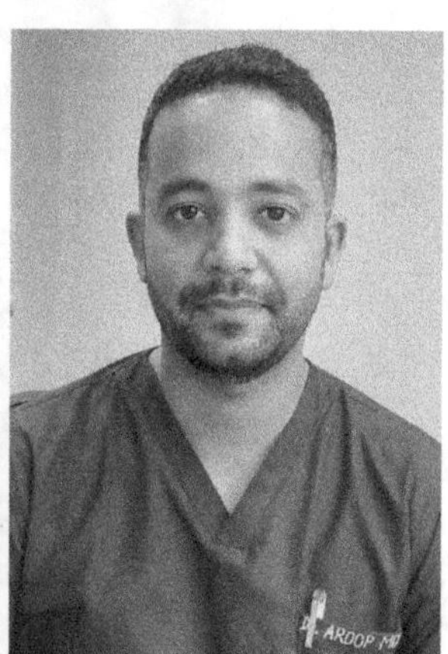

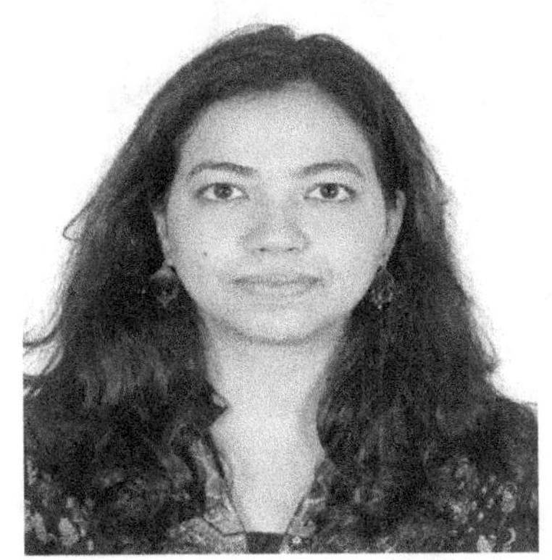
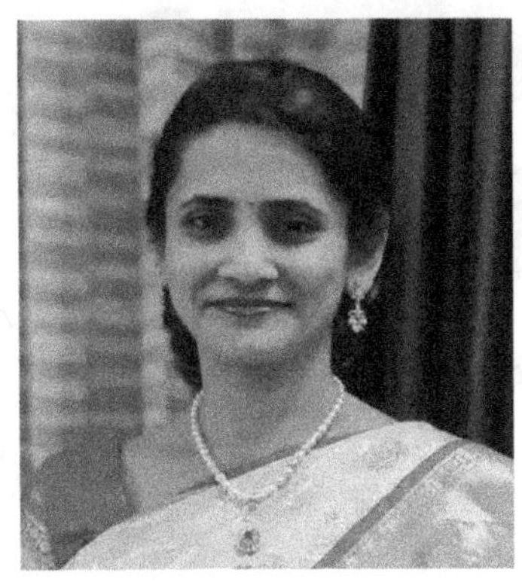
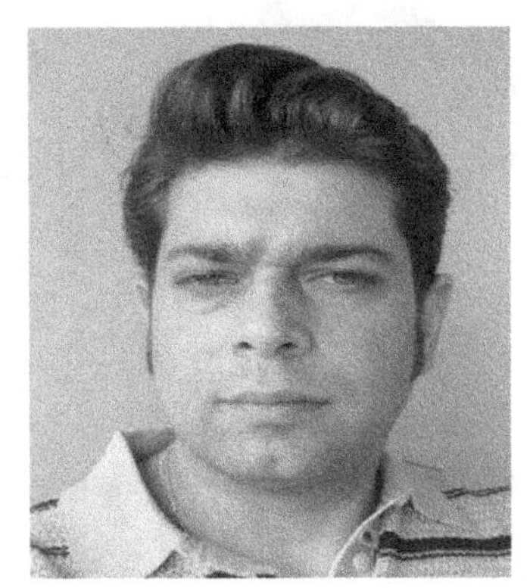
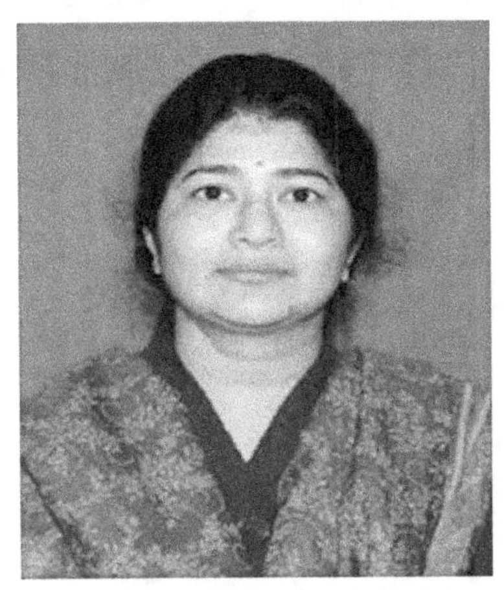
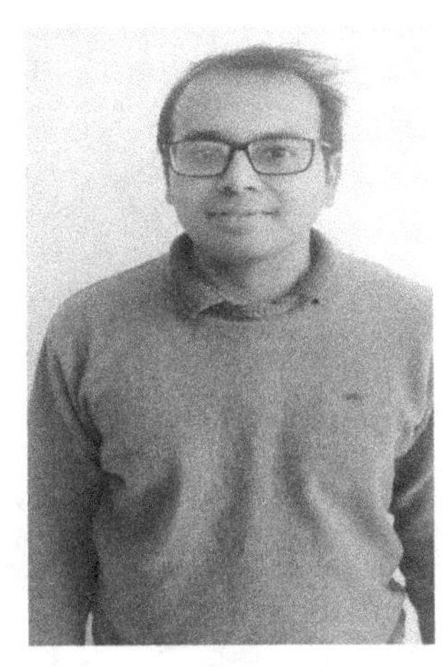
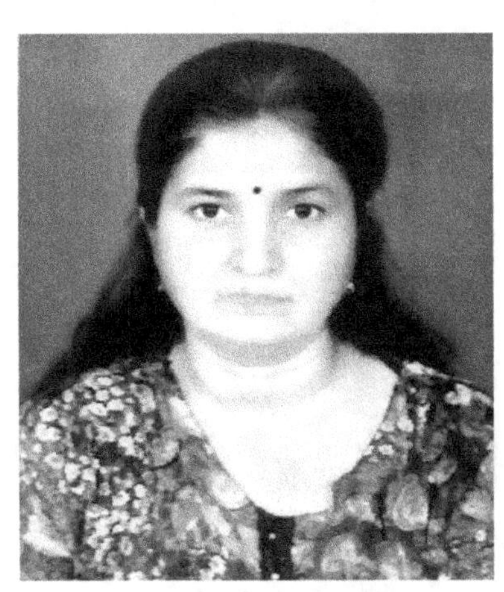
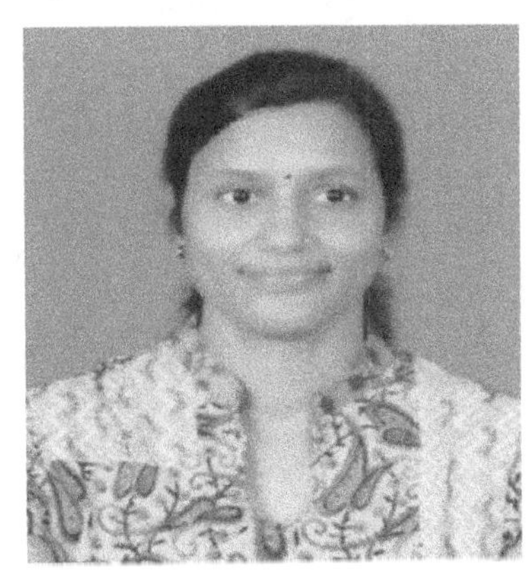
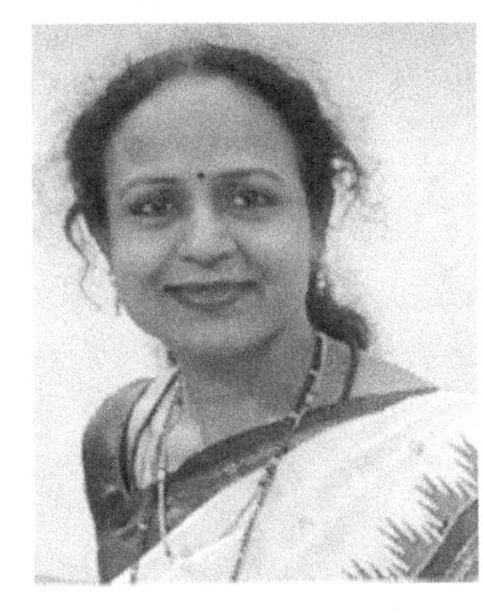
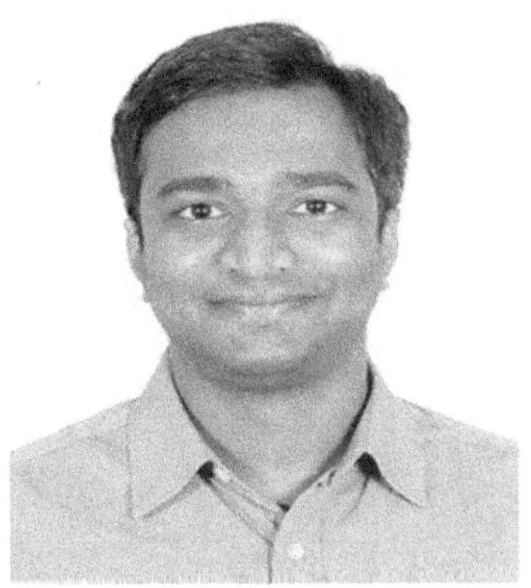
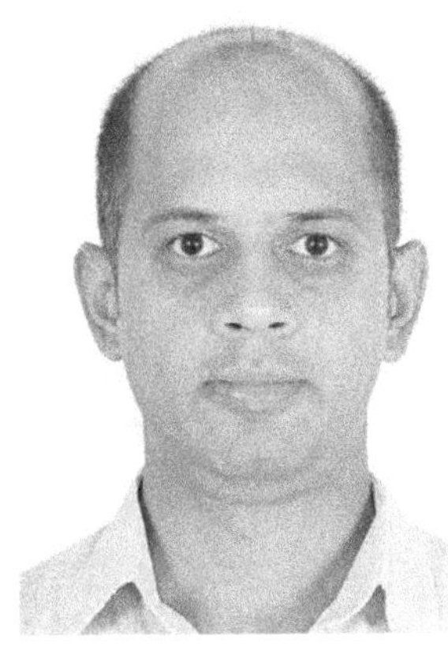
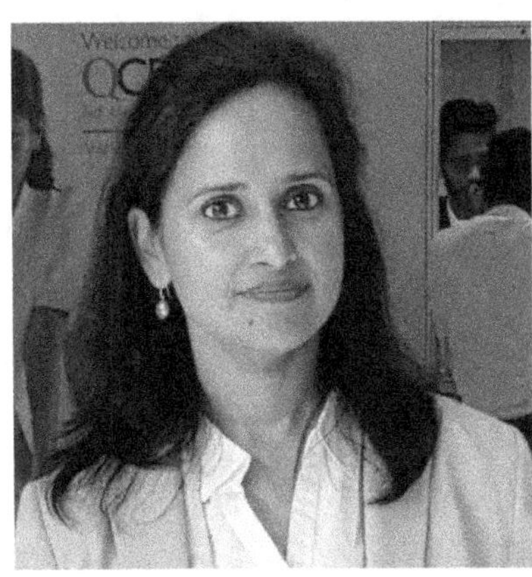
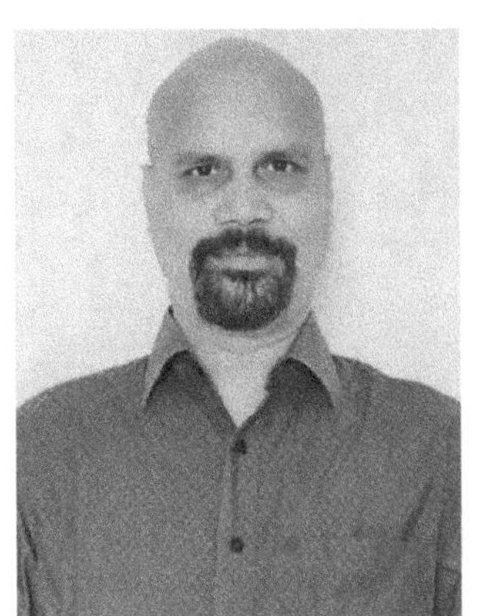